Bariatric Endocrinology

J. Michael Gonzalez-Campoy
Daniel L. Hurley • W. Timothy Garvey
Editors

Bariatric Endocrinology

Evaluation and Management of Adiposity, Adiposopathy and Related Diseases

Springer

Editors
J. Michael Gonzalez-Campoy
MNCOME
Eagan, MN
USA

Daniel L. Hurley
Mayo Clinic
Rochester, MN
USA

W. Timothy Garvey
University of Alabama - Birmingham
Birmingham, AL
USA

The Birmingham VA Medical Center
Birmingham, AL
USA

ISBN 978-3-030-07077-9 ISBN 978-3-319-95655-8 (eBook)
https://doi.org/10.1007/978-3-319-95655-8

This Springer imprint is published by the registered company Springer Nature Switzerland AG
The registered company address is: Gewerbestrasse 11, 6330 Cham, Switzerland

To our colleagues, especially our predecessors, whose inquisitive minds, work, and dedication to the advancement of science have led to the publication of this textbook.

To our patients with overweight, obesity, and adiposopathy, for whom we continue this work – they inspire and motivate us.

And to our families, for their unwavering love and support – they allow us to pursue our scientific and medical endeavors, for the common good.

Preface

At its annual meeting in 2017 the United Nations Educational, Scientific and Cultural Organization (UNESCO) inscribed the Caves and Ice Age Art in Swabian Jura, Germany on the World Heritage List. The caves have Aurignacian layers which date from 43,000 to 33,000 years ago. Among the items found in these ancient layers is a 6 cm tall statuette of a woman, carved out of mammoth ivory. This is the oldest known statue depicting a human being, and the woman clearly has obesity. Known as the Venus of Hohle Fels, the statuette helps us understand that for as long as there has been humanity, there have been individuals who can accumulate adipose tissue. Ancient civilizations, including the Egyptians and the Greek, came to regard obesity as a disease, a concept which was forgotten and which up until recently was still the subject of intense debate.

Over the years the condition of having excess adipose tissue has been named obesity, fatness, adiposity, overweight, corpulence, plumpness, chubbiness, stoutness, portliness, heaviness, tubbiness, flabbiness, largeness, chunkiness, heftiness, and bulkiness. Obesity was considered a reflection of success and wealth – those with the means could afford the regular ingestion of excess calories, and perhaps the service of others, leading to the accumulation of fat mass. Historical figures like King Henry VIII of England exemplified obesity as a disease – he was known to be ill from his obesity, and his gout attacks are chronicled for posterity.

With wars and worldwide famine, with infectious diseases that limited longevity, with limitations of the food supply, and with lifestyles that demanded physical activity, the historical prevalence of obesity had been limited. Individuals with obesity were featured attractions in traveling circuses, including Jack "The Happy Fat Man" Eckert and the "Humongous Circus Fat Man 'Tom Ton'", both of whom achieved notoriety at the turn of the nineteenth century.

With the industrialization of the world, humanity changed. Over the second half of the twentieth century, the food supplies of industrialized nations started to provide a steady stream of nutrients. There also developed myriads of disincentives for physical activity. With the advent of public health interventions, including waste disposal and water purification, the burden of infectious diseases significantly abated. And with the implementation of pasteurization, sterile techniques, and antibiotic treatments, the lifespan of human beings has been significantly prolonged. This all has allowed for the development of chronic diseases, including overweight and obesity, over the extended years of life for modern day humans.

We now understand that overweight and obesity represent a continuum of a complex, multifactorial disease that leads to the loss of health for most individuals who have it. Further, we now also realize that adiposity (the accumulation of fat mass) is but one aspect of the disease. The discovery that adipose tissue is an endocrine organ, and that the adipocyte is an endocrine cell, established that there are changes in anatomy and function that are at the genesis of metabolic diseases. Adiposopathy and "sick fat" are terms that are now engrained in the literature which encompass these pathophysiological changes. For some of our colleagues, these terms are not acceptable (they cannot take ownership of what they did not conceive), and this has led to scientific discordance. We respectfully agree to disagree. Yet, for a new generation of physicians and scientists, familiarity with these terms has opened a new frontier in medicine.

This textbook has been written with an adipocentric perspective. Not only is it a thorough review of obesity medicine, it also helps the reader understand the importance of adipose tissue dysfunction in the genesis of the metabolic complications of overweight and obesity. Bariatric endocrinology is thus born, paving the way for a new generation of physicians to diagnose and treat adiposopathy.

Eagan, MN, USA J. Michael Gonzalez-Campoy
Rochester, MN, USA Daniel L. Hurley
Birmingham, AL, USA W. Timothy Garvey

Contents

Editors and Contributors

Editors

J. Michael Gonzalez-Campoy, MD, PhD Minnesota Center for Obesity, Metabolism and Endocrinology, PA (MNCOME), Eagan, MN, USA

W. Timothy Garvey, MD, FACE Department of Nutrition Sciences, The University of Alabama at Birmingham, University of Alabama Hospital, Birmingham, AL, USA

The Birmingham VA Medical Center, Birmingham, AL, USA

Daniel L. Hurley, MD Mayo Graduate School of Medicine, Mayo Clinic, Division of Endocrinology, Diabetes, Metabolism, and Nutrition, Rochester, MN, USA

Contributors

Elise M. Brett, MD, FACE, CNSC, ECNU Icahn School of Medicine at Mount Sinai, Division of Endocrinology, Diabetes, and Bone Disease, New York, NY, USA

Elena A. Christofides, MD Endocrinology Associates, Inc., Columbus, OH, USA

Israel Hartman, MD, FACE University of Texas Southwestern Medical School, Department of Endocrinology, Dallas, TX, USA

Caroline M. Houston, MD The Brody School of Medicine at East Carolina University, Division of Endocrinology, Diabetes, and Metabolism, Greenville, NC, USA

Scott D. Isaacs, MD, FACP, FACE Atlanta Endocrine Associates, Atlanta, GA, USA

Jila Kaberi-Otarod, MD, CNSC Geisinger System – North East, Department of Nutrition and Weight Management, Scranton, PA, USA

Quang T. Nguyen, DO, FACE, FACP, FTOS Las Vegas Endocrinology, Clinical Education, AZCOM, TUNCOM, Henderson, NV, USA

Raymond A. Plodkowski, MD University of California San Diego, Division of Endocrinology and Metabolism, Scripps Clinic, San Diego, CA, USA

Domenica M. Rubino, MD Washington Center for Weight Management and Research, Arlington, VA, USA

Jeffrey Sicat, MD, FACE Virginia Weight and Wellness, Glen Allen, VA, USA

Yi-Hao Yu, MD, PhD Weight Loss and Diabetes Center, Department of Endocrinology, Stamford, CT, USA

Greenwich Hospital and Endocrinology Associates of Greenwich, Northeast Medical Group, Yale-New Haven Health, Greenwich, CT, USA

Farhad Zangeneh, MD Endocrinology, Diabetes and Osteoporosis Clinic, Sterling, VA, USA

Abbreviations

11ß-HSD	11-beta-hydroxysteroid dehydrogenase
2-AG	Endocannabinoid 2-arachidonoylglycerol
5-HT	5-hydroxytryptamine, serotonin
A1C	Hemoglobin A1c
AA	Amino acid
AACE	American Association of Clinical Endocrinologists
ACC	American College of Cardiology
ACE	American College of Endocrinology
ACEi	Angiotensin-converting enzyme inhibitor
ACTH	Adrenocorticotropic hormone
AD	Adiposis dolorosa
ADA	American Diabetes Association
ADA	Americans with Disabilities Act
ADHD	Attention deficit hyperactivity disorder
AG	Acylated ghrelin
AGB	Adjustable gastric band
AGPAT	Acylglycerophosphate acyltransferase
AgRP	Agouti-related protein
AHA	American Heart Association
AHI	Apnea-hypopnea index;
AHSD	α-hydroxysteroid dehydrogenase
AICR	American Institute for Cancer Research
ALA	Alpha-linolenic acid
ALLHAT	Antihypertension and Lipid-Lowering treatment to prevent Heart Attack Trial
AMA	American Medical Association
AMP	Adenosine monophosphate
AMPK	Adenosine monophosphate-activated protein kinase
AN	Anterior nucleus of the hypothalamus
AP	Area postrema
Apo E	Apolipoprotein E

apo	Apolipoprotein
ARB	Angiotensin receptor blocker
ARC	Arcuate nucleus of the hypothalamus
ART	Assisted reproductive technologies
ASBP	American Society of Bariatric Physicians
ASBS	American Society for Bariatric Surgery
ASMBS	American Society for Metabolic and Bariatric Surgery
ASP	Acylation-stimulating protein
ASSIST	Appetite Suppression Induced by Stimulation Trial
ATP	Adenosine triphosphate
ATP	Adult Treatment Panel
AUD	Alcohol use disorder
BA	Bile acids
BAT	Brown adipose tissue
BBB	Blood-brain barrier
BDI	Beck Depression Inventory
BDNF	Brain-derived neurotrophic factor
BE	Barrett's esophagus
BED	Binge eating disorder
BHSD	β-hydroxysteroid dehydrogenase
BIA	Bioelectrical impedance analysis
BID	Twice daily
BMI	Body mass index
BMOD	Behavior modification
BP	Blood pressure (S = systolic and D = diastolic)
BPD	Biliopancreatic diversion
BPD-DS	Biliopancreatic diversion with duodenal switch
BRFSS	Behavioral Risk Factor Surveillance System
bT	Bioavailable testosterone
BWL	Behavioral weight loss
CABG	Coronary artery bypass grafting
cAMP	Cyclic adenosine monophosphate
CARDIA	Coronary Artery Risk Development in Young Adults study
CART	Cocaine- and amphetamine-related transcript
CB	Cannabinoid receptor
CBT	Cognitive behavioral treatment
CBTgsh	Cognitive behavioral therapy with guided self-help
CCB	Calcium channel blocker
CCK	Cholecystokinin
CDC	Centers for Disease Control and Prevention
CETP	Cholesteryl ester transfer protein
CI	Confidence interval
CKD	Chronic kidney disease
cm	Centimeters
CNPS	Cardiac natriuretic peptide system

CNS	Central nervous system
CO	Cardiac output
COR	Contrave Obesity Research
CPAP	Continuous positive airway pressure therapy
CRC	Colorectal cancer
CRH	Corticotropin-releasing hormone
CRP	C-reactive protein
CS	Cushing's syndrome
CT	Computerized tomography
CTR	Calcitonin receptor
CV	Cardiovascular
CVA	Cerebrovascular accident;
CVD	Cardiovascular disease
CVO	Circumventricular organs
CY	Cytochrome
DA	Dopamine
DASH	The Dietary Approaches to Stop Hypertension
DBP	Diastolic blood pressure
DEXA	Dual-energy X-ray absorptiometry
DGAT	Diacylglycerol acyltransferase
DHA	Docosahexaenoic acid
DHEA	Dehydroepiandrosterone
DJB	Duodenojejunal bypass
dL	Deciliter
DM	Diabetes mellitus
DMN	Dorsomedial nucleus of the hypothalamus
DMPA	Depot medroxyprogesterone acetate
DNA	Deoxyribonucleic acid
DPP	Dipeptidyl peptidase
DPP-4	Dipeptidyl peptidase 4
DPP-4I	Dipeptidyl-peptidase-4 inhibitors
DXA	Dual Energy X-ray absorptiometry
E_2	Estradiol
EAC	Esophageal adenocarcinoma
EASO	European Association for the Study of Obesity
ECG	Electrocardiogram
ED	Erectile dysfunction
EEC	Enteroendocrine cells
eGFR	Estimated glomerular filtration rate
EH	Energy homeostasis
EKG	Electrocardiogram
eNOS	Endothelial nitric oxide synthase
ENS	Enteric nervous system
EPA	Eicosapentaenoic acid
ER	Estrogen receptor

ES	Endoluminal sleeve(s)
EWL	Excess weight loss
FA	Food addiction
FBG	Fasting blood glucose
FDA	Food and Drug Administration
FFA	Free fatty acids
FFM	Fat-free mass
FGF15/FGF19	Fibroblast growth factor 15/19
FH	Familial hypercholesterolemia
FM	Fibromyalgia
FMI	Fat mass index
FML	Familial multiple lipomatosis
fMRI	Functional magnetic resonance imaging
FOURIER	Further Cardiovascular Outcomes Research with PCSK9 Inhibition in Subjects with Elevated Risk
FPG	Fasting plasma glucose
FSH	Follitropin or follicle-stimulating hormone
fT	Free testosterone
FTO	Fat mass and obesity associated (gene)
FXR	Farnesoid X receptor
G6P	Glucose-6-phosphate
GABA	Gamma-aminobutyric acid
GBS	Gastric bypass surgery
GC	Glucocorticoid
GCGR	G-protein-coupled glucagon receptor
GERD	Gastroesophageal reflux disease
GES	Gastric electrical stimulation
GH	Growth hormone
GHRL	Growth hormone secretagogue receptor ligand
GHSR	Ghrelin/growth hormone secretagogue receptor
GIP	Glucose-dependent insulinotropic peptide
GK	Glucokinase
GLP-1	Glucagon-like peptide-1
GLP-1R	Glucagon-like peptide-1 receptor
GLUT	Glucose transporter
GLUT4	Glucose transporter 4
GM	Gut microbiota
Gn	Gonadotropin
GnRH	Gonadotropin-releasing hormone
GOAT	Ghrelin O-acyltransferase
GPAT	Glycerol-3-phosphate acyltransferase
GPCR	G-protein-coupled receptor
GRPP	Glicentin-related pancreatic peptide
GWAS	Genome-wide association studies
H&E	History and examination
H&P	History and physical examination

HbA_{1c}	Hemoglobin A1C
HBV	Hepatitis B virus
HCC	Hepatocellular carcinoma
HCFA	Healthcare Financing Administration
HCG	Human chorionic gonadotropin
HCV	Hepatitis C virus
HDL	High-density lipoprotein
HDL-C	High-density lipoprotein cholesterol
HFD	High-fat diet
HIF1	Hypoxia-inducible factor 1
HMG-CoA	3-Hydroxy-3-methyl-glutaryl-coenzyme A
HMGCR	3 Hydroxy-3-methyl-glutaryl-coenzyme A reductase
HOMA	Homeostasis model assessment
HOMA-IR	Homeostasis model assessment of insulin resistance
HP	Highly palatable
HPA	Hypothalamic-pituitary-adrenal
HPAA	Hypothalamic-pituitary-adrenal axis
HR	Hazard ratio
HRT	Hormone replacement therapy
HS-CRP	Highly sensitive C-reactive protein
HSL	Hormone-sensitive lipase
HTN	Hypertension
IAP	Intra-abdominal pressure
ICD	International Classification of Diseases
IFG	Impaired fasting glucose
IGB	Intragastric balloons
IGF	Insulin-like growth factor
IGF-1R	Insulin-like growth factor-1 receptor
IGS	Implantable gastric stimulator
IGT	Impaired glucose tolerance
IIEF-5	International Index of Erectile Function 5
IL	Interleukin
IMPROVE-IT	Improved Reduction of Outcomes: Vytorin Efficacy International Trial
INS	Insulin
IPT	Individual psychotherapy
IR	Insulin receptor
ISH	Isolated systolic hypertension
ITT	Intention to treat
IU	International units
IWB	Internalized weight bias
JIB	Jejunoileal bypass
JNC	Joint National Committee
JUPITER	Justification for the Use of Statins in Prevention: an Intervention Trial Evaluating Rosuvastatin
Kcal	Kilocalories

kg	Kilogram
kg/m^2	kilograms/meter^2
LAR	Leptin-to-adiponectin ratio
lbs	Pounds
LCFA	Long-chain fatty acids
LDJB-SG	Loop duodenojejunal bypass with sleeve gastrectomy
LDL	Low-density lipoprotein
LDL-C	Low-density lipoprotein cholesterol
LEARN	Lifestyle, Exercise, Attitude, Relationships and Nutrition
LEP	Leptin
LEPR	Leptin receptor
LGA	Left gastric artery
LGAE	Left gastric artery embolization
LH	Lutropin or luteinizing hormone
LHA	Lateral hypothalamic area
LOCF	Last observation carried forward
LOFI	Lean-on-the-outside-fat-on-the-inside
LP(a)	Lipoprotein (a)
LPL	Lipoprotein lipase
LRYGB	Laparoscopic Roux-en-Y gastric bypass
LUTS	Lower urinary tract symptoms
LVSG	Laparoscopic vertical sleeve gastrectomy
m	Meter
MAOI	Monoamine oxidase inhibitor
MAP kinase	Mitogen-activated protein kinase
MC	Melanocortin
MC4R	Melanocortin 4 receptor
MCFA	Medium-chain fatty acid
MCH	Melanin-concentrating hormone
MCP	Monocyte chemoattractive protein
MCR4	Melanocortin receptor 4
MDD	Major depressive disorder
METs	Metabolic equivalents
mg	Milligram
MGB	mini gastric bypass
MI	Myocardial infarction
mITT	Modified intention-to-treat
mmHg	Millimeters of mercury
MN	Mammillary nucleus of the hypothalamus
MNT	Medical nutrition therapy
MRFIT	Multiple Risk Factor Intervention Trial
MRI	Magnetic resonance imaging
mRNA	Messenger ribonucleic acid
MSH	Melanocyte-stimulating hormone
mTOR	Mammalian target of rapamycin

MTTP	Microsomal triglyceride transfer protein
MUFA	Monounsaturated fatty acids
Myf5	Myogenic factor 5
NA	Nucleus accumbens
NAASO	North American Association for the Study of Obesity
NAFLD	Nonalcoholic fatty liver disease
NASH	Nonalcoholic steatohepatitis
NB	Naltrexone-bupropion
NCEP ATP	National Cholesterol Education Program Adult Treatment Panel
NCEP	National Cholesterol Education Program
NCHS	National Center for Health Statistics
NEFA	Non-esterified fatty acid
NES	Night-eating syndrome
NHANES	National Health and Nutrition Examination Survey
NHLBI	National Heart, Lung and Blood Institute
NIH	National Institutes of Health
non-SHBG-bound T	Non-sex hormone-binding globulin-bound testosterone
NPC1L1	Niemann-Pick C1-Like 1
NPY	Neuropeptide Y
NTS	Nucleus tractus solitarius
OA	Osteoarthritis
OAGB	One anastomosis gastric bypass
OGTT	Oral glucose tolerance test
OMA	Obesity Medical Association
OR	Odds ratio
OSA	Obstructive sleep apnea
OVRD	Oral volume restricting device
OX	Orexin receptor
OXM	Oxyntomodulin
P_4	Progesterone
PAI-1	Plasminogen activator inhibitor-1
PAP	Phosphatidic acid phosphorylase
PCI	Percutaneous coronary intervention
PCOS	Polycystic ovary syndrome
PCS	Pain Catastrophizing Scale
PCSK9	Proprotein convertase subtilisin/kexin type 9
PE	Pulmonary embolus;
PFC	Prefrontal cortex
PG	Percutaneous gastrostomy
PGC-1α	PPAR gamma coactivator 1-alpha
PHEN/TPM	Phentermine-topiramate
PI3K	Phosphatidylinositol 3-kinase
PKA	Protein kinase A
PN	Posterior nucleus of the hypothalamus

POMC	Pro-opiomelanocortin
PON	Preoptic nucleus of the hypothalamus
PP	Pancreatic polypeptide
PPAR	Peroxisome proliferator-activated receptor
PPG	Postprandial glucose
PPNAD	Primary pigmented nodular adrenocortical disease
PR	Peripheral resistance
PRL	Prolactin
PSA	Prostate-specific antigen
PSCK1	Prohormone convertase 1
PTCA	Percutaneous transluminal coronary angioplasty
PTSD	Post-traumatic stress disorder
PUFA	Polyunsaturated fatty acid
PVN	Paraventricular nucleus of the hypothalamus
PYY	Peptide YY
QD	Daily
QOL	Quality of Life
RA	Retinoic acid
RAAS	Renin-angiotensin-aldosterone system
RAMPs	Receptor activity-modifying proteins
RBP	Retinol-binding protein
REE	Resting energy expenditure
REMS	Risk evaluation and mitigation strategies
RNS	Reactive nitrogen species
ROS	Reactive oxygen species
ROS	Review of systems
RR	Relative risk
RR	Risk ratio
RXR	Retinoid X receptors
RYGB	Roux-en-Y gastric bypass
SADI	Single anastomosis duodenoileostomy
SAGI	Single anastomosis gastroileostomy
SASI	Single anastomosis sleeve ileostomy
SBP	Systolic blood pressure
SCALE	Satiety and Clinical Adiposity-Liraglutide Evidence
SCFA	Short-chain fatty acid
SCN	Suprachiasmatic nucleus of the hypothalamus
Sct	Secretin
SctR	Secretin receptor
SD	Standard deviation
SGLT-1	Sodium-dependent glucose transporter 1
SGLT-2	Sodium-dependent glucose transporter-2
SH2B1	Src homology 2B adaptor protein 1
SHAPE	Screened Health Assessment and Pacer Evaluation trial
SHBG	Sex hormone-binding globulin

SIPS	Stomach intestinal pylorus sparing surgery
SL	Symmetrical lipomatosis
SMC	Smooth muscle cell
SNP	Single nucleotide polymorphism
SNRI	Serotonin norepinephrine reuptake inhibitor
SON	Supraoptic nucleus of the hypothalamus
SSRI	Selective serotonin reuptake inhibitor
SVR	Systemic vascular resistance
T	Testosterone
T2DM	Type 2 diabetes mellitus
T3	Triiodothyronine
T4	Tetraiodothyronine or thyroxine
TC	Total cholesterol
TEE	Total energy expenditure
TES	The Endocrine Society
TFA	Trans-fatty acids
TG	Triacylglycerol
TG	Triglycerides
TGR5	The G-protein coupled receptor 5
TID	Three times daily
TKA	Total knee arthroplasty;
TNF	Tumor necrosis factor
TOGA	Transoral gastroplasty
TOS	The Obesity Society
TRH	Thyrotropin-releasing hormone
TRT	Testosterone replacement therapy
TRUS	Transrectal ultrasound
TSH	Thyroid-stimulating hormone
TT	Total testosterone
TWIST	Twist-related protein
TZDs	Thiazolidinediones
UAG	Unacylated ghrelin
UCP	Uncoupling protein
UDCA	Ursodeoxycholic acid;
UK	United Kingdom
US	United States
USA	United States of America
USDA	United States Department of Agriculture
UTI	Urinary tract infection;
VAN	Vagal afferent neurons
VBG	Vertical banded gastroplasty
VEGF	Vascular endothelial growth factor
VLC	Very low-calorie
VLCMP	Very low-calorie meal plan
VLDL	Very low-density lipoprotein

VLDL-C	Very low-density lipoprotein cholesterol
VMN	Ventromedial nucleus of the hypothalamus
VSG	Vertical sleeve gastrectomy
VTA	Ventral tegmental area
WAT	White adipose tissue
WC	Waist circumference
WCRF	World Cancer Research Fund
WHI	Women's Health Initiative
WHO	World Health Organization
WHR	Waist-to-hip ratio
WHtR	Waist-to-height ratio
YFAS	Yale Food Addiction Scale

Chapter 1
Bariatric Endocrinology

J. Michael Gonzalez-Campoy

Pearls of Wisdom

- Bariatric endocrinology developed from the knowledge that adipose tissue is an endocrine organ that actively participates in the regulation of metabolism and that it may become diseased (adiposopathy), thus contributing to the development of metabolic diseases.
- Adipose tissue may develop both anatomical and pathophysiological changes which lead to derangements of structure and function, collectively termed adiposopathy.
- Adipocytes both produce hormones with varied end-organ targets, and have receptors for many circulating hormones, establishing an active cross talk that maintains metabolic homeostasis. Adiposopathy leads to dysregulation of metabolic homeostasis, forcing other tissues to compensate, and leading to metabolic diseases when compensation is inadequate.
- Overweight, obesity, and adiposopathy are caused by both a genetic predisposition and environmental factors, and must be treated like any other chronic disease.
- The goals of bariatric endocrinology are to help individual patients decrease the burden of increased fat mass (treatment of adiposity) and to return adipose tissue function to normal (treatment of adiposopathy).

J. M. Gonzalez-Campoy
Minnesota Center for Obesity, Metabolism and Endocrinology, PA (MNCOME),
Eagan, MN, USA
e-mail: drmike@mncome.com

J. M. Gonzalez-Campoy et al. (eds.), *Bariatric Endocrinology*,
https://doi.org/10.1007/978-3-319-95655-8_1

1.1 Introduction

Bariatric endocrinology first became a subject at the 2014 meeting of the American Association of Clinical Endocrinologists (AACE) in Las Vegas, Nevada. The co-editors of this textbook held a scientific session that defined obesity as an endocrine disease, adipose tissue as an endocrine organ, and the adipocyte as an endocrine cell. As such, obesity became not just a disease of excessive fat mass but rather a treatment target for clinical endocrinologists, a major goal of treatment becoming the correction of underlying adipose tissue dysfunction. This emerging position has been difficult to understand and accept by the vast majority of physicians who still think of success in the treatment of obesity as merely a reduction in poundage. This textbook of bariatric endocrinology was conceived after the 2014 AACE meeting to set the stage for future generations of clinicians who will have learned that adipose tissue dysfunction is a viable target of medical interventions, in addition to the traditional goal of decreasing fat mass. A brief history of how we got here is important.

In 1903, Dr. Perry published a paper entitled "The Nature and Treatment of Obesity" in the *California State Journal of Medicine*. He described obesity as "20 per cent to 40 per cent excess of weight over the normal of 2.05 pounds per inch of height, or 300 grammes per centimeter." In his paper, he explained that corpulence must be due to excessive muscular development, excessive fatty tissue, excessive water, myxedema, or pseudo-muscular hypertrophy. Prior to his publication, there are no indexed papers with obesity in the title in the National Library of Medicine. For the next half century, the view of adipose tissue became one of a storage organ. Yet the concept that obesity is a risk to health dates back to the writings of Hippocrates. And over this half century, progress was made identifying obesity as a disease.

In 1963, the emerging field of lipidology defined the role that adipose tissue had to play in lipid metabolism. Dr. Martha Vaughan and colleagues at the National Institutes of Health (NIH) documented that there is a hormone-sensitive triglyceride-splitting enzyme activity in adipose tissue. Hormone-sensitive lipase was shown to respond to epinephrine, leading to increased lipolysis and defining adipose tissue as a target of circulating hormones. Insulin was subsequently shown to inhibit this same enzyme, being strongly antilipolytic. In 1976, Dr. Lewis Williams and colleagues identified beta-adrenergic receptors in adipocytes, confirming that the adipocyte was indeed under hormonal control.

The first hints of a circulating factor that could affect fat mass came earlier. In 1959, parabiosis experiments done by Dr. Hervey at the University of Cambridge, in which paired rats were made to exchange blood and plasma by being surgically conjoined at the hip, provided an important clue to the presence of a circulating factor that could regulate energy stores. Damage to the ventromedial hypothalamus leads to obesity caused by overeating in rats. The damage prevents the ventromedial hypothalamus from responding to physiological signals that suppress appetite. When a rat with a ventromedial hypothalamus lesion is conjoined to a normal rat, the rat with the lesion overeats and gains weight. The normal rat without a lesion, on the other hand, significantly decreases its caloric intake, losing weight and declining food even when made available. When both paired rats have damage to the ventromedial hypothalamus, both overfeed and gain weight. This was strong evidence of a circulating factor that decreases caloric intake by stimulating a hypothalamic target, thus decreasing fat mass. And it was also evidence that there is central regulation of energy balance.

In the late 1980s, adipose tissue was found to produce estrogen. Aromatase, the enzyme responsible for the synthesis of estrogen from testosterone, was identified in adipose tissue. This established the adipocyte as an endocrine cell capable of synthesizing estrogen. The degree of adiposity was subsequently related to the amount of estrogen in the circulation of patients with obesity and reproductive tract cancer. But aromatase and estrogen were not exclusive to adipose tissue.

In 1949, mice homozygous for the ob mutation (ob/ob mice) were first identified at the Jackson Laboratory. These mice exhibit uncontrolled feeding and develop obesity. In 1990, the ob gene was mapped. Subsequently, the gene product of the ob gene was identified as a hormone. When the gene product was given to ob/ob mice, it suppressed excessive feeding and promoted weight loss. Accordingly, this protein was named leptin, a derivative of the Greek root for "thin," *lepto*. Leptin was the first adipocyte-derived hormone (adipokine) to be discovered. A search of the Medi-Span database as of 2016 includes over 13,000 references with the word leptin in the title.

When leptin was characterized as a hormone made exclusively in adipose tissue, the search for other adipocyte products intensified. Adipocytes were also shown to produce adiponectin (which improves insulin sensitivity), adipsin (which is deficient in obesity), resistin (which causes insulin resistance), and visfatin (which has plasma glucose-lowering effects). Additionally, adipose tissue was shown to produce inflammatory cytokines including interleukin-6, tumor necrosis factor-alpha, and macrophage and monocyte chemoattractant protein-1, documenting its potential for macrophage infiltration and the development of inflammation.

By the late 1990s, the view of adipose tissue as a mere storage organ had been replaced by the contemporary perspective that it actively participates in the signaling that regulates the body's energy needs. The concept that adipose tissue may become diseased, or that adiposopathy may develop, was introduced into the medical literature by Dr. Harold Bays in 2004. Adiposopathy is now a treatment target in clinical endocrinology.

With a recognized worldwide obesity epidemic, there were over 64,000 publications on the subject by the end of 2015 (Fig. 1.1). This chapter reviews the epidemiology of obesity, its economic impact, its differential effect in different ethnic groups, the public health efforts to address it, and the principles of bariatric endocrinology that will help treat this disease.

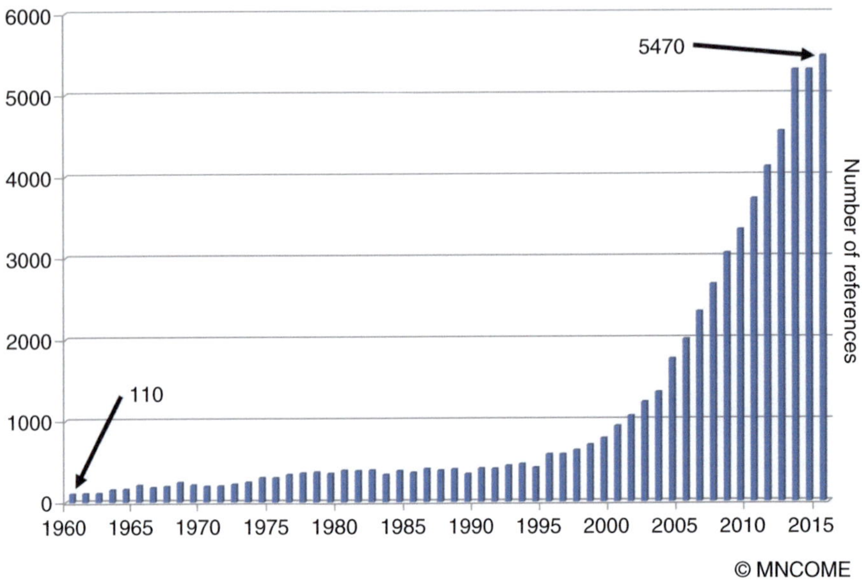

Fig. 1.1 Number of publications with "obesity" in the title by year (1960–2015); Copyright MNCOME

1.2 The Obesity Epidemic in the United States of America (USA)

1.2.1 Adult USA Population

The National Health and Nutrition Examination Survey (NHANES) is a program of studies designed to assess the health and nutritional status of adults and children in the United States. It is funded by the Centers for Disease Control (CDC), through the National Center for Health Statistics (NCHS). The survey is unique in that it combines interviews and physical examinations. All counties in the United States are divided into 15 groups based on their characteristics. One county is selected from each large group, and together, they form the 15 counties in the NHANES surveys for each year. Within each of these 15 counties, smaller groups, with a large number of households in each group, are formed. Between 20 and 24 of these small groups are then selected. In each small group, all the houses and apartments are identified, and a sample of about 30 households is selected for interviewers to visit. A computer algorithm randomly selects some, all, or none of the household members.

NHANES data for USA adults ages 20 or higher from 1962 documented that 30.5% of the population had a body mass index (BMI) in the range of 25–29.9 kg/m^2, and 12.8% had a BMI of 30 kg/m^2 or more. By 2012, these numbers had risen to 33.9% and 35.1%, respectively. For this period, there was a 1.7-fold increase in the prevalence of people with a BMI of 30 kg/m^2 or more.

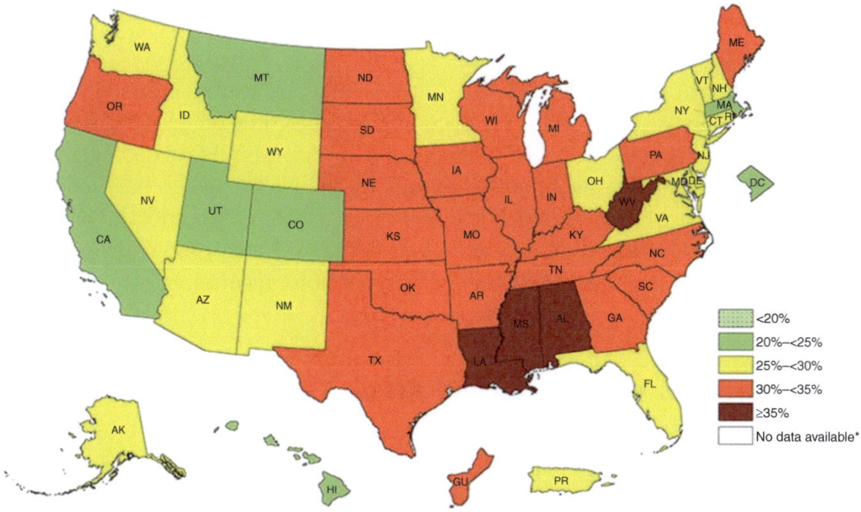

Fig. 1.2 Prevalence of self-reported obesity among USA adults by state and territory, BRFSS, 2015. (From Centers for Disease Control. https://www.cdc.gov/obesity/data/prevalence-maps.html (accessed 9/5/2016))

The Behavioral Risk Factor Surveillance System (BRFSS) is a system of health-related telephone surveys that collect state data about USA residents regarding their health-related risk behaviors, chronic health conditions, and the use of preventive services. It also is funded by the CDC. BRFSS was established in 1984 with 15 states and has expanded to collect data in all 50 states, the District of Columbia, and three USA territories. BRFSS completes more than 400,000 adult interviews each year, making it the largest continuously conducted health survey system in the world.

Figure 1.2 shows the 2015 BRFSS data on the prevalence of self-reported obesity among adults in the USA by state and territory. BRFSS USA data show that in 2015:

- No state had a prevalence of obesity less than 20%.
- In six states (California, Colorado, Hawaii, Massachusetts, Montana, and Utah) and the District of Columbia, obesity ranged from 20% to less than 25%.
- Nineteen states and Puerto Rico had a prevalence of obesity between 25% and less than 30%.
- Obesity prevalence in 21 states and Guam was from 30% to less than 35%.
- Four states (Alabama, Louisiana, Mississippi, and West Virginia) had an obesity prevalence of 35% or greater.
- The south had the highest prevalence of obesity (31.2%), followed by the Midwest (30.7%), the northeast (26.4%), and the west (25.2%).

Using the NHANES 2011–2012 database, the prevalence of obesity is higher among middle-age adults age 40–59 years (40.2%) and older adults age 60 and over (37.0%) than among younger adults age 20–39 (32.3%).

1.2.2 Children and Adolescent USA Population

The prevalence of obesity in 2011–2014 was 17.0%, and extreme obesity (defined as a BMI at or above 120% of the sex-specific 95th percentile on the CDC BMI-for-age growth charts) was 5.8%. Childhood obesity has also been documented to become more prevalent since the first reports by the NCHS using the 1988–1994 NHANES database. This textbook focuses on adult bariatric endocrinology, but these data are included because youth with obesity will swell the ranks of adults having the disease at a much younger age than previous generations.

1.3 Obesity in USA Racial and Ethnic Groups

Using data from 9120 participants in the 2011–2012 nationally representative NHANES database, in the USA non-Hispanic blacks have the highest age-adjusted rates of obesity (48.1%), followed by Hispanics (42.5%), non-Hispanic whites (34.5%), and non-Hispanic Asians (11.7%). Among non-Hispanic black and Mexican-American men, those with higher incomes are more likely to have obesity than those with low incomes. To the contrary, higher-income women are less likely to have obesity than low-income women.

1.4 Obesity in Geographical Regions of the World

In 1988, Gurney and Gorstein published initial data compiled by the World Health Organization (WHO) on the prevalence of obesity in many countries. The publication validated that, for adults, the body mass index is reasonably easy to obtain and correlates well with mortality and morbidity risk. For children, "overweight" is indicated by a weight-for-height ratio above the median NCHS value plus two standard deviations. By 1999, the prevalence of obesity around the world was estimated to exceed 250 million people. The first formal WHO Consultation on obesity concluded that the global obesity epidemic was a consequence of modernization, economic development, urbanization, and other societal changes. These led to widespread reductions in spontaneous and work-related physical activity and to excessive consumption of energy dense foods. The International Obesity Task Force launched a global initiative for coherent action to tackle the epidemic of obesity. Despite increased awareness and attempts to intervene at the public health level, the prevalence of obesity around the world has continued to rise.

Reports on the prevalence of obesity in both adults and children from countries around the world continue to highlight both potential causes and opportunities for intervention. In 2008, the prevalence of obesity (using estimated mean BMI in a regression model to predict overweight and obesity prevalence by age, country, year, and sex) in women ranged from 1.4% (0.7–2.2%) in Bangladesh and 1.5%

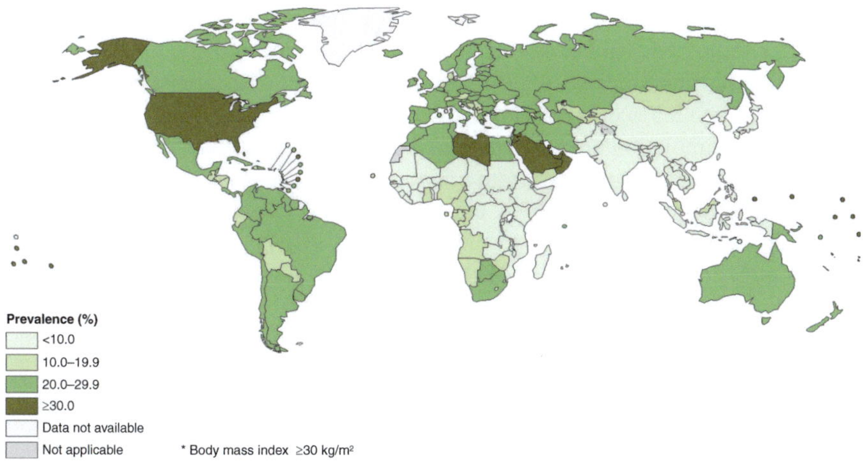

Fig. 1.3 Worldwide prevalence of obesity by BMI*, ages 18+, both sexes, 2014. (From World Health Organization. http://gamapserver.who.int/mapLibrary/Files/Maps/Global_Obesity_2014_BothSexes.png (27/Mar/2015 post; accessed 9/5/2016))

(0.9–2.4%) in Madagascar to 70.4% (61.9–78.9%) in Tonga and 74.8% (66.7–82.1%) in Nauru. Obesity in men was below 1% in Bangladesh, Democratic Republic of the Congo, and Ethiopia and was the highest in Cook Islands (60.1%, 52.6–67.6%) and Nauru (67.9%, 60.5–75.0%). Figure 1.3 shows the latest data on the prevalence of obesity compiled by WHO, as of 2015.

The WHO data have also clearly established the rising rates of diabetes worldwide, parallel to the development of obesity. Some populations around the world seem particularly susceptible to the twin epidemics of obesity and diabetes. In India, for example, defining obesity as a BMI of 25 kg/m^2 or higher, the incidence of obesity rose from 2% to 17.1% of the population between 1989 and 2003. This represented a 750% increase in the incidence of obesity. Over the same period, the incidence of diabetes rose from 2.2% to 6.4% of the population, a 191% increase. At the CDC, Ali Mokdad and colleagues documented the same parallel rise in the incidence of obesity and diabetes in the USA. Between 1998 and 2012, there was a 96% increase in the incidence of obesity, defined as a BMI of 30 kg/m^2 or higher, with a 43% concomitant increase in the incidence of diabetes. It has also been established that the incidence of hypertension, dyslipidemia, and diabetes rises with BMI thresholds from normal to overweight to obesity.

1.5 The Economic Impact of Obesity

Awareness of the increasing prevalence of obesity from data generated by the CDC in the 1980s and 1990s led to significant concern about the financial impact of this disease. Early projections based on the prevalence of obesity of 34 million adults in the USA in 1980 led to the estimate of 1986 expenditures of $11.3 billion for diabetes, $22.2 billion for cardiovascular disease, $2.4 billion for gallbladder disease, $1.5 billion for hypertension, and $1.9 billion for breast and colon cancers—$39.3 billion or around 5.5% of the costs of illnesses in 1986.

In 2011, a simulation model, to project the probable health and economic consequences in the next two decades from a continued rise in obesity in the USA and the United Kingdom (UK), estimated 65 million and 11 million more adults with obesity in the USA and the UK, respectively, by 2030. The projections were for an additional 6–8.5 million cases of diabetes, 5.7–7.3 million cases of heart disease and stroke, 492,000–669,000 additional cases of cancer, and 26–55 million quality-adjusted life years forgone for the USA and the UK combined. The combined medical costs associated with the treatment of these preventable complications of obesity were estimated to increase by $48–66 billion/year in the USA and by £1.9–2 billion/year in the UK by 2030.

By the end of 2014, the National Center for Weight and Wellness at George Washington University placed the cost of obesity at more than $300 billion annually in direct medical and nonmedical services, decreased worker productivity, disability, and premature death.

There are now projections that weight loss reduces lifetime health-care costs. Using claims data for 2.1 million beneficiaries in the federal government in 2008, there were 857,200 patients with overweight and 521,800 patients with obesity, all aged 18–64 years. Among federal beneficiaries who have overweight or obesity, lifetime expenditures decline by $440 (3% discount rate) for each permanent 1% reduction in body weight. This includes $590 in savings from improved health, offset by $150 in additional expenditures from prolonged life. Estimates range from a $660 reduction for adults aged <45 years with obesity to a $40 gain for adults aged 55–64 years with obesity, where expenditures from increased longevity exceed savings from improved health. If weight loss is temporary and regained after 24 months, lifetime expenditures decline by $40 per 1% reduction in body weight. The long-term benefits from weight loss are substantially greater than the short-term benefits.

There are additional economic correlates to the epidemic of obesity. Obesity results in increased medical expenditures and absenteeism among full-time employees. Approximately 30% of the total costs to employers result from increased absenteeism. Employees with stage 3 obesity represent about 3% of the employed population but account for 21% of the costs of obesity. These costs do not include the additional loss of income to employers from disability and presenteeism (loss of productivity during the time present at work). Physical disabilities magnify the costs of obesity. The combination of physical disabilities and obesity costs employers around $23.9 billion/year or roughly 50% of the total costs attributable to obesity in the USA. Using data on medical expenditures and body weight from the National Health and Interview Survey and the Medical Expenditure Panel Survey, it is estimated that, in a health plan with a coinsurance rate of 17.5%, obesity imposes a welfare cost of about $150 per capita on health insurance costs. The welfare loss to health insurance companies can be reduced by technological change that lowers pecuniary and nonpecuniary costs of losing weight and also by increasing the coinsurance rate for people with obesity. The workplace has become a venue of active obesity prevention and treatment as a means to decrease health-care costs to employers and to increase productivity. Regardless, the rates of personal bankruptcy have risen along with the incidence of obesity. Using the National Longitudinal Survey of Youth 1979, a duration model was used to investigate the relative importance of obesity on the timing of bankruptcy. Even after accounting for possible endogeneity of BMI and controlling for a wide variety of individual and aggregate-level confounding factors, having obesity puts a person at a greater risk of filing for bankruptcy. Thus, obesity has an impact on the individual employee and also on the employers.

Older adults with obesity are twice as likely to be admitted to a nursing home. Many have comorbidities such as type 2 diabetes mellitus. Older adult patients with obesity and diabetes incurred one in every four nursing home days. Besides the costs of early entrance into nursing facilities, caring for residents with obesity is different than caring for residents who do not have obesity. Residents with obesity need additional equipment, supplies, and staff costs. Unlike emergency rooms and hospitals, nursing homes do not have federal requirements to serve all patients. Some nursing homes are not prepared to deal with patients with stage 2 or higher obesity, having to decline their care. The epidemic of obesity makes this gap in nursing home care a public health concern.

In addition to all the financial considerations mentioned above, an estimated 15 million adults in the USA took prescription medications concurrently with herbal remedies and/or high-dose vitamins in 1997. Alternative medicine professional services in 1997 were estimated at $21.2 billion, with at least $12.2 billion paid out-of-pocket. The total 1997 out-of-pocket expenditures on alternative therapies, estimated at $27 billion, matched the 1997 out-of-pocket expenditures for all USA physician services. Alternative therapies for weight management incurred the American public a $30 billion expenditure in 2003 without documentable long-term benefit.

Medical tourism is a relatively new phenomenon. Facing increasing health-care costs and the dilemma that obesity care is frequently excluded from coverage, many find it cheaper to have medical interventions abroad. This is certainly true for both bariatric surgery procedures and cosmetic surgeries following weight loss. The debate about safety, efficacy, and overall cost of care continues, but there is an increasing call for the globalization of medicine. With cheaper medical consultation, pharmacotherapy, and surgical costs abroad, many patients cross borders to secure medical care at a lower cost.

1.6 Obesity and Mortality

Actuarial tables from insurance companies provided the first data that overweight and obesity conveyed a higher risk of death. In 1972, Ancel Keys and colleagues coined the term BMI and published the formula for calculating it. For most people,

BMI is a reflection of fat mass. But individuals may have changes in BMI that are not related to fat mass—especially when body weight changes due to water (edema or dehydration) or muscularity (muscle hypertrophy or sarcopenia). Yet, data correlating BMI to death have continued to document a higher mortality risk for people at higher BMIs. In an analysis of pooled data from 19 prospective studies including 1.46 million white adults age 19–84, Cox regression was used to estimate hazard ratios and 95% confidence intervals for an association between BMI and all-cause mortality, adjusting for age, study, physical activity, alcohol consumption, education, and marital status. The median age was 58 years. The median baseline BMI was 26.2 kg/m^2. During a median follow-up period of 10 years (range, 5–28 years), 160,087 deaths were identified. In white adults, overweight and obesity are associated with increased all-cause mortality. All-cause mortality is lowest within the BMI range of 20.0–24.9 kg/m^2. Similar findings were published by the Prospective Studies Collaboration in the UK. Analysis of data from almost 900,000 adults in 57 prospective studies, documents that overall mortality is lowest at a BMI between 22.5 and 25 kg/m^2 in both genders and at all ages after adjustment for smoking status. Table 1.1 lists the cause-specific mortality versus baseline BMI in the ranges of 15–25 and 25–50 kg/m^2.

Table 1.1 Cause-specific mortality versus baseline BMI in the ranges 15–25 kg/m^2 and 25–50 kg/m^2

	15–25 kg/m^2		25–50 kg/m^2	
BMI range -->	Deaths	HR (95% CI)	Deaths	HR (95% CI)
Ischemic heart disease	7461	1.22 (1.13–1.32)	10,783	1.39 (1.34–1.44)
Stroke	2964	0.92 (0.82–1.03)	3164	1.39 (1.31–1.48)
Other vascular disease	2648	0.84 (0.75–0.95)	3396	1.47 (1.39–1.56)
Diabetes	171	0.96 (0.59–1.55)	393	2.16 (1.89–2.46)
Kidney disease (non-neoplastic)	197	1.14 (0.74–1.77)	217	1.59 (1.27–1.99)
Liver disease (non-neoplastic)	489	0.69 (0.52–0.91)	603	1.82 (1.59–2.09)
Lung cancer	2959	0.71 (0.63–0.79)	2040	0.98 (0.88–1.09)
Upper aerodigestive cancer	685	0.49 (0.39–0.61)	471	0.90 (0.79–1.20)
Other specified cancer	6134	0.94 (0.87–1.02)	6190	1.12 (1.06–1.18)
Respiratory disease[a]	2426	0.31 (0.28–0.35)	1344	1.20 (1.07–1.34)
Other specified disease	2049	0.62 (0.54–0.71)	1823	1.20 (1.10–1.31)
External cause	2112	0.82 (0.71–0.95)	1720	1.19 (1.08–1.32)
Unknown cause[b]*n*	4961	0.72 (0.66–0.79)	5349	1.22 (1.16–1.28)
All causes	35,256	0.79 (0.77–0.82)	37,493	1.29 (1.27–1.32)

From: Prospective Studies C et al. (2009)
Hazard ratio (HR) per 5 kg/m^2 higher BMI (HR): HR less than 1 if BMI inversely associated with risk. Analyses exclude the first 5 years of follow-up and adjust for study, sex, age at risk (in 5-year groups), and baseline smoking status
BMI body mass index, *Kg* kilogram, *m* meter, *HR* hazard ratio, *CI* confidence interval
[a]HR 0.37 (95% CI: 0.30–0.44) in the range 15–25 kg/m^2 after exclusion of the first 15 years of follow-up (leaving 956 deaths)
[b]Includes 4113 deaths from cancer of unspecified site

The concept that increasing BMI conveys increased mortality was challenged by observations of improved survival for patients undergoing hemodialysis, or with heart failure, at increasing BMIs. This obesity paradox has been clarified. It is individuals who have low cardiorespiratory fitness and inactivity that have the greater health threat. And in 2014, Cerhan and colleagues published the observation that in white adults a higher waist circumference is positively correlated with a higher mortality at all levels of BMI from 20 to 50 kg/m^2. Therefore, BMI alone is inadequate to assess mortality risk, and the waist circumference should be assessed even for those with a normal BMI.

1.7 Obesity Clinical Practice Guidelines: Overcoming a Century of Discrimination Against Patients with Obesity

In July 1965, President Lyndon Johnson signed into law the creation of Medicare under Title XVIII of the Social Security Act. Medicare was created to provide health insurance to people age 65 and older, regardless of income or medical history. In 1965, there was no awareness of obesity as a disease. Coverage for obesity care was not considered under Medicare, a situation that largely remains the same. In 2010, Lee and colleagues did a state-by-state analysis of Medicaid for adult and pediatric obesity care. Very few states ensured coverage of recommended treatments for obesity through Medicaid or private insurance. On the other hand, most states allowed obesity to be used to adjust rates in the small-group and individual markets and to deny coverage in the individual market.

In my state of Minnesota, statute 256B.0625 (Covered Services), Subdivision 13d (Drug formulary), specifically states that "the state's formulary shall not include drugs used for weight loss, except that medically necessary lipase inhibitors be covered for a recipient with type 2 diabetes." The genesis of this language comes from an obsolete notion that medications for the treatment of obesity are not safe or have the potential for abuse.

Overcoming the historical barriers to health care access for patients with obesity, given how deeply rooted they are, will require a major socioeconomic change. Fortunately, on many different fronts this is coming.

The following chronology outlines some of the recent developments that have advanced the social, political, and economical agendas to allow patients with overweight, obesity, and adiposopathy access to the medical care they need.

1916 The Association for the Study of Internal Secretions is founded.

1950 The National Obesity Society is organized.
[This is the first professional organization dedicated to the study and treatment of patients with obesity and associated conditions. It was named in succession the National Glandular Society, The American College of Endocrinology and Nutrition, The American Society of Bariatrics, and The American Society of Bariatric Physicians (ASBP)].

1952 The Association for the Study of Internal Secretions changes its name. The Endocrine Society (TES) begins operations.
1959 FDA approves phentermine for the short-term treatment of obesity.
1977 The Healthcare Financing Administration (HCFA) rules that obesity is not a disease.
1982 North American Association for the Study of Obesity (NAASO) is formed.
1983 American Society for Bariatric Surgery (ASBS) is formed.
[A surgical society to advance the art and science of metabolic and bariatric surgery].
1986 European Association for the Study of Obesity (EASO) is created.
1991 American Association of Clinical Endocrinologists (AACE) is founded.
1998 National Heart, Lung, and Blood Institute (NHLBI)—in collaboration with NAASO publishes.
Clinical Guidelines on the Identification, Evaluation, and Treatment of Overweight and Obesity.
[These guidelines recognized obesity as a chronic disease].
1999 WHO publishes a consultation on obesity.
[Highlights the benefits of weight loss].
2001 Surgeon General David Satcher. The Surgeon General's Call to Action to Prevent and Decrease Overweight and Obesity.
[Recognizes overweight and obesity as a nationwide epidemic. Calls to both prevent and treat overweight and obesity but fails to incorporate pharmacotherapy].
2002 Internal Revenue Service (IRS) issues a ruling on obesity.
[Expenses for the treatment of obesity qualify as deductible medical expenses].
2002 NHLBI—National Cholesterol Education Program (NCEP), Adult Treatment Panel (ATP) III.
Detection, Evaluation, and Treatment of High Blood Cholesterol in Adults.
[Incorporated measurement of waist circumference as a component of the dysmetabolic syndrome].
2002 WHO issues BMI thresholds for Asian populations.
2003 American Medical Association (AMA) publishes Roadmaps for Clinical Practice.
[First comprehensive primer on Assessment and Management of Adult Obesity in 10 booklets authored by Dr. Robert F Kushner and colleagues, including tools to implement effective treatment of obesity].
2004 Harold Bays, MD, introduces the term "adiposopathy," or "sick fat".
2004 TES publishes A Handbook on Obesity in America.
2004 AMA Obesity Summit held.
[Medical practice, Schools, Worksite, and Community workgroups issued recommendations to address the epidemic of obesity].
2004 Centers for Medicare and Medicaid Services (CMS) remove the phrase "obesity is not an illness".
2005 NAASO changes its name to The Obesity Society (TOS).
2006 CMS issues a ruling on coverage for bariatric surgery.
[Establishes a national coverage policy for bariatric/metabolic surgery].

2007 ASBS changes its name to the American Society for Metabolic and Bariatric Surgery (ASMBS).

2008 TOS published a white paper on evidence that obesity is a disease.

2010 AACE holds the first Adipose Tissue Pathophysiology Scientific Conference.
[Proceedings not published due to the lack of funding and support from AACE leadership at the time].

2011 The American Board of Obesity Medicine (ABOM) is established.
Joined the American Board of Bariatric Medicine and the Certified Obesity Medicine Physician into a single certification process. The effort was led by Dr. Robert F. Kuchner.
[Established to serve the public and the field of obesity medicine through the establishment and maintenance of criteria and procedures for examination and certification of candidate physicians who seek recognition of their accomplishments in obesity medicine].

2012 AACE Position Statement on Obesity and Obesity Medicine.
[AACE views obesity as a disease].

2013 AACE and TOS issue Clinical Practice Guideline:
Healthy eating for the prevention and treatment of metabolic and endocrine diseases in adults.
[First-ever evidence-based, reference-graded clinical practice guideline on healthy eating].

2013 AMA ends the debate about obesity being a disease.
[Resolution 420 recognizes obesity as a disease requiring a range of medical interventions to advance obesity treatment and prevention].

2013 ASBP Obesity Algorithm: Adult Adiposity Evaluation and Treatment.
[Includes that adiposopathy or "sick fat" is part of the obesity disease complex].

2013 NIH-NHLBI Management of Overweight and Obesity in Adults.
[The guideline was issued with evidence-based recommendations before new obesity medications were released—focused on behavior modification interventions].

2014 EASO Position Statement on Multidisciplinary Obesity Management in Adults.
[Obesity management cannot focus only on weight and BMI reduction. Emphasizes comprehensive approach to obesity management].

2014 Veteran's Administration and Department of Defense.
Evidence-based Clinical Practice Guidelines for Screening and Management of Overweight and Obesity.
[The first government agency in the USA to call for pharmacotherapy and bariatric surgery as adjuncts to comprehensive lifestyle intervention].

2014 AACE/ACE holds Consensus Conference on Obesity Pillar Participants.
[Reiterates that obesity is a chronic disease—incorporated as a clinical component in addition to an anthropometric component in the definition of obesity].

2014 AACE and American College of Endocrinology (ACE).

Position Statement on the 2014 Advanced Framework for a New Diagnosis of Obesity as a Chronic Disease.
[Redefined obesity at a BMI of 25 kg/m^2 in the presence of one or more obesity-related complications].

2014 J. Michael Gonzalez-Campoy, MD, PhD, FACE introduces "*Bariatric Endocrinology*" to the medical literature.
[Establishes that adipose tissue is an endocrine organ that may have derangements of structure and function which may affect other organs, contributing to, or precipitating, metabolic diseases, and calls for endocrinologists to make it a treatment goal to return adipose tissue to normal by applying the same model of chronic disease management that is applied to other chronic diseases].

2014 AACE holds the first session on Bariatric Endocrinology at its annual meeting.

2015 TES—Pharmacological Management of Obesity: An Endocrine Society Clinical Practice Guideline.
[Formally establishes pharmacotherapy for overweight and obesity as the standard of care].

2016 ASBP changes its name to Obesity Medicine Association (OMA).

2016 AACE-ACE Clinical Practice Guidelines for Comprehensive Medical Care of Patients with Obesity.
[The first comprehensive guideline incorporating all aspects of clinical care, including pharmacotherapy — evidence based, and reference graded].

1.8 Role of Adipose Tissue: Adiposity Versus Adiposopathy

Bariatric endocrinology was born from the need to address adipose tissue as an endocrine organ and to study the role of adiposopathy in the etiology of metabolic diseases. Further, bariatric endocrinology focuses on the development of medical interventions that return adipose tissue to normal. Whereas the loss of adipose tissue mass improves the complications of adiposity, the treatment of adiposopathy, independent of fat mass, is now a primary treatment target for clinical endocrinologists.

As with any other chronic disease, the continuum of overweight and obesity, with or without adiposopathy, may be treated, managed, controlled, and even put into remission. But it cannot be cured. Patients need to understand this premise, because the treatment of obesity is life-long. The implementation of models of chronic disease management for the treatment of obesity provides the appropriate framework for success. Thus, obesity treatment should include all available treatment modalities, from lifestyle changes that include better nutrition and more physical activity (NOT diet and exercise) to pharmacotherapy, to the use of devices, and to surgery for weight loss.

1.9 Principles of Bariatric Endocrinology

The principles of bariatric endocrinology also include:

- Every patient who has overweight or obesity should be initially evaluated for causes and complications of weight gain, including adiposopathy.
- Every patient who has overweight or obesity should have periodic risk re-stratification.
- The application of the same principles of chronic disease management to overweight and obesity, with or without adiposopathy.
- Behavior modification must be at the core of treatment for every patient. Small incremental and sustained changes are the best approach to achieve success long term.
- The team approach should be offered to all patients with overweight or obesity to achieve improved nutrition and increased physical activity.
- Pharmacotherapy must be an integral part of treatment for all patients who have overweight or obesity, with or without adiposopathy.
- Failure of monotherapy to achieve treatment goals should not lead to discontinuation of the agent. Rather causes for an inability to lose weight should be sought, and combination therapy should be used. In the absence of clinical trials to validate combinations of obesity medications, as is the case always in clinical medicine, the interests of the patient come first. Combination therapy frequently results in ongoing success with treatment.
- Bariatric surgery should be reserved for patients who are truly refractory to medical management.

1.10 Conclusion

The combined efforts of the many physicians and scientists who have studied adipose tissue, the adipocyte, and obesity as a disease, have helped shape the emerging field of bariatric endocrinology. As an endocrine cell, the adipocyte fits in the domain of clinical endocrinology. As a tissue with active cross talk, capable of modulating the function of other organs and contributing to the development of metabolic diseases, adipose tissue dysfunction is now a treatment target for the clinical endocrinologist and for bariatric endocrinology. Moving forward, the goals of treatment must be to decrease the burden of fat mass for the physical complications of obesity but also to return adipose tissue function to normal, for adiposopathy.

Reading List

Adams KT. Managing the high cost of obesity. Manag Care. 2015;24:42–4.

Andres R. The obesity-mortality association: where is the nadir of the U-shaped curve? Trans Assoc Life Insur Med Dir Am. 1980;64:185–97.

Bays HE. Current and investigational antiobesity agents and obesity therapeutic treatment targets. Obes Res. 2004;12:1197–211.
Bays H. Adiposopathy: role of adipocyte factors in a new paradigm. Expert Rev Cardiovasc Ther. 2005;3:187–9.
Bays HE, Gonzalez-Campoy JM. Adiposopathy. In: Friedberg E, Castrillon DH, Galindo RL, Wharton K, editors. New-opathies. Hackensack: World Scientific; 2012. p. 105–68.
Bays HE, Gonzalez-Campoy JM, Henry RR, et al. Is adiposopathy (sick fat) an endocrine disease? Int J Clin Pract. 2008;62:1474–83.
Berrington de Gonzalez A, Hartge P, Cerhan JR, et al. Body-mass index and mortality among 1.46 million white adults. N Engl J Med. 2010;363:2211–9.
Bhattacharya J, Sood N. Health insurance and the obesity externality. Adv Health Econ Health Serv Res. 2007;17:279–318.
Bray GA. Harvey Cushing and the neuroendocrinology of obesity. Obes Res. 1994;2:482–5.
Cerhan JR, Moore SC, Jacobs EJ, et al. A pooled analysis of waist circumference and mortality in 650,000 adults. Mayo Clin Proc. 2014;89:335–45.
Chalupka S. Workplace obesity prevention. AAOHN J Off J Am Assoc Occup Health Nurses. 2011;59:236.
Colditz GA. Economic costs of obesity. Am J Clin Nutr. 1992;55:503S–7S.
Dall TM, Zhang Y, Zhang S, et al. Weight loss and lifetime medical expenditures: a case study with TRICARE prime beneficiaries. Am J Prev Med. 2011;40:338–44.
Eisenberg DM, Davis RB, Ettner SL, et al. Trends in alternative medicine use in the United States, 1990–1997: results of a follow-up national survey. JAMA. 1998;280:1569–75.
Finkelstein E, Fiebelkorn l C, Wang G. The costs of obesity among full-time employees. Am J Health Promot. 2005;20:45–51.
Flegal KM, Kruszon-Moran D, Carroll MD, Fryar CD, Ogden CL. Trends in obesity among adults in the United States, 2005 to 2014. JAMA. 2016;315:2284–91.
Ford ES, Mokdad AH, Giles WH, Galuska DA, Serdula MK. Geographic variation in the prevalence of obesity, diabetes, and obesity-related behaviors. Obes Res. 2005;13:118–22.
Gill TP, Antipatis VJ, James WP. The global epidemic of obesity. Asia Pac J Clin Nutr. 1999;8:75–81.
Gonzalez-Campoy JM. The birth of bariatric endocrinology and the coming of age of obesity medicine. USA Endocrinol. 2016:10–1. https://doi.org/10.17925/USE.2016.12.01.10.
Gonzalez-Campoy JM, Richardson B, Richardson C, et al. Bariatric endocrinology: principles of medical practice. Int J Endocrinol. 2014;2014:917813.
Guettabi M, Munasib A. The impact of obesity on consumer bankruptcy. Econ Hum Biol. 2015;17:208–24.
Gurney M, Gorstein J. The global prevalence of obesity—an initial overview of available data. World Health Stat Q. 1988;41:251–4.
Hall JA, French TK, Rasmusson KD, et al. The paradox of obesity in patients with heart failure. J Am Acad Nurse Pract. 2005;17:542–6.
Haslam D. Obesity: a medical history. Obes Rev. 2007;8(Suppl 1):31–6.
Heber D. Herbal preparations for obesity: are they useful? Prim Care. 2003;30:441–63.
Hervey GR. The effects of lesions in the hypothalamus in parabiotic rats. J Physiol. 1959;145:336–52.
Keys A, Fidanza F, Karvonen MJ, Kimura N, Taylor HL. Indices of relative weight and obesity. J Chronic Dis. 1972;25:329–43.
Khoo JC, Steinberg D, Thompson B, Mayer SE. Hormonal regulation of adipocyte enzymes. The effects of epinephrine and insulin on the control of lipase, phosphorylase kinase, phosphorylase, and glycogen synthase. J Biol Chem. 1973;248:3823–30.
Lee JS, Sheer JL, Lopez N, Rosenbaum S. Coverage of obesity treatment: a state-by-state analysis of Medicaid and state insurance laws. Public Health Rep. 2010;125:596–604.
Lunt N, Hardey M, Mannion R. Nip, tuck and click: medical tourism and the emergence of web-based health information. Open Med Inform J. 2010;4:1–11.

Marihart CL, Brunt AR, Geraci AA. The high price of obesity in nursing homes. Care Manag J: J Case Manag; J Long Term Home Health Care. 2015;16:14–9.
Marks HH. Influence of obesity on morbidity and mortality. Bull N Y Acad Med. 1960;36:296–312.
Masters RK, Powers DA, Link BG. Obesity and USA mortality risk over the adult life course. Am J Epidemiol. 2013;177:431–42.
McAuley PA, Blair SN. Obesity paradoxes. J Sports Sci. 2011;29:773–82.
Mokdad AH, Serdula MK, Dietz WH, Bowman BA, Marks JS, Koplan JP. The spread of the obesity epidemic in the United States, 1991–1998. JAMA. 1999;282:1519–22.
Ogden CL, Carroll MD, Kit BK, Flegal KM. Prevalence of childhood and adult obesity in the United States, 2011–2012. JAMA. 2014;311:806–14.
Ogden CL, Carroll MD, Lawman HG, et al. Trends in obesity prevalence among children and adolescents in the United States, 1988–1994 through 2013–2014. JAMA. 2016;315:2292–9.
Perry AW. Nature and treatment of obesity. Calif State J Med. 1903;1:356–9.
Peterson MD, Mahmoudi E. Healthcare utilization associated with obesity and physical disabilities. Am J Prev Med. 2015;48:426–35.
Prospective Studies C, Whitlock G, Lewington S, et al. Body-mass index and cause-specific mortality in 900 000 adults: collaborative analyses of 57 prospective studies. Lancet. 2009;373:1083–96.
Ramachandran A, Snehalatha C, Baskar AD, et al. Temporal changes in prevalence of diabetes and impaired glucose tolerance associated with lifestyle transition occurring in the rural population in India. Diabetologia. 2004;47:860–5.
Schmidt DS, Salahudeen AK. Obesity-survival paradox-still a controversy? Semin Dial. 2007;20:486–92.
Sheppard CE, Lester EL, Chuck AW, et al. Medical tourism and bariatric surgery: who pays? Surg Endosc. 2014;28:3329–36.
Stevens GA, Singh GM, Lu Y, et al. National, regional, and global trends in adult overweight and obesity prevalences. Popul Health Metrics. 2012;10:22.
Strand O, Vaughan M, Steinberg D. Rat adipose tissue lipases: hormone-sensitive lipase activity against triglycerides compared with activity against lower glycerides. J Lipid Res. 1964;5:554–62.
Unti JA. Medical and surgical tourism: the new world of health care globalization and what it means for the practicing surgeon. Bull Am Coll Surg. 2009;94:18–25.
Vaughan M, Steinberg D. Effect of hormones on lipolysis and esterification of free fatty acids during incubation of adipose tissue in vitro. J Lipid Res. 1963;4:193–9.
Wang YC, McPherson K, Marsh T, Gortmaker SL, Brown M. Health and economic burden of the projected obesity trends in the USA and the UK. Lancet. 2011;378:815–25.
Williams LT, Jarett L, Lefkowitz RJ. Adipocyte beta-adrenergic receptors. Identification and subcellular localization by (−)-[3H]dihydroalprenolol binding. J Biol Chem. 1976;251:3096–104.
Yang Z, Zhang N. The burden of overweight and obesity on long-term care and Medicaid financing. Med Care. 2014;52:658–63.

Chapter 2
The Adipocyte

Elena A. Christofides

Pearls of Wisdom

- Adipose tissue is the largest organ by weight in the human body. The adipocyte is the predominant functional cell in adipose tissue, and it is an endocrine cell.
- Adipose tissue is heterogeneous; its function is determined by the type of adipocytes that form it and other cells that may infiltrate it.
- The fat vacuole in adipocytes is the site where most triglyceride storage occurs.
- Adipose tissue is an endocrine organ. It can make autocrine, paracrine, and, endocrine factors; all of which play a major role in metabolism homeostasis, including leptin and adiponectin.
- Adipose tissue has receptors for many different hormones, putting it at the crossroads of metabolism and offering the promise of therapeutic options for overweight, obesity, and metabolism.

E. A. Christofides
Endocrinology Associates, Inc., Columbus, OH, USA
e-mail: christofides@endocrinology-associates.com

J. M. Gonzalez-Campoy et al. (eds.), *Bariatric Endocrinology*,
https://doi.org/10.1007/978-3-319-95655-8_2

2.1 Introduction

The concept that adipose tissue is just for storage of energy in the form of lipids has long been discarded. The functional unit of adipose tissue, the adipocyte, has been defined as an active endocrine cell. It has receptors that respond to hormones made by other organs, and it too makes hormones that help regulate metabolism. In addition to this, numerous paracrine and autocrine factors are known to regulate adipocyte function across its cell cycle. The adipocyte therefore plays an integral role in maintaining metabolic homeostasis. The adipocyte, as any other cell, has the potential for becoming dysfunctional, which then contributes to metabolic disorders. This chapter describes the adipocyte (and adipose tissue) as a crucial player in the regulation of metabolism.

2.2 Teleology

Adipose stem cells reside as peroxisome proliferator-activated receptor (PPAR)-γ–positive mural cells in a vascular niche within adipose tissue. Maintenance of adipose tissue in adult humans is a dynamic process that involves stem cell commitment, quiescence, and eventual proliferation. Differentiation may be in the form of early recruitment, or of late lipid filling. These processes, which define the life cycle of adipocytes, are under the influence of environmental stimuli, which include the composition of meals, caloric load, medications, and tissue injury.

From their common precursor cell, the development of adipocytes is not uniform. Adipose cell development is dependent on its functional destiny. Our current understanding is that there are predominantly three types of adipocytes: white, brown, and beige.

White adipose tissue (WAT) arises from stem cells of mesodermal origin. It primarily serves as an energy repository to protect the needs of animals during times of prolonged caloric deficit. This is compared to the liver, which stores and releases calories readily to meet our immediate energy needs in times of acute energy shifts. WAT is detectable by the midpoint of gestation and is capable of increasing over time. It was previously believed that WAT was metabolically inert but is now appreciated to be as significant as brown adipose tissue (BAT) in the overall hormonal control of metabolism. WAT plays a key role in the control of the thyroid, thymus, and reproductive organs. Indeed the integration of energy management for the sustainability of an organism and future generations of humans makes healthy WAT a basic necessity.

Brown adipose tissue (BAT) is the subject of intense interest and research. BAT arises from stem cells of mesodermal origin as well and is only apparent in mammals. It has a genetic fingerprint similar to that of skeletal muscle tissue. Both have cell surface marker myogenic factor 5 (Myf5), which is lacking in all other adipose tissue lines. BAT is responsible for nonshivering thermogenesis as opposed to shivering-induced thermogenesis of muscle tissue. Although the repository of BAT is thought to be fixed and stable, it is clear that the absolute volume of BAT decreases as an animal ages and is inversely correlated to body mass index (BMI). Energy consumption by BAT for thermoregulation is via the activation of uncoupling protein (UCP)-1 present in the mitochondria.

Beige adipose tissue arises from a similar but distinct preadipocyte precursor stem cell line as WAT. Partial induction of WAT into beige adipose tissue is possible, but a separate and stable population of beige adipocytes does exist. Induction of beige adipose tissue increases the expression of UCP1 and nonshivering thermogenesis. The fate of an adipocyte into WAT or beige is determined by environmental pressures such as exposure to cold or beta-adrenergic stimuli. Beige adipose tissue is easily induced by these various forms of stimuli, which suggests an evolutionarily protective need for a flexible mode of thermogenesis.

2.3 Adipocyte Cytology

The adipocyte has a fibroblast morphology but is distinct from skin fibroblasts reflective of its mesodermal origin. Perilipin proteins mark the cell surface of all adipocytes and the phosphorylation of these proteins is a key requirement of lipid mobilization.

WAT and beige adipocytes are characterized by globularly shaped cells consisting of a single, large lipid droplet with the nucleus and a few mitochondria eccentrically placed. WAT hormone receptor density on the cell surface is greater than that of BAT. The connective tissue supportive structure is vascular and innervated. Key features that distinguish WAT are the presence of PPARγ, glucose transporter 4 (GLUT4) and leptin receptors on the cell surface, and the absence of UCP1 capable mitochondria. Beige adipocytes share all the key features of WAT with the exception that they have UCP1 capable mitochondria.

BAT is characterized by a polygonal-shaped cell with multiple, smaller lipid droplets and numerous mitochondria located in a more uniform fashion. The connective tissue supportive structures are more vascular than that of WAT, and the innervation is predominantly β-adrenergic. Key features that distinguish BAT are the presence of PPAR-ϒ and GLUT4 and the absence of leptin receptors on the cell surface. The mitochondria of BAT are UCP1 capable and are more densely packed with cristae lending BAT its name and characteristic coloration.

2.4 Adipocyte Physiology

The role of adipose tissue varies based on type and location. Although hormone receptor density is greater with WAT than with BAT, functional outcome is ultimately determined by activation and the relationships between the various hormonal control messengers. The following is a brief review of enzymes and hormones that adipose tissue makes, and those that have effects on adipose tissue, thus helping to maintain metabolic homeostasis.

WAT is located in the subcutaneous tissue layer with concentrated depots in the thighs, buttocks, and abdomen. Smaller depots exist around the kidneys, intestines, and omentum. The basic role of WAT is to take up unesterified fatty acids from the circulation and esterify them using diacylglycerol acyltransferase (DGAT), allowing for storage into triglyceride-containing lipid droplets. These depots represent the greatest repository of triglycerides in mammalian tissue with coupled oxidative phosphorylation to produce adenosine triphosphate (ATP) as the primary product.

BAT is concentrated centrally in the cervical, supraclavicular, and axillary areas. The basic role of BAT is the utilization of triglycerides in uncoupled oxidative phosphorylation, which produces thermal energy as the primary product.

Fat storage and fat breakdown in adipocytes are under control by lipoprotein lipase (LPL) and hormone-sensitive lipase (HSL), which is modulated by epinephrine and insulin. In the fasting state, HSL is active, leading to the hydrolysis of triglycerides. This generates fatty acids and glycerol, which become a substrate for gluconeogenesis. After feeding, HSL activity is suppressed and LPL activity increases.

2.4.1 Intracellular Signals

Within the cellular processes of the adipocyte, adenosine monophosphate (AMP)-activated protein kinase (AMPK) is a key regulator of glucose metabolism, as it is directly responsible for the phosphorylation of acetyl-CoA. AMPK indirectly stimulates fatty acid oxidation and cellular glucose uptake by facilitating translocation of GLUT4 to the cell surface of the adipocyte with subsequent downregulation of gluconeogenesis gene transcription. AMPK increases with prolonged fasting via an alteration of the ratio of AMP/ATP rather than an absolute change in the concentration of either compound. AMPK is activated by adiponectin and leptin. In BAT, AMPK acts as a regulator of chronic thermogenic potential and not an acute activator of nonshivering thermogenesis. This effect of cold exposure is mediated via the activation of the β-adrenergic system. Physical activity, particularly endurance physical activity, can induce AMPK via muscle-derived interleukin (IL)-6.

DGAT1 is one of the most recognizable enzymes of a functioning adipocyte. It produces triacylglycerol (TG) from diacylglycerol (retinol) and is stimulated by feeding. The highest concentration of DGAT1 is in adipose tissue. DGAT1 is also present in the lumen of the intestines, where it contributes to the uptake of fatty acids for transport into the plasma, and in the liver, where it is involved in lipid synthesis.

The PPAR family has numerous well-described subtypes that have varied but critically integrated functions. They are all stimulated by prolonged fasting (greater than 24 h) and serve to activate fatty acid oxidation. Various polyunsaturated fats

(PUFA) such as arachidonic acid are natural endogenous ligands. All PPARs form heterodimers with retinoid X receptors (RXR) in order to bind to deoxyribonucleic acid (DNA) and induce transcription. PPAR-α is activated by energy deprivation. It is necessary for ketogenesis, and its activation leads to the upregulation of genes involved in fatty acid transport and breakdown. On the other hand, PPAR-δ and PPAR-β are activated by all-trans retinoic acid (RA), which subsequently recruits RXR. This complex integration is a key step in the adipocyte uptake of FFA, production of lipid droplets, and adipogenesis via recruitment and differentiation.

PPAR-ϒ coactivator 1-alpha (PGC-1α) is a major integrator of the external cell signals to the nucleus in the interior. It serves as a cofactor to PPAR-ϒ, thyroid hormone, and AMPK. The main stimuli for PGC-1α are cold, cellular stress signals, endurance exercise, and prolonged fasting. It coordinates the signal between PPAR-ϒ and thyroid hormone to induce UCP action for thermogenesis. Reactive oxygen species (ROS) and reactive nitrogen species (RNS) are key inducers of PGC-1α via IL-1RN. When stimulated by endurance exercise or other cellular stress signals, PGC-1α establishes a lactate threshold by determining mitochondrial biogenesis as well as inducing muscle fiber fuel pathway switching. Specifically, PGC-1α has been shown to be able to switch cardiac muscle utilization away from a glycolytic fuel source to a fatty acid oxidation fuel source. PGC-1α activation in the fasting state is via glucagon and cyclic AMP, which induce gluconeogenesis in the liver and fatty acid oxidation by downregulating insulin signaling. PGC-1α increases the expression of GLUT4 in the fed state. There is a subsequent increase in glucose uptake in the skeletal muscle predominantly.

2.4.2 Hormone Receptors in Adipocytes

There are numerous receptors that have been identified in adipose tissue. Some are clearly established to be in adipocytes, and others are located in other cell types within adipose tissue. The expression of receptors varies between adipose tissue location and type.

2.4.2.1 Insulin Receptor Stimulation Leads to Lipogenesis

Insulin is likely the most recognizable anabolic hormone signal. The insulin receptor is a cell surface tyrosine kinase receptor embedded in the plasma membrane of adipose tissue and is composed of two alpha subunits in the extracellular space, which serve as the hormone-binding site, and two beta subunits in the intracellular space. Insulin receptor activation causes an increased rate of glycolysis through increased hexokinase and 6-phosphofructokinase activities. Insulin also stimulates glycogen synthesis. Movement of glucose and FFA requires the activation of GLUT4 by insulin in all tissues except for the brain and liver. Insulin facilitates the uptake of glucose and free fatty acids (FFA) by adipocytes. By increasing the rate of glucose transport across the cell membrane, insulin increases fatty acid and triglyceride uptake in adipocytes, stimulating the growth of the lipid droplet.

2.4.2.2 Epinephrine Receptor Stimulation Leads to Lipolysis

Epinephrine has long been known to cause a rapid increase in lipolysis. There are at least five adrenergic receptors in adipose tissue: α1, α2, β1, β2, and β3. Binding of β-adrenergic receptors by epinephrine causes an immediate rise in cyclic adenosine monophosphate (cAMP). The rise in cAMP activates cAMP protein kinase. This enzyme phosphorylates various target proteins in adipocytes. Epinephrine binding of the β-adrenergic receptors activates HSL and causes lipolysis. On the other hand, the activation of α2 receptors has the opposite effect, lowering cAMP and decreasing the rate of lipolysis.

Epinephrine has a higher affinity for α2- than the β-adrenergic receptors. The level of expression of β-adrenergic and α2-adrenergic receptor subtypes differs depending on the anatomic location of fat deposits. The higher net effect of epinephrine to cause lipolysis is therefore a function of differential receptor stimulation.

2.4.2.3 Thyroid Hormone Receptor Stimulation Causes Lipolysis

Thyroid hormones are capable of free movement in and out of all cells. Thyroid hormones stimulate nuclear receptors (which exist in several isoforms) and also bind thyroid response elements in target genes. The thyroid hormone concentrations in adipose tissue are modulated by deiodinases.

Thyroid hormones activate many genes in adipocytes and have effects on adipocyte proliferation, adipocyte differentiation, adipocyte gene expression, and ultimately adipocyte function. Thyroid hormone stimulation of the adipocyte leads to increased mobilization of free fatty acids (FFA) in WAT, which stimulates oxidative phosphorylation. In BAT, thyroid hormone stimulates UCP1 via β-adrenergic stimulation, increasing thermogenesis.

As an example of how thyroid hormone acts in the adipocyte, triiodothyronine stimulates the adiponutrin gene. Adiponutrin is a triacylglycerol lipase whose upregulation by triiodothyronine results in the hydrolysis of triacylglycerol. Thyroid hormone effects are in turn modulated by other hormones. For example, lipoprotein lipase is downregulated by triiodothyronine but upregulated by triiodothyronine with norepinephrine.

2.4.2.4 Steroid Hormone Receptors

There are numerous steroid hormone receptors present on adipose tissue which are responsive primarily to circulating sex steroids. These are members of the ligand-dependent transcription factor family of steroid receptors. The adipocyte produces enzymes that modulate steroid hormone activity (i.e., hydroxysteroid dehydrogenases) in response to individual steroid hormone signals. The expression and action of these steroid enzymes are adipose tissue-type specific but primarily serve to antagonize the actions of insulin.

17-β-hydroxysteroid dehydrogenase (BHSD) mediates the conversion of weak androgens or estrogens into their more potent counterparts, specifically androstenedione to testosterone and estrone to estradiol. The enzyme aromatase in adipocytes converts androgens to estrogens, specifically androstenedione to estrone and testosterone to estradiol. The ratio of the expression of 17-BHSD to aromatase is inversely related to adipose tissue location (subcutaneous versus visceral) and is correlated with central adiposity. Both are cytochrome P450-dependent aromatases.

3-BHSD and its allosteric 3α counterpart are the only members of the steroid enzyme family that are not dependent on cytochrome P450. 3-BHSD mediates the conversion of progesterone from pregnenolone, 17-hydroxypregnenolone from 17-hydroxyprogesterone, and androstenedione from dehydroepiandrosterone (DHEA), creating active sex steroids from precursor molecules.

11-BHSD is highly expressed in visceral adipose tissue. It is responsible for the local conversion of hormonally inactive 11β-ketoglucocorticoid metabolites (cortisone) to hormonally active 11β-hydroxylated metabolites (cortisol). The cortisol produced does not contribute to circulating levels of cortisol. Locally produced and circulating cortisol each contributes to net lipolysis.

Estrogen receptor (ER)-α stimulation protects adipose tissue against inflammatory damage and allows for subcutaneous adipocyte number expansion. On the other hand, a state of estrogen deficiency promotes adipocyte hypertrophy, ectopic fat deposition, and decreased subcutaneous adipocyte number expansion. Estrogen deficiency leads to a proinflammatory milieu, adipose tissue fibrosis, and adiposopathy.

Table 2.1 summarizes some of the adipocyte receptors that have been characterized to date.

2.4.3 The Adipocyte as an Endocrine Cell

While all adipose tissue is hormonally active, WAT produces an astounding array of protein products that have far-reaching actions. Many of the products of adipose tissue are structurally similar to cytokines and are thus called adipokines. These are better termed adipose tissue hormones.

2.4.3.1 Adipsin

Adipsin was first described in 1987 and became the first adipose tissue hormone identified. Adipsin is a serine protease made by mature WAT and is a critical component of acylation-stimulating protein (ASP), which regulates adipocyte function

Table 2.1 Adipocyte receptors

Adipocyte receptor	Effect of receptor stimulation in adipocytes
Adenosine	Antilipolytic
Adrenergic receptor α1	Antilipolytic, glycogenolysis, lactate production
Adrenergic receptor α2	Antilipolytic, activation of mitogen-activated protein kinases
Adrenergic receptor β1	HSL activation, lipolysis, glycogenolysis
Adrenergic receptor β2	HSL activation, lipolysis, phosphorylation of GLUT 4 with inhibition of insulin-induced glucose transport
Adrenergic receptor β3	HSL activation, lipolysis
Angiotensin I	Antilipolytic
Angiotensin II	Lipogenesis
Estrogen receptor α	Anti-inflammatory, promotes expansion of the subcutaneous adipose tissue
Glucocorticoid receptor	Lipolytic
Insulin receptor	Lipogenesis, antilipolytic, activation of GLUT 4 receptors
Natriuretic peptide receptor	Lipolysis, increased adiponectin release
Neuropeptide Y receptor	Antilipolytic, increased leptin release
Peptide YY receptor	Antilipolytic, increased leptin release
Prostaglandin E2 (paracrine factor) receptor	Antilipolytic

HSL Hormone-sensitive lipase, *GLUT* Glucose transporter type 4

via a G-protein receptor. ASP specifically increases lipoprotein lipase action, which improves the clearance of FFA and the production of triglycerides. Adipsin helps maintain beta cell function in people with diabetes by generating C3a, a peptide that is a potent insulin secretagogue. Adipsin levels are paradoxically decreased in obesity, which contributes to the development of hyperglycemia. Adipsin is also involved in the suppression of infection.

2.4.3.2 Leptin

Leptin is likely the most well known of the adipose tissue hormones. Leptin is a 167-amino acid protein whose gene is located on chromosome 7 in humans. The leptin gene is expressed not only in WAT but also in BAT, stomach, liver, placenta, and mammary glands. It has a tertiary structure that fits into the cytokine family, for which the term adipokine was used. Leptin circulates in the serum both in free form and bound to carrier proteins. Leptin levels increase with increasing fat mass as well as nutrient sufficiency. Hyperleptinemia is a hormonal derangement found almost universally in humans with obesity.

The original description of the function of leptin was that it induces weight loss in leptin-deficient animals with obesity. Subsequently, obesity has been characterized as a state of increasing leptin levels with increasing fat mass. Therefore, in humans with obesity, a slimming effect of leptin is not apparent. This has given rise to the concept of leptin resistance. Another way of interpreting the role of leptin is that it is a signal from adipose tissue to the central nervous system (CNS) about how much energy the body has in storage.

Neuropeptide Y (NPY) is produced by the gut and the hypothalamus. Stimulation of central NPY neurons leads to feeding. Leptin has receptors in the lateral hypothalamus, where it inhibits hunger by counteracting the effects of NPY. Leptin also counteracts tetrahydrocannabinol receptors in the lateral hypothalamus, leading to further inhibition of hunger. α-melanocyte-stimulating hormone (MSH) has effects opposite to those of NPY; it suppresses feeding. Stimulation of leptin receptors in the medial hypothalamus promotes the synthesis of α-MSH; hence, leptin indirectly suppresses hunger.

Women have higher serum leptin concentrations than men, so gender is a modulator of leptin. There is also a diurnal variation in circulating leptin levels, with the highest levels between midnight and early morning. Patients with obesity and obstructive sleep apnea have reductions in circulating leptin levels with institution of treatment with continuous positive airway pressure. In lean people, leptin levels rise with 8–12 h of unbroken sleep. Conversely, sleep deprivation causes a drop in leptin levels. Estrogen, testosterone, emotional stress, dexamethasone, and insulin all raise leptin levels. Regular physical activity decreases leptin levels independent of fat mass.

Leptin levels are most significantly impacted by acute changes to caloric intake. Leptin serum concentrations may decrease up to 30% after a 72-h fast. This drop in leptin is sensed by the brain as an acute stress and results in the decreased production of sex steroids and thyroid hormone and a rise in cortisol and insulin-like growth factor (IGF)-1. The same fasting with leptin replacement does not lead to these changes in pituitary axis hormones.

Leukocytosis is associated with hyperleptinemia. Acute infection increases leptin as well as other inflammatory cytokines. Thus, leptin also functions as an acute phase reactant to activate the immune system.

2.4.3.3 Adiponectin

Adiponectin is a 244-amino acid protein that belongs to the collagen superfamily. It is made by mature adipocytes and is primarily produced by subcutaneous WAT. Adiponectin is also made by the placenta. Circulating adiponectin levels are lower in males than females. Levels of adiponectin are inversely correlated to fat mass and insulin resistance, with declining levels being predictive of the clinical onset of type 2 diabetes mellitus. Interestingly, adiponectin levels also correlate with the degree of inflammation associated with endocrine and rheumatologic autoimmune diseases. The metabolites of adiponectin are biologically active, and the specificity of their actions is tissue specific. The metabolites can alternately activate proinflammatory macrophages or deactivate them into anti-inflammatory monocytes. These actions have been linked to decreased foam cell formation.

There are two major adiponectin receptors identified: adiponectin receptor 1 and adiponectin receptor 2. They are members of the progestin and adipoQ receptor family, therefore also known as PAQR1 and PAQR2, respectively; each has seven transmembrane domains, and they are G protein-coupled receptors. The adiponectin receptors bind globular and full-length adiponectin and mediate increased AMPK and PPAR-α activity, fatty acid oxidation, and glucose uptake. They are expressed mainly in the liver and muscle but also in the heart, adipose tissue, osteoblasts, pancreas, leukocytes, and brain. Adiponectin receptor activation translates into improved insulin sensitivity via fatty acid oxidation and increased energy expenditure, diminished hepatic glucose production and decreased oxidized low-density lipoprotein-induced endothelial proliferation.

2.4.3.4 Resistin

Resistin is an amino acid chain encoded by the RETN gene. It was discovered in 2001 and named because it causes insulin resistance when injected into mice. Resistin is a product of WAT and is predominantly expressed by visceral adipose tissue. Resistin levels increase with obesity, although this is not a universal finding. Increasing fat mass causes the upregulation of resistin, with further adipocyte differentiation. Mice lacking resistin have reduced hepatic glucose production and low blood glucose levels after fasting. In the liver, resistin increases the production of low-density lipoprotein and degrades the LDL receptors.

2.4.4 Other Adipose Tissue-Circulating Factors

Adipose tissue releases into the circulation hormones and other chemicals that do not originate in the adipocytes. Rather they come from cells that reside in the stroma and the vasculature of adipose tissue. Many of these circulating factors significantly contribute to the regulation of metabolism. Table 2.2 contains many of the identified adipose tissue factors and their role, and the discussion that follows highlights some of them.

2.4.4.1 Angiotensinogen

Angiotensinogen is classically discussed in relationship to the renin-angiotensin-aldosterone system (RAAS), the control of blood pressure, and vascular volume. All components of RAAS are capable of being produced by adipose tissue, but visceral adipose tissue is a significant contributor to angiotensinogen levels. Local levels of angiotensinogen do directly contribute to overall blood pressure regulation. Further, locally produced angiotensin II causes lipogenesis through the stimulation of the angiotensin II receptor while blocking lipolysis through the angiotensin I receptor, thus contributing to the accrual of fat mass.

Table 2.2 Adipose tissue products

Adipose tissue product	Process it is involved in
α1-acid glycoprotein	Immune system, acute-phase reactants, and inflammation
Acylation-stimulating protein	Lipid and lipoprotein metabolism; insulin sensitivity of the muscle, hepatocyte, and adipocyte
Adiponectin	Metabolism and energy homeostasis; insulin sensitivity of the muscle, hepatocyte, and adipocyte
Adipsin	Immune system, acute-phase reactants, and inflammation; insulin sensitivity of the muscle, hepatocyte, and adipocyte
Adrenomedullin	Blood vessel control and angiogenesis
Amyloid A3	Immune system, acute-phase reactants, and inflammation
Angiopoietin-2	Blood vessel control and angiogenesis
Angiotensinogen	Blood vessel control and angiogenesis
Angiotensin II	Blood vessel control and angiogenesis
Apelin	Blood vessel control and angiogenesis; insulin sensitivity of the muscle, hepatocyte, and adipocyte
Asproxin	Metabolism and energy homeostasis; insulin sensitivity of the muscle, hepatocyte, and adipocyte
Autotaxin	Lipid and lipoprotein metabolism
Cathepsin L	Immune system, acute-phase reactants, and inflammation
Cathepsin S	Immune system, acute-phase reactants, and inflammation
Cholesterol ester transport protein	Lipid and lipoprotein metabolism
Collagen type 6	Metabolism of extracellular matrix
Complement factor B	Immune system, acute-phase reactants, and inflammation
Complement factor C3	Immune system, acute-phase reactants, and inflammation
Complement factor D	Immune system, acute-phase reactants, and inflammation
Cortisol	Immune system, acute-phase reactants, and inflammation; lipid and lipoprotein metabolism
Epidermal growth factor 8	Metabolism of extracellular matrix
Estradiol	Adipose tissue development; metabolism and energy homeostasis; insulin sensitivity of the muscle, hepatocyte, and adipocyte
Haptoglobin	Immune system, acute-phase reactants, and inflammation
Insulin-like growth factor 1	Adipose tissue development
Interleukin-1β	Immune system, acute-phase reactants, and inflammation
Interleukin-1 receptor antagonist	Immune system, acute-phase reactants, and inflammation
Interleukin-6	Metabolism and energy homeostasis; immune system, acute-phase reactants, and inflammation; insulin sensitivity of the muscle, hepatocyte, and adipocyte
Interleukin-8	Metabolism and energy homeostasis; immune system, acute-phase reactants, and inflammation
Interleukin-10	Immune system, acute-phase reactants, and inflammation

(continued)

Table 2.2 (continued)

Adipose tissue product	Process it is involved in
Leptin	Food intake and activation of the sympathetic nervous system; metabolism and energy homeostasis; blood vessel control and angiogenesis; insulin sensitivity of the muscle, hepatocyte, and adipocyte
Lipocalin 24p3	Immune system, acute-phase reactants, and inflammation
Lipoprotein lipase	Lipid and lipoprotein metabolism
Macrophage inflammatory protein 1β	Immune system, acute-phase reactants, and inflammation
Metallothionein	Immune system, acute-phase reactants, and inflammation
Metalloproteases	Metabolism of extracellular matrix
Mitogen factor	Adipose tissue development
Monobutyrin	Blood vessel control and angiogenesis
Monocyte chemoattractant protein-1	Immune system, acute-phase reactants, and inflammation
Nerve growth factor	Adipose tissue development
Omentin-1	Insulin sensitivity of the muscle, hepatocyte, and adipocyte
Pentraxin-3	Immune system, acute-phase reactants, and inflammation
Plasminogen activator inhibitor-1	Metabolism of extracellular matrix
PPAR-ϒ angiopoietin-related protein	Blood vessel control and angiogenesis
Prostacyclin	Lipid and lipoprotein metabolism
Prostaglandin E2	Lipid and lipoprotein metabolism
Prostaglandin F2α	Lipid and lipoprotein metabolism
Resistin	Metabolism and energy homeostasis; insulin sensitivity of the muscle, hepatocyte, and adipocyte
Retinol-binding protein 4	Lipid and lipoprotein metabolism; metabolism and energy homeostasis
Thrombopoietin	Blood vessel control and angiogenesis; adipose tissue development
Tissue inhibitor of metalloproteases 1	Metabolism of extracellular matrix
Tissue inhibitor of metalloproteases 2	Metabolism of extracellular matrix
Tissue inhibitor of metalloproteases 3	Metabolism of extracellular matrix
Tumor necrosis factor α	Immune system, acute-phase reactants, and inflammation
Vaspin	Insulin sensitivity of the muscle, hepatocyte, and adipocyte
Vascular endothelium growth factor	Blood vessel control and angiogenesis; adipose tissue development
Visfatin	Insulin sensitivity of the muscle, hepatocyte, and adipocyte

PPAR-ϒ Peroxisome proliferator-activated receptor-ϒ

2.4.4.2 TNF-α

TNF-α is produced by macrophages residing in adipose tissue and has effects on adipocytes and thc liver. In adipocytes TNF-α deactivates the insulin receptor, suppresses lipogenesis, induces lipolysis, and increases the uptake of glucose and non-esterified fatty acids. It is capable of suppressing adiponectin and has been shown to be synergistic to elevated levels of plasminogen activator inhibitor-1.

2.4.4.3 Interleukin-6

Interleukin (IL)-6 is an adipokine whose receptor is homologous to leptin. It is preferentially expressed by visceral adipose tissue. IL-6, as an adipokine, is a potent trigger of the hepatic acute phase reaction. Circulating levels in the periphery correlate to adiposity and diabetes, whereas the inverse is true of the levels in the CNS. IL-6 functions to decrease food intake and increase energy expenditure through catabolic pathways, thereby decreasing adipogenesis. IL-6 inhibits adiponectin and insulin receptor function.

2.4.4.4 Plasminogen Activator Inhibitor-1 (PAI-1)

PAI-1 is produced predominantly by visceral adipose tissue, and circulating levels are strongly correlated to the degree of visceral adiposity. The levels of PAI-1 are predictive of the development of diabetes and cardiovascular disease.

2.4.4.5 Omentin

Omentin is the first fat depot-specific secretory protein to be identified. It was discovered through the sequencing of expressed sequence tags from a human omental fat cDNA library. Omentin mRNA encodes a peptide of 313 amino acids, containing a secretory signal sequence and a fibrinogen-related domain. Omentin mRNA is predominantly expressed in visceral adipose tissue and is barely detectable in subcutaneous fat in humans. The source of omentin is the stromal-vascular cells and not adipocytes themselves. Omentin has a vasodilation effect in isolated blood vessels. Addition of recombinant omentin in vitro increases insulin-stimulated glucose uptake.

2.5 Epigenetic Changes Which Can Influence the Function of the Adipocyte

Epigenetics is an emerging field in pathophysiology. It is defined as "the study of changes in organisms caused by modification of gene expression rather than alteration of the genetic code itself." These changes have been described as DNA methylations, histone acetylations, and chromatin alterations. DNA methylation occurs when a methyl group (CH_3) is added to the cytosine or adenine nucleotides of DNA. The addition of a methyl group can create either a gain of function or loss of function within a gene group and may be permanent. Some epigenetic changes are heritable particularly if they occur in the oocyte prior to fertilization. Many of the methylations occur due to environmental pressures either in utero or during postnatal growth.

One of the most significant epigenetic changes seen in humans has been the alteration of the circadian clock. Maternal health during the peripartum period has acute and chronic epigenetic influences on the fetal circadian clock. Circadian dysrhythmia is known to negatively impact energy balance and long-term health maintenance.

A significant body of evidence on epigenetics exists in animal studies owing to the ease of rapid generational manipulations and observations. Unsurprisingly, manipulation of dietary macronutrient composition has been the most impactful on the health of the adipocyte. Female animals made overweight by the feeding of a high-fat diet tend to produce offspring that have an increase in body mass at birth which persists into adulthood. However, if the female is fed a high-fat diet where the ratio of PUFA to saturated fat intake is increased, the substitution of saturated fat by PUFA appears to ameliorate some of those epigenetic pressures on the offspring, with a decreased adipocyte mass at birth. Animals fed high-fat and high-sugar meals during gestation give birth to offspring that have altered growth hormone regulation. Methylation of IGF genes induces a gain of function which leads to higher birth weight, higher glucose, and higher leptin levels, all of which contribute to subsequent increased overall insulin resistance. Animals fed high-fat meals alone during gestation develop an upregulated methylation of PPAR-ϒ and give birth to offspring with lower bone density due to reduced osteocyte populations. Poor protein intake before and during gestation induces histone methylation, which silences skeletal muscle GLUT4 action. Poor protein intake during gestation also leads to a gain of function DNA methylation in IGF-2 and Zinc transport proteins. This is accentuated with high-fat feeding in the offspring, which is partially reversible with offspring folate supplementation.

2.6 How Aging Influences the Adipocyte-Adipocyte Cross Talk

The most significant change that occurs in the aging person is the progressive loss of BAT. The inability to maintain the most thermogenically active repository of adipocytes creates a metabolic mismatch. There is recruitment of smaller adipocytes by larger adipocytes with a transfer of lipid droplets. Increasing recruitment creates a more inflammatory adipocyte. Decreased expression of PPAR-ϒ in the visceral adipose tissue drives increases in regulatory T-cell numbers, IL-6, monocyte chemoattractive protein (MCP)-1, and palmitate which increase TNF-α. There is an inverse correlation that occurs in the bone marrow with an increased expression of PPAR-ϒ. This leads to a shift away from osteoblast formation to adipocyte formation owing to a common progenitor cell line. Markers of bone formation decrease accordingly.

2.7 Other Functions of Adipose Tissue

2.7.1 Thermogenesis and Insulation

Brown adipose tissue is capable of generating heat in mammals, but this process is limited in humans. Beta-adrenergic receptor stimulation by norepinephrine causes a rise in cAMP, which then stimulates HSL. The ensuing production of free fatty acids from triglycerides provides the substrate for mitochondria to generate heat. UCP (also called thermogenin) is a 33-kDa inner-membrane mitochondrial protein exclusive to brown adipocytes. UCP functions as a proton transporter, allowing protons to bypass the ATP synthase channel. The dissipation of the energy generated by the proton gradient produces heat. Nonshivering thermogenesis is regulated by thyroid hormone, epinephrine, and leptin through the activation of the sympathetic nervous system. The induction of brown fat differentiation and the stimulation of thermogenesis remain areas of interest as potential treatment targets for obesity.

The subcutaneous distribution of adipose tissue allows it to serve as a layer of insulation. In humans, this role of subcutaneous fat is limited. Blubber in animals, on the other hand, is required for survival in some climates.

2.7.2 Padding

Adipose tissue serves the role of padding for other organs. In the subcutaneous space, it protects nerves and blood vessels from trauma. Loss of subcutaneous fat increases the risk of extravasation of the blood. In the internal cavities of the body, adipose tissue also provides padding. This is especially true of the intra-abdominal organs.

2.7.3 Contouring

Adipose tissue provides substance that shapes and contours the body. Adipose tissue is indispensable to shape the female breasts, the facial features, and the hips. Abnormal fat mass quantity and distribution results in distortions of contour.

2.8 Adipose Tissue Circulation and Nerve Supply

As is the case for every tissue in the body, adipose tissue has its blood supply and innervation. This was first recognized in 1948, but an active investigation into these components of adipose tissue has only recently yielded clues to their importance in adipose tissue physiology and pathophysiology.

2.9 Conclusion

Adipose tissue is the largest organ by weight in humans. Adipose tissue physiology remains an emerging field of medicine. Adipose tissue is now known to have many major roles in maintaining metabolic homeostasis. In addition to serving as a reservoir for triglycerides, the adipocyte both secretes paracrine and endocrine factors and has receptors for many hormones, putting it at the crossroad of metabolism. Understanding the physiology of the adipocyte, and of adipose tissue, helps us define their pathophysiology. This in turn will provide therapeutic options for the treatment of overweight, obesity, and adiposopathy.

Reading List

Ahima RS. Metabolic actions of adipocyte hormones: focus on adiponectin. Obesity (Silver Spring). 2006;14(Suppl 1):9S–15S. Epub 2006/04/29.

Armani A, Marzolla V, Fabbri A, Caprio M. Cellular mechanisms of MR regulation of adipose tissue physiology and pathophysiology. J Mol Endocrinol. 2015;55:R1. Epub 2015/08/15

Berry DC, Stenesen D, Zeve D, Graff JM. The developmental origins of adipose tissue. Development. 2013;140(19):3939–49. Epub 2013/09/21.

Chan JL, Mantzoros CS. Role of leptin in energy-deprivation states: normal human physiology and clinical implications for hypothalamic amenorrhoea and anorexia nervosa. Lancet. 2005;366(9479):74–85. Epub 2005/07/05.

Coelho M, Oliveira T, Fernandes R. Biochemistry of adipose tissue: an endocrine organ. Arch Med Sci AMS. 2013;9(2):191–200. Epub 2013/05/15.

Daval M, Foufelle F, Ferre P. Functions of AMP-activated protein kinase in adipose tissue. J Physiol. 2006;574(Pt 1):55–62. Epub 2006/05/20.

Flier JS, Cook KS, Usher P, Spiegelman BM. Severely impaired adipsin expression in genetic and acquired obesity. Science. 1987;237(4813):405–8. Epub 1987/07/24.

Fonseca-Alaniz MH, Takada J, Alonso-Vale MI, Lima FB. Adipose tissue as an endocrine organ: from theory to practice. J Pediatr. 2007;83(5 Suppl):S192–203. Epub 2007/11/09.

Gimeno RE, Klaman LD. Adipose tissue as an active endocrine organ: recent advances. Curr Opin Pharmacol. 2005;5(2):122–8. Epub 2005/03/23.

Goldberg AP, Fantuzzi G, Fried SK, Mazzone T. Adipose tissue and adipokines in health and disease. Totowa: Humana Press; 2007.

Izzi Engbeaya C, Salem V, Atkar RS, Dhillo WS. Insights into Brown adipose tissue physiology as revealed by imaging studies. Adipocytes. 2015;4(1):1–12. Epub 2015/07/15.

Lafontan M. Historical perspectives in fat cell biology: the fat cell as a model for the investigation of hormonal and metabolic pathways. Am J Physiol Cell Physiol. 2012;302(2):C327–59. Epub 2011/09/09.

Lafontan M, Barbe P, Galitzky J, Tavernier G, Langin D, Carpene C, et al. Adrenergic regulation of adipocyte metabolism. Hum Reprod. 1997;12(Suppl 1):6–20. Epub 1997/12/24.

Luscher TF. Mechanisms of disease: paracine effects of adipose tissue, progenitor cell function, and epigenetics of diabetic vascular disease. Eur Heart J. 2015;36(13):765–7. Epub 2015/04/04.

Martinez JA, Milagro FI, Claycombe KJ, Schalinske KL. Epigenetics in adipose tissue, obesity, weight loss, and diabetes. Adv Nutr. 2014;5(1):71–81. Epub 2014/01/16.

Min HY, Spiegelman BM. Adipsin, the adipocyte serine protease: gene structure and control of expression by tumor necrosis factor. Nucleic Acids Res. 1986;14(22):8879–92. Epub 1986/11/25.

Mohamed-Ali V, Pinkney JH, Coppack SW. Adipose tissue as an endocrine and paracrine organ. Int J Obes Relat Metab Disord. 1998;22(12):1145–58. Epub 1999/01/07.

Obregon MJ. Adipose tissues and thyroid hormones. Front Physiol. 2014;5:479. Epub 2015/01/08.

Proenca AR, Sertie RA, Oliveira AC, Campana AB, Caminhotto RO, Chimin P, et al. New concepts in white adipose tissue physiology. Braz J Med Biol Res. 2014;47(3):192–205. Epub 2014/03/29.

Shapiro B, Wertheimer E. The synthesis of fatty acids in adipose tissue in vitro. J Biol Chem. 1948;173(2):725–8. Epub 1948/04/01.

Thompson D, Karpe F, Lafontan M, Frayn K. Physical activity and exercise in the regulation of human adipose tissue physiology. Physiol Rev. 2012;92(1):157–91. Epub 2012/02/03.

Trayhurn P, Beattie JH. Physiological role of adipose tissue: white adipose tissue as an endocrine and secretory organ. Proc Nutr Soc. 2001;60(3):329–39. Epub 2001/10/30.

Wertheimer E, Shapiro B. The physiology of adipose tissue. Physiol Rev. 1948;28(4):451–64. Epub 1948/10/01.

Wozniak SE, Gee LL, Wachtel MS, Frezza EE. Adipose tissue: the new endocrine organ? A review article. Dig Dis Sci. 2009;54(9):1847–56. Epub 2008/12/05.

Yang RZ, Lee MJ, Hu H, Pray J, Wu HB, Hansen BC, et al. Identification of omentin as a novel depot-specific adipokine in human adipose tissue: possible role in modulating insulin action. Am J Physiol Endocrinol Metab. 2006;290(6):E1253–61. Epub 2006/03/15.

Yvan-Charvet L, Quignard-Boulange A. Role of adipose tissue renin-angiotensin system in metabolic and inflammatory diseases associated with obesity. Kidney Int. 2011;79(2):162–8. Epub 2010/10/15.

Chapter 3
Hormonal Regulation of Energy Balance and Energy Stores

J. Michael Gonzalez-Campoy

Pearls of Wisdom

- The human body has fuel sensors that engage a complex network of hormonal and neural regulation of food intake and energy stores.
- Adipose tissue is a target for insulin, adrenalin, and other circulating hormones and is the major site for energy storage in the human body.
- Adipose tissue directly signals the brain through leptin receptors, which are integrated with other stimuli in the regulation of food intake.
- Adipose tissue actively signals other organs involved in energy homeostasis, including the pancreas, liver, and muscle.
- Adiposopathy leads to alterations in the function of other organs, including the liver, muscle, brain, and endocrine pancreas. This cross talk from adipose tissue translates into clinical hyperglycemia, dyslipidemia, hypertension, systemic inflammation, and vasculopathy.

3.1 Introduction

Humans sustain life by ingesting nutrients at regular intervals. There are biological drivers of food intake that get triggered during energy deprivation. Conversely, these biological drivers are turned off with the provision of energy. The integrated regulation of energy balance and energy stores involves the sensing of nutrients; the generation of signals from organs involved, which reflect their current

J. M. Gonzalez-Campoy
Minnesota Center for Obesity, Metabolism and Endocrinology, PA (MNCOME), Eagan, MN, USA
e-mail: drmike@mncome.com

J. M. Gonzalez-Campoy et al. (eds.), *Bariatric Endocrinology*,
https://doi.org/10.1007/978-3-319-95655-8_3

energetic state; and the translation of these signals into action. The afferent limbs of the nervous system provide input to the brain from the periphery, but there is a rich hormonal signaling as well. The brain generates signals of hunger or satiety based on the integration of both neural and humoral signals. Within the brain, the hypothalamus is the major determinant of the body's action to maintain or change the current energy status. The hypothalamus is integrated into neural circuits that regulate its activity with input from other areas of the brain. The hypothalamus is also the major regulator of pituitary function leading to the neurohormonal regulation of metabolism. Neurohormonal regulation also occurs through the efferent limbs of the nervous system and the innervation of the organs involved in energy homeostasis. Acute changes in energy status are a part of daily living. Progressive changes in energy status cause changes in energy reserves. These chronic changes affect energy homeostasis and lead to adaptations to compensate for them. The neuroendocrine responses to food deprivation include decreasing fertility by inhibiting the hypothalamic–pituitary–gonadal axis, slowing of the metabolic rate by decreasing the activity of the thyroid axis, increasing the activity of cortisol through the production of adrenocorticotropic hormone, increasing insulin sensitivity, and decreasing the leptin to adiponectin ratio from adipose tissue. Conversely, chronic positive energy balance leads to the re-establishment of normal pituitary function, insulin resistance, and an increased leptin to adiponectin ratio from adipose tissue. This chapter will review the sensing and signaling mechanisms involved in energy homeostasis. Chapter 4 in this textbook will review their integration in the brain.

3.2 Fat Metabolism

3.2.1 Cholecystokinin (CCK)

Over 90% of ingested fats enter the small intestine as triglycerides (TG). The entrance of TG into the duodenum stimulates the release of CCK. CCK is synthesized and released by entero-endocrine I cells in the mucosal lining of the small intestine (mostly in the duodenum and jejunum). CCK is also released from the neurons of the enteric nervous system and the brain. CCK is synthesized as a 115-amino acid preprohormone. In the central nervous system (CNS), there are several isoforms of CCK, of which sulfated octapeptide is the most common. Peripherally, CCK is released rapidly into the circulation in response to a meal and has a relatively short half-life of 2.5 min.

The greatest stimulus for CCK release is the presence of fatty acids in the chyme entering the duodenum. CCK is also released in response to amino acids released from protein digestion, monitor peptide from pancreatic acinar cells, CCK-releasing peptide (via paracrine signaling mediated by enterocytes in the gastric and intestinal mucosa), and acetylcholine (from the vagus nerve). A decrease in the amount of luminal free fatty acids, somatostatin, and pancreatic peptide, each cause a decrease in CCK secretion. CCK production is also decreased when trypsin released by the exocrine pancreas inactivates CCK-releasing peptide and monitor peptide.

CCK has many recognized actions, including the following:

- Slowing gastric emptying
- Stimulation of pancreatic acinar cells, resulting in the release of pancreatic digestive enzymes, through the CCK A receptor
- Increased production of bile
- Contraction of the gallbladder and biliary tree
- Relaxation of the sphincter of Oddi
- Mediation of satiety stimulating its receptors in the central nervous system (CNS)
- Triggering anxiety by the stimulation of multiple CNS centers through the CCKB receptor
- Triggering panic (CCK tetrapeptide fragment) by stimulating neurons in the anterior cingulate gyrus, the cerebellar vermis, and the claustrum-insular-amygdala

3.2.2 Intestinal Fat Transport

Both pancreatic and intestinal lipases hydrolyze TG to diglycerides and monoglycerides and then to glycerol and free fatty acids (FFA). Bile acids emulsify these FFA into micelles, which allow for the intestinal transport of fats. Micelles interact with the brush border of the small intestine, and this allows for the transport of glycerol and FFA into enterocytes. Once inside enterocytes, glycerol and free fatty acids are re-esterified into TG. TG is packaged along with re-esterified cholesterol into apolipoprotein B48-containing chylomicrons.

Chylomicrons are secreted into mesenteric lymph vessels and eventually into the venous circulation through the thoracic duct. There is no first-pass hepatic metabolism of fats, since the first large capillary bed that lipids pass is that of the lungs. Circulating chylomicrons pass into the left side of the heart and are sent into the peripheral arterial system for delivery to organs, including the liver.

3.2.3 Fat Storage

Chylomicrons deliver triglycerides to adipose tissue, which is the major storage site for fats. There are large genetic variations that predispose individuals to increase regional fat deposits. However, accrual of adipose tissue mass from chronic storage of fat happens in all adipose tissue. For most people, the storage takes place in intra-abdominal fat.

In adipocytes, the storage of triglycerides in the fat vacuole is under hormonal regulation. Epinephrine rapidly stimulates the transport of long-chain fatty acids (LCFA) across the plasma membrane. The epinephrine-stimulated rates are fivefold to tenfold higher than the basal rate of influx or efflux. The stimulatory effect of epinephrine on transport is mediated by β-adrenergic receptor binding, and the generation of intracellular cyclic adenosine monophosphate (cAMP), and correlates to hormone-sensitive lipase activation and lipolysis.

Insulin at physiological concentrations completely blocks the epinephrine effect. The insulin effect is on the LCFA transport process is in both directions—influx and efflux. In addition to counteracting lipolysis, insulin action also suppresses lipid mobilization, leading to lipogenesis.

Chylomicrons also deliver lipids to the liver via the arterial circulation. Increased saturated fats delivered to the liver may increase hepatosteatosis and increase very low-density lipoprotein (VLDL) secretion. Omega-3 fatty acids may decrease hepatosteatosis and may substantially decrease hepatic VLDL secretion.

During fasting and when fatty acids are needed for energy, stored fatty acids in adipocytes are released into the circulation through increased activity of hormone-sensitive lipase. Fatty acids undergo beta-oxidation to form acetyl CoA, which enters the citric acid cycle in the muscle, liver, and other tissues.

3.2.4 Adipose Tissue Signaling

Chapters 2 and 6 of this textbook describe the adipocyte as an endocrine cell, adipose tissue as an endocrine organ, and the pathophysiology that develops in adiposopathy. The signals generated by adipose tissue play a major role in energy homeostasis.

3.2.4.1 Leptin

Leptin is a humoral signal from adipose tissue to the CNS about energy stores. Although leptin is now known to be synthesized in the placenta, ovaries, skeletal muscle, stomach, mammary epithelial cells, bone marrow, and stomach, white adipose tissue is by and large the primary source in humans. As adipose tissue mass increases, the production of leptin by adipocytes goes up. Conversely, with loss of fat mass, leptin levels drop. Thus, sensing of leptin levels by the CNS represents sensing of energy stores. The major CNS target for leptin is the hypothalamus.

Leptin inhibits the production of neuropeptide Y (NPY) and agouti-related protein (AgRP) in neurons of the arcuate nucleus. NPY activity increases food intake (orexigenic). Therefore, leptin inhibition of NPY activity leads to decreased food intake (anorexigenic). Leptin also stimulates the synthesis of α-melanocyte-stimulating hormone (MSH) in pro-opiomelanocortin (POMC) neurons of the hypothalamus. MSH is anorexigenic, and stimulation by leptin causes suppression of

Table 3.1 Effects of leptin

Target	Action	Effect
Hypothalamus	Inhibits neuropeptide Y and agouti-related protein neurons Stimulates α-melanocyte-stimulating hormone Reverses starvation-induced inhibition of the hypothalamic–pituitary–gonadal and hypothalamic–pituitary–thyroid axes (indirect effect) Stimulates gonadotropin-releasing hormone Causes parasympathetic-induced increased hepatic insulin sensitivity with inhibition of glucose production (arcuate nucleus projections to the nucleus of tractus solitarius)	Anorexigenic effect Hypoglycemic effect Reproductive effect
Skeletal muscle	Increases glucose uptake Increases glucose and fatty acid oxidation	Catabolic effect
Liver	Decreases gluconeogenesis	Hypoglycemic effect
Adipocyte (autocrine activity)	Promotes glucose and fatty acid oxidation Promotes lipolysis Decreases leptin gene expression	Catabolic effect
Pancreatic Islets	Inhibits insulin release Decreases glucagon release	Glucoregulatory effect (adipoinsular axis)
Adrenal cortex	Decreases adrenocorticotropic hormone-stimulated glucocorticoid release	Decreased insulin antagonism Catabolic effect
Immune system cells (permissive effect)	Enhances phagocytic activity of macrophages Stimulates cytokine and chemotaxin production	Immunoprotective effect
Bone (permissive)	Increases bone mineral density Increases hematopoiesis	Anabolic skeletal effect

hunger. These combined effects of leptin cause weight loss, which led to the naming of this hormone. Paradoxically, in overweight and obesity, there is hyperleptinemia, but the CNS effects of leptin are blunted, a condition commonly referred to as leptin resistance. Table 3.1 summarizes the known effects of leptin.

3.2.4.2 Adiponectin

Adiponectin is a hormone secreted by adipocytes. The only other tissue known to produce it in significant amounts is the placenta. However, adiponectin is now considered to be an active autocrine–paracrine hormone, and there is local production by many other tissues. Adiponectin levels in the blood are decreased in obesity, insulin resistance, and type 2 diabetes. Caloric restriction causes adiponectin levels to rise despite decreasing fat mass. Adiponectin receptor 1 is expressed in the skeletal muscle. Adiponectin receptor 2 is expressed in the liver. Adiponectin has hypoglycemic and anti-atherogenic effects. Its insulin-sensitizing effect is mediated by increased fatty acid oxidation through the activation of adenosine monophosphate kinase (AMPK) and peroxisome proliferator-activated receptor (PPAR)-α. The actions of adiponectin include decreased gluconeogenesis, increased glucose uptake, and triglyceride clearance.

3.2.4.3 Leptin to Adiponectin Ratio (LAR)

Leptin levels rise with increasing fat mass, whereas adiponectin levels fall. Both hyperleptinemia and hypoadiponectinemia are present in overweight and obesity, and the relationship between them is a clinical measure of adipose tissue health. In the lean state, the ratio of leptin to adiponectin is a fraction. As fat mass accrues, the ratio of these two adipose tissue hormones reaches identity, and eventually, there is more leptin than adiponectin (Fig. 3.1). An increasing LAR reflects progressive adiposopathy and is a better predictor of increased arterial stiffness assessed by pulse wave velocity than either leptin or adiponectin alone, metabolic risk, and eventual vascular disease. In the practice of bariatric endocrinology, trending the LAR documents the progressive state of adipose tissue health, the goal of treatment being to affect a reduction in LAR over time (Fig. 3.2).

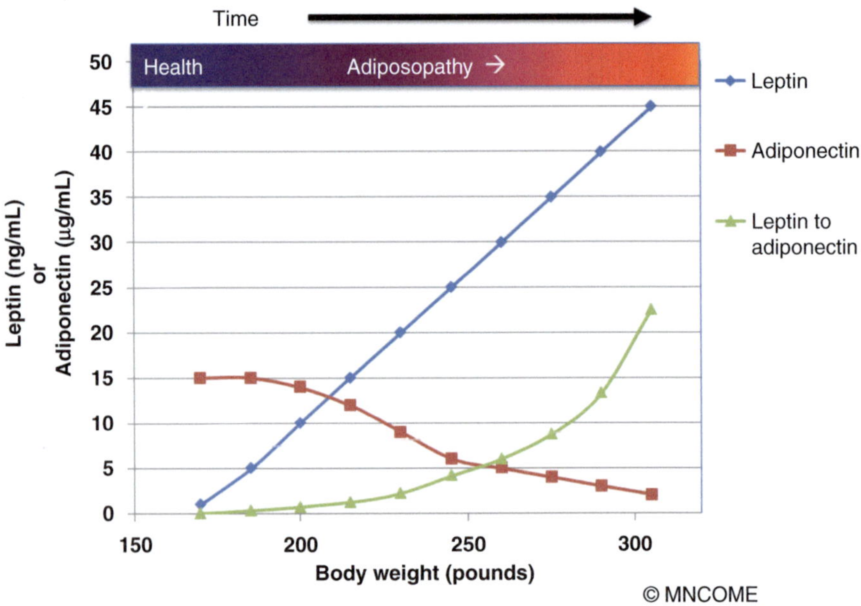

Fig. 3.1 Leptin to adiponectin ratio. The accumulation of fat mass leads to a directly proportional increase in circulating leptin levels. On the other hand, adiponectin levels decrease with increasing fat mass. The leptin to adiponectin ratio reaches identity and becomes progressively higher as fat mass continues to increase and adipose tissue function declines. Abbreviations: ng nanogram, mL milliliter, µg microgram, MNCOME Minnesota Center for Obesity, Metabolism and Endocrinology, PA. (Reproduced with permission from MNCOME)

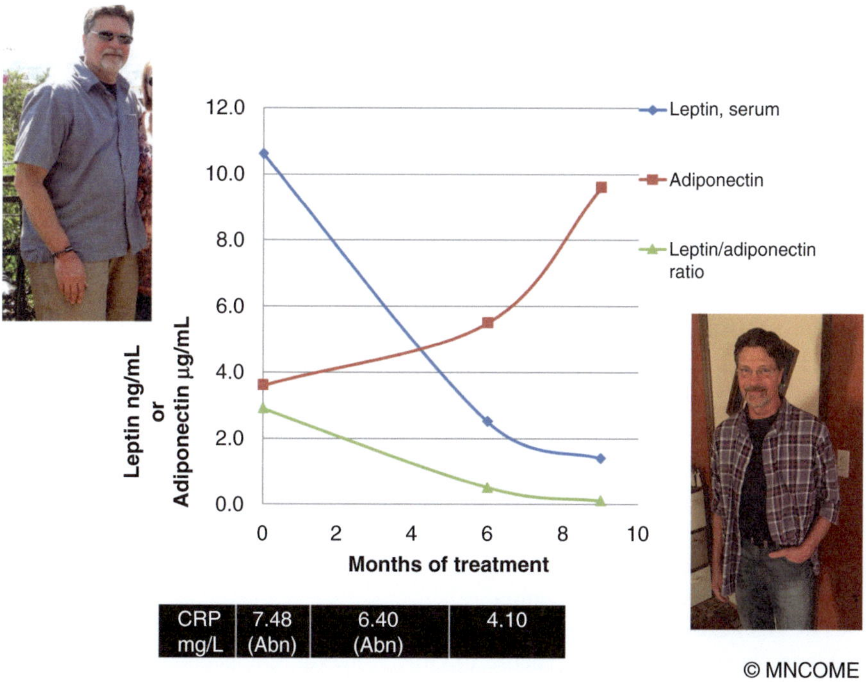

CRP mg/L	7.48 (Abn)	6.40 (Abn)	4.10

Fig. 3.2 Leptin to adiponectin ratio trending. Serial measurements of the leptin to adiponectin ratio over time reflect adipose tissue health. A progressively higher leptin to adiponectin ratio indicates worsening adipose tissue health. Conversely, a decreasing leptin to adiponectin ratio indicates improvements in adipose tissue health. Abbreviations: ng nanogram, mL milliliter, µg microgram, CRP C-reactive protein, Abn abnormal, MNCOME Minnesota Center for Obesity, Metabolism and Endocrinology, PA. (Reproduced with permission from MNCOME)

3.3 Protein Metabolism

Ingested proteins are rapidly digested in the stomach (by gastric pepsin) and the duodenum (by pancreatic trypsin and chymotrypsin). The initial digestion of proteins renders polypeptides that are further broken down by exopeptidases and dipeptidases of the intestine into simple amino acids. Amino acids are taken up by all tissues to synthesize the myriad proteins that regulate metabolism and contribute to the structure of cells and the extracellular matrix.

Amino acid metabolism takes place mostly in the liver. Surplus amino acids delivered to the liver undergo deamination, and through gluconeogenesis, are converted into glucose (e.g., alanine cycle). The nitrogen derived from the removal of the amine group of amino acids is converted to urea (e.g., urea cycle). Most of the urea that is generated by the urea cycle is ultimately excreted by the kidneys. Amino acids may also be used to generate keto acids, giving rise to acetyl CoA and, then through lipogenesis, the creation of fat.

Different proteins in the meal plan may have varying effects upon insulin secretion, adipocyte hypertrophy, circulating free fatty acids, and lipotoxicity on the liver and muscle. As an example, compared to a casein-rich meal plan (milk and dairy products), soy protein (from soybeans) may decrease adiposity and lower glucose levels.

3.4 Glucose Metabolism

3.4.1 Glucokinase

Glucokinase (GK) catalyzes the phosphorylation of glucose to glucose-6-phosphate (G6P). This chemical reaction is the first step of both glycogen synthesis and glycolysis. GK is expressed in only four types of mammalian cells (hepatocytes, β-cells, enterocytes, and glucose-sensitive neurons). GK acts as a glucose sensor, triggering shifts in metabolism or cell function in response to rising or falling levels of glucose in the circulation. GK gene mutations are known to cause secondary forms of diabetes, or hypoglycemia.

GK is a hexokinase. There are least three other hexokinases, each of which can mediate phosphorylation of glucose to G6P. However, GK is coded by a separate gene, and its distinctive kinetic properties give it a lower affinity for glucose than the other hexokinases. GK is localized to a few cell types and, under usual physiological conditions, its activity varies substantially according to the concentration of glucose.

In the fed state, carbohydrate is broken down by the enzymatic activity of salivary and pancreatic amylases. The resulting monosaccharides and disaccharides are acted on by intestinal brush border disaccharidases, leading to the generation of glucose and other simple sugars like fructose (from sucrose) and galactose (from lactose).

Glucose absorbed from the intestine enters the venous circulation of the gut and is delivered to the liver, which is the first major organ to receive it. Under the influence of insulin, which is stimulated by the rise in circulating glucose, there is glycogenesis in the liver, resulting in the storage of complex glucose chains as glycogen. This process also requires the activation of GK in hepatocytes by the increased concentration of circulating glucose.

3.4.2 Insulin

3.4.2.1 Insulin Secretion

The structure and function relationships of the pancreatic islets are important in their overall function. Arterial blood flow to the pancreatic islets is a major determinant of the overall ratio of insulin to glucagon. Blood entering the pancreatic islets circulates through the β-cells that make insulin first, and downstream, the α-cells that make glucagon.

β-cells have constitutively expressed glucose transporter (GLUT) 2. GLUT2 is the only glucose transporter expressed in β-cells. For practical purposes, GLUT2 is the first glucose sensor, since it allows for facilitated diffusion of glucose into the β-cells. Mobilization of GLUT2 to the plasma membrane of β-cells is insulin independent. GLUT2 has a low substrate affinity, ensuring high glucose influx into the β-cells, along its concentration gradient. By contrast, GLUT4, which is primarily expressed in the muscle and fat cells, is insulin dependent.

After entering β-cells, glucose is phosphorylated by GK. GK has a lower affinity for glucose than other hexokinases. Its Michaelis constant (substrate concentration for half the maximum velocity of the enzyme) is 6 mmol/L, which is in the middle of the normal blood glucose range (4–10 mmol/L). By contrast, other hexokinases function at full maximal velocity at this glucose concentration. GK is not inhibited by its product, G6P, which enables its continued activity in spite of glycolysis load on the β-cell.

The net result of the influx of glucose into β-cells is an increase in the adenosine triphosphate (ATP) to adenosine diphosphate ratio. An increase in this ratio results in closure of cell membrane ATP-sensitive potassium channels which causes depolarization of the cell membrane. This depolarization in turn leads to calcium influx into the cell through voltage-gated membrane calcium channels. Finally, the calcium influx into the β-cell leads to exocytosis of the insulin secretory vesicles and hence insulin secretion. In the process of releasing insulin into the circulation, the prohormone proinsulin is cleaved, resulting in equimolar release of insulin and c-peptide.

In the pancreatic islets of Langerhans, there are other cell types. The δ-cells make somatostatin, which inhibits both insulin and glucagon release. The F-cells make pancreatic polypeptide, which suppresses gastric secretion, gastric emptying, pancreatic enzyme secretion, and hunger. The ε-cells make ghrelin (the major site of production for which is the stomach), which suppresses insulin release.

β-cell insulin release is also stimulated by amino acids (which rise after the ingestion of proteins) in a synergistic way. Ingestion of mixed amino acids stimulates insulin release more than the ingestion of a single amino acid. Similarly, in the fed state, FFA enhances glucose-stimulated insulin release from the β-cells. Paradoxically, chronic elevations in FFA that develop with adiposopathy inhibit glucose-stimulated insulin release and lead to insulin resistance.

Gut peptides including glucagon-like peptide-1 (GLP-1) made by the intestinal L-cells, and glucose-dependent insulinotropic polypeptide (made by the intestinal K cells) also stimulate insulin release during the fed state. The role of gut peptides and intestinal signaling in overweight, obesity, and adiposopathy has been defined over the past decade. Deficiencies in the production of these gut hormones lead to impaired insulin secretion and hyperglycemic states.

In addition to somatostatin and ghrelin, inhibition of β-cell insulin release also is caused by circulating adrenalin and norepinephrine stimulation of the α-2 adrenergic receptors. The powerful suppression of insulin release by adrenalin is the major mechanism to prevent hypoglycemia in patients with diabetes. Insulin suppression adds to the hyperadrenergic symptoms that lead patients to seek food during hypoglycemia.

3.4.2.2 Pancreatic Islet Blood Flow and Regulation of Insulin and Glucagon Release

The blood flow entering the pancreatic islets after a meal carries a high glucose content and stimulates the β -cells to increase insulin secretion, leading to a high insulin concentration. This blood then reaches the α-cells, where insulin inhibits glucagon release. Past the α-cells, in the fed state, the outflow of blood from the pancreas has a high glucose concentration and a high insulin to glucagon ratio. This venous flow from the pancreas reaches the portal circulation and enters the liver. The majority of the insulin made by the pancreas in the fed state binds receptors in hepatocytes, stimulating glycogenesis and inhibiting gluconeogenesis.

Insulin that goes beyond the pancreas enters the systemic circulation and targets other organs. In the muscle, insulin allows for the incorporation of GLUT4 transporters into cell membranes, entrance of glucose, and the formation of glycogen in the muscle. In adipose tissue, insulin stimulates the incorporation of GLUT4 into the adipocyte cell membranes, allowing the influx of glucose. Glucose serves to form glycerol, which is then incorporated into the synthesis of triglycerides. At the adipocyte, insulin also promotes the activity of the extracellular lipoprotein lipase that hydrolyzes circulating triglycerides to free fatty acids that may enter the cell. This promotes the influx of fats into adipocytes. At the same time, insulin inhibits hormone-sensitive lipase, and this stops the efflux of fats from adipocytes. The net effect of insulin on the adipocyte, in the fed state, is lipogenic—insulin helps to trap FFA within adipose tissue.

In the fasting state, the blood flow through the pancreatic islets enters with a normal (i.e., not high) glucose concentration. There is no increased uptake of insulin by the β-cells, and insulin production decreases. Moving beyond the β-cells, the blood carries normal glucose and low insulin levels onto the α-cells of the islets. Without the high insulin levels to inhibit glucagon release by the α-cells, glucagon now enters the blood stream freely. The blood coming out of the pancreas in the fasting state now carries a normal glucose concentration, low insulin level, and high glucagon levels. This blood enters the portal circulation and arrives at the liver. Without insulin, glucagon stimulates hepatocytes, causing glycogenolysis and stimulating gluconeogenesis after prolonged fasting.

3.4.2.3 Insulin Effects in the Brain

Insulin receptors (IRs) are widely distributed throughout the body. Table 3.2 summarizes the major effects of insulin. In the integration of metabolism and the regulation of food intake, the activity of insulin on its CNS receptors plays an important role.

Insulin enters the CNS through the blood–brain barrier by a receptor-mediated transport. IRs are located in various regions of the brain. IR activation by insulin

Table 3.2 Effects of insulin

Target	Action	Effect
Adipocytes	Induces lipoprotein lipase activity (influx of FFA into adipocytes) Inhibits hormone-sensitive lipase (stops efflux of FFA) Increases glucose uptake (GLUT4)	Lipogenesis
Hepatocytes	Inhibits glycogenolysis and gluconeogenesis Inhibits conversion of fatty acids and amino acids to keto acids Promotes glycogenesis (inhibits phosphorylase; stimulates glucokinase, and glycogen synthase) Increases triglyceride synthesis and very low-density lipoprotein formation	Glycogenesis
Brain	Causes satiety Increases energy expenditure	Anorexigenic effect
Muscle	Increases amino acid transport and protein synthesis Increases glucose uptake (GLUT4) and glycogen synthase activity Inhibits phosphorylase	Glycogenesis Anabolic effect
Pancreas	Inhibits glucagon release	Hypoglycemic effect

Abbreviations: *FFA* free fatty acids, *GLUT* glucose transporter

helps to regulate food intake, sympathetic activity, and peripheral insulin action. Along with leptin, insulin activates phosphatidylinositol 3-kinase (PI3K), which is crucial to its biological effects. Decreased activity of PI3K is now linked to insulin resistance and explains the lack of insulin effect in adiposopathy.

Tau protein is a highly soluble microtubule-associated protein. Excessive or abnormal phosphorylation of tau results in the transformation of normal adult tau into paired helical filament tau and neurofibrillary tangles of tau. Insulin regulates phosphorylation of tau, and deficient insulin activity leads to the formation of these abnormal tau protein variants. Insulin resistance is therefore etiological in the pathophysiology of Alzheimer's disease. The abnormal phosphorylation of tau is also a hallmark of several other related neurodegenerative disorders. For example, the density of neurofibrillary tangles in the neocortex correlates with dementia. Insulin also regulates the metabolism of amyloid precursor protein and the clearance of β-amyloid from the brain. Insulin signaling links energy homeostasis and protection from the development of neurodegenerative diseases.

3.5 Gut Hormones

In the normal digestive process, the intestine not only provides for the breakdown of foods and absorptive capacity; rather, it is an important modulator of metabolism through both neural and hormonal signaling. In brief, as food enters the digestive tract, the gut actively signals other organs. The signaling helps to regulate food intake by the brain and to activate hormonal systems that help process the energy. Chapter 5 in this textbook provides an in-depth review of the role of the gut in metabolic homeostasis. This section is a summary of the subject with a focus on the integration of metabolism.

3.5.1 Ghrelin

The stomach is the major organ for food breakdown through a combination of its grinding action, secretion of acid, and activation of digestive enzymes. There is active communication between the stomach and the brain. The vagal afferent and efferent nerves are a major signaling mechanism. Nesfatin (which is made by the hypothalamus, pancreatic islets, gastric endocrine cells, and adipocytes), the gastric endocannabinoid system, and ghrelin are part of the hormonal signaling between the CNS and the stomach.

In 1996, a heterotrimeric receptor coupled to guanosine-5′-triphosphate-binding protein was described in the pituitary and the arcuate ventromedial and infundibular hypothalamus. The receptor was cloned and shown to be the target of growth hormone secretagogues. In 1999, the ligand for this receptor was reported, and named ghrelin, based on its role as growth hormone-releasing peptide. Ghrelin is also known as lenomorelin.

Ghrelin is mostly produced by the Gr cells of the stomach. It is also produced in the duodenum, jejunum, lungs, pancreatic islets, gonads, adrenal cortex, placenta, kidneys, and locally in the brain. Ghrelin is secreted when the stomach is empty, away from meals. Circulating levels of ghrelin are highest immediately before ingestion of a meal. Conversely, stretching of the stomach halts the secretion of ghrelin. Circulating ghrelin levels drop immediately after the consumption of a meal. The postprandial drop in ghrelin is stronger in response to ingested protein and carbohydrate, compared to the ingestion of lipids.

The growth hormone secretagogue receptor ligand (*GHRL)* gene encodes for ghrelin. *GHRL* first produces preproghrelin, a 117-amino acid chain which is homologous to promotilin, both members of the motilin family of peptides. Preproghrelin is cleaved to generate the prohormone proghrelin. In turn, proghrelin is cleaved to form ghrelin, which is an unacylated 28-amino acid chain. Cleavage of proghrelin also produces c-ghrelin, which is an acylated form. C-ghrelin is further cleaved to produce obestatin, which antagonizes ghrelin.

Ghrelin is activated by ghrelin O-acyltransferase (GOAT), an enzyme that links caprylic (octanoic) acid to the serine at the third position. GOAT is located on the cell membrane of Gr cells. Ghrelin which is not activated in this way is unable to activate the ghrelin-growth hormone secretagogue receptor (GHSR). Inactivated ghrelin antagonizes activated ghrelin, stimulates appetite, and inhibits hepatic glucose output.

Ghrelin levels are lower in people with obesity, compared to people who are lean. An exception to this physiological adjustment to increased fat mass is the Prader-Willi syndrome, where ghrelin levels are high, leading to increased food intake.

On the other hand, people with low energy stores, as is the case in anorexia nervosa and the cachexia of cancer, have high levels of ghrelin. This again suggests a physiological adaptation to counteract the loss of fat mass.

With aging, the ghrelin levels increase. This represents a pathophysiological role of ghrelin in the accrual of fat mass with advancing age. Patients who undergo weight loss surgery that involves gastric reduction, either a Roux-N-Y procedure or a gastric sleeve procedure, have marked reductions of ghrelin levels. These patients lose the normal ghrelin cycling, and the loss of hunger that follows is a major mechanism for postsurgical weight loss.

The biological effects of activated ghrelin make it a major regulator of energy balance and metabolism and are summarized in Table 3.3. In the brain, ghrelin receptors are found in the same neurons that also express the leptin receptor. Ghrelin

Table 3.3 Effects of ghrelin

Target	Action	Effect
Stomach	Increases gastric acid secretion Increases gastric motility Decreases the mechanosensitivity of gastric vagal afferent nerves (makes them less sensitive to gastric distention)	Prepares the stomach for food intake
Intestine	Promotes intestinal cell proliferation Inhibits intestinal cell apoptosis during inflammation Suppresses proinflammatory mechanisms Augments anti-inflammatory mechanisms Stimulates regeneration of gastric mucosa	Intestinal healing and anti-inflammatory effect
Pancreatic islets of Langerhans	Inhibits glucose-stimulated insulin secretion by β-cells (indirect effect) Stimulates somatostatin release by δ-cells (direct effect)	Hypoglycemic effect
Hippocampus	Regulates neurotrophy Alters neuronal connections	Stimulates learning and memory
Pituitary	Stimulates growth hormone release Stimulates ACTH release	Stimulates growth and development Antidepressant effect Anxiolytic effect
Hypothalamic arcuate nucleus	Stimulates orexigenic neuropeptide Y and agouti-related protein neurons Increases hunger Inhibits gonadotropin-releasing hormone	Orexigenic effect Increase body weight and fat mass Decreases fertility
Dopamine neurons that link ventral tegmental area to nucleus accumbens	Produces sensations of reward and reinforcement Contributes to the development of addictions	Hedonism with regard to foods and drugs like alcohol
Endothelium	Activates nitric oxide synthase	Vasodilator
Lung	Promotes lung growth early in fetal life	Lung growth

is a true orexigenic neuropeptide in the CNS, causing energy intake. Peripherally, ghrelin determines the proportion of energy that is directed to the production of ATP or is sent to storage as triglyceride in adipose tissue or as glycogen in the liver. Ghrelin also helps determine short-term heat loss. Thus, ghrelin helps regulate energy distribution and rate of use.

As of 2016, ghrelin was not approved for therapeutic use. However, research is under way to develop ghrelin receptor blockers as a treatment to prevent or treat obesity. Ghrelin agonists or analogs may play a role in the treatment of anorexia nervosa or cachexia and are used as a gastric prokinetic treatment. Studies are also under way for these uses.

3.5.2 Obestatin

Obestatin was first identified in the year 2005. The same GHRL gene that encodes for ghrelin also encodes for obestatin, which is created by the cleavage of C-ghrelin. Thus, obestatin is mostly produced in the stomach. Obestatin is also produced in the duodenum, jejunum, colon, large and small intestines, pancreas, thyroid, lung, mammary gland, Leydig cells of the testis, spleen, muscle, and adipocytes. Amidation of a flanking conserved glycine residue at the C-terminal of obestatin is necessary for it to acquire biological activity. The enzyme that causes amidation of obestatin has not yet been identified.

In humans, plasma obestatin levels do not vary with fixed energy meals. People with obesity have lower obestatin levels than people who are lean. Obestatin may therefore play a role in the long-term regulation of fat mass. Binding sites for obestatin have been identified in the pancreas, heart, and white adipose tissue. The obestatin receptor is still to be fully identified. However, obestatin is bound by the adipocyte and pancreatic β-cell GLP-1 receptor (GLP-1R).

In the pancreas, obestatin is co-localized with ghrelin in the ghrelin-producing ε-cells at the periphery of the islets of Langerhans. Obestatin and ghrelin act in concert as local regulators of β-cell function. Somatostatin, glucagon, and insulin do not co-localize with obestatin, indicating that α- and β-cells do not produce obestatin. Thus, obestatin has local autocrine/paracrine roles in the pancreatic islets, in addition to its actions as an endocrine hormone.

Obestatin receptors are found in adipose tissue. Obestatin is able to regulate growth, proliferation, differentiation, and survival of adipocytes. Obestatin also regulates genes that stimulate cell proliferation and protect against apoptosis mediated by proinflammatory cytokines.

In summary, obestatin is involved in improving memory, regulating sleep and food intake, affecting cell proliferation and promoting survival of pancreatic β-cells and adipocytes, inhibiting glucose-induced insulin secretion, and regulating gastrointestinal tract functions.

3.5.3 Ghrelin to Obestatin Ratio

Individuals with obesity have an elevated preprandial ghrelin to obestatin ratio compared to people who are lean. A change in the ghrelin to obestatin ratio may be etiological in the development of overweight, obesity, and adiposopathy.

3.5.4 GLP-1

The proglucagon gene is expressed in the α-cells of the pancreatic islets of Langerhans, the L-cells of the intestine, and the CNS neurons of the caudal brainstem and hypothalamus. Proglucagon processing yields different products in the pancreas than in the gut or CNS. In the pancreas, the α-cells generate glucagon. In the intestine and CNS, proglucagon yields glicentin, GLP-1, and GLP-2. Glicentin in turn gives rise to glicentin-related pancreatic peptide (GRPP) and oxyntomodulin.

GLP-1 is a 30-amino acid hormone secreted by intestinal enteroendocrine L-cells and neurons in the nucleus of the tractus solitarius in the brainstem. The ingestion of a meal is the major stimulus for secretion of GLP-1. The initial product GLP-1(1–37) undergoes amidation and proteolytic cleavage. Two truncated and equipotent biologically active forms, GLP-1 (7–36) amide and GLP-1 (7–37), are formed from GLP-1 (1–37). GLP-1 is an incretin—it amplifies the release of insulin in the presence of hyperglycemia. GLP-1 also:

- Decreases the quantity and frequency of food consumption
- Decreases the hedonic (pleasurable) aspect of food intake
- Decreases the motivation to eat
- Decreases general levels of motor activity
- Increases hippocampus-related function
- Increases acquisition/strength of conditioned taste aversions
- Increases anxiety
- Increases nausea or visceral malaise (illness)
- Increases insulin sensitivity in both α- and β-cells of the islets of Langerhans
- Increases β-cell mass
- Increases insulin expression, post-translational modification, and secretion
- Inhibits acid secretion and gastric emptying in the stomach
- Decreases insulin resistance
- Decreases glucagon secretion from the pancreas via G-protein-coupled receptor binding

Endogenous GLP-1 is rapidly degraded by dipeptidyl peptidase-4 (DPP-4). Neutral endopeptidase 24.11 also degrades GLP-1. Only 10–15% of GLP-1 produced by the L-cells reaches the circulation intact. GLP-1 is cleared from the circulation by the kidneys. The half-life of GLP-1 is approximately 2 min.

In addition to the actions outlined above, GLP-1 and its metabolites may have effects on adipose tissue. GLP-1 promotes preadipocyte proliferation and inhibits apoptosis. On the other hand, loss of GLP-1R expression causes a reduction in adipogenesis through the induction of apoptosis in preadipocytes.

GLP-1 (9–36) is generated by DPP4 cleavage of GLP-1 (7–36). GLP-1 (9–36) has a very low affinity for GLP-1R. However, in human adipose stem cells, GLP-1 (9–36) inhibits cell proliferation, glucose uptake, and adipogenesis. It also induces cell apoptosis. GLP-1 (9–36) effects are not reverted by the receptor antagonist exendin (9–39), which does revert the effects of GLP-1 (7–36).

3.6 Other Endocrine Regulation of Metabolism

Under the control of the hypothalamus and the anterior pituitary gland, there is further hormonal regulation of metabolism. Chapters 15 and 16 of this textbook address the role of gonadal hormones. This section will deal with the role of the thyroid and adrenal hormones in the regulation of energy balance.

3.6.1 Triiodothyronine

The thyroid hormones tetraiodothyronine (thyroxine, T4) and triiodothyronine (T3) are made by the follicular cells of the thyroid gland. T4 is the major circulating form of thyroid hormone. In the blood, the ratio of T4 to T3 is 14:1–20:1. T4 is converted to T3 in the thyroid gland and in every tissue of the human body by deiodinase (5′-iodinase). T3 is up to five times more potent than T4 and is the major thyroid hormone in humans.

There are T3 receptors throughout the human body. They act to increase the basal metabolic rate by sensitizing the tissues to catecholamines. T3 is essential for the proper development and differentiation of all cells of the human body. T3 regulates vitamin, protein, fat, and carbohydrate metabolism. Some of the physiological effects of T3 also include:

- An increase in the heart rate, which then causes an increase in cardiac output
- Increased ventilatory rate
- Increased basal metabolic rate
- Increased sympathetic activity
- Increased catabolism of proteins and carbohydrates
- Decreased transit time for food through the digestive tract (shortened time of digestion)
- Increased muscle contractility

- Regulation of differentiation of adipocytes, promoting the reactivation of the brown adipose tissue and inducing beige ("brite") adipocyte formation
- Increased nonshivering thermogenesis

Thyroid gene expression in adipocytes is reduced in obesity. This is true in both subcutaneous and visceral fat. Thyroid gene expression rises with major weight loss. The relevance of these observations still needs to be refined.

3.6.2 Adrenal Hormones

The adrenal hormones, both the cortical steroids and the medullary catecholamines, are each known as antagonists of insulin. This certainly holds true in adipose tissue. Whereas insulin is lipogenic, epinephrine and cortisol are lipolytic. This section will briefly review the role of adrenal hormones in the integration of metabolism.

3.6.2.1 Glucocorticoids

Cortisol is the main glucocorticoid in the human body and is produced by the zona fasciculata cells of the adrenal cortex. Cortisol has immune regulatory, metabolic, and developmental effects in the body. The metabolic effects of cortisol include:

- Stimulation of hormone-sensitive lipase in adipocytes, causing lipolysis
- Antagonism of insulin in myocytes and adipocytes, decreasing glucose uptake
- Inhibition of adiponectin release by white adipose tissue
- Stimulation of gluconeogenesis in the liver by enhancing the expression of enzymes involved in it
- Mobilization of amino acids from extrahepatic tissues to serve as substrates for gluconeogenesis

Leptin receptors are present in adrenocortical cells. Leptin decreases the corticotropin-stimulated release of steroid hormones. Leptin also appears to have effects at higher levels of the hypothalamic–pituitary–adrenal axis. Leptin deficiency leads to increased activity of this axis. This leads to the conclusion that leptin decreases the activity of the hypothalamic-pituitary-adrenal axis.

Adiponectin receptors are also present in all layers of the adrenal cortex and medulla. Adiponectin downregulates key enzymes of steroidogenesis, resulting in decreased corticosterone and aldosterone production.

Thus, adipose tissue regulates adrenal cortical function. The adipose–adrenal interactions need further physiological and pathophysiological definitions. However, these known interactions highlight the link between metabolism and stress regulation in humans.

3.6.2.2 Epinephrine (Adrenalin)

The adrenal medulla secretes catecholamine hormones, primarily epinephrine, under the control of the sympathetic nervous system. Epinephrine is also known as adrenalin. Adrenergic receptors are present throughout the body, and the effect of receptor activation depends on location and subtype. Some of the metabolic effects of adrenalin include:

- Inhibition of insulin release from the β-cells of the pancreas (α-adrenergic receptor)
- Stimulation of glycogenolysis in the liver and muscle (α-adrenergic receptor)
- Stimulation of glycolysis in the muscle (α-adrenergic receptor)
- Inhibition of insulin-mediated glycogenesis in the muscle (α-adrenergic receptor)
- Stimulation of glucagon release from the α-cells of the pancreas (β-adrenergic receptor)
- Stimulation of adrenocorticotropic hormone from the pituitary gland (β-adrenergic receptor)

The β-adrenergic receptor was the first hormone receptor identified in adipocytes. Adrenalin has potent lipolytic effects on adipose tissue by stimulating hormone-sensitive lipase.

There is a cross talk between catecholamines and adipose tissue. Activation of leptin receptors in the adrenal medulla leads to catecholamine release. Resistin, on the other hand, suppresses medullary catecholamine secretion. There is an adrenal–adipose feedback loop, since catecholamines promote the expression of proinflammatory cytokines by adipocytes and reduce the production of both leptin and resistin.

3.7 Conclusion

Figure 3.3 summarizes this chapter. Adipose tissue is an active participant in the regulation of metabolism. Receptors in adipocytes and other cells in adipose tissue allow it to actively receive signals from other tissues involved in fuel sensing. The response of adipose tissue to this signaling depends on the ratio of anabolic to catabolic input. The major anabolic signal to the adipocyte is insulin, which promotes the storage of energy as triglycerides in the fat vacuole of each adipocyte. There are several catabolic signals to adipocytes, including the adrenal hormones adrenalin and cortisol, which promote lipolysis. In return, adipose tissue actively signals other tissues both directly and indirectly. The major hormonal signals from adipose tissue are leptin, which signals the brain about energy reserves, and adiponectin, which signals adipose tissue function. The ratio of leptin to adiponectin has emerged as a strong measure of adipose tissue health over time.

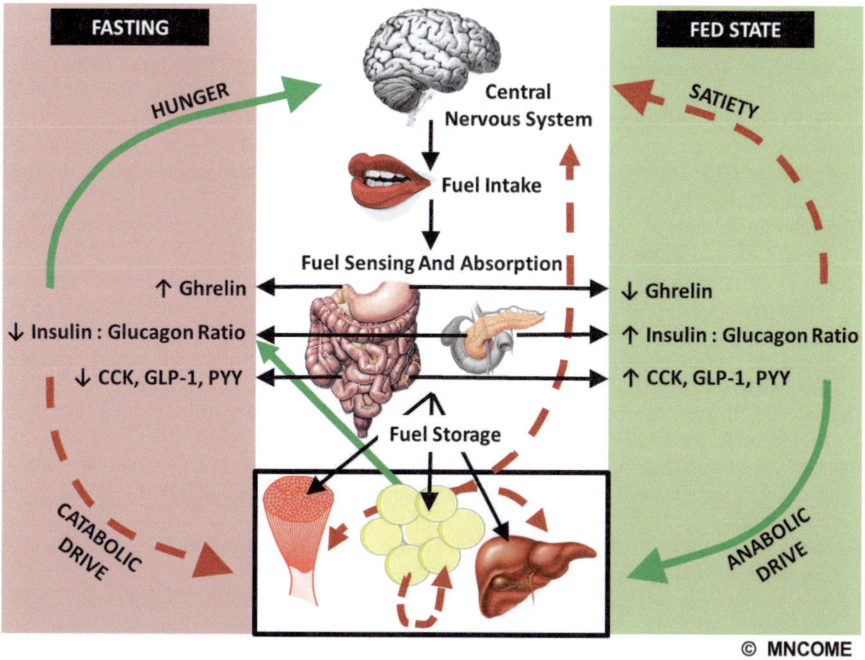

Fig. 3.3 Acute energy balance regulation. Solid green arrows signify a positive or stimulatory effect. Dashed red arrows signify a negative or inhibitory effect. The ingestion of a meal leads to signaling that inhibits feeding (satiety; fuel intake is stopped) and stimulates the storage of energy (fuel storage is promoted; there is an anabolic drive). As time passes from a meal, the signaling changes to regenerate a hunger signal (fuel intake is eventually achieved) and to promote the release of stored energy (fuel storage is inhibited; there is a catabolic drive). Leptin signaling from adipose tissue has an anorexigenic effect on the central nervous system. In the liver, it decreases gluconeogenesis, and in the muscle, it increases glucose and fatty acid oxidation. Leptin has a catabolic effect on adipocytes, promoting lipolysis and decreasing its own gene expression. The major effect of leptin in the pancreas is to inhibit insulin release, decreasing the insulin to glucagon ratio. Acutely, the adipocyte contributes to stopping each feeding event and maintaining circulating fuels between meals. Abbreviations: CCK cholecystokinin, GLP-1 glucagon-like peptide-1, PYY Peptide YY, MNCOME Minnesota Center for Obesity, Metabolism and Endocrinology, PA. (Reproduced with permission from MNCOME)

Reading List

Abu-Hamdah R, Rabiee A, Meneilly GS, Shannon RP, Andersen DK, Elahi D. Clinical review: the extrapancreatic effects of glucagon-like peptide-1 and related peptides. J Clin Endocrinol Metab. 2009;94(6):1843–52. Epub 2009/04/02.

Bays HE, Gonzalez-Campoy JM. Adiposopathy. In: Friedberg E, Castrillon DH, Galindo RL, Wharton K, editors. New-Opathies: World Scientific; 2012. p. 105–68.

Breen DM, Rasmussen BA, Cote CD, Jackson VM, Lam TK. Nutrient-sensing mechanisms in the gut as therapeutic targets for diabetes. Diabetes. 2013;62(9):3005–13. Epub 2013/08/24.

Broeders EP, Vijgen GH, Havekes B, Bouvy ND, Mottaghy FM, Kars M, et al. Thyroid hormone activates brown adipose tissue and increases non-shivering thermogenesis—a cohort study in a Group of Thyroid Carcinoma Patients. PLoS One. 2016;11(1):e0145049. Epub 2016/01/20.
Brubaker PL. Minireview: update on incretin biology: focus on glucagon-like peptide-1. Endocrinology. 2010;151(5):1984–9. Epub 2010/03/23.
Cantini G, Di Franco A, Mannucci E, Luconi M. Is cleaved glucagon-like peptide 1 really inactive? Effects of GLP-1(9–36) on human adipose stem cells. Mol Cell Endocrinol. 2017;439:10–5. Epub 2016/10/30.
Chakraborti CK. Role of adiponectin and some other factors linking type 2 diabetes mellitus and obesity. World J Diabetes. 2015;6(15):1296–308. Epub 2015/11/12.
Challa TD, Beaton N, Arnold M, Rudofsky G, Langhans W, Wolfrum C. Regulation of adipocyte formation by GLP-1/GLP-1R signaling. J Biol Chem. 2012;287(9):6421–30. Epub 2011/12/31.
D'Aquila T, Hung YH, Carreiro A, Buhman KK. Recent discoveries on absorption of dietary fat: presence, synthesis, and metabolism of cytoplasmic lipid droplets within enterocytes. Biochim Biophys Acta. 2016;1861(8 Pt A):730–47. Epub 2016/04/25.
DePaoli AM. 20 years of leptin: leptin in common obesity and associated disorders of metabolism. J Endocrinol. 2014;223(1):T71–81. Epub 2014/06/29.
Esfahani M, Movahedian A, Baranchi M, Goodarzi MT. Adiponectin: an adipokine with protective features against metabolic syndrome. Iranian J Basic Med Sci. 2015;18(5):430–42. Epub 2015/07/01.
Farooqi IS, O'Rahilly S. 20 years of leptin: human disorders of leptin action. J Endocrinol. 2014;223(1):T63–70. Epub 2014/09/19.
Glasow A, Bornstein SR. Leptin and the adrenal gland. Eur J Clin Investig. 2000;30(Suppl 3):39–45. Epub 2001/04/03.
Gurriaran-Rodriguez U, Al-Massadi O, Roca-Rivada A, Crujeiras AB, Gallego R, Pardo M, et al. Obestatin as a regulator of adipocyte metabolism and adipogenesis. J Cell Mol Med. 2011;15(9):1927–40. Epub 2010/10/30.
Htike ZZ, Zaccardi F, Papamargaritis D, Webb DR, Khunti K, Davies MJ. Efficacy and safety of glucagon-like peptide-1 receptor agonists in type 2 diabetes: a systematic review and mixed-treatment comparison analysis. Diabetes Obes Metab. 2017;19(4):524–36. Epub 2016/12/17.
Kargi AY, Iacobellis G. Adipose tissue and adrenal glands: novel pathophysiological mechanisms and clinical applications. Int J Endocrinol. 2014;2014:614074. Epub 2014/07/16.
Kawwass JF, Summer R, Kallen CB. Direct effects of leptin and adiponectin on peripheral reproductive tissues: a critical review. Mol Hum Reprod. 2015;21(8):617–32. Epub 2015/05/13.
Lacquaniti A, Donato V, Chirico V, Buemi A, Buemi M. Obestatin: an interesting but controversial gut hormone. Ann Nutr Metab. 2011;59(2–4):193–9. Epub 2011/12/14.
Liao YC, Liang KW, Lee WJ, Lee WL, Lee IT, Wang JS, et al. Leptin to adiponectin ratio as a useful predictor for cardiac syndrome X. Biomarkers: Biochem Indicators Exposure Response Susceptibility Chem. 2013;18(1):44–50. Epub 2012/10/17.
Liu R, Li L, Chen Y, Yang M, Liu H, Yang G. Effects of glucagon-like peptide-1 agents on left ventricular function: systematic review and meta-analysis. Ann Med. 2014;46(8):664–71. Epub 2014/08/20.
Lopez-Jaramillo P, Gomez-Arbelaez D, Lopez-Lopez J, Lopez-Lopez C, Martinez-Ortega J, Gomez-Rodriguez A, et al. The role of leptin/adiponectin ratio in metabolic syndrome and diabetes. Horm Mol Biol Clin Invest. 2014;18(1):37–45. Epub 2014/11/13.
Mantzoros CS, Magkos F, Brinkoetter M, Sienkiewicz E, Dardeno TA, Kim SY, et al. Leptin in human physiology and pathophysiology. Am J Physiol Endocrinol Metab. 2011;301(4):E567–84. Epub 2011/07/28.
Muller MJ, Enderle J, Bosy-Westphal A. Changes in energy expenditure with weight gain and weight loss in humans. Curr Obes Rep. 2016;5(4):413–23. Epub 2016/10/16.
Nayak S, Bhaktha G, Mohammed S. Adiponectin in diabetic subjects without any micro- or macrovascular complications: a review. J Diabetes Sci Technol. 2015;9:1160. Epub 2015/04/26

Nerup N, Ambrus R, Lindhe J, Achiam MP, Jeppesen PB, Svendsen LB. The effect of glucagon-like peptide-1 and glucagon-like peptide-2 on microcirculation: a systematic review. Microcirculation. 2017; Epub 2017/03/08.

Obregon MJ. Adipose tissues and thyroid hormones. Front Physiol. 2014;5:479. Epub 2015/01/08.

Park JT, Yoo TH, Kim JK, Oh HJ, Kim SJ, Yoo DE, et al. Leptin/adiponectin ratio is an independent predictor of mortality in nondiabetic peritoneal dialysis patients. Perit Dial Int. 2013;33(1):67–74. Epub 2012/08/03.

Pruszynska-Oszmalek E, Szczepankiewicz D, Hertig I, Skrzypski M, Sassek M, Kaczmarek P, et al. Obestatin inhibits lipogenesis and glucose uptake in isolated primary rat adipocytes. J Biol Regul Homeost Agents. 2013;27(1):23–33. Epub 2013/03/16.

Sayegh AI. The role of cholecystokinin receptors in the short-term control of food intake. Prog Mol Biol Transl Sci. 2013;114:277–316. Epub 2013/01/16.

Seim I, Walpole C, Amorim L, Josh P, Herington A, Chopin L. The expanding roles of the ghrelin-gene derived peptide obestatin in health and disease. Mol Cell Endocrinol. 2011;340(1):111–7. Epub 2011/04/05.

Sun F, Chai S, Li L, Yu K, Yang Z, Wu S, et al. Effects of glucagon-like peptide-1 receptor agonists on weight loss in patients with type 2 diabetes: a systematic review and network meta-analysis. J Diabetes Res. 2015;2015:157201. Epub 2015/02/18.

Tang SQ, Jiang QY, Zhang YL, Zhu XT, Shu G, Gao P, et al. Obestatin: its physicochemical characteristics and physiological functions. Peptides. 2008;29(4):639–45. Epub 2008/03/08.

Vega GL, Grundy SM. Metabolic risk susceptibility in men is partially related to adiponectin/leptin ratio. J Obes. 2013;2013:409679. Epub 2013/03/28.

Vilsboll T, Christensen M, Junker AE, Knop FK, Gluud LL. Effects of glucagon-like peptide-1 receptor agonists on weight loss: systematic review and meta-analyses of randomised controlled trials. BMJ. 2012;344:d7771. Epub 2012/01/13.

Zhang JV, Ren PG, Avsian-Kretchmer O, Luo CW, Rauch R, Klein C, et al. Obestatin, a peptide encoded by the ghrelin gene, opposes ghrelin's effects on food intake. Science. 2005;310(5750):996–9. Epub 2005/11/15.

Chapter 4
Central Nervous System Regulation of Energy Balance and Energy Stores

J. Michael Gonzalez-Campoy

Pearls of Wisdom
- The adipocyte is an endocrine cell which generates hormonal signals that provide the central nervous system with information on the state of the body's energy reserves.
- The hypothalamus is the major area of the brain where integration of afferent and efferent signals for the regulation of hunger and satiety takes place.
- The core homeostatic role of the hypothalamus in maintenance of energy balance is heavily modulated by input from all areas of the brain.
- Adiposopathy, overweight, and obesity result from a condition of long-term positive energy balance where orexigenic signals are upregulated and anorexigenic signals are downregulated, including a state of leptin resistance.
- Bariatric endocrinology includes an understanding of the energy homeostatic systems in the body, including the role of the hypothalamus and the rest of the central nervous system, and how derangements in function contribute to overweight, obesity, and adiposopathy.

J. M. Gonzalez-Campoy
Minnesota Center for Obesity, Metabolism and Endocrinology, PA (MNCOME), Eagan, MN, USA
e-mail: drmike@mncome.com

J. M. Gonzalez-Campoy et al. (eds.), *Bariatric Endocrinology*,
https://doi.org/10.1007/978-3-319-95655-8_4

4.1 Introduction

In 1840, Mohr first described hypothalamic obesity. The autopsy of a 57-year-old woman who gained significant weight within a year prior to death revealed a large hypophyseal tumor that deformed the sella. The tumor was large enough to distort and compress the base of the brain, including the cerebral peduncles, optic nerves, optic chiasm, and the region of the hypothalamus. Multiple reports of obesity in association of hypophyseal lesions followed.

In 1904, Erdheim noted that compression of the base of the brain was always present when excess adiposity developed. Then, in 1913, Camus and Roussy showed that hypophysectomy in dogs did not cause an increase in weight gain unless the base of the brain was damaged during the procedure.

Beginning in the 1940s, over the course of two decades, Brobeck and colleagues at Yale University were able to define that bilateral destructive lesions made to the lateral hypothalamus of rats or cats result in complete cessation of eating. Unilateral lesions did not have this effect. On the other hand, bilateral lesions placed more centrally in the hypothalamus, avoiding the lateral areas, produced hyperphagia and obesity. Further, they noted that animals that developed obesity from medial lesions of the hypothalamus could be made to cease feeding by subsequently making bilateral lesions of the lateral hypothalamus (Fig. 4.1). They thus referred to the lateral

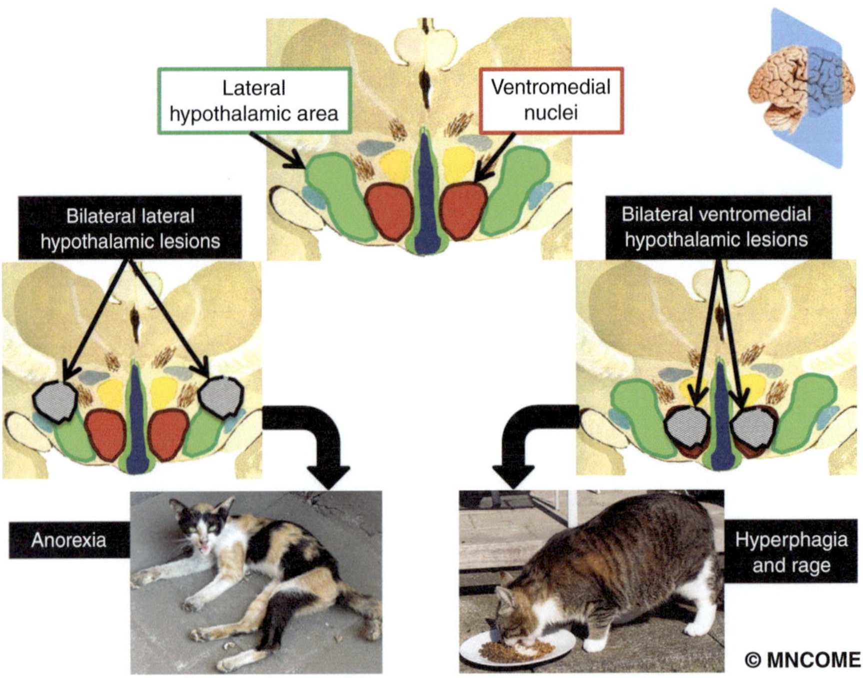

Fig. 4.1 Lesions of the hypothalamus affect feeding behaviors. The lateral hypothalamic area drives hunger and feeding. Damage to this area causes anorexia and weight loss. The ventromedial nuclei drive satiety and cessation of feeding. Lesions in this area cause hyperphagia and rage. (Copyright, Minnesota Center for Obesity, Metabolism and Endocrinology, PA (MNCOME))

areas of the hypothalamus as a "feeding center." They also noted that the ventromedial nuclei are capable of exerting an inhibitory control on feeding through nerve fibers which run laterally into the lateral hypothalamic area (LHA).

The anatomical, hormonal, neuronal, and biochemical pathways that underlie the observations from decades ago have been clarified. Much of this knowledge has come from recognition of specific mutations associated with monogenic obesity (see Chap. 9 in this textbook). This chapter offers an overview of the role of the central nervous system (CNS) in the regulation of energy balance and energy stores.

4.2 Brain Appetite Circuitry and Homeostatic Systems

The neural circuitry controlling food intake and energy metabolism extends throughout the brain. Afferent signals originate in the sensory organs and reach the CNS through the cranial nerves. Direct neural connections to the brain from throughout the gastrointestinal tract are relayed by the vagus and sympathetic nerves and convey information about the fed state and nutrient availability. The brain integrates all these neural inputs with hormonal signals that arrive through the circulation. Hormonal signals originate in many organs involved with energy homeostasis, including adipose tissue. Extensive cross-signaling of various CNS centers then leads to efferent signals from the brain back to the periphery. Neural output through both the sympathetic and parasympathetic nervous systems and hormonal output through the pituitary gland control all aspects of metabolism (Fig. 4.2).

4.2.1 The Hypothalamus

The hypothalamus is located inferior to the thalamus, at the base of the brain. It is part of the limbic system. The hypothalamus forms the ventral part of the diencephalon in all vertebrates. Each half of the hypothalamus is made up of nuclei, each of which has defined functions (Table 4.1).

The hypothalamus is largely responsible for the regulation of metabolic processes. One of its most important functions is to link the nervous system to the endocrine system. The hypothalamus has receptors for circulating hormones which convey signals from all organs involved in energy homeostasis. The hypothalamus in turn synthesizes and secretes neurohormones, which are released into the portal circulation between the hypothalamus and the pituitary gland. These neurohormones regulate the release of anterior pituitary hormones. The hypothalamus also controls body temperature, hunger, satiety, parenting and attachment behaviors, emotion (rage), short-term memory, thirst, fatigue, blood pressure, heart rate, gastrointestinal tract peristalsis, arousal, and circadian rhythms.

Peripheral hormones must pass through the blood–brain barrier (BBB) to reach the hypothalamus. The hypothalamus is connected to brain regions where the BBB is not intact. These regions, which include the neurohypophysis and the median

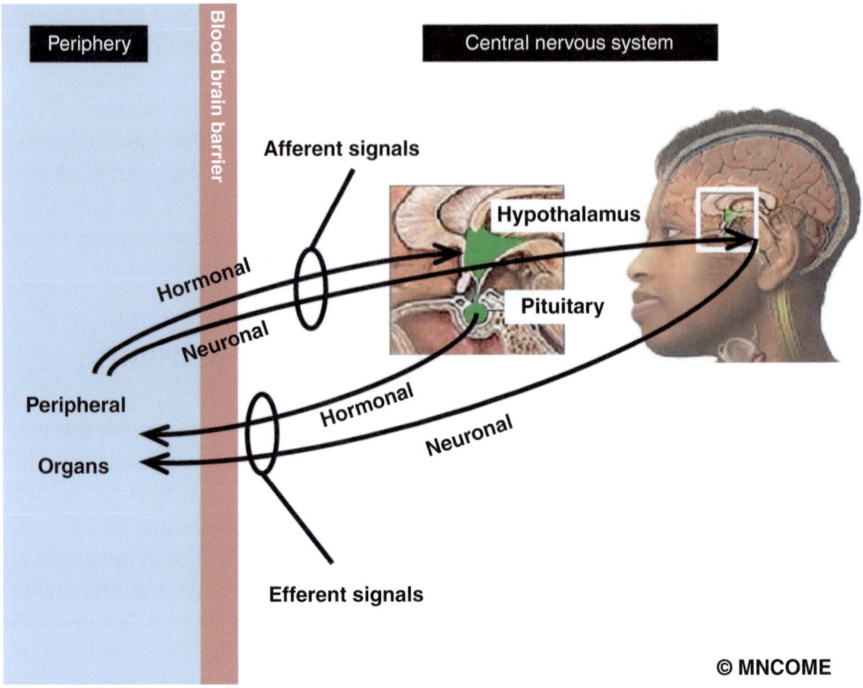

Fig. 4.2 Afferent and efferent CNS pathways for metabolic regulation. The brain regulates energy balance and energy stores. There are afferent and efferent hormonal and neuronal signals that allow the central nervous system to control all metabolic processes. The hypothalamus is the major CNS center for this integration, and it receives most of the hormonal signaling from peripheral organs. Both sympathetic and parasympathetic fibers provide afferent signals to the brain and receive efferent signals from the brain. The hypothalamus regulates efferent hormonal signals released from the pituitary gland. (Copyright, Minnesota Center for Obesity, Metabolism and Endocrinology, PA (MNCOME))

eminence, where neurosecretion takes place, have a capillary endothelium that is fenestrated and allows free passage of large proteins.

The hypothalamus is also connected to other brain regions at which the brain samples the composition of the blood. The circumventricular organs (CVO; subfornical organ and the organum vasculosum of the lamina terminalis) have neurons in contact with both the blood and cerebrospinal fluid. They have an extensive vascular supply. Neurons in the CVO have osmoreceptors and sodium sensors. These neurons control drinking, vasopressin release, sodium excretion, and sodium appetite. Neurons in the CVO have receptors for angiotensin, atrial natriuretic factor, endothelin, and relaxin. These circulating peptides contribute to fluid and electrolyte balance. CVO neurons project to the supraoptic nucleus (SON), paraventricular nucleus (PVN), and preoptic nucleus (PON) of the hypothalamus. CVO neurons are also the site of action of interleukins. Through activation of CVO neurons and their projections to the PVN, interleukins cause fever and adrenocorticotropic hormone (ACTH) secretion.

Table 4.1 Hypothalamic nuclei

Nucleus/(abbreviation)	Functions	Zone(s)	Region(s)
Preoptic nucleus (PON)	Thermoregulation GnRH (from sexually dimorphic nucleus)	Medial Lateral	Anterior
Anterior nucleus (AN)	Thermoregulation (through parasympathetic heat loss) TSH inhibition	Medial	Anterior
Suprachiasmatic nucleus (SCN)	Circadian rhythm regulation	Medial	Anterior
Supraoptic nucleus (SON)	Vasopressin release (fluid balance) Oxytocin release (milk let-down, parturition)	Medial Lateral	Anterior
Paraventricular nucleus (PVN)	Vasopressin release (fluid balance), Oxytocin release (milk let-down, parturition) Anterior pituitary control (TRH, CRH, somatostatin) Autonomic nervous system regulation Fullness by NTS activation	Periventricular Medial	Anterior Tuberal
Lateral hypothalamic area (LHA)	Hunger center (orexin release leads to arousal, hunger) Body weight control	Lateral	Tuberal
Dorsomedial nucleus (DMN)	Emotion (rage) Blood pressure and heart rate Gastrointestinal stimulation	Medial	Tuberal
Ventromedial nucleus (VMN)	Satiety center Body weight control Insulin regulation	Medial	Tuberal
Arcuate nucleus (ARC)	Anterior pituitary control (GHRH) Dopamine (prolactin inhibition) Hunger and feeding (NPY) Satiety (α-MSH)	Periventricular Medial	Tuberal
Posterior nucleus (PN)	Thermoregulation (through sympathetic heat conservation)	Medial	Posterior
Mammillary nucleus (MN)	Emotion Short-term memory Cortical activation of arousal Learning Sleep Energy balance	Medial	Posterior

Other abbreviations: *CRH* corticotropin-releasing hormone, *GHRH* gonadotropin-releasing hormone, *GnRH* gonadotropin-releasing hormone, *α-MSH* α-melanocyte-stimulating hormone, *NPY* neuropeptide Y, *NTS* nucleus tractus solitarius, *TRH* thyrotropin-releasing hormone, *TSH* thyroid-stimulating hormone

The functional anatomy of the hypothalamus continues to be uncovered. The role that the hypothalamus plays in energy homeostasis, and the crosstalk with adipose tissue and other peripheral organs, should be in the realm of comfort for bariatric endocrinologists.

4.2.1.1 PVN and Satiety

The PVN lies adjacent to the third ventricle, within the periventricular zone of the hypothalamus. It has a rich vascular supply but is protected by the BBB. Neuroendocrine cells of the PVN have projections that reach outside the BBB, to the median eminence and the posterior pituitary. The PVN contributes to neurohormonal integration by regulating both anterior pituitary hormone release and the direct release of vasopressin and oxytocin from the posterior pituitary. PVN has descending projections to the brainstem and spinal cord sympathetic centers, including the rostral ventrolateral medulla and the intermediolateral column of the spinal cord. Thus, PVN coordinates autonomic homeostatic responses (Table 4.1). There are glutamate and gamma-aminobutyric acid (GABA) neurons that are active in the PVN and modulate its intrinsic functions.

The PVN receives projections from other hypothalamic nuclei. The projections from the arcuate nucleus of the hypothalamus (ARC) will be reviewed below. The PVN also receives projections from the hindbrain, including the medulla oblongata, nucleus tractus solitarius (NTS), sympathetic premotor area, and dorsal motor nucleus of the vagus nerve. These hindbrain centers receive sensory feedback from the digestive organs, which helps to regulate food, water, and salt intake.

In turn, neurons from the PVN project to the brainstem, including NTS, dorsal motor nucleus of the vagus (from which parasympathetic preganglionic cells originate), and the intermediolateral cell column of the spinal cord (from which sympathetic preganglionic cells originate).

The reciprocal innervation of the hindbrain centers and PVN allows direct communication to and from the adipose tissue, pancreas, gut, and liver via the autonomic nervous system. The PVN thus directs pancreatic secretion, adipose storage, thermogenesis, peripheral glucose uptake, and hepatic glucose flux. Direct projections of the PVN to the NTS increase the response of the NTS to afferent signals arriving through the vagus, including gastric distention. The PVN projections to the NTS have the net effect of inhibiting food intake.

4.2.1.2 Lateral Hypothalamic Area (LHA), Orexin, and Hunger

The LHA drives food intake and has been referred to as the "hunger center" or "feeding center." The mechanisms that drive to feeding are slowly being defined. Orexin, or hypocretin, was discovered in 1998. It is produced in the neurons of the perifornical nucleus, the LHA, and the dorsomedial nucleus (DMN). These neurons have projections throughout the nervous system, including the olfactory bulb, cerebral cortex, thalamus, other hypothalamic nuclei, brainstem, and all levels of the spinal cord.

There are two isoforms of orexin (orexin-A and orexin-B) and two G-protein-coupled orexin receptors (OX1 and OX2). Orexin-A binds to both receptors with equal affinity. Orexin-B binds predominantly to OX2 and is 20% as potent in binding to OX1.

Orexin increases the craving for food and increases meal size by suppressing inhibitory postprandial signals from the gut. Orexin also causes arousal, and increased food intake may also be due to longer wake times with more opportunities for food ingestion. In the absence of orexin, there is narcolepsy, hypophagia, and, paradoxically, obesity. Orexin production is inhibited by leptin and hyperglycemia. Orexin production is stimulated by ghrelin, fasting (hunger), and hypoglycemia.

Orexin neurons project to the ARC and innervate neuropeptide Y (NPY) cell bodies, stimulating the release of NPY. There are reciprocal projections from NPY neurons in the ARC back to orexin neurons in the LHA. NPY neurons in the ARC also project to the PVN, and orexin-containing nerve fibers have projections in close association. NPY receptor activation of PVN neurons causes a potent inhibition of the fullness signal. By inhibiting the generation of fullness signals from the PVN, NPY becomes a strong orexigenic peptide. Since arcuate NPY neurons are excited by orexins, orexin-stimulated feeding occurs at least in part through the inhibition of satiety by NPY projections to the PVN. This is corroborated by a reduction in orexin-stimulated feeding with NPY receptor blockade. Figure 4.3 summarizes the principal orexigenic signals in the hypothalamus.

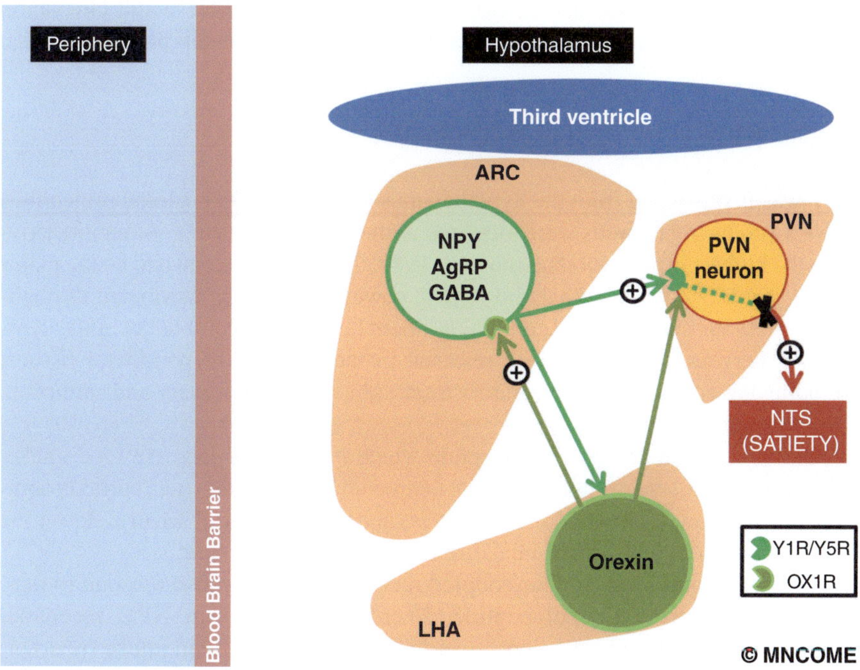

Fig. 4.3 Major orexigenic signals in the hypothalamus. NPY is the principal orexigenic signal in the hypothalamus. NPY neurons from the ARC project to the PVN and stimulate Y1R and Y5R. This causes the PVN neurons to turn off the satiety signal to the NTS (dashed line; black cross), leading to hunger and feeding. Orexin projections from the LHA stimulate NPY secretion in the ARC. Abbreviations: AgRP Agouti-related protein, ARC arcuate nucleus, NPY neuropeptide Y, NTS nucleus of the tractus solitarius, OX1R orexin 1 receptor, PVN paraventricular nucleus, Y1R neuropeptide Y1 receptor, Y5R neuropeptide Y5 receptor. (Copyright, Minnesota Center for Obesity, Metabolism and Endocrinology, PA (MNCOME))

4.2.1.3 ARC and Homeostasis of Hunger: Satiety Signaling

The ARC is located in the mediobasal hypothalamus. It is adjacent to the third ventricle and the median eminence. The ARC contains several populations of neurons. They include centrally projecting neurons that contain NPY, agouti-related protein (AgRP), and the inhibitory neurotransmitter GABA. NPY-AgRP-GABA neurons are located in the most ventromedial part of the ARC. These neurons project to the PVN and the LHA. When NPY-AgRP-GABA neurons are activated, they produce hunger, which leads to feeding, by blocking the satiety signals of the PVN. In addition to orexin, discussed above, NPY-AgRP-GABA neurons are activated by ghrelin. These neurons are inhibited by leptin, insulin, and peptide YY (PYY).

The ARC also has neurons that contain peptide products of pro-opiomelanocortin (POMC) and cocaine- and amphetamine-regulated transcript (CART). These neurons have widespread projections throughout the brain. POMC-CART cells inhibit feeding when activated. These neurons are activated by circulating leptin and insulin. NPY-AgRP-GABA neurons within the ARC inhibit POMC-CART neurons.

Dopaminergic neurons in the ARC release dopamine into the portal circulation between the hypothalamus and the pituitary gland. Dopamine inhibits prolactin release.

4.2.1.4 NPY

NPY was first isolated from the hypothalamus in 1982. In 1983, axonal projections of NPY-producing neurons were localized to the PVN, where NPY immunoreactivity is the highest in the hypothalamus. By 1989, the ARC was known to be the major source of NPY in the hypothalamus. NPY, however, is widely distributed throughout the nervous system. NPY-containing fibers originate in cell bodies in the sympathetic nervous system. NPY is released in the majority of peripheral tissues, including the gut, pancreas, respiratory tract, skin, and genitourinary and cardiovascular systems.

NPY is a 36-amino acid neuropeptide which is known to increase food intake, promote storage of energy as fat, regulate neuroendocrine function (i.e., corticotropin-releasing hormone production), reduce stress and anxiety, control seizures, lower the blood pressure, reduce alcohol intake, and reduce pain perception.

NPY receptors are G-protein-coupled receptors, and they also respond to peptide YY and pancreatic polypeptide. There are five known NPY receptors. Blockade of the Y1 and Y5 receptors in the PVN decreases food intake (anorexigenic signal from PVN to NTS is turned off). On the other hand, NPY stimulation of PVN Y1 and Y5 receptors leads to feeding (anorexigenic signal from PVN to NTS is turned on).

The Y2 receptor in NPY-AgRP-GABA neurons serves for NPY to turn off its own production (automodulation by presynaptic processing). Circulating PYY stimulates Y2 receptors in NPY-AGRP-GABA neurons, inhibiting the release of NPY.

4.2.1.5 AgRP

AgRP is a neuropeptide which is synthesized by the hypothalamic NPY-AgRP-GABA cell bodies. It was first discovered in 1997 and consists of 112 amino acids. AgRP is a paracrine signal which causes hunger by antagonism of the hypothalamic melanocortin (MC) receptors MC3-R and MC4-R. It also lowers energy expenditure. AgRP expression is stimulated by ghrelin during periods of fasting and suppressed by leptin. AgRP also stimulates the release of ACTH and prolactin and enhances the ACTH response to inflammatory cytokines. AgRP decreases the release of thyrotropin-releasing hormone (TRH) from the PVN, helping to conserve energy during starvation. When AgRP levels in the hypothalamus decrease during the fed state, TRH levels rise. TRH-secreting neurons from the PVN then have a stimulatory effect on AgRP release.

4.2.1.6 GABA

GABA was first described in 1883. It was not until 1950 that it was discovered in the mammalian nervous system. GABA is present throughout the nervous system. It reduces neuronal excitability by causing a negative change in the transmembrane potential of target neurons (hyperpolarization). There are two GABA receptors, $GABA_A$ and $GABA_B$. In the hypothalamus, GABA activity leads to feeding.

GABA immunoreactivity is present in the NPY/AgRP neurons of the ARC. GABA is also present in approximately one-third of POMC-expressing neurons, but they are unable to release it. Both NPY and AgRP stimulate food intake when infused into the brain. The weight loss seen when NPY-AgRP-GABA neurons in the ARC are destroyed is recapitulated by targeted deletion of their ability to release GABA, rather than NPY or AgRP. The synaptic release of GABA by NPY-AgRP-GABA neurons in the ARC is required to maintain a critical level of appetite stimulation by NPY.

4.2.1.7 POMC

POMC is a 241-amino acid polypeptide synthesized from the 285-amino acid-long polypeptide precursor pre-pro-opiomelanocortin (pre-POMC), by the removal of a 44-amino acid-long signal peptide sequence during translation. POMC is cleaved to produce several peptide hormones released by exocytosis. POMC is the source of ACTH in the anterior pituitary gland. POMC gene expression is present in the pancreas, stomach, appendix, kidney, testis, prostate, placenta, skin, adipose tissue, skeletal muscle, lymph node, brain, adrenal, and lung. POMC expression in the brain is localized to the ARC and the NTS. POMC-CART neurons of the ARC produce α-melanocyte-stimulating hormone (MSH), one of the several members of this family, also known as the melanotropins or intermedins.

There are five MC receptors. MC2R is specific for ACTH and is also known as the ACTH receptor. MC3R and MC4R are present in the hypothalamus and contribute to energy homeostasis. MC4R is expressed by PVN neurons. MC3R is expressed by NPY-AgRP-GABA neurons in the ARC. α-MSH released from POMC-CART neurons in the ARC causes stimulation of MC4R on PVN neurons, which triggers fullness. AgRP blocks MC4R and causes hunger. Simulation of the MC3R receptor in NPY-AgRP-GABA neurons in the ARC by α-MSH from POMC-CART neighbor neurons inhibits AgRP and NPY release, which leads to fullness. Figure 4.4 summarizes these major hypothalamic anorexigenic signals.

4.2.1.8 CART

CART is a neuropeptide protein that mediates reward, feeding, and stress. It is considered an endogenous psychostimulant. CART is expressed throughout the central and peripheral nervous systems, with high levels in the hypothalamus. It is expressed in the same hypothalamic neurons that generate POMC and its products. CART is also found in the pituitary gland, the adrenal medulla, somatostatin cells in the pancreas, and gastrin cells in the stomach. CART inhibits food intake and blocks the feeding

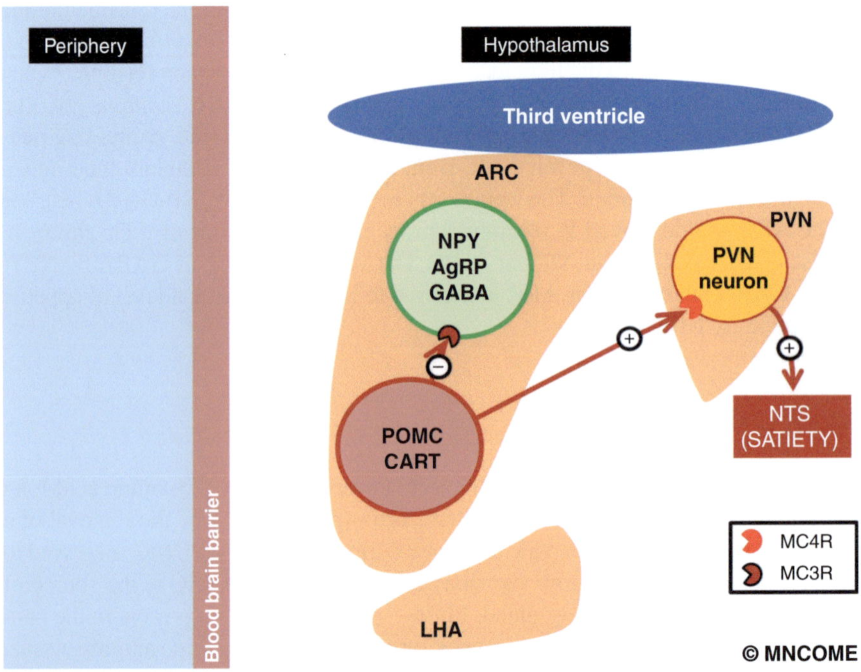

Fig. 4.4 Major anorexigenic signals in the hypothalamus. POMC neurons in the ARC project to the PVN and neighboring NPY-AgRP-GABA neurons. α-MSH stimulation of MC4R causes a strong satiety signal from PVN to NTS. MC3R stimulation by α-MSH inhibits the major orexigenic signals from ARC. Abbreviations: ARC arcuate nucleus, CART cocaine- and amphetamine-regulated transcript, MC3R melanocortin 3 receptor, MC4R melanocortin 4 receptor, MSH melanocyte-stimulating hormone, NPY neuropeptide Y, NTS nucleus of the tractus solitarius, OX1R orexin 1 receptor, POMC pro-opiomelanocortin, PVN paraventricular nucleus. (Copyright, Minnesota Center for Obesity, Metabolism and Endocrinology, PA (MNCOME))

response induced by NPY. Decreased activity of CART in the hypothalamus is seen in depression and is associated with hyperphagia and weight gain.

4.2.1.9 Cannabinoids

Endocannabinoids are endogenous lipid-based retrograde neurotransmitters. There are two major cannabinoid receptors (CBs), CB_1 and CB_2, expressed throughout the central and peripheral nervous systems. Endocannabinoids regulate fertility, pregnancy, prenatal and postnatal development, appetite, pain sensation, mood, and memory. CBs also mediate the pharmacological effects of cannabis.

In the hypothalamus, the amount of endocannabinoid produced is inversely proportional to the amount of leptin in the blood. In leptin deficiency, hypothalamic endocannabinoids reach abnormally high levels. POMC-CART neurons express the OX-1 receptor and CB_1 on the plasma membrane. Orexin-A simulation of OX-1 in POMC-CART neurons promotes the biosynthesis of the endocannabinoid 2-arachidonoylglycerol (2-AG), which acts at CB_1. 2-AG stimulation by orexin-A causes hyperphagia and weight gain by blunting α-MSH production. Pharmacological blockade of OX-1 causes a reduction in food intake and loss of body weight. Hypothalamic CB_1 stimulation thus leads to increased hunger and food-seeking behavior.

4.2.1.10 Melanin-Concentrating Hormone (MCH)

MCH is a hypothalamic cyclic 19-amino acid neuropeptide hormone. MCH neurons are located in the LHA and zona incerta. These neurons have projections throughout the brain. MCH is a potent orexigen. MCH causes an increase in food intake acutely. MCH leads to an increase in fat mass chronically. A lack of MCH prevents diet-induced obesity. MCH antagonists reduce food intake acutely and prevent body weight gain when given chronically, so they are the subject of clinical research.

4.2.1.11 Serotonin

5-hydroxytryptamine (5-HT), or serotonin, is not produced in the hypothalamus. It reaches several hypothalamic nuclei through the ascending projections from the raphe nuclei in the brainstem. Serotonin receptor activation in the hypothalamus leads to suppression of food intake.

There are at least 18 identified serotonin receptors. The 5HT2C receptor is highly expressed in the hypothalamus. Stimulation of the 5HT2C receptor in the hypothalamus causes fullness.

4.2.1.12 Brain-Derived Neurotrophic Factor (BDNF)

BDNF is a member of the neurotrophin family. Mutations in the genes for BDNF and its receptor, TrkB, result in hyperphagia and severe obesity in humans.

BDNF mRNA is present in the LHA, PVN, and NTS among other CNS sites. BDNF immunoreactive fibers are present in the ARC and PVN of the hypothalamus and the NTS and dorsal raphe nucleus.

4.3 Peripheral Afferent Signals

Chapter 2 in this textbook provides an overview of adipose tissue and its role as an active participant in regulating metabolism. Chapter 3 in this textbook addresses the neurohormonal integration of metabolism and discusses the major hormonal signals that regulate energy balance and energy stores. Chapter 5 reviews the gut–brain axis. The reader is referred to these chapters for this material. Table 4.2 summarizes the major orexigenic and anorexigenic signals that are integrated in the hypothalamus. Figure 4.5 provides an overview of integrated hypothalamic signaling.

There are additional discrete signals from adipose tissue that also contribute to the regulation of energy balance and energy stores.

Table 4.2 Major orexigenic and anorexigenic molecules

Orexigenic molecules	Anorexigenic molecules
Agouti-related peptide	Amino acids
Cannabinoids	Amylin
Cortisol	Bombesin
Dynorphin	Brain-derived neurotrophic factor
Galanin	Cholecystokinin
Ghrelin	Cocaine- and amphetamine-regulated transcript peptides
Melanin-concentrating hormone	Corticotropin-releasing hormone
Neuropeptide Y	Fatty acids
Omentin-1	Glucagon
Orexins (A,B)	Glucagon-like peptide 1
	Glucose
	Insulin
	Leptin
	(α[alpha],β,γ)-melanocyte-stimulating hormones (melanocortins)
	Norepinephrine
	Oxyntomodulin
	Oxytocin
	Pancreatic polypeptide
	Peptide YY
	Serotonin
	Vagal afferent neurotransmitters (i.e., glutamate)
	Vaspin

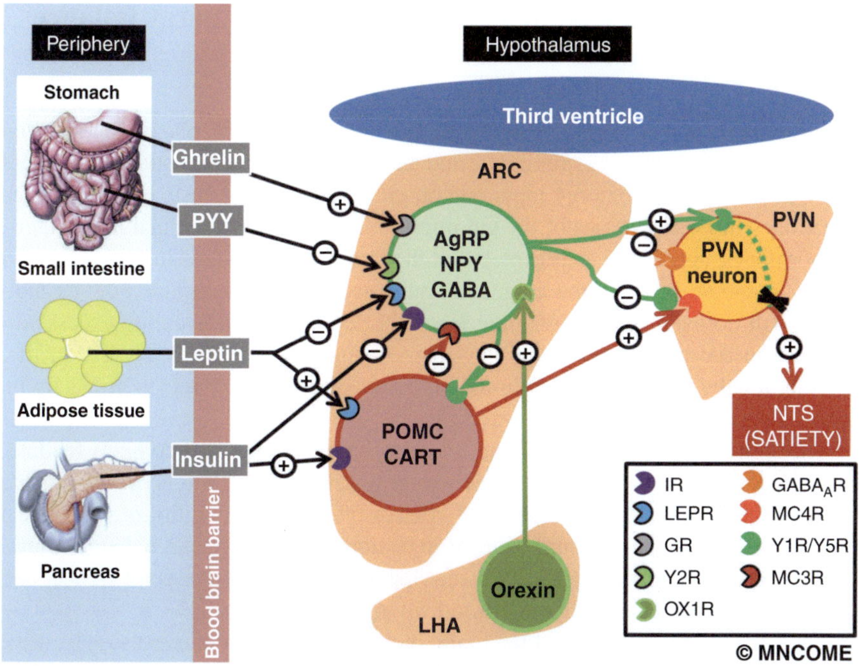

Fig. 4.5 Integrated major hypothalamic signaling in the regulation of food intake. The hypothalamus is the CNS site for the integration of metabolic signaling. The balance of these signals determines whether hunger or satiety signals predominate. In adiposopathy, overweight, and obesity, the orexigenic signaling is predominant over the anorexigenic signaling, leading to a positive energy balance over time. Abbreviations: AgRP Agouti-related protein, ARC arcuate nucleus, CART cocaine- and amphetamine-regulated transcript, GABA gamma-aminobutyric acid, GABAAR gamma-aminobutyric acid A receptor, GR ghrelin receptor, IR insulin receptor, LEPR leptin receptor, MC3R melanocortin 3 receptor, MC4R melanocortin 4 receptor, NPY neuropeptide Y, NTS nucleus of the tractus solitarius, OX1R orexin 1 receptor, POMC pro-opiomelanocortin, PVN paraventricular nucleus, PYY peptide YY, Y1R neuropeptide Y1 receptor, Y2R neuropeptide Y2/PYY(3–36) receptor. (Copyright, Minnesota Center for Obesity, Metabolism and Endocrinology, PA (MNCOME))

4.3.1 Omentin-1

Omentin-1, a visceral fat depot-specific secretory protein, is inversely correlated with obesity and insulin resistance. Omentin-1 has an orexigenic effect, which is due to decreased CART and CRH gene expression and increased norepinephrine synthesis and release in the hypothalamus. Omentin-1 does not affect hypothalamic POMC, AgRP, NPY, or orexin-A.

4.3.2 Vaspin

Visceral adipose tissue-derived serine protease inhibitor (Vaspin) improves glucose tolerance and insulin sensitivity. Vaspin triggers anorexic pathways in the hypothalamus, where reduction of NPY and increase of POMC signals lead to satiety and feeding cessation.

4.4 Extra Hypothalamic CNS Modulation of Energy Balance and Food Stores

The hypothalamus is a homeostatic system which controls energy balance and fat stores tightly by balancing orexigenic and anorexigenic input and output. There are many other aspects of energy input and output that affect the basic energy balance equation. The contributions of the gut microbiome, other intraluminal messengers, gut hormones, and the myenteric plexus of the intestine are covered in Chaps. 3 and 5 of this textbook. Genetic and epigenetic influences largely determine how an individual will do over time maintaining lean muscle mass and preventing excess adipose tissue accrual. The prenatal environment and imprinting from early in life, whether a baby is breast- or bottle-fed, and the environment a person grows up in, are all determinants of fat mass over time.

The sight and smell of foods lead to activation of hunger and compels feeding. The olfactory cortex, brainstem nuclei, ventral striatum, and the NTS, all provide input to the hypothalamic centers that control feeding. Availability of food, meal timing, meal size, the pleasure of meal ingestion (palatability and hedonic input), energy expenditure, wake time, circadian patterns, reproductive competence, and social cues, all affect the volume of food we ingest.

The corticolimbic circuits of the brain, in the presence of a nutrient supply, drive food intake, and there is a lack of inhibition for the acquisition of calories. The ingestion of food in modern day America is largely driven by the mesolimbic (dopamine) system, which is referred to as a reward system. It includes the ventral tegmental area, the nucleus accumbens, and the frontal cortex. It is palatability rather than energy needs that drives food intake.

The limbic system, which is resident in the amygdala, hypothalamus, and mesocorticolimbic system, contributes to the accumulation of adipose tissue. Perceived stress leads to hypercortisolism and a hyperadrenergic state. There is insulin resistance and hyperinsulinism which cause hypothalamic leptin resistance. Without the tonic inhibition of leptin an increased appetite develops, and caloric intake goes up. Hypercortisolism, insulin resistance, hyperinsulinemia, and hyperleptinemia make chronic stress a significant contributor to adiposopathy and metabolic derangements.

4.5 Conclusion

The hypothalamus has emerged as the major regulatory center of hunger and satiety in the CNS. The hypothalamus is able to sense afferent circulating signals that interact mostly with neurons in the ARC. Afferent signals coming through the autonomic nervous system reach the hypothalamus through the hindbrain and its ascending projections. There are several populations of neurons in the hypothalamus, each with multiple connections. Over time many hypothalamic neurotransmitters have been identified as being orexigenic or anorexigenic. The relative strength of hunger and satiety signals that reach the hypothalamus at any given point in time determines the output of the hypothalamic neurons that regulate feeding. Hunger and fullness are generated through specific hypothalamic nuclei and their output, through the autonomic nervous systems in the hindbrain. Integration of the hypothalamic signaling sets the feeding behavior. This is a very dynamic signaling process that helps maintain energy homeostasis. The hypothalamus further regulates metabolism by an efferent hormonal signaling system through the pituitary gland.

In adiposopathy, overweight, and obesity, there is a tonic upregulation of orexigenic signaling and downregulation of anorexigenic signaling. The chronic positive energy balance leads to the storage of excess calories, frequently to the detriment of the organism. Identification of orexigenic and anorexigenic signaling has provided opportunities for pharmacological interventions for the treatment of adiposopathy, overweight, and obesity.

Reading List

Abdel-Magid AF. Melanin-concentrating hormone receptor 1 antagonists for treatment of obesity. ACS Med Chem Lett. 2015;6(4):367–8. Epub 2015/05/06.

Adam CL, Mercer JG. Appetite regulation and seasonality: implications for obesity. Proc Nutr Soc. 2004;63(3):413–9. Epub 2004/09/18.

Allen JM, Adrian TE, Tatemoto K, Polak JM, Hughes J, Bloom SR. Two novel related peptides, neuropeptide Y (NPY) and peptide YY (PYY) inhibit the contraction of the electrically stimulated mouse vas deferens. Neuropeptides. 1982;3(2):71–7. Epub 1982/12/01.

Anand BK, Brobeck JR. Hypothalamic control of food intake in rats and cats. Yale J Biol Med. 1951;24(2):123–40. Epub 1951/11/01.

Backberg M, Hervieu G, Wilson S, Meister B. Orexin receptor-1 (OX-R1) immunoreactivity in chemically identified neurons of the hypothalamus: focus on orexin targets involved in control of food and water intake. Eur J Neurosci. 2002;15(2):315–28. Epub 2002/02/19.

Blevins JE, Baskin DG. Hypothalamic-brainstem circuits controlling eating. Forum Nutr. 2010;63:133–40. Epub 2009/12/04.

Brobeck JR, Tepperman J, Long CN. The effect of experimental obesity upon carbohydrate metabolism. Yale J Biol Med. 1943;15(6):893–904. Epub 1943/07/01.

Brobeck JR. Hypothalamus, appetite, and obesity. Physiol Pharmacol Physicians. 1963;18:1–6. Epub 1963/11/01.

Brunetti L, Orlando G, Ferrante C, Recinella L, Leone S, Chiavaroli A, et al. Orexigenic effects of omentin-1 related to decreased CART and CRH gene expression and increased norepinephrine synthesis and release in the hypothalamus. Peptides. 2013;44:66–74. Epub 2013/03/30.

Challis BG, Yeo GS, Farooqi IS, Luan J, Aminian S, Halsall DJ, et al. The CART gene and human obesity: mutational analysis and population genetics. Diabetes. 2000;49(5):872–5. Epub 2000/07/25.

Chamorro S, Della-Zuana O, Fauchere JL, Feletou M, Galizzi JP, Levens N. Appetite suppression based on selective inhibition of NPY receptors. Int J Obes Relat Metab Disord. 2002;26(3):281–98. Epub 2002/03/16.

Cheng X. Elucidating the pathophysiological significance of circulating omentin levels: is higher better? Atherosclerosis. 2016;251:522–4. Epub 2016/07/09.

Chretien M, Benjannet S, Gossard F, Gianoulakis C, Crine P, Lis M, et al. From beta-lipotropin to beta-endorphin and 'pro-opio-melanocortin. Can J Biochem. 1979;57(9):1111–21. Epub 1979/09/01.

Delgado TC. Glutamate and GABA in appetite regulation. Front Endocrinol. 2013;4:103. Epub 2013/08/24.
Dockray GJ. Cholecystokinin and gut-brain signalling. Regul Pept. 2009;155(1–3):6–10. Epub 2009/04/07.
Donovan MH, Tecott LH. Serotonin and the regulation of mammalian energy balance. Front Neurosci. 2013;7:36. Epub 2013/04/02.
Geerling JC, Shin JW, Chimenti PC, Loewy AD. Paraventricular hypothalamic nucleus: axonal projections to the brainstem. J Comp Neurol. 2010;518(9):1460–99. Epub 2010/02/27.
Gibson WT, Ebersole BJ, Bhattacharyya S, Clayton P, Farooqi IS, Sealfon SC, et al. Mutational analysis of the serotonin receptor 5HT2c in severe early-onset human obesity. Can J Physiol Pharmacol. 2004;82(6):426–9. Epub 2004/09/24.
Hanley NR, Van de Kar LD. Serotonin and the neuroendocrine regulation of the hypothalamic—pituitary-adrenal axis in health and disease. Vitam Horm. 2003;66:189–255. Epub 2003/07/11.
Harrold JA, Halford JC. The hypothalamus and obesity. Recent Pat CNS Drug Discov. 2006;1(3):305–14. Epub 2008/01/29.
Keller PA, Compan V, Bockaert J, Giacobino JP, Charnay Y, Bouras C, et al. Characterization and localization of cocaine- and amphetamine-regulated transcript (CART) binding sites. Peptides. 2006;27(6):1328–34. Epub 2005/11/29.
King PJ. The hypothalamus and obesity. Curr Drug Targets. 2005;6(2):225–40. Epub 2005/03/22.
Kristensen P, Judge ME, Thim L, Ribel U, Christjansen KN, Wulff BS, et al. Hypothalamic CART is a new anorectic peptide regulated by leptin. Nature. 1998;393(6680):72–6. Epub 1998/05/20.
Kumar D, Mains RE, Eipper BA. 60 YEARS OF POMC: from POMC and alpha-MSH to PAM, molecular oxygen, copper, and vitamin C. J Mol Endocrinol. 2016;56(4):T63–76. Epub 2015/12/17.
Kym PR, Iyengar R, Souers AJ, Lynch JK, Judd AS, Gao J, et al. Discovery and characterization of aminopiperidinecoumarin melanin concentrating hormone receptor 1 antagonists. J Med Chem. 2005;48(19):5888–91. Epub 2005/09/16.
Lau J, Farzi A, Qi Y, Heilbronn R, Mietzsch M, Shi YC, et al. CART neurons in the arcuate nucleus and lateral hypothalamic area exert differential controls on energy homeostasis. Molecul Metab. 2018;7:102–18. Epub 2017/11/18.
Liao GY, An JJ, Gharami K, Waterhouse EG, Vanevski F, Jones KR, et al. Dendritically targeted Bdnf mRNA is essential for energy balance and response to leptin. Nat Med. 2012;18(4):564–71. Epub 2012/03/20.
Lin S, Boey D, Herzog H. NPY and Y receptors: lessons from transgenic and knockout models. Neuropeptides. 2004;38(4):189–200. Epub 2004/09/01.
Loh K, Herzog H, Shi YC. Regulation of energy homeostasis by the NPY system. Trends Endocrinol Metab. 2015;26(3):125–35. Epub 2015/02/11.
Meister B. Control of food intake via leptin receptors in the hypothalamus. Vitam Horm. 2000;59:265–304. Epub 2000/03/14.
Morton GJ, Schwartz MW. The NPY/AgRP neuron and energy homeostasis. Int J Obes Relat Metab Disord. 2001;25(Suppl 5):S56–62. Epub 2002/02/13.
Presse F, Conductier G, Rovere C, Nahon JL. The melanin-concentrating hormone receptors: neuronal and non-neuronal functions. Int J Obesity Suppl. 2014;4(Suppl 1):S31–6. Epub 2014/07/01.
Pritchard LE, Turnbull AV, White A. Pro-opiomelanocortin processing in the hypothalamus: impact on melanocortin signalling and obesity. J Endocrinol. 2002;172(3):411–21. Epub 2002/03/05.
Pritchard LE, White A. Neuropeptide processing and its impact on melanocortin pathways. Endocrinology. 2007;148(9):4201–7. Epub 2007/06/23.
Schaffler A, Neumeier M, Herfarth H, Furst A, Scholmerich J, Buchler C. Genomic structure of human omentin, a new adipocytokine expressed in omental adipose tissue. Biochim Biophys Acta. 2005;1732(1–3):96–102. Epub 2006/01/03.
Schousboe A. Metabolic signaling in the brain and the role of astrocytes in control of glutamate and GABA neurotransmission. Neurosci Lett. 2018.; Epub 2018/01/30.

Shen WJ, Yao T, Kong X, Williams KW, Liu T. Melanocortin neurons: multiple routes to regulation of metabolism. Biochim Biophys Acta. 2017;1863(10 Pt A):2477–85. Epub 2017/05/14.

Singru PS, Wittmann G, Farkas E, Zseli G, Fekete C, Lechan RM. Refeeding-activated glutamatergic neurons in the hypothalamic paraventricular nucleus (PVN) mediate effects of melanocortin signaling in the nucleus tractus solitarius (NTS). Endocrinology. 2012;153(8):3804–14. Epub 2012/06/16.

Sperling M, Grzelak T, Pelczynska M, Jasinska P, Bogdanski P, Pupek-Musialik D, et al. Concentrations of omentin and vaspin versus insulin resistance in obese individuals. Biomed Pharmacother. 2016;83:542–7. Epub 2016/07/28.

Tao YX. Melanocortin receptors. Biochim Biophys Acta. 2017;1863(10 Pt A):2411–3. Epub 2017/08/13.

Timper K, Bruning JC. Hypothalamic circuits regulating appetite and energy homeostasis: pathways to obesity. Dis Model Mech. 2017;10(6):679–89. Epub 2017/06/09.

Trayhurn P. The biology of obesity. Proc Nutr Soc. 2005;64(1):31–8. Epub 2005/05/10.

Turtzo LC, Lane MD. NPY and neuron-adipocyte interactions in the regulation of metabolism. EXS. 2006;95:133–41. Epub 2005/12/31.

Valassi E, Scacchi M, Cavagnini F. Neuroendocrine control of food intake. Nutr Metab Cardiovasc Dis. 2008;18(2):158–68. Epub 2007/12/07.

Vanevski F, Xu B. Molecular and neural bases underlying roles of BDNF in the control of body weight. Front Neurosci. 2013;7:37. Epub 2013/03/23.

Volkoff H. The role of neuropeptide Y, orexins, cocaine and amphetamine-related transcript, cholecystokinin, amylin and leptin in the regulation of feeding in fish. Comp Biochem Physiol A Mol Integr Physiol. 2006;144(3):325–31. Epub 2005/12/06.

Yu Y, Deng C, Huang XF. Obese reversal by a chronic energy restricted diet leaves an increased Arc NPY/AgRP, but no alteration in POMC/CART, mRNA expression in diet-induced obese mice. Behav Brain Res. 2009;205(1):50–6. Epub 2009/07/21.

Yulyaningsih E, Zhang L, Herzog H, Sainsbury A. NPY receptors as potential targets for anti-obesity drug development. Br J Pharmacol. 2011;163(6):1170–202. Epub 2011/05/07.

Zhou JY, Chan L, Zhou SW. Omentin: linking metabolic syndrome and cardiovascular disease. Curr Vasc Pharmacol. 2014;12(1):136–43. Epub 2012/06/26.

Chapter 5
Role of the Gut in the Regulation of Energy Balance and Energy Stores

Jila Kaberi-Otarod and Yi-Hao Yu

Pearls of Wisdom

- The gut plays an important role in the regulation of food intake and energy absorption, and therefore the body's energy reserves and the size of the fat mass. The gut produces orexigenic and anorexigenic hormones which communicate with the central nervous system directly via endocrine pathways or indirectly via vagal afferent neurons. Some of the gut hormones influence the long-term energy status by participating in the brain's metabolic and hedonic neuroendocrine networks.
- "Taste buds" are not only located on the tongue but also throughout the gut as enteroendocrine cells. These chemosensors "taste" the lumen content of the gut and play an important role in the secretion and regulation of gut hormones and in energy homeostasis.
- The vagus nerve, as a part of the autonomic nervous system of the gut, mediates physiological responses to stimuli originating from sensation of nutrients by enteroendocrine cells in the gut. Afferent neurons of the vagus nerve express receptors of orexigenic and anorexigenic gut hormones, and the expression of these receptors reflects nutrient status. The interrelationship between gut motility and gut hormones, mediated by vagal neurons, significantly affects energy homeostasis.

J. Kaberi-Otarod (✉)
Geisinger System – North East, Department of Nutrition and Weight Management, Scranton, PA, USA
e-mail: jkaberiotarod@geisinger.edu

Y.-H. Yu
Weight Loss and Diabetes Center, Department of Endocrinology, Stamford, CT, USA

Greenwich Hospital and Endocrinology Associates of Greenwich, Northeast Medical Group, Yale-New Haven Health, Greenwich, CT, USA

J. M. Gonzalez-Campoy et al. (eds.), *Bariatric Endocrinology*,
https://doi.org/10.1007/978-3-319-95655-8_5

- Bile acids, in addition to acting as emulsifiers that facilitate lipid absorption, are signaling molecules that help regulate glucose and lipid metabolism. They play an important role in energy homeostasis by affecting gut hormone release.
- Food composition strongly influences the diversity of gut microbiota. The interplay between ingested food, gut microbiota, and bile acid composition ultimately affects gut hormones and energy homeostasis.

5.1 Introduction

As the largest endocrine organ, the gut secretes more than 20 hormones. These hormones, directly, or indirectly through the vagus nerve, signal the brain to regulate appetite and food intake (Fig. 5.1). Traditionally regarded as hormones involved in meal initiation/termination, meal size, and meal frequency via their actions on the brainstem, many of these hormones may have a role in long-term energy homeostasis (EH), as increasing evidence has shown that they act on the hypothalamus and the mesolimbic system. The orexigenic and anorexigenic hormones involved in the gut-brain communication and EH are listed in Table 5.1. The gut-brain axis is a

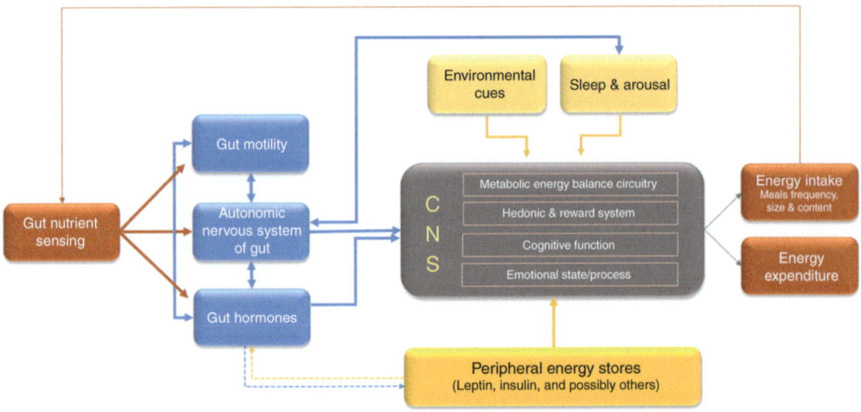

Fig. 5.1 Gut-brain-adiposity crosstalk. The gut participates in body weight regulation by virtue of its primary function on food intake. Food intake is a complex process. It is coordinated through various feedback signaling mechanisms, involving the gut chemosensors and mechanosensors/"taste" receptors, gut hormones, and the autonomic nervous system of the gut. These functions of the gut crosstalk with the central nervous system (CNS), which directs energy intake and energy expenditure, involving both conscious and subconscious processes in the CNS. Gut hormones levels oscillate between fasting and fed states and are involved in meal initiation and termination. They regulate short-term energy balance, and some of the gut hormones can also influence the long-term energy balance and body weight via their actions through the "energy balance circuitry" and the "hedonic and reward system" in the CNS. These actions are potentiated/diminished by the signals coming from the adipose tissue and other peripheral tissues that function to inform the size of body's energy stores (e.g., leptin and insulin)

Table 5.1 The gut hormones

Hormones	Cell(s) of origin	Stimuli for release	Receptor	Function on energy balance and GI motility	Effects via		Hormone levels	
					Vagus	Endocrine	Obesity	Post-GBS
Ghrelin	X/A-cells, stomach	Fasting	GHS-R1a	↑food intake ↑increase gastric motility ↑GH	Y	Y	↓↑ Different type of obesity? UAG/AG ratio?	↑↓↔ Different assays?
CCK (cholecystokinin)	I-cells, Dduodenum and Jejunum	FA > AA	CCK-R1 (predominantly) and CCK-R2	Anorexigenic ↑GB emptying Slows gastric emptying ↑SB transit	Y		Unknown	↔
Secretin	S-cells/ duodenum	Low pH–AA	Sct-R	Anorexigenic ↓LES contractility ↓gastric emptying and acid	Y	Y		
Insulin	**β**-cells, pancreas	Hyperglycemia	IR	Anorexigenic ↓ food intake		Y	↑	↓
Glucagon (proglucagon cleavage product)	**α**-cells, pancreas	Hypoglycemia	GCGR	↓food intake and meal size ↑energy expenditure		Y		↑↔
GLP-1 (glucagon-like peptide) Proglucagon cleavage product	L-cells, small and large bowel	CHO >FA, AA	GLP-1R	Anorexigenic Ileal brake ↓gastric emptying Slows small bowel transit (probably) ↑colonic transit	Y	Y	↓	↑↑
GIP (glucose-dependent insulinotropic peptide)	K-cells, small bowel	CHO, FA, AA	GIP receptor	↓gastric emptying and acid secretion ↓ghrelin secretion		Y		↓↔

(continued)

Table 5.1 (continued)

Hormones	Cell(s) of origin	Stimuli for release	Receptor	Function on energy balance and GI motility	Effects via		Hormone levels	
					Vagus	Endocrine	Obesity	Post-GBS
Amylin (procalcitonin peptide family)	**β**-cells, pancreas	?Unknown	CTR RAMPs	Anorexigenic Delay gastric emptying ↓motility Enhances the effect of CCK, PYY, insulin, GLP-1, and leptin on eating	Y		↓	
Oxyntomodulin (proglucagon cleavage product)	L-cells, small-large intestine	FA	GLP-1R and GCGR Dual agonist?	Anorexigenic ↑energy expenditure ↓gastric acid secretion and emptying		Y		↑
Obestatin Preproghrelin family	P/D1-like cells, stomach-duodenum	?Unknown	GLP-1R? Other receptors? Does not bind to GHS-R1a	Anorexigenic Delay gastric emptying		Y	↑Ghrelin/Obestatin ratio ↓Obestatin?	
PYY (peptide tyrosine-tyrosine) PYY_{3-36}	L-cells, small and large bowel	AA>CHO	Y2R (neuropeptide Y 2 receptor)	Anorexigenic ↓gastric emptying Ileal brake ↓small bowel transit ↓colonic transit (in mice)	Y	Y	↓	↑↑
Pancreatic polypeptide (PP-fold family)	PP cells, pancreas	Meal intake	Y4R (neuropeptide Y 4 receptor)	Anorexigenic Delay gastric emptying ↓motility, ↑Energy expenditure (animal studies)	Y		Blunted postprandial response	

↑-Increased ↑↑-Significantly increased ↓-Decreased ↔-No change

AG: acylated ghrelin, *UAG* unacylated ghrelin, *GB* gallbladder, *GH* growth hormone, *SB* small bowel, *LES* lower esophageal sphincter, *CHO* carbohydrates, *FA* fatty acids, *AA* amino acids, *GCGR* G-protein-coupled glucagon receptor, *CTR* calcitonin receptor core, *RAMPs* receptor activity-modifying proteins, *GBS* gastric bypass surgery

complex signaling network that begins with the arrival of food in the gut. Nutrients are sensed by mechanosensors and chemosensors, which release gut hormones that act in a paracrine and endocrine fashion to regulate EH. There is evidence that bile acids (BA) are also signaling molecules that affect gut hormones and gut microbiota (GM). Recent studies show that GM is an important regulator of EH through its influences on several relevant organ systems.

This chapter is an overview of the role of the gut in this complex and integrated signaling network that regulates energy metabolism (Fig. 5.1).

5.2 Orexigenic Gut Hormones

Ghrelin Cleaved from preproghrelin, ghrelin is a 28-amino acid (AA) peptide. It is synthesized predominantly in X/A-like cells in the stomach. In circulation, ghrelin is present in acylated (AG) and unacylated (UAG) forms. Post-translational acylation is required for ghrelin to bind to its receptor, GHS-R1a, which is found in the pancreas, liver, intestine, heart, reproductive system, pituitary gland, and spinal cord. The acylation is catalyzed by ghrelin-O-acyltransferase (GOAT), which regulates ghrelin bioactivity and affects the relative abundance of the two isoforms. Contrary to previous belief, evidence suggests that UAG is also biologically active and that both isoforms have independent effects and may compete at the receptor level. It is possible that the ratio of the isoforms is more important than the total ghrelin levels. Ghrelin levels are increased by fasting and fall rapidly in response to feeding or oral glucose administration. The pulsatile secretion of ghrelin suggests that it may signal feeding initiation. There is evidence to support the role of ghrelin in long-term regulation of energy homeostasis in addition to its short-term control of food intake. In humans, ghrelin levels correlate inversely with the degree of adiposity. Ghrelin levels are chronically elevated in individuals with weight loss (i.e., exercise-induced weight loss, weight loss due to decreased calorie intake), which likely contribute to the increased appetite to promote food intake in these individuals. Ghrelin levels fall with overfeeding. Subjects with obesity have a less noticeable fall in ghrelin after meal ingestion. In patients with Prader-Willi syndrome, plasma ghrelin levels are higher than in normal subjects and do not decrease after a meal. This may partially explain the insatiable appetite and hyperphagia in these patients. Ghrelin and leptin may be essential for survival during starvation. Ghrelin can counter energy deficiency by stimulating growth hormone release, which results in protection against hypoglycemia, and further by reducing spontaneous physical activity and therefore decreasing energy expenditure. Increased ghrelin in prolonged starvation increases appetite and food-seeking behavior and, in close relationship with leptin and insulin, contributes to transitioning from carbohydrate to fatty acid oxidation. In physiological conditions with limited food availability, ghrelin acts as a regulator of energy balance by increasing food intake, storing energy, and reducing energy expenditure. In contrast, impaired ghrelin secretion due to ingestion of specific nutrients and genetic or environmental factors can promote the excessive accumulation of fat and the development of insulin resistance and metabolic derangements. It was hypothesized that satiety after restrictive bariatric surgery may be caused by removing ghrelin-producing cells from the stomach. However, data so far reveal that ghrelin's role in weight loss after the surgery is marginal.

5.3 Anorexigenic Gut Hormones

5.3.1 Cholecystokinin

Derived from a 115-AA precursor, cholecystokinin (CCK) is produced in the I-cells of the proximal intestine. A number of post-translational molecular forms of CCK are recognized, and CCK-58 is the most common form. CCK receptors are expressed in the pancreas, gallbladder, stomach, and afferent vagal nerve, and they are widely distributed in the brain. CCK has two receptors: CCK-1R and CCK-2R. Aside from its known effect on stimulation of gallbladder contraction, pancreatic exocrine secretion, and inhibition of gastric emptying, CCK also regulates appetite and reduces meal size. CCK-1R is the predominant receptor involved in food intake and satiety and mediates the action of CCK in stimulation of vagus afferent neurons (VAN) (Fig. 5.2). Peripheral administration of CCK stimulates cocaine- and amphetamine-related transcript (CART)-expressing neurons in the paraventricular nucleus (PVN) of the hypothalamus via vagal innervations. The VAN-expressing CCK-1R demonstrates neurochemical plasticity according to nutrient status. In animal studies, lack of food intake induces the expression of nodose ganglion neurons of orexigenic signaling, while reducing expression of CART and neuropeptide Y receptor 2 (Y2R) and inhibiting anorexigenic signaling. These effects can be reversed by CCK-1R activation. There is an interaction between CCK and leptin in regulating the expression of CART by VAN, and it appears that leptin determines the magnitude of CCK-mediated stimulation of CART expression (Fig. 5.2). Hence, the neurochemical phenotype of VAN is dependent on the integration of signals from adipose tissue and recent nutrient status. Obesity diminishes the satiety effect of CCK by decreasing the activation of nucleus tractus solitarius (NTS) and splanchnic sympathetic nerve discharge. Leptin resistance in VAN and a diminished CCK-1R responsiveness with a high-fat diet (HFD) also result in increased ghrelin-mediated suppression of CART expression, which leads to the stimulation of food intake.

5.3.2 Secretin

Secretin (Sct), a 27-AA peptide hormone, belongs to the vasoactive intestinal peptide/Sct/glucagon/ GHRH family and is produced from duodenal S cells. Sct is long known to provide an optimal milieu for food digestion by regulating gastric secretion and by emptying and stimulating the release of bicarbonate-rich fluid from the pancreas and bile from the liver. Sct is also proposed to act as an incretin in a

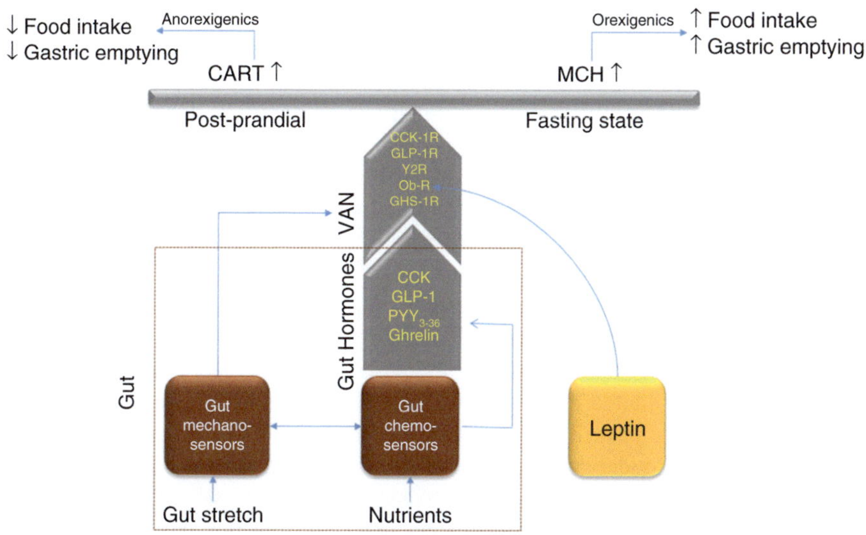

Fig. 5.2 Illustration of CCK signaling via vagal afferent neurons (VAN) in regulating food intake and gastric emptying. Postprandial release of cholecystokinin (CCK) activates neuropeptide cocaine- and amphetamine-related transcript (CART) in VAN via CCK action on its receptor in VAN. This in turn attenuates food intake and decreased gastric emptying, fulfilling a negative feedback loop. In the fasting state, CCK level is suppressed and ghrelin level is increased, resulting in the suppression of anorexigenic peptides and activation of orexigenic neuropeptides such as melanin concentrating hormone (MCH) in VAN, which in turn stimulates appetite and promotes gastric emptying. The effect of CCK on VAN is potentiated by leptin. Other gut hormones may stimulate/suppress food intake and gastric emptying via their respective receptors in VAN in a similar fashion; some of these gut hormones and their receptors are also included in this illustration. While gut chemosensors mediate the release of gut hormones, gut mechanosensors also have independent actions on VAN. CCK-1R Cholecystokinin-1 receptor, GHS-1R Ghrelin receptor, GLP-1 Glucagon-like peptide-1, GLP-1R Glucagon-like peptide-1 receptor, Ob-R Leptin receptor, PYY Polypeptide YY, Y2R PYY receptor

prolonged glycemic stimulation. Sct has a lipolytic action during starvation via a hormone-sensitive lipase-mediated mechanism. The Sct level increases postprandially. The peripheral and central administration of Sct has recently been shown to reduce food intake. Sct receptor (SctR) proteins are detected in arcuate nucleus (ARC), PVN, and VAN connecting to NTS. The anorexigenic effect of Sct demonstrated in mice may occur through the activation of pro-opiomelanocortin (POMC). Sct crosses the blood-brain barrier (BBB) to directly activate the neurons in the CNS and also exert its effect through the vagal nerve.

5.3.3 Insulin

Insulin, a 51-AA peptide hormone, is secreted from the **β**-cells of the pancreas and is best known for its peripheral action of reducing circulating glucose levels. Insulin increases glucose uptake, glycogen synthesis, inhibits gluconeogenesis, and glycogenolysis in the liver, stimulates lipid uptakes into adipocytes, and inhibits release of free fatty acids from adipocytes. Insulin can increase cellular uptake of amino acids into the skeletal muscle. There is a basal, constitutive secretion of insulin and an increased secretion that is stimulated by feeding. Both basal and stimulated insulin secretion are in direct proportion to adiposity. Hence, insulin is a hormonal marker of peripheral adiposity. Insulin receptors (IRs) are widely expressed in different areas of the CNS, including the ARC, cerebral cortex, cerebellum, hippocampus, and the lower brain stem. Insulin passes the BBB and exerts its function by interacting with IRs. In the CNS, insulin and leptin act as satiety hormones. Infusion of insulin into the brain in animals affects EH by inhibiting neuropeptide Y (NPY)/Agouti-related protein (AgRP) and stimulating POMC, resulting in decreased food intake and increased energy expenditure. The central action of insulin is affected by obesity induced by a high caloric intake. Overnutrition and HFD cause insulin resistance in the brain attributable to increased proinflammatory cytokines, oxidative stress, and local inflammation in the hypothalamus, which impairs the anorexigenic effects of insulin. In leptin-sensitive individuals, leptin inhibits insulin synthesis from the pancreas, while insulin increases the secretion of leptin from adipose tissue. In the CNS, the effect of insulin is dependent on an intact leptin signaling system. Hence, leptin resistance results in insulin resistance in the CNS.

5.3.4 *Glucagon*

Glucagon, a 29-AA peptide, is the second principal pancreatic hormone and is the product of post-translational processing of proglucagon. This cleavage and production of glucagon is tissue specific (Fig. 5.3). Glucagon has catabolic effects on fuel metabolism, stimulates hepatic gluconeogenesis and gylcogenolysis, and inhibits glycogenesis, resulting in increased hepatic glucose release. Additionally, glucagon can delay gastric emptying causing satiety, inhibit food intake, cause lipolysis and fatty acid oxidation, and increase thermogenesis and energy expenditure. It exerts its

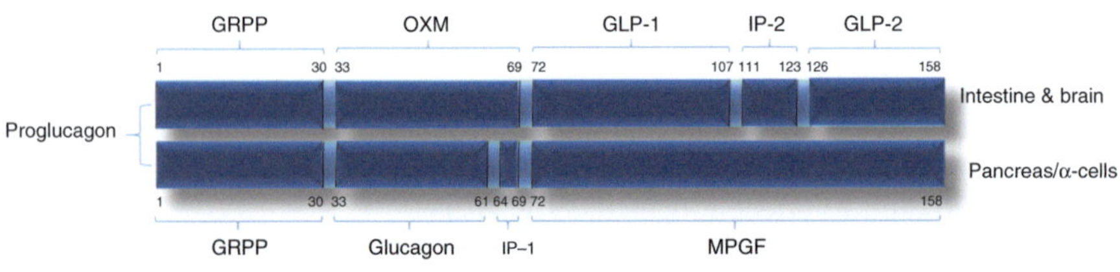

Fig. 5.3 The preproglucagon family: The processing of proglucagon is tissue specific. Proglucagon in pancreatic **α**-cells is mainly cleaved by prohormone convertase-2 to produce glucagon and the other peptides as shown. In the intestine and brain, this propeptide is predominantly cleaved by prohormone convertase-1/3 to produce GLP-1, GLP-2, glicentin-related polypeptide (GRPP), and oxyntomodulin. GRPP, Intervening peptide-1 (IP-1), and intervening peptide-2 (IP-2) and major proglucagon fragment are biologically inactive

effect by binding to G-protein-coupled glucagon receptor (GCGR) expressed in the liver and thebrain, which suggests that glucagon passes the BBB and could exert part of its biological effects through a central pathway. A study of rodent models has shown an increase in energy expenditure through thc activation of brown adipose tissue (BAT). Compared to the wild-type mice, *Gcgr*$^{-/-}$ mice have markedly decreased fat mass, which is compensated by increased lean mass. When exposed to HFD, they demonstrated a decreased fat intake, 30% less weight gain, and protection from hepatic steatosis. The effect of central glucagon action is anorexigenic, similar to that of insulin, in contrast to their opposite peripheral effects, but the mechanism mediating its central effect(s) is mainly unknown. However, there is a possibility that central glucagon activates corticotropin-releasing factor and the hypothalamus-pituitary-adrenal axis to suppress food intake, as was shown in chicks.

5.3.5 Incretin Hormones

The incretins are gut hormones released from enteroendocrine cells (EEC) that augment nutrient-induced insulin secretion from pancreatic **β**-cells in response to meal intake. The incretin effect on insulin secretion is glucose dependent, which is important in preventing the oversecretion of insulin in the absence of hyperglycemia.

5.3.5.1 Glucagon-Like Peptide-1

Glucagon-like peptide-1 (GLP-1) is a 31-AA polypeptide derived from the proglucagon gene (Fig. 5.3). It is cosecreted with peptide tyrosine-tyrosine (PYY) from L-cells, predominantly in the ileum and colon. In response to food intake, GLP-1 level rises in 10–15 min after food ingestion. This is followed by a longer second phase that peaks at 30–60 min. The early phase is likely mediated by the autonomic nervous system, and the second phase is mediated by the direct contact of EEC with nutrients. GLP-1 exerts its function by binding to GLP-1 receptor (GLP-1R) expressed in the pancreas, lung, brain, pituitary, stomach, heart, kidney, liver, and vagal neurons. This widespread placement is consistent with its pleiotropic effects, such as appetite regulation, inhibition of gastric acid production and gastric emptying, regulation of hepatic glucose production, and regulation of cardiac function and bone resorption. GLP-1 regulates food intake and energy hemostasis. Endogenous GLP-1 delays gastric emptying and intestinal motility, promotes a feeling of fullness, and contributes to the ileal brake, an inhibitory feedback mechanism to optimize nutrient digestion and absorption. The effects of GLP-1 on energy hemostasis are likely accomplished by both peripheral and central actions of GLP-1 through mechanisms which are complex and not completely understood. However, neuronal and humeral responses to peripheral GLP-1 must activate areas in the brain that are known to regulate food intake. Both peripheral and central injections of GLP-1 induce *c-fos* in the PVN, but only central injection of GLP-1 induces *c-fos* in the ARC, suggesting different mechanisms for effects of central versus peripheral GLP-1. There is evidence that GLP-1 also interacts with leptin, ghrelin, and glucagon to influence energy homeostasis. Overall, GLP-1 promotes a negative energy balance by decreasing food intake and increasing energy expenditure, probably in part by stimulating thermogenesis in the brown adipose tissue. Circulating levels of GLP-1 and responses to food intake are diminished in subjects with obesity. Diet-induced and surgical weight loss are associated with increases in GLP-1 levels. The mechanism of the increase in GLP-1 levels associated with gastric bypass surgery (GBS) is not entirely understood. This exaggerated response could be the result of decreased degradation of GLP-1 due to a decrease in dipeptidyl peptidase-4 (DPP-4) activity, resolution of insulin resistance, changes in BA and GM, or redirecting the nutrients to the distal intestine where the L-cells are densely located.

5.3.5.2 Glucose-Dependent Insulinotropic Peptide

Glucose-dependent insulinotropic peptide (GIP) is released from K-cells in the upper intestine in response to food intake. The release of GIP is in proportion to the caloric load. GIP stimulates food intake-mediated insulin secretion, resulting in lipid storage in adipocytes. GIP-knockout mice are resistant to diet-induced obesity, suggesting a possible role of GIP in energy metabolism. Nevertheless, GIP has no known direct effects on satiety or hunger in humans.

5.3.6 *Amylin*

Amylin is a 37-AA peptide related to the calcitonin peptide family. Amylin is mainly synthesized by the pancreatic β-cells. In response to nutrients, amylin is cosecreted with insulin. Amylin reduces gastric acid secretion, gastric emptying, and pancreatic glucagon secretion. Its actions seem to be complementary to the function of insulin. Amylin decreases food intake by reducing meal sizes. Amylin receptors are expressed in the area postrema (AP) where amylin demonstrates strong binding affinity. Amylin and glucose coactivate AP neurons and reduce the fasting-induced *c-fos* expression in these neurons. Studies have shown that the injection of the amylin receptor antagonist AC187 in the AP or the use of electrolytic lesions of the AP results in a reduction of the effect of peripheral amylin. Also, the local injection of amylin into the AP inhibits eating and reduces meal sizes. These results suggest that AP neurons play an essential role in generating the anorexigenic action of amylin. Amylin receptors are composed of a calcitonin receptor core (CTR) and one of the receptor activity-modifying proteins (RAMPs). Amylin interacts with other hormones, such as CCK, PYY, GLP-1, and leptin. Like CCK, amylin produces an acute satiating effect, but unlike CCK, the effect of amylin with continuous infusion is not reduced and there is no compensatory increase in meal frequency. Furthermore, CCK affects AP via a paracrine mechanism by activating adjacent vagal afferent nerves projecting to the NTS, whereas amylin acts through a humoral pathway. Amylin enhances the anorexigenic effect of PYY_{3-36} and continuous administration of both results in a synergistic effect. The increase in insulin secretion induced by GLP-1 also increases the release of amylin significantly, which may contribute to some degree to the anorexigenic effect of GLP-1. Peripheral or central infusion of amylin reduces the fat mass. Central, but not peripheral, actions of amylin increase energy expenditure or at least prevent weight loss-induced decreases in energy expenditure. Amylin and leptin seem to act synergistically; effects of leptin are reduced in amylin-deficient mice. Amylin also affects the central processing of leptin signaling and sensitivity. In animal studies, combined amylin/leptin treatment caused reduced eating and adiposity and prevented the decrease in energy expenditure in weight-reduced animals. Evidence suggests that this interaction occurs in the hypothalamus since acute injection of amylin upregulates hypothalamic leptin receptor expression. As such, combining amylin and leptin could be a potentially effective treatment of obesity. Clinical trials have been conducted but terminated before completion because of the development of antileptin neutralizing antibodies.

5.3.7 Oxyntomodulin

Oxyntomodulin (OXM) is a 37-AA peptide and a product of proglucagon gene (Fig. 5.3) secreted from L-cells in proportion to food ingestion. OXM is a dual agonist of the GLP-1R and GCGR. Increased postprandial levels of OXM diminish gastric acid secretion and delay stomach emptying. OXM also stimulates glucose-dependent insulin secretion from **β**-cells. Peripheral administration of OXM results in increased *c-fos* in the ARC and may act on the POMC neurons to inhibit feeding. OXM decreases food intake and increases energy expenditure and results in weight loss in individuals with obesity. The central anorexigenic effect of OXM seems to be mediated in part by the GLP-1R. Additionally, OXM may exert its appetite suppressing effect in part by reducing circulating levels of ghrelin. Other effects of OXM, such as promoting energy expenditure and stimulation of heart rate, appear to be independent of GLP-1R. Since there is no known OXM receptor, it is hypothesized that the GLP-1R-independent effects of OXM, such as the activation of thermogenesis in the BAT, could be mediated via GCGR. However, the possibility of the existence of an OXM receptor has not been absolutely dismissed, since OXM still produced a small weight loss effect in the presence of a GCGR antagonist in GLP-1$R^{-/-}$ mice.

5.3.8 Obestanin

A member of the preproghrelin gene-derived peptide family, obestatin is a 23-AA amidated peptide with the ability to inhibit food intake in mice when injected peripherally. Obestatin levels are lower in obesity, and this observation in children suggests its association with childhood obesity. Like ghrelin, obestatin is predominantly produced in the stomach. However, its expression is also demonstrated in the pancreas, adipose tissue, skeletal muscle, and liver. In contrast to ghrelin, obestatin has positive effects on insulin sensitivity and β-cell function and works against the effects of ghrelin on food intake and GH stimulation. Moreover, animal studies have shown a ghrelin-independent effect of obestatin on delaying gastric emptying and blunting weight gain. Identification of obestatin receptor has been challenging and its central effects are undefined, but it seems clear that obestatin's effects are not via GHS-R1a. Demonstration of obestatin affecting different signaling pathways and the presence of different binding sites for obestatin in different cells, in addition to recent findings that obestatin binds to GLP-1R in pancreatic β-cells and adipocytes, suggest that obestatin is a multifunctional hormone affecting a variety of cells and tissues, not merely a ghrelin antagonist as it was initially assumed.

5.3.9 Peptide Tyrosine-Tyrosine

Peptide tyrosine-tyrosine (PYY) is secreted from L-cells and belongs to the pancreatic polypeptide (PP) family, along with pancreatic peptide (PP) and NPY. These peptides are 36 AA in length and mediate their effects through the NPY receptors. There are several subtypes of these receptors (Y1, Y2, Y4, and Y5). There are two main endogenous forms of human PYY: PYY_{1-36} and PYY_{3-36}. PYY_{1-36} binds to and activates all NPY receptor subtypes, whereas PYY_{3-36} has high affinity for Y2 receptor (Y2R). PYY_{3-36} is produced by cleavage of the tyrosine-proline amino terminal residues of PYY_{1-36} by the enzyme DPP-4.

In response to food ingestion, PYY_{3-36} levels rise in plasma. The peak level is proportional to the ingested calories. PYY levels are low and progressively fall during the fasting state. These responses are blunted in individuals with obesity with an intact anorexigenic effect of PYY_{3-36}, suggesting that PYY deficiency may contribute to the pathogenesis of obesity. PYY levels increase with weight loss and decline with weight gain, and the higher baseline levels correlate with greater weight loss in subjects with obesity who assume a weight-reducing lifestyle modification program. Hence, PYY levels may predict long-term changes in body weight. In a study of patients with obesity in a 10-week weight loss program on a very low-calorie food intake, there was a reduction of postprandial and fasting plasma levels of PYY, which persisted after 1 year and did not return to preintervention levels. These changes are believed to encourage weight regain, suggesting the higher body weight is being defended through the blunting of PYY response. Thus, obesity may involve a higher intervention point and a maladaptive response of energy-regulating hormones, including PYY, to weight loss. PYY responses after GBS are in contrast with those with severe obesity who lost weight as a result of low calorie intake, consistent with the long(er) lasting weight loss effect of the surgery. Study of transgenic mice overexpressing PYY showed a reduced food intake and protection against obesity. Conversely, the knockout mice were prone to obesity and insulin resistance. PYY_{3-36} or Y2R agonists attenuated body weight gain in obesity-prone rodents, and the gene deletion of the Y2R in mice resulted in increased food intake and body weight. Collectively, these findings make the PYY_{3-36} and Y2R promising targets for treatment of obesity.

5.3.10 Pancreatic Polypeptide

Pancreatic polypeptide (PP) is an amidated 36-AA peptide, released from PP cells in the pancreas islets of Langerhans and EEC in the gut. It is a part of the PP family and is formed through duplication of the PYY gene. It acts at the Y4 receptor (Y4R), which is expressed in the AP, NTS, dorsal motor nucleus of vagus, ARC, and PVN. PP is released in response to meal ingestion, and its level is proportional to caloric intake. The levels remain elevated up to 6 h postprandially. This response to meal is blunted in subjects with obesity, while it is exaggerated in patients with anorexia nervosa. Studies on the effect of PP in leptin-deficient *ob/ob* mice have demonstrated decreased weight gain and improved insulin resistance and hyperlipidemia. Overexpression of PP in transgenic mice, as well as infusion of PP in humans, has resulted in decreased food intake. The anorexigenic effect of PP is suggested to be mediated through Y4R in the brain stem and the hypothalamus. PP administration in mice resulted in increased oxygen consumption and increased sympathetic release innervating the BAT and the adrenal gland. This suggests that PP plays a role in increased energy expenditure.

5.4 Nutrient Sensing and Signaling

5.4.1 Gut Hormones, Mechanosensory, and Chemosensory Mechanism

The enteroendocrine system is the primary sensor of nutrient and is responsible for secretion of different hormones that act as mediators for gut motility and secretion, glucose homeostasis, appetite, and food intake. There is a complex neuroendocrine relationship between gut motility and hormone secretion.

The mechanosensitive and chemosensitive actions of the VAN have been long demonstrated. The mechanosensory stimuli are generated by food entering the gut lumen, the transit of the bolus, and stretching of gut mucosa. Two types of mechanoreceptors are mucosal and tension receptors. The transit of gut contents impacts the degree of hormonal secretion due to nutrient sensing. On the other hand, the control of food intake, gastric emptying, and gallbladder emptying require the activation of the vagal nerve by gut peptides released from the mucosal epithelium (Fig. 5.4).

Chemosensing is rather an indirect process and is thought to depend on pre- or postabsorptive mechanisms. The EEC function as chemosensory transducers between

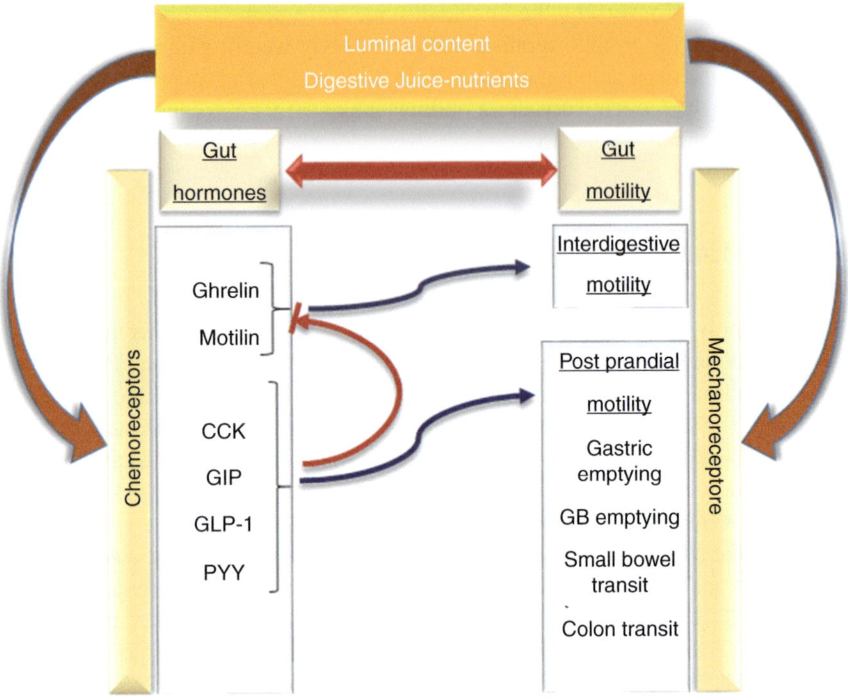

Fig. 5.4 Complex neuroendocrine relationship between gut motility and hormone secretion. Gastric distention limits food intake by creating a feeling of fullness, mediated by vagal afferent nerves (VAN). The gut hormones ghrelin and motilin, released from the stomach, control the interdigestive motility, and gastric emptying, forwarding the food to the lower intestine. Gut hormones released from the lower intestine oppose ghrelin and motilin's effect via paracrine and endocrine effects on mechanoreceptors and chemoreceptors. PYY Peptide tyrosine-tyrosine, GLP-1 Glucagon-like peptide, GIP Glucose-dependent insulinotropic peptide, CCK cholecystokinin

the intestinal lumen content and the afferent nerve terminals. While EEC represent a small number of intestinal epithelial cells, their function is critical to normal digestive physiology and EH. EEC are located throughout the gut, including the taste buds on the tongue, as part of the gustatory system (Fig. 5.5). EEC detect changes in luminal condition, such as pH and osmolality, nutrient, and microflora. They signal their arrival by triggering the release of regulatory peptides (Fig. 5.6) in an endocrine or paracrine fashion. Nutrition in the lumen affects differentiation of EEC and hence the variations in gut hormone profile. For instance, fiber in food enhances the differentiation of L-cells and thus the GLP-1 production. VAN express several gut hormone receptors, such as GLP-1, CCK 1 and 2, GHS-1R, and Y2 receptors. Released hormones in a paracrine fashion attach to their receptors on VAN. VAN fibers converge in the NTS of the brain stem. The neuronal projection from NTS carries signals to the hypothalamus. There is some evidence that the expression of these receptors in VAN can be altered by nutritional status.

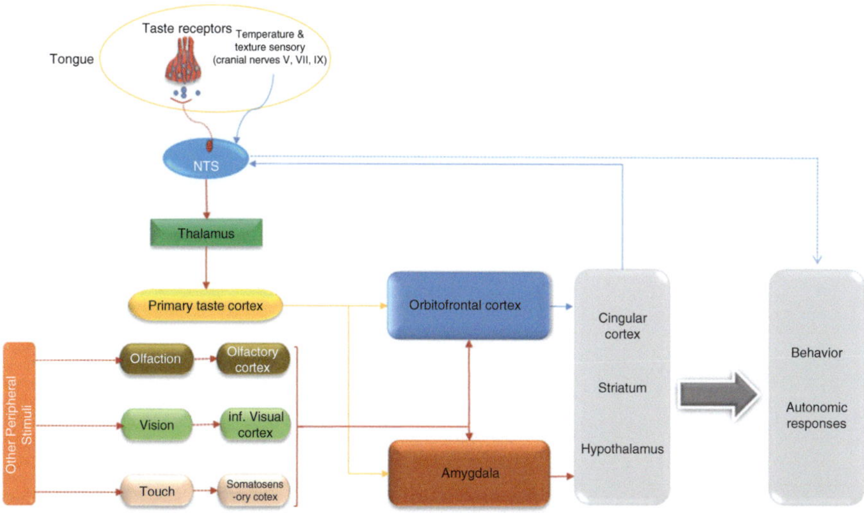

Fig. 5.5 The gustatory-reward pathway. Taste perception has two components: taste sensitivity and hedonic value or preference and palatability. The quality of food, in addition to taste, also depends on other properties such as texture, odor, and temperature of food. Accordingly, there are other sensory inputs in the mouth as well as peripheral cues (somatosensory) and olfactory stimuli, and the final integration of these sensory stimuli with gustatory stimuli occurs in reward cortex and result in ingestive behaviors. The gustatory system originates from the taste receptors in mouth-GPCR (G-protein-coupled receptor) for sweet, salty, bitter, sour, and umami tastes as prototypes—which relay the signals to nucleus tractus solitarius (NTS) and thalamus. Thalamic afferents project to the primary taste cortex. The primary taste cortex projects to the central nucleus of amygdala and orbitofrontal cortex (OFC) and the secondary taste cortex projects from where gustatory information reaches the lateral hypothalamus (modulation of taste by satiety state) and dopaminergic reward system. OFC also receives projections from the primary olfactory cortex, and this integration results in flavor perception. Cortical taste areas send afferent neurons to NTS as well, resulting in modulation of taste in the brain stem

5.4.2 Bile Acid Signaling

It is now apparent that BA have functions beyond their classic role in fat absorption. It is recognized that BA are also signaling molecules (Fig. 5.6) that can activate BA receptors including farnesoid X receptor (FXR) and the G-protein-coupled receptor 5 (TGR5) to initiate signaling pathways and control gene expressions to regulate BA homeostasis and the modulation of lipids, glucose, and EH.

The key receptor TGR5 is highly expressed in liver cells, BAT, muscle cells, small intestine, and colonic L-cells that produce GLP-1. BA signaling through TGR5 is cell-type specific and can result in gallbladder relaxation, anti-inflammatory effects, increased small intestine motility, increased energy expenditure, improved glucose metabolism, and insulin sensitivity. The incretin effect of BA occurs through TGR-5 stimulation of GLP-1 production. In the gut, BA also bind to FXR, which activates fibroblast growth factor 19 (FGF-19) expression (Fig. 5.6), resulting in

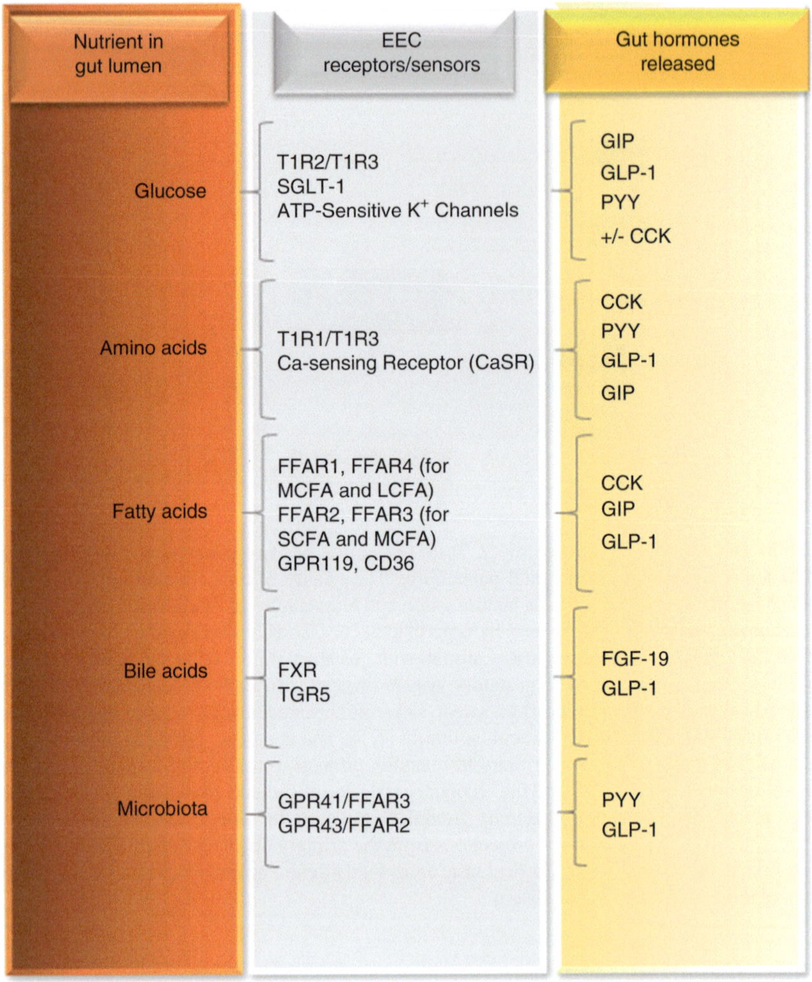

Fig. 5.6 Nutrient sensing via enteroendocrine cells (EEC). Luminal macronutrients such as glucose, amino acids, and fatty acids (left column) are sensed by EEC via their specific receptors/sensors (middle column), leading to the release of specific gut hormones (right column) from the basolateral side of the cells. Luminal glucose potently stimulates the release of glucose-dependent insulinotropic peptide (GIP), glucagon-like peptide-1 (GLP-1), and peptide tyrosine-tyrosine (PYY) and, less consistently, of cholecystokinin (CCK). Glucose is sensed by a number of mechanisms via T1R2/T1R3, the sodium-dependent glucose transporter 1 (SGLT-1), and through the cellular glucose metabolism and closure of ATP-sensitive K+ channels. Dietary protein is a strong stimulant of CCK. It also can stimulate GLP1 and GIP, and probably PYY. Amino acids activate EECs via taste receptors (T1R1/T1R3) and Gq-coupled calcium-sensing receptor (CaSR). Luminal fat stimulates the secretion of CCK, GIP, and GLP-1 via nonesterified fatty acid. Fatty acid receptors, FFA1 and FFA4, are sensitive to medium-chain (MCFA) and long-chain (LCFA) fatty acids. FFA2 and FFA3 receptors respond to medium- and short-chain FA. G-protein-coupled receptor 119 (GPR119) is activated by lipid derivatives and correlates with increased concentrations of GIP and GLP-1. Cluster of differentiation/fatty acid translocase (CD36) may indirectly facilitate the release of FA-induced CCK and secretin. Bile acids and microbiota may directly and indirectly influence EEC and their hormone release as well. For example, microbiota affects EEC hormonal secretion by producing SCFA, which signal via FFA2 and FFA3 receptors and induce the production of GLP-1 and PYY

increased BA production. BA signaling pathways inhibit diet-induced obesity and prevent the development of insulin resistance. The BA-TGR5-dependent effect on weight reduction is due to enhanced energy expenditure and not due to reduced caloric intake.

The effect of BA on GLP-1 and their role on GBS outcomes have been studied. Increased BA signaling after bariatric surgery via TGR-5 receptor enhances GLP-1 production. However, there is a lag of several months between the increase in BA and GLP-1 after the surgery, and although the increased GLP-1 is most likely one mediator, the exact mechanism is not completely understood.

5.5 Gut Microbiota

The human gut is colonized by large numbers of microbiota. The majority of GM are anaerobes and mostly from Firmicutes phylum (64%) and Bacteroidetes phylum (23%). The GM are involved in a number of physiological functions, such as the prevention of colonization of pathogens, immunomodulation, digestion, metabolism and the absorption of nutrients, and synthesis of vitamins. New evidence points to the contribution of microbiota to the regulation of EH (Fig. 5.7), the mechanism of which is not well understood. The fecal transplant from ob/ob mice to germ-free

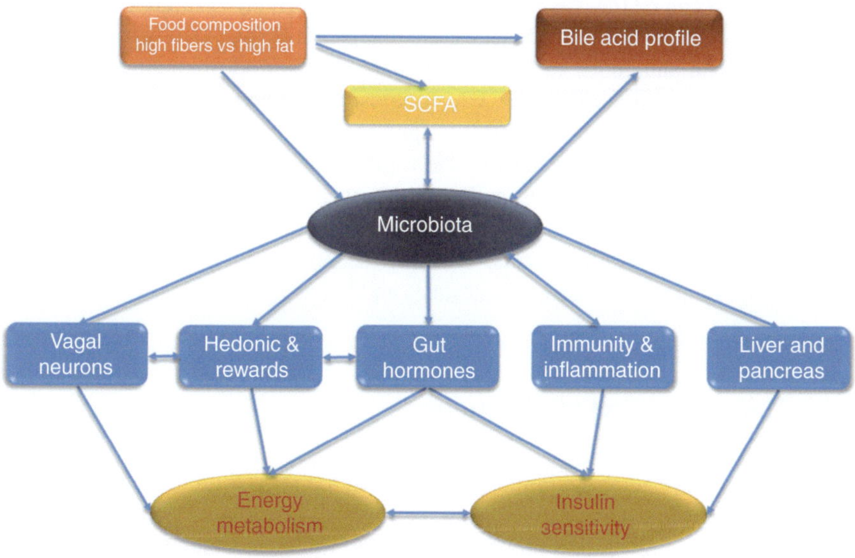

Fig. 5.7 Microbiota and energy metabolism. On the top, possible interplays among food composition, short-chain fatty acids (SCFA), bile acid composition, and microbiota are depicted. Microbiota may affect energy metabolism directly by converting "indigestible" fibers in the colon to SCFA that may be absorbed, but they may also influence energy metabolism indirectly via its effect on bile acid profile (top), as well as via various organ systems that affect insulin sensitivity and energy metabolism, as depicted in the bottom half of the figure

mice caused significantly greater adiposity in the recipient than the fecal transplant of a lean donor. Obesity seems to be associated with the changes in relative abundance of the bacterial groups and diversity of GM. The studies of animal models of obesity followed by studies of humans with obesity revealed a significant reduction in Bacteroidetes and increase in Firmicutes phylum. The alteration in the relative abundance in these phyla in obesity is associated with increased capacity to harvest food energy (Firmicutes phylum harvests greater energy than Bacteroidetes phylum). Short-chain fatty acids (SCFA), principally acetate, propionate, and butyrate, are produced by intestinal bacteria from food-derived fibers, and the composition of GM is significantly influenced by food composition. SCFA can be used as a source of energy for intestinal cells, are transported via the portal vein, and are converted to triglycerides in the liver. SCFA function as signaling molecules (Fig. 5.6), as ligands to receptors FFAR2 and FFAR3 in the intestine, immune cells, liver, and adipocytes. FFAR2 regulates the uptake of energy in white adipocytes and affects energy expenditure in muscles. FFAR3 stimulates sympathetic nerves and regulates energy expenditure. SCFA bind to gut receptors to induce PYY and GLP-1 production, decrease gut motility and intestinal transit, and induce satiety. SCFA may also modulate the immune response by reducing the intestinal permeability due to their effect on the tight junction functions and mucus production. The microbiota can modulate hepatic BA production, and the level of a particular BA can in turn change the profile of the GM. The change in BA profile can affect BA signaling function and the ability to activate BA receptors or even display an antagonistic action on the receptors. This can be the reason that germ-free mice displayed limited BA receptor activation. This was shown in a recent study that increased production of muricholic acid acted as an antagonist to FXR and FGF15 receptors despite an enlarged BA pool. Furthermore, the change in BA composition affects their hydrophobicity, which alters nutrient absorption and BA signaling.

There is evidence that GM activate the vagus nerve signaling to the brain. Early studies on infected animals with pathogens showed decreased *c-fos* expression in the PVN after subdiaphragmatic vagotomy. Later studies in nonpathogenic microbiota demonstrated similar results. Overall, the gut-microbiome-brain axis may play an important role in energy hemostasis and behaviors.

5.6 Hedonic Effect of Hormones

The neuronal and endocrine influences on eating are very complex. Food intake is rewarding and reinforcing. Homeostatic factors can be deluged by environmental cues related to the rewarding properties of food (nonhomeostatic factors). Obesity may be the consequence of the hedonic effect and reward-driven feeding, especially with food abundance. However, the reward pathway is essential for the minimal food intake required to survive, and the mesolimbic reward system has evolved to strengthen behaviors which assist achieving the rewards essential for survival (natural reward). This system closely relates to the hemostatic control system (Fig. 5.1).

A major neurotransmitter of the reward system is dopamine. Dopamine neurons arise from the substantia nigra and ventral tegmental area (VTA) of the midbrain and project to nucleus accumbens (NA) and the medial prefrontal cortex. There is evidence that the gut hormones participate in the regulation of food reward. The reward-processing areas of the brain express receptors for the gut peptides ghrelin, PYY, CCK, and GLP-1, amylin, insulin, and the adipokine, leptin.

Ghrelin has evolved to enforce adequate food intake during starvation. Foods high in energy are favored for survival. There is less evidence on ghrelin and reward in humans than in animals. However, functional magnetic resonance imaging (fMRI)s in subjects exposed to images of palatable foods have shown increased ghrelin responses in the area of reward system. Ghrelin seems to play a role in motivation to ingest sweet, palatable, and energy-dense foods over bland foods. These palatable foods increased dopamine response in NA, which was not seen in GHS-R1A knockout mice. Ghrelin appears to play a role in overeating and promoting overconsumption of energy dense and palatable foods. The effect of ghrelin in reward is not limited to natural reward and may contribute to motivation and reward disorders in drug abuse and addiction. Animal models have shown an anxiolytic effect of ghrelin with stress. Although there is less evidence in humans, it is proposed that increased ghrelin in chronic stress, as an adaptive response to control excessive anxiety and prevent depression, may increase emotional eating by acting on the hedonic/reward system. In obesity, possible central ghrelin resistance in hedonic areas may result in an inability to control anxiety and increased depression. In response, depressed subjects may have an altered hedonic/reward response to ghrelin, which makes them susceptible to obesity and eating disorders.

Although the suppressive effect of PYY_{3-36} on the reward system is not clear, studies using fMRI have shown that PYY_{3-36} modulates activities of nonhomeostatic areas in VTA and amygdala. It has been suggested that PYY_{3-36} increases discrimination of rewarding foods and reduces reward-motivated drives to eat in the fed state.

Central CCK signaling has not been shown to change food reward behaviors, although there are some links between CCK signaling and suppressed reward from the substance of abuse such as alcohol. CCK also is linked to increased anxiety.

The central GLP-1 is the only anorexigenic gut hormone that has a clear role in suppressing food reward behaviors and is linked to decreased food palatability. The hindbrain neurons can produce GLP-1; hence, it can directly act on the reward system. GLP-1 appears to lessen the cocaine and amphetamine-induced behaviors, which is in contrast to the effect of ghrelin.

It has been shown that post-GBS patients have changes in food preferences and eating behaviors. They find the sweet and high-fat foods less palatable, and they show healthier eating behaviors. In a study using fMRI, subjects exhibited markedly different hedonic responses to food after GBS compared to a band surgery. Post-GBS subjects showed reduced activation of several hedonic regions of the brain to high-calorie foods. It seems that the brain hedonic reward system may respond acutely and chronically to the exaggerated postprandial increase in PYY and GLP-1 and the increased level of BA. Learned conditioned aversion due to nausea and symptoms of dumping syndrome may contribute to less hedonic responses to high-calorie food. However, it is not clear whether the mechanisms contributing to these hedonic changes are due to altered taste receptors; the change in the central processing of taste perception; or changes in signaling by the altered gut hormones, vagal neurons, BA, or microbiota.

5.7 Conclusion

Body weight (particularly fat mass) in an adult is relatively constant due to multiple energy homeostatic mechanisms. Imbalance of energy intake and energy expenditure results in weight loss or weight gain. The gut is where food is taken in, digested, and absorbed. The gut is directly responsible for the body's energy intake, one of the two arms of energy homeostasis. The neuroendocrine system of the gut serves to maintain normal functions of food intake on a daily basis but also interact with the homeostatic energy balance system and the reward system in the CNS to regulate long-term energy balance. Gut hormones are categorized as orexigenic and anorexigenic hormones, and the potential role of many of these hormones in the long-term energy balance is being increasingly elucidated, and some hormones (e.g., GLP-1 and amylin) have been demonstrated in clinical settings associated with clinically significant weight loss. Various nutrients passing through the gut, as well as BA secreted in response to food intake, can also serve (sometimes indirectly) as signals that are integrated into the energy homeostatic and nonhomeostatic (the reward system) pathways, affecting body weight. Finally, the gut microbiota has emerged as a significant player in long-term energy regulation, probably via its modulation of the gut signaling, in addition to affecting energy absorption in the colon. Further understanding of the gut neuroendocrine system in controlling energy intake promises future developments of more effective treatment modalities to fight against obesity.

Reading List

Adamska E, Ostrowska L, Gorska M, Kretowski A. The role of gastrointestinal hormones in the pathogenesis of obesity and type 2 diabetes. Przeglad Gastroenterol. 2014;9(2):69–76. Epub 2014/07/26.

Asakawa A, Inui A, Yuzuriha H, Ueno N, Katsuura G, Fujimiya M, et al. Characterization of the effects of pancreatic polypeptide in the regulation of energy balance. Gastroenterology. 2003;124(5):1325–36. Epub 2003/05/06.

Batterham RL, Cowley MA, Small CJ, Herzog H, Cohen MA, Dakin CL, et al. Gut hormone PYY(3–36) physiologically inhibits food intake. Nature. 2002;418(6898):650–4. Epub 2002/08/09.

Boey D, Lin S, Enriquez RF, Lee NJ, Slack K, Couzens M, et al. PYY transgenic mice are protected against diet-induced and genetic obesity. Neuropeptides. 2008;42(1):19–30. Epub 2008/01/01.

Boey D, Lin S, Karl T, Baldock P, Lee N, Enriquez R, et al. Peptide YY ablation in mice leads to the development of hyperinsulinaemia and obesity. Diabetologia. 2006;49(6):1360–70. Epub 2006/05/09.
Chabot F, Caron A, Laplante M, St-Pierre DH. Interrelationships between ghrelin, insulin and glucose homeostasis: physiological relevance. World J Diabetes. 2014;5(3):328–41. Epub 2014/06/18.
Charron MJ, Vuguin PM. Lack of glucagon receptor signaling and its implications beyond glucose homeostasis. J Endocrinol. 2015;224(3):R123–30. Epub 2015/01/09.
Cho YM, Fujita Y, Kieffer TJ. Glucagon-like peptide-1: glucose homeostasis and beyond. Annu Rev Physiol. 2014;76:535–59. Epub 2013/11/20.
De Silva A, Bloom SR. Gut hormones and appetite control: a focus on PYY and GLP-1 as therapeutic targets in obesity. Gut Liver. 2012;6(1):10–20. Epub 2012/03/01.
Depoortere I. Taste receptors of the gut: emerging roles in health and disease. Gut. 2014;63(1):179–90. Epub 2013/10/18.
Dockray GJ. Cholecystokinin. Curr Opin Endocrinol Diabetes Obes. 2012;19(1):8–12. Epub 2011/12/14.
Dockray GJ. Enteroendocrine cell signalling via the vagus nerve. Curr Opin Pharmacol. 2013;13(6):954–8. Epub 2013/09/26.
Filippi BM, Abraham MA, Yue JT, Lam TK. Insulin and glucagon signaling in the central nervous system. Rev Endocr Metab Disord. 2013;14(4):365–75. Epub 2013/08/21.
Forsythe P, Bienenstock J, Kunze WA. Vagal pathways for microbiome-brain-gut axis communication. Adv Exp Med Biol. 2014;817:115–33. Epub 2014/07/06.
Gesmundo I, Gallo D, Favaro E, Ghigo E, Granata R. Obestatin: a new metabolic player in the pancreas and white adipose tissue. IUBMB Life. 2013;65(12):976–82. Epub 2013/11/13.
Gueugnon C, Mougin F, Nguyen NU, Bouhaddi M, Nicolet-Guenat M, Dumoulin G. Ghrelin and PYY levels in adolescents with severe obesity: effects of weight loss induced by long-term exercise training and modified food habits. Eur J Appl Physiol. 2012;112(5):1797–805. Epub 2011/09/13.
Hussain SS, Bloom SR. The regulation of food intake by the gut-brain axis: implications for obesity. Int J Obes. 2013;37(5):625–33. Epub 2012/06/20.
Kitamura A, Tsurugizawa T, Uematsu A, Uneyama H. The sense of taste in the upper gastrointestinal tract. Curr Pharm Des. 2014;20(16):2713–24. Epub 2013/07/28.
Lacquaniti A, Donato V, Chirico V, Buemi A, Buemi M. Obestatin: an interesting but controversial gut hormone. Ann Nutr Metab. 2011;59(2–4):193–9.
Li T, Chiang JY. Bile acids as metabolic regulators. Curr Opin Gastroenterol. 2015;31(2):159–65. Epub 2015/01/15.
Lutz TA. The interaction of amylin with other hormones in the control of eating. Diabetes Obes Metab. 2013;15(2):99–111. Epub 2012/08/07.
Madsbad S. The role of glucagon-like peptide-1 impairment in obesity and potential therapeutic implications. Diabetes Obes Metab. 2014;16(1):9–21. Epub 2013/04/27.
Manning S, Batterham RL. The role of gut hormone peptide YY in energy and glucose homeostasis: twelve years on. Annu Rev Physiol. 2014;76:585–608. Epub 2013/11/06.
Moran CP, Shanahan F. Gut microbiota and obesity: role in aetiology and potential therapeutic target. Best Pract Res Clin Gastroenterol. 2014;28(4):585–97. Epub 2014/09/10.
Munzberg H, Laque A, Yu S, Rezai-Zadeh K, Berthoud HR. Appetite and body weight regulation after bariatric surgery. Obesity Rev: Off J Int Assoc Study of Obesity. 2015;16(Suppl 1):77–90. Epub 2015/01/24.
Naveilhan P, Hassani H, Canals JM, Ekstrand AJ, Larefalk A, Chhajlani V, et al. Normal feeding behavior, body weight and leptin response require the neuropeptide Y Y2 receptor. Nat Med. 1999;5(10):1188–93. Epub 1999/09/30.
Neary MT, Batterham RL. Gaining new insights into food reward with functional neuroimaging. Forum Nutr. 2010;63:152–63. Epub 2009/12/04.

Nieuwdorp M, Gilijamse PW, Pai N, Kaplan LM. Role of the microbiome in energy regulation and metabolism. Gastroenterology. 2014;146(6):1525–33. Epub 2014/02/25.

Page AJ, Symonds E, Peiris M, Blackshaw LA, Young RL. Peripheral neural targets in obesity. Br J Pharmacol. 2012;166(5):1537–58. Epub 2012/03/22.

Pinkney J. The role of ghrelin in metabolic regulation. Curr Opin Clin Nutr Metab Care. 2014;17(6):497–502. Epub 2014/08/12.

Pocai A. Action and therapeutic potential of oxyntomodulin. Molecula Metab. 2014;3(3):241–51. Epub 2014/04/22.

Pocai A. Unraveling oxyntomodulin, GLP1's enigmatic brother. J Endocrinol. 2012;215(3):335–46. Epub 2012/09/29.

Pols TW, Noriega LG, Nomura M, Auwerx J, Schoonjans K. The bile acid membrane receptor TGR5: a valuable metabolic target. Dig Dis. 2011;29(1):37–44. Epub 2011/06/22.

Psichas A, Reimann F, Gribble FM. Gut chemosensing mechanisms. J Clin Invest. 2015;125(3):908–17. Epub 2015/02/11.

Scholtz S, Miras AD, Chhina N, Prechtl CG, Sleeth ML, Daud NM, et al. Obese patients after gastric bypass surgery have lower brain-hedonic responses to food than after gastric banding. Gut. 2014;63(6):891–902. Epub 2013/08/22

Seeley RJ, Chambers AP, Sandoval DA. The role of gut adaptation in the potent effects of multiple bariatric surgeries on obesity and diabetes. Cell Metab. 2015;21(3):369–78. Epub 2015/02/11

Sekar R, Chow BK. Metabolic effects of secretin. Gen Comp Endocrinol. 2013;181:18–24. Epub 2012/12/19.

Simpson KA, Bloom SR. Appetite and hedonism: gut hormones and the brain. Endocrinol Metab Clin N Am. 2010;39(4):729–43. Epub 2010/11/26.

Sjostrom L. Review of the key results from the Swedish obese subjects (SOS) trial—a prospective controlled intervention study of bariatric surgery. J Intern Med. 2013;273(3):219–34. Epub 2012/11/21.

Skibicka KP, Dickson SL. Enteroendocrine hormones—central effects on behavior. Curr Opin Pharmacol. 2013;13(6):977–82. Epub 2013/10/05.

Speakman JR, Levitsky DA, Allison DB, Bray MS, de Castro JM, Clegg DJ, et al. Set points, settling points and some alternative models: theoretical options to understand how genes and environments combine to regulate body adiposity. Dis Model Mech. 2011;4(6):733–45. Epub 2011/11/09.

Steinert RE, Beglinger C. Nutrient sensing in the gut: interactions between chemosensory cells, visceral afferents and the secretion of satiation peptides. Physiol Behav. 2011;105(1):62–70. Epub 2011/03/08

Sumithran P, Prendergast LA, Delbridge E, Purcell K, Shulkes A, Kriketos A, et al. Long-term persistence of hormonal adaptations to weight loss. N Engl J Med. 2011;365(17):1597–604. Epub 2011/10/28.

Suzuki K, Jayasena CN, Bloom SR. Obesity and appetite control. Exp Diabetes Res. 2012;2012:824305. Epub 2012/08/18.

Sweeney TE, Morton JM. Metabolic surgery: action via hormonal milieu changes, changes in bile acids or gut microbiota? A summary of the literature. Best Pract Res Clin Gastroenterol. 2014;28(4):727–40. Epub 2014/09/10.

Teubner BJ, Bartness TJ. PYY(3–36) into the arcuate nucleus inhibits food deprivation-induced increases in food hoarding and intake. Peptides. 2013;47:20–8. Epub 2013/07/03.

Yu YH, Vasselli JR, Zhang Y, Mechanick JI, Korner J, Peterli R. Metabolic vs. hedonic obesity: a conceptual distinction and its clinical implications. Obesity Rev: Off J Int Assoc Study Obesity. 2015;16(3):234–47. Epub 2015/01/16.

Chapter 6
Adiposopathy

Elena A. Christofides and J. Michael Gonzalez-Campoy

Pearls of Wisdom

- Adipose tissue, like any other tissue of the body, may develop disease. Adiposopathy (or sick fat) is akin to retinopathy, dermopathy, nephropathy, neuropathy, encephalopathy, and other tissue or organ diseases.
- Adiposopathy includes changes to adipose tissue function and adipose tissue anatomy.
- Adiposopathy contributes to the development of other metabolic diseases.
- There are defined disorders of regional fat distribution.
- A goal of treatment for clinical endocrinologists is to treat adiposopathy, returning adipose tissue function to normal and addressing disorders of regional fat distribution as appropriate.

6.1 Introduction

Adipose tissue may become diseased by changes in size, distribution, or function (Table 6.1). Adiposopathy is defined as derangements of adipose tissue function and/or anatomy that result in a pathological state. It is important to distinguish between the accumulation of fat mass (adiposity) and adiposopathy (disorders of

E. A. Christofides (✉)
Endocrinology Associates, Inc., Columbus, OH, USA
e-mail: christofides@endocrinology-associates.com

J. M. Gonzalez-Campoy
Minnesota Center for Obesity, Metabolism and Endocrinology, PA (MNCOME), Eagan, MN, USA

J. M. Gonzalez-Campoy et al. (eds.), *Bariatric Endocrinology*,
https://doi.org/10.1007/978-3-319-95655-8_6

Table 6.1 Anatomical and functional changes of adipose tissue in adiposopathy

Anatomical changes	Functional changes

Adipocyte hypertrophy
Growth of adipose tissue beyond its vascular supply
Increased number of adipose tissue immune cells
  Macrophage ring structures surrounding dying adipocytes
Ectopic fat deposition (in other body tissues)
Heterogeneous adipose tissue distribution
  Visceral adiposity linked to metabolic diseases
	Impaired adipogenesis and adipocyte hypertrophy
	Adipocyte lipolysis in excess of lipogenesis
	  Increased free fatty acids
	Pathogenic adipose tissue endocrine responses
	  Hypoadiponectinemia
	  Hyperleptinemia
	Pathogenic adipose tissue immune responses
	  High levels of inflammatory markers
	Pathogenic crosstalk between fat and other organs

function and structure of adipose tissue). One may exist without the other, but most often adiposity and adiposopathy go hand in hand.

It is not in dispute that excess adiposity can be detrimental to the health of a person. The difficulty has been to characterize the features of adipose tissue dysfunction which clinically correlate to the degree of adiposopathy. Numerous studies have shown that adipocytes can be diseased even when not in excess, and clinically lean individuals can have features of the metabolic syndrome. This lean-on-the-outside-fat-on-the-inside (LOFI) phenotype has created a paradox for the term "excess adiposity." Therefore the term, "obesity" or "excess adiposity" can no longer be used to adequately describe the process of adipocyte disease that occurs regardless of adipose mass. The term "adiposopathy" best characterizes the multiplicity of effects that the diseased adipocyte can have on the organism as a whole. The ability to name this entity more concisely allows educational material to be organized around a central theme that is not contradictory or confusing.

6.2 Anatomical Changes in Adiposopathy

Healthy adipocytes are characterized by lipid droplets of a particular size such that the lipid content represents approximately 90% of the total adipocyte cell volume. In adipose tissue, the supportive structures taken collectively (collagen matrix, vasculature, immune cells etc.) should equal 50% of the total mass. Collectively, the adipose mass is approximately 20% visceral white adipose tissue (WAT) and 80% peripheral WAT. Stimulation for adipose tissue deposition in visceral versus peripheral fat stores is predetermined primarily at birth. Throughout life, ongoing stimulation for differential deposition in these two fat stores is directed by environmental pressures, sex steroids (independently of gender), age, and epigenetic changes. Women typically have visceral adipocytes that are smaller than their peripheral adipocytes. In obesity, this ratio is not preserved and women with obesity have a more uniform distribution of adipocyte size. Men have a more uniform distribution of adipocyte size throughout their lives.

The distribution of excess nutrient intake is dependent on the difference between caloric intake and expenditure over time. Initially, the liver serves as the primary target of excess nutrients, followed by the muscle. Both however have a limited capacity for energy storage. Excess nutrient intake over prolonged periods of time leads to the recruitment of preadipocytes through peroxisome proliferator-activated receptor (PPAR)-γ. Lipid droplet transfer from mature adipocytes into newly formed immature adipocytes allows for storage of excess energy over time. Dysfunctional PPAR-γ activation impairs this process and prevents the mature adipocyte from shedding additional lipid droplets leading to hypertrophy and further dysfunction.

Under the influence of androgenic hormone predominance, excess caloric intake is preferentially shunted to the peripheral adipose tissue. Men have a decreased capacity for adipogenesis, therefore increased demand places great strain on the peripheral adipocyte and hypertrophy ensues. The loss of testosterone activity in a man shifts the burden of free fatty acid (FFA) uptake to the visceral adipose tissue, which has a lower capacity to store triglycerides. If the excess caloric intake occurs under the influence of estrogen hormone predominance the visceral adipose tissue is bypassed in favor of deposition in the peripheral adipocytes, which favors adipogenesis and increased adipose mass via recruitment of preadipocytes rather than hypertrophy. During times of great psychosocial stress, nutrient intake has a different fate. Excess nutrient intake in the presence of elevated glucocorticoid levels preferentially shunts calories to visceral adipose tissue for storage. The visceral adipocyte is stimulated to hypertrophy in part due to the downregulation of adipocyte recruitment in the periphery. If the nutrient excess is prolonged, then the peripheral adipocyte is also induced to hypertrophy. Other factors may affect this differential accretion of adipose tissue. For example, in the presence of isolated hypertension, without other clinical features of obesity, there is suppression of peripheral adipocyte recruitment due to elevated levels of angiotensinogen. Thus, the development of excess adipose mass (adiposity) exerts variable hormonal effects and is in turn affected by the hormonal milieu that creates it. Peripheral adiposity is significantly less inflammatory than intra-abdominal adiposity. All things considered, health risk assessment strictly based on body mass index (BMI) criteria is inaccurate.

Visceral adipose tissue is more metabolically active in regard to adipokine production and thus more sensitive to perturbations of metabolic stress than peripheral adipose tissue. Visceral adipose tissue is more limited in its capacity for triglyceride storage. Visceral adipocytes have a higher turnover of lipid metabolism. The epicardial fat layer is the most metabolically active fat depot, but all visceral fat contributes to fat metabolism. As such, the visceral adipose mass is not a major energy repository but rather represents a mediator of energy pass through. In the presence of continuous nutrient intake excess, the visceral adipocytes are less capable of adipogenesis. Engorgement of mature visceral adipocytes ensues, and adipocyte hypertrophy then promotes an inflammatory milieu.

6.3 Pathophysiological Changes in Adiposopathy

Adipose tissue develops inflammation when hypertrophied. The hypertrophied adipocyte outgrows its oxygen supply. Once the adipocyte grows beyond the passive diffusion distance of oxygen, it triggers hypoxia-inducible factor 1 (HIF1) and this initiates cell death (Fig. 6.1). HIF1 recruits proinflammatory macrophages that act as scavengers. Macrophages suppress adipogenesis directly and indirectly. There is downregulation of uncoupling protein (f)-2, PPARγ,and glucose transporter 4 (GLUT4). Nutrient uptake is hindered, and preadipocyte recruitment is prevented. Hypoxia-induced macrophage infiltration of WAT, as it hypertrophies, may be considered a sentinel event to the development of adiposopathy. Total macrophage mass within WAT is directly correlated to adipose mass and production of tumor necrosis factor (TNF)-α. Adiponectin is a well-recognized hormone produced by healthy adipose tissue. It heralds insulin sensitivity and has an anti-inflammatory effect. Adiponectin secretion is inhibited by HIF1. A decrease in adiponectin levels correlates with the hypoxic inflammatory environment created by adipocyte hypertrophy.

Plasma levels of interleukin-6 (IL-6) correlate to adiposity and the development of diabetes and cardiovascular disease. This adipokine has been shown to decrease adiponectin levels, inhibit adipogenesis, and downregulate insulin receptors. Interestingly, the inverse is true in the central nervous system (CNS) fluid. Elevated levels of IL-6 in the CNS promote energy catabolism and decrease food intake. One potential mechanism of impaired signaling in adiposopathy may well be the inability of the plasma IL-6 to communicate with the CNS.

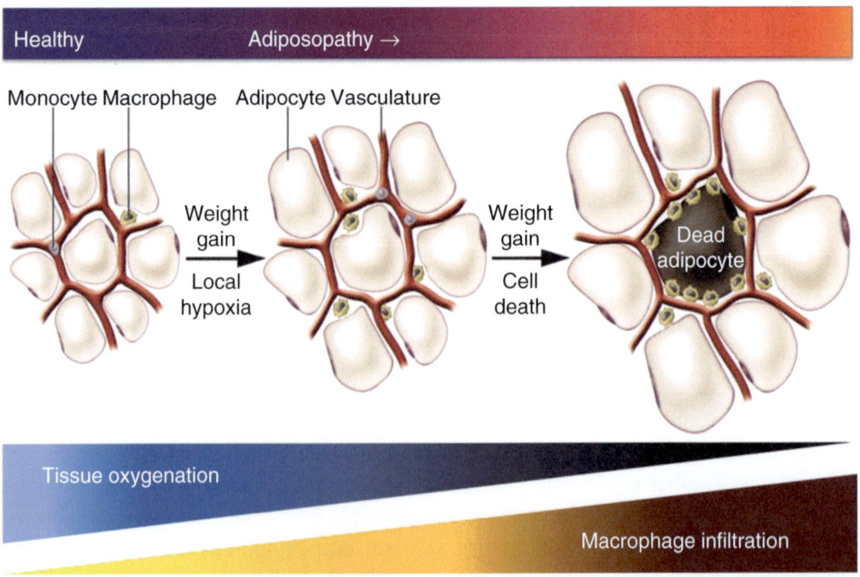

Fig. 6.1 Adipose tissue changes which develop with the progression of adiposopathy

Adipocytes undergoing oxidative stress produce plasminogen-activator inhibitor (PAI)-1 in excess. Plasma levels of PAI-1 correlate with hyperinsulinemia, obesity, and the presence of dysmetabolic syndrome. PAI-1 is a procoagulant and a potent inducer of fibrosis. Fibrosis of the supportive structures surrounding the adipocyte further increases the burden of hypoxia.

Healthy adipocytes use adenosine monophosphate-activated protein kinase (AMPK) as a key step in glucose metabolism under the influence of adiponectin and leptin. Insulin inhibits AMPK function, which in turn downregulates preadipocyte differentiation. Metformin has been shown to activate AMPK. Hyperinsulinemia and excess exogenous insulin may play a role in preventing healthy adipocyte recruitment to attenuate nutrient excess.

Leptin levels are directly proportional to total fat mass. Leptin may be considered a signal from adipose tissue to the brain about total energy storage. Leptin levels correlate with hypertrophied adipose mass but not adipocyte number. This is counter-intuitive to the usual functions of leptin. Leptin is stimulated by negative caloric balance and has a potent lipolytic effect via stimulation of release of FFA into the circulation. In adiposopathy, there is classic leptin resistance, where the leptin level is no longer bound by the negative nutrient intake. Leptin continues to induce lipolysis with unmitigated release of FFA into the circulation. Rising levels of leptin have also been shown to induce hypertension.

Adiposopathy relates to overall nutritional status through retinol-binding protein (RBP)-4 levels. RBP-4 transports vitamin A in the retinol form and appears to be stimulated by declining glucose levels. The RBP-4-vitamin A complex binds with retinoid X receptors (RXR) in combination with transthyretin to induce glycolysis in the liver and downregulation of GLUT4 in the periphery. RBP-4 levels correlate with visceral adiposity. RBP-4 levels decline as visceral adipose mass declines. RBP-4 levels are unchanged with alterations of the peripheral adipose mass. Declining levels of RBP-4 are highly predictive of success at long-term weight loss maintenance regardless of method (i.e., bariatric surgery or nutrition and physical activity).

Brown adipose tissue (BAT) is much less than WAT in humans. Regulation of BAT by PPARγ coactivator 1-alpha (PGC1α) binding with twist-related protein 1 (TWIST1) is more closely tied to subcutaneous adipose mass and induced by PPARδ. Promotion of thermogenic fatty acid oxidation declines with increasing peripheral adiposity. In WAT, macrophage infiltration downregulates the PGC1α-TWIST1 protein complex through the production of TNF-α and IL-6.

Adipose tissue dysfunction and adipose tissue distribution are tightly coupled. Although it is possible for adipose tissue dysfunction to develop independent of adipose tissue mass, for most patients, the accumulation of intra-abdominal fat, or visceral fat, is directly responsible for the changes in function that cause adiposopathy (Table 6.1). There is a strong genetic component involved. There are many patients who accumulate significant amounts of visceral fat but who do not have markers of adipose tissue dysfunction or metabolic diseases in association. Adiposopathy, on the other hand, may happen with only modest increases in visceral fat, as is the case in populations with gene pools originating in the Asian subcontinent or Southeast Asia.

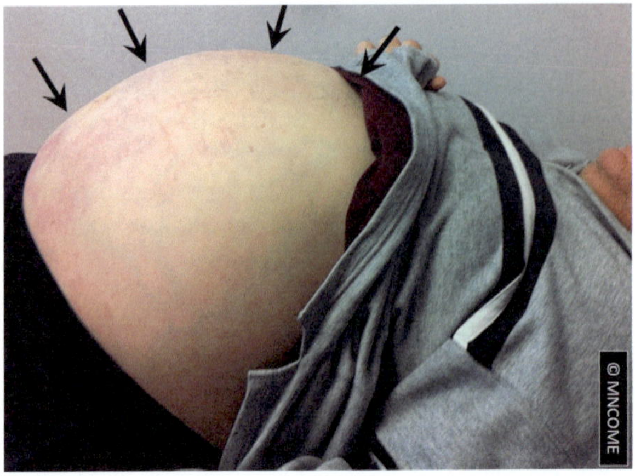

Fig. 6.2 Visceral adiposity

Intra-abdominal or visceral fat is considered to be a tumor, and its mass effect may be significant (Fig. 6.2). The intra-abdominal space is finite, and the accumulation of visceral fat produces a significant mass effect. In addition to affecting systemic vascular tone by the generation of a vast vascular network that increases peripheral resistance, increased adipose tissue mass raises the intra-abdominal pressure (IAP). An elevation of IAP leads to mechanical problems such as acid reflux disease, urinary incontinence, and the development of hernias. It also affects the function of other organs in the abdominal cavity and the retroperitoneal space.

6.4 Adipocyte Disruptors

Adipocyte function may be affected by hormonal and neural inputs. The environment in which we exist modulates the expression of genes. Other than the availability and palatability of foods, and disincentives for physical activity, there are other adipocyte disruptors, which are amenable for clinical intervention.

6.4.1 Circadian Dysrhythmia

Circadian dysrhythmia has long been suspected of creating metabolic havoc. Identification of the clock nuclei in the hypothalamus and their integrated functions has proved a boon to our understanding of the influence of the day-night cycle. Humans evolved to require set periodicity in light-dark cycles of particular lengths. Disruptions come in many forms of our own doing. The most common disruption for modern man is the invention of the light bulb. With the capability of generating light after dark, the human brain can no longer rely on the natural light-dark rhythms of the earth's 24-h cycle. Failure to ensure complete darkness for a set period of time disrupts the CNS clock. Further disruptions come in the form of blue-light-emitting electronics that are utilized during expected periods of darkness. Blue light entering the retina has been shown to disrupt melatonin secretion causing a phase delay in sleep cycle. Delayed and disrupted sleep cycles impair CNS control centers from the task of correct nutrient intake timing and delivery.

Pro-opiomelanocortin (POMC) and cocaine- and amphetamine-regulated transcript (CART) proteins exist in the hypothalamus specifically to coordinate light-dark and sleep-wake cycles. They entrain the hypothalamic-pituitary-adrenal (HPA) axis and the ghrelin/leptin signaling timing. Ghrelin and leptin are secreted in accordance with food intake. Correct stimulation and suppression of these hormones in the course of a 24-h day are important to ensure correct timing of FFA uptake in the gut and thermoregulation by BAT. In addition, beige adipocytes are recruited for additional thermogenesis as needed to dissipate caloric excess. The drive to consume calories is also timed to meet thermoregulatory demands beyond basic metabolic needs. Alterations from the expected day-night cycle impair nutrient intake timing and delivery of nutrients. Thus, circadian rhythm also applies to the gastrointestinal system. Expectation of nutrient intake is not random but timed after sleep, interspersed throughout the day and not expected at night.

Glucagon-like peptide (GLP)-1 has emerged as a critical hormone for the control of postprandial glucose disposal. GLP1 is also entrained to the circadian clock and if it loses periodicity, it loses the ability to stimulate GLUT4 for the transport of glucose into cells. The disordered FFA metabolism that ensues if circadian disruption occurs further alters the leptin response to glucose stimulation. Perhaps, one of the most critical components of the circadian clock is the HPA axis. Disordered sleep-wake cycles alter the HPA axis with disordered cortisol secretion. Loss of periodicity of cortisol secretion simulates Cushing's syndrome (pseudo-Cushing's) with subsequent shifting of FFA uptake away from the peripheral and into the visceral adipose tissue.

6.4.2 *Nutrients*

Nutrient density is more than just caloric content. Multiple aspects of the health or dysfunction of the adipocyte are a direct result of the vitamin content of meals or the digestive capability of the gut. Vitamin A upregulates RBP-4 when intake is inadequate. RBP-4 has direct and indirect effects on cellular capacity for glucose metabolism. RBP-4 impairs GLUT4, which decreases glucose uptake. RBP-4 has also been shown to indirectly suppress adipogenesis.

Vitamin D deficiency is a key player in glucose regulation based on its role in binding to RXR, which as a complex is critical to gene transcription of insulin (in the pancreas). The downregulation of proinflammatory macrophages is also influenced by adequate vitamin D levels. It has been postulated that despite correcting for socioeconomic factors, the increased cardiovascular disease mortality of minority populations, particularly African-Americans, is related to a more significant degree of vitamin D deficiency than the Caucasian population.

6.4.3 *The Gut and Gut Microbiome*

The mass of the gastrointestinal epithelium may be second only to the adipose mass in sheer volume and hormonal functionality. Failure to maintain a healthy gut has wide-ranging implications for the adipocyte. The gut microbiome is comprised of tens of trillions of bacteria with more than 150 times more genes than our own bodies. Gut dysbiosis is an emerging risk factor for adiposopathy. Nutrient delivery to the microbiome is necessary for a healthy population of gut bacteria. Alteration of the population of gut bacteria, which shifts the population balance and disrupts the functions needed to maintain a healthy gut endothelium, has been described. Tetracycline has been implicated in the downregulation of mitochondrial activity. It is believed that gut bacteria are responsible for the interaction of ingested fats such as polyunsaturated fatty acids (PUFAs) in stimulating GLP1. It is known that several species of gut bacteria are capable of producing serotonin as well as stimulating localized serotonin production in the gastrointestinal track independent of the CNS. It is possible that this neurotransmitter release has an effect on the central CNS with subsequent downstream consequences on the adipocyte. Indeed, perturbations of gut-brain neural communication have been demonstrated to impact adipocyte function. These effects on adipocyte function are mediated by the HPA axis, POMC disruptions due to altered serotonin function, and improper handling of FFA by the gut. Fecal transplantation in human and animal trials suggests that adipocytes can be manipulated by merely shifting the population of gut bacteria, with some species being obesogenic and others inducing weight loss.

6.5 Adiposopathy and Crosstalk with Other Organs

Other chapters in this textbook will address many of the interactions between adipose tissue and other organ systems, including the effects of adiposopathy. This section will discuss other crosstalk effects of adipose tissue and adiposopathy.

6.5.1 *Nervous System*

Adipokine measurements in plasma reflect adipose tissue function in obesity. The levels of adipokines and other signaling molecules are not the same when CNS fluid is sampled. Adipokines in the plasma have been shown to alter CNS permeability. The CNS is responsive to ratios of signaling hormones rather than absolute values of individual adipokines. Thus, attempts to manipulate peripheral adipokine levels in order to control metabolism may not proceed as predicted.

Adipose tissue is intensely innervated and the adrenergic system is a potent controller of thermogenesis in BAT. Loss of β-adrenergic neurons decreases UCP-1 activation with subsequent diminishment of FFA consumption by thermogenesis. Progressive loss of peripheral β-adrenergic innervation of adipose tissue decreases recruitment of WAT into beige adipocytes further decreasing metabolic flexibility to dispose of excess caloric intake.

There is emerging evidence that adiposopathy plays a role in the development of dementia. The presence of adipokines and other inflammatory markers in brain tissue samples of dementia victims indicates a correlation at minimum. Given that there is no consistent finding of other adiposopathy-associated illnesses present with dementia, perhaps there is a sentinel event or epigenetic change that predisposes a patient to proceed down this particular path. The apolipoprotein E (Apo E) gene is a known lipid metabolism gene. It is responsible for lipid movement across cell membranes; in particular, it appears to be responsible for lipid movement in and out of the CNS. Epidemiologic studies have shown a consistent correlation with the development of dementia as well as the decade of onset based on the number of ApoE 4 alleles versus the ApoE 3 alleles present. The presence of the ApoE 3/4 heterozygosity or ApoE 4/4 homozygosity and the associated increased risk of developing of dementia suggests a relationship between adiposopathy and dementia that needs exploring more fully.

6.5.2 Toxic Effects of Free Fatty Acids

Initial deposition of excess energy in the form of parenteral-derived FFA is presented to the liver and the muscle tissue. If positive caloric balance continues beyond capacity, then those FFAs are shunted to the adipocyte. If the adipocyte is incapable of accepting the excess nutrients, then the FFAs are freely circulating. Excess circulating FFAs are directly toxic to all cells. Indirectly, they activate reactive oxygen species (ROS), suppress nitric oxide production in the vascular endothelium, and cause vasoconstriction. An excess of ROS is known to be present in adiposopathy. ROS are directly toxic to neurologic tissue. Much of the ROS in adiposopathy occur locally during hypoxia of hypertrophied adipose tissue.

6.5.3 Effect on Bone Mineral Density

The bone marrow contains a common progenitor cell of both osteoblasts and adipocytes. Recruitment and differentiation is need-based and responds to hormone signaling. A correlation between increased adipogenesis and decreased bone mineral density has been observed in humans. The exact mechanism is unclear, but it is postulated that excessive demand on the bone marrow for adipogenesis depletes the population of progenitor cells that could be targeted for differentiation into osteoblasts. Provided that adipogenesis pressures are not prolonged, the bone marrow has the ability to replenish the stem cell depot. If adipogenesis pressures are excessive or prolonged, the aging bone marrow may not be able to maintain adequate osteoblast recruitment from the progenitor depot in order to maintain healthy bone mineral density.

6.5.4 Heart and Vasculature

The heart historically has been assigned a passive role in the discussion about adiposopathy. In fact, the epicardial fat depot is the most biologically active adipose tissue. Epicardial fat exhibits the highest rate of lipid turnover of any adipose tissue type. It accounts for up to 20% of the weight of the heart and is responsible for maintaining ventricular function, cardiac vessel health, and autonomic innervation. The presence of an epicardial layer of fat signals a very important interplay of the endocrine system and the myocardium. The thickness of the epicardial fat is independently correlated to the degree of overall obesity as well as the degree of myocardial dysfunction. Increasing amounts of epicardial fat correlate with increasing features of adiposopathy, metabolic syndrome (particularly hypertension), and adipokine production. HIF1 activation in epicardial fat correlates with the degree of cardiomyopathy present. This suggests that the heart, or at least epicardial fat, is an active contributor to adiposopathy.

The epicardial fat is known to be especially innervated. A potentially new categorization of cardiovascular disease as a function of a neuro-endocrine-vascular dysfunction should be considered as a consequence of adiposopathy. Interventional and observational studies have repeatedly shown that aggressive medical management is more effective for cardiovascular disease outcomes than invasive procedures such as percutaneous transluminal coronary angioplasty (PTCA) or percutaneous coronary intervention (PCI). Interestingly, transposition of a vessel without the associated vascular fat as in coronary artery bypass graft (CABG) is the only cardiac intervention proven to be more effective than medical therapy in patients with diabetes. Addressing adiposopathy in patients with diabetes appears to be more relevant to cardiac outcomes than the manipulation of the vascular lumen via internal catheters.

The vasculature and supportive structures make up the largest volume of tissue affected by adiposopathy. Elevated levels of proinflammatory cytokines blunt endothelial nitric oxide synthase (eNOS) production. Inflammatory macrophages secrete vascular endothelial growth factor (VEGF), which induces vascular remodeling with smooth muscle cell (SMC) proliferation. Prostaglandin secretion is also elevated in these circumstances, which causes further vasoconstriction and fibrosis, culminating in hypertension. Hypertension alone has been shown to inhibit adipogenesis. If the inflammation is accompanied by elevated levels of circulating FFAs, then an increase in ROS is seen. ROS damage the vascular endothelium allowing for the formation of characteristic atherosclerotic plaque. Once a vessel is damaged, it signals and recruits adipocytes locally in order to absorb the excess FFA. These perivascular adipocytes are fully functioning WAT. If there is a continuous elevation of circulating FFA, the perivascular adipocytes begin to hypertrophy due to ongoing suppression of adipogenesis. Hypertrophic adipocytes become progressively more hypoxic with localized damage. Hypoxia locally increases ROS which increase SMC remodeling and fibrosis, as evidenced by increased collagen V levels in diseased vessels. Ongoing vessel exposure to excess FFA clearly creates a systemic reaction in the vasculature and periorgan adipose layers. The organs with the highest oxygen demand, such as the heart, brain, and kidneys, are the most susceptible to dysfunction.

The presence of hypertension in the setting of overweight or obesity is sufficient to assume that adiposopathy is occurring. The impairment of healthy adipogenesis that occurs in the setting of hypertension will clearly lead to the progression of vascular disease if neither the hypertension nor the excess caloric intake is addressed. Numerous antihypertensive agents in the renin-angiotensin-aldosterone system (RAAS) family have shown particular affinity toward blocking SMC remodeling and fibrosis of the vasculature. RAAS blockade should be given initial consideration for treatment of hypertension in all patients. Suppression of angiotensinogen, in particular, has the potential to be the most potent treatment for adiposopathy, as it relates to hypertension.

6.6 Disorders of Regional Fat Distribution

6.6.1 Lypodystrophy

The absence of subcutaneous fat is characteristic of lipodystrophy syndromes. Lipoatrophy is a rare condition. The loss of the WAT depots in the subcutaneous fat stimulates an induction of visceral adipose tissue. The loss of subcutaneous fat depots with maintenance of visceral adiposity correlates with low levels of leptin and adiponectin. Leptin levels rise with increasing fat mass. In lipodystrophy, despite an increase in intra-abdominal mass, the loss of subcutaneous fat makes overall fat mass decrease. Leptin levels are therefore decreased. At the same time, adiposopathy develops in the intra-abdominal space, causing adiponectin levels to also drop. Thus, the absence of WAT in the subcutaneous space produces inappropriately low levels of adiponectin and leptin. In lipodystrophy, there is a paradoxically high level of insulin resistance due to an additive effect of FFA oxidation which results from low leptin and adiponectin levels. Replacement of leptin and adiponectin individually, or in combination, in animal models as well as in humans, has shown reversal of the excess FFA oxidation with subsequent decrease in insulin resistance features.

Whereas lipodystrophy is rare, accrual of fat mass affects two-thirds of the American population. There are recognized disorders of regional fat distribution (Table 6.2). Some of these disorders are also rare, and some are exceedingly common (visceral adiposity). The location of adipose tissue growth seems to be largely genetically driven. For some of these disorders, the genetic factors involved have been identified.

Table 6.2 Adiposopathy conditions

Adiposopathy condition	Characteristics	ICD-10 code
Localized adipose tissue accumulation (regional)		
Abdominal obesity (intra-abdominal) Adiposity, localized (i.e., dorsal arm, thighs, and flanks) Buffalo hump (Dowager's hump) Panniculus (subcutaneous abdominal)		E65
Specified localized adipose tissue accumulation (regional)		
Hoffa's fat pad disease	Infrapatellar fat pad	E88.89
Gynecomastia	Glandular breast growth in men	N62
Lipedema (lipoedema)	Lower extremity distribution	R60.9
Liposarcoma Malignant lipomatous tumor		C49.9
Lipodystrophies		
Acquired generalized lipodystrophy Acquired lipoatrophic diabetes Lawrence syndrome Lawrence-Seip syndrome *Acquired partial lipodystrophy* Barraquer syndrome Barraquer-Simons disease Simons syndrome Partial lipoatrophy Partial lipodystrophy Progressive cephalothoracic lipodystrophy Progressive partial lipodystrophy *Congenital generalized lipodystrophy, types 1, 2, 3, and 4* Berardinelli-Seip syndrome Lipodystrophy of Berardinelli Seip syndrome *(Congenital) familial partial lypodystrophy, types 1, 2, 3, 4, 5, and 6* Kobberling-Dunnigan syndrome Lipoatrophic diabetes	Lipoatrophy is associated with low circulating leptin and osteosclerosis	E88.1

Table 6.2 (continued)

Adiposopathy condition	Characteristics	ICD-10 code
Fat wasting Lupus panniculitis *Lipoatrophia annularis* Ferreira-marques Lipoatrophia *Centrifugal abdominal lipodystrophy* Lipodystrophia centrifugalis abdominalis infantilis		E88.1
AIDS-related lipoatrophy Fat redistribution syndrome Highly active antiretroviral therapy (HAART)-induced lipodystrophy Lipoatrophy due to HIV infection		B20
Lipohypertrophy	Subcutaneous adipose tissue hypertrophy is usually seen at insulin injection sites	E65
	Lipomatosis	
Lipoma (single; may form from periorgan fat anywhere in the body) *Lipomatosis* (multiple)	Each is circumscribed or encapsulated Each reaches a relatively static size after the initial growth period Size does not regress, even with starvation Become hard with the application of ice. Cytological staining is positive for leptin and reticulin, which surrounds adipocytes. Cytogenetically, 55–75% of solitary lipomas have rearrangements of the high-mobility group A T-hook 2 gene. Multiple lipomas usually have a normal phenotype.	D17.*xy* (*x* and *y* = digits to define anatomical location)
Epidural lipomatosis		D17.79
Adiposis dolorosa Adiposalgia Adiposis tuberosa simplex (fatty degeneration occurring in nodular masses) Adipose tissue rheumatism Ander's disease Dercum's disease Lipomatosis dolorosa Morbus dercum	Lipomas are encapsulated Lipomas are tender to touch Pain is unresponsive to common analgesic medications May be a lymphovascular disorder—Abnormal adipose tissue deposition has been correlated to abnormal lymphatic structure and function The preferred treatment is excision of the affected lesion Recurrence is common	E88.2

(continued)

Table 6.2 (continued)

Adiposopathy condition	Characteristics	ICD-10 code
Symmetric(al) lipomatosis (SL) Benign symmetric(al) lipomatosis Diffuse symmetrical lipomatosis Multiple symmetrical lipomatosis (a) SL type 1 (cervical region and face) Familial benign cervical symmetric lipomatosis Madelung's disease Madelung-Launois-Bensaude syndrome (b) SL type 2 (shoulders, upper arms, and chest) Launois (Lanois)-Bensaude syndrome Lipomastia (c) SL type 3 (gynecoid) Steatopygia (d) SL type 4 (palmar or plantar)	Nonencapsulated Affects patients who are 30–70 years old Prevalence of 1 in 25,000 Male-to-female ratio of 15–30:1. Lipomas measure from 1 to 20 cm and may cause local compression symptoms affecting the airway and thoracic outlet in 15–20% of patients. Dysphagia, obstructive apnea, hoarseness, and irregular breathing have all been described with progressive fat mass accrual. Limitations of joint mobility and joint pain (especially the cervical spine and shoulders), paresthesias due to nerve damage, and gait disturbance frequently are a part of the syndrome. Most patients also have visceral adiposity with insulin resistance, hepatomegaly, and hyperglycemia	E88.2
Familial multiple lipomatosis Familial multiple symmetric lipomatosis Multiple familial lipomatosis	Encapsulated Characterized by painless lipomas of the neck, arms, abdomen, and thighs that most commonly appear in the third decade of life Most affected individuals have generalized adiposity and insulin resistance Lipomas may be multiple and large	E88.2
Encephalocutaneous lipomatosis *Haberland syndrome* *Hemihyperplasia-multiple lipomatosis syndrome* *Neurolipomatosis* *Roch-Leri mesosomatous lipomatosis*		E88.2
Fat necrosis Fatty degeneration Lipoid degeneration *Lipomatosis gigantea* *Lipomatosis renis* *Nodular circumscribed lipomatosis*		E78.89

Table 6.2 (continued)

Adiposopathy condition	Characteristics	ICD-10 code
	Generalized adiposity	
Drug-induced obesity		E66.1
Obesity hypoventilation syndrome Cardiopulmonary obesity syndrome Obesity with alveolar hypoventilation Pickwickian syndrome		E66.2
Overweight	Race-defined BMI thresholds	E66.3
Obesity	Race-defined BMI thresholds Redefined based on burden of disease attributable to accrued fat mass and adiposopathy	E66.9
Obesity (classes 1 and 2; BMI 30–39.9) Exogenous obesity	Race-defined BMI thresholds	E66.09
Obesity with morbidity Morbid obesity *Extreme obesity (classes 3 and higher; BMI 40 kg/m² or higher)* *Morbid obesity with spermatogenic failure*	Excess fat mass with any associated metabolic or physical complication or comorbid condition	E66.01
Familial obesity Obesity due to specific mutations Mutation of CART gene Mutation of MC4R gene Mutation of NR0B2 gene Mutation of POMC gene Mutation of SIM1 gene *Endogenous obesity* *Hypogonadal obesity*		E66.8
Adiposity (generalized) *Obesity due to cancer therapy* *Obesity of nonendocrine origin*		E66.9
Adiponectin deficiency *Obesity due to leptin deficiency*		E88.9
Hypothalamic obesity		E34.8
Obesity of endocrine origin		E34.9

6.6.2 *Lipomas*

A lipoma is a benign tumor composed of adipose tissue, which is mostly fat. Lipomas literally translate as a tumor of fat. Lipomas have been described everywhere in the human body, since adipose tissue is distributed wherever the vasculature reaches.

Lipomas have a defined mass, which is circumscribed or encapsulated, and are composed of mature adipocytes. Lipomas cause medical problems by their mass effect when they grow in constrained spaces. Examples of this include retro-orbital lipomas, spinal canal lipomas, and angiomyolipomas.

6.6.3 *Adiposis Dolorosa*

AD was first described in 1892 by Dr. Francis Xavier Dercum to describe the growth of encapsulated lipomas anywhere in the subcutaneous fat, from small nodules to large masses, many becoming painful, and being tender to touch. Dercum's disease, as AD is commonly named in the literature, represents a small percentage of patients affected with lipomas.

6.6.4 *Familial Multiple Lipomatosis (FML)*

FML is an autosomal dominant disease which can be traced over generations in an affected family. Affected individuals have numerous individual lipomas throughout the body. Chromosome 12, locus q15, which encodes the high-mobility group protein isoform I-C, is translocated with the lipoma preferred partner gene on chromosome 3. Other translocation partners have been described in chromosomes 1, 2, 4, 5, 6, 7, 10, 11, 13, 15, 17, 21, and X.

6.6.5 *Symmetrical Lipomatosis (SL)*

In 1846, the British surgeon, Sir Benjamin Collins Brodie, described an individual with the abnormal symmetrical accumulation of adipose tissue in the upper body. His patient had nuchal lipomas. In 1888, Madelung, in Germany, and in 1898, Launois and Bensaude, in France, each reported patients with upper body SL. Four distinct SL phenotypes can now be distinguished based on the predominant distribution of adipose tissue.

- Type 1 is located primarily in the cervical and upper back region giving a "horse collar" appearance. This is associated with alcohol use (Fig. 6.3).
- Type 2 is located on the shoulders, upper arms, and chest causing a "pseudo-athletic" look. This is not associated with alcohol use. It may cause lipomastia (Fig. 6.4).
- Type 3 is located in the waist and pelvic area and has a "gynecoid" appearance. The term "steatopygia" is used to describe this when the accumulation is mostly around the buttocks, typically in women of African ancestry (Fig. 6.5).
- Type 4 affects the hands and the soles of the feet.

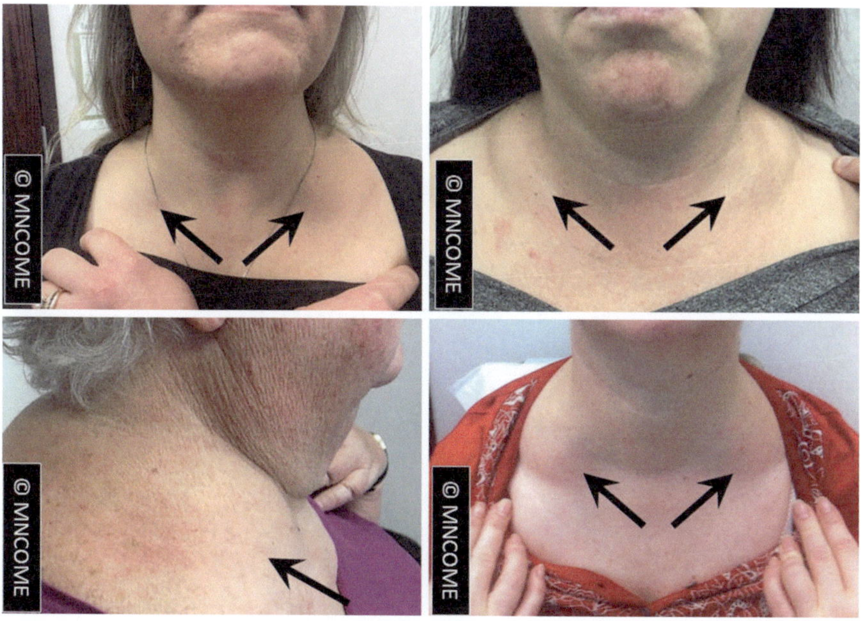

Fig. 6.3 Symmetrical lipomatosis, type 1

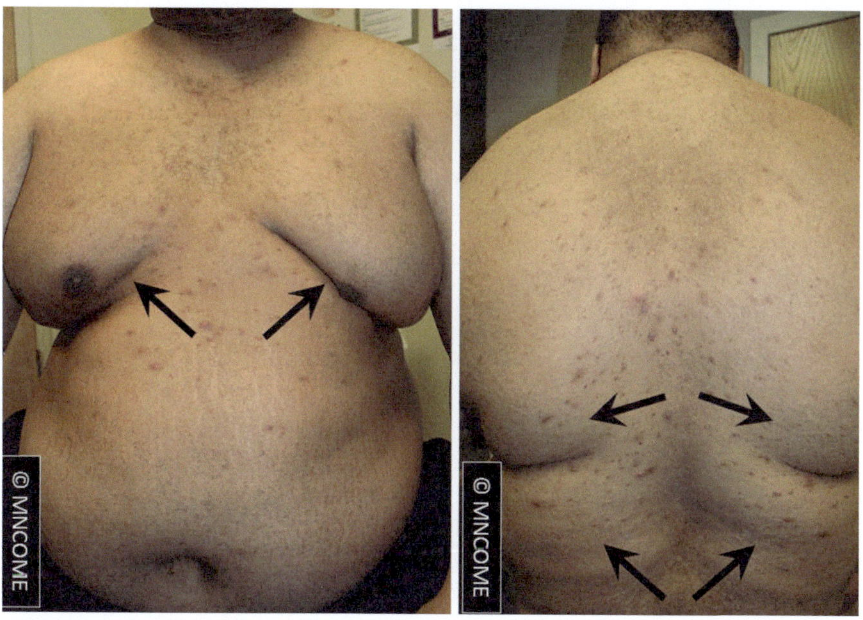

Fig. 6.4 Symmetrical lipomatosis, type 2

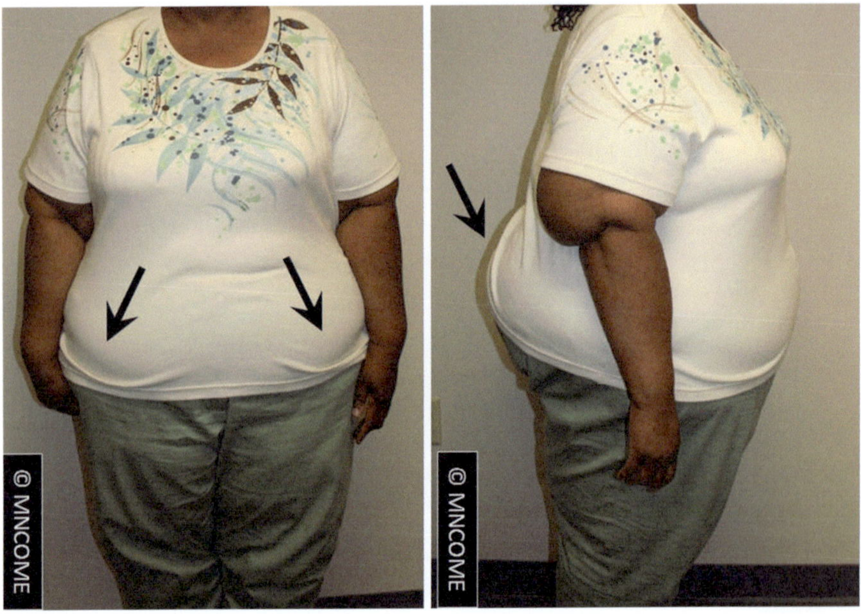

Fig. 6.5 Symmetrical lipomatosis, type 3

Mitochondrial gene mutations and/or deletions are known to cause many cases of SL. Adipose tissue from lipomas in SL is not different in the morphologic appearance and the surface marker profile compared to normal adipose tissue. Compared to individual lipomas, where the mass is easily circumscribed and identified (Fig. 6.6), in SL the lipomas do not bear this characteristic. In SL, the adipose tissue organizes and grows to a considerable size. In SL, stem cells from lipomas have marked changes in genes associated with proliferation, hormonal regulation, and mitochondria, assessed by polymerase chain reaction arrays.

6.6.6 *Other Disorders of Regional Fat Distribution*

Table 6.2 lists many of the disorders that together represent the spectrum of adiposopathy. Lipohypertrophy refers to a reversible increase in adipose tissue volume that develops under the influence of insulin when it is repeatedly injected in the same site (Fig. 6.7). This process, by definition, is reversible upon discontinuation of the repeated injections at that site. Gynecomastia should be distinguished from lipomastia. In gynecomastia, there is a glandular breast tissue that develops, and this is in response to a change in the ratio of estrogens to androgens in males. A decrease in testosterone and an increase in estrogen, as is seen in obesity, predisposes men to develop gynecomastia. Lipomastia, on the other hand, is purely adipose tissue in the anatomical area of the breasts. Lipomastia may be due to SL, type 2 (Fig. 6.4).

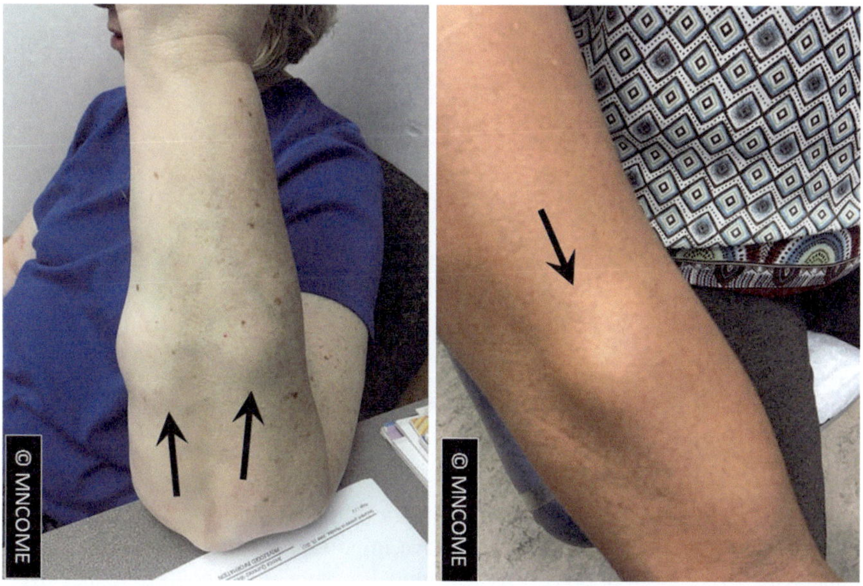

Fig. 6.6 Lipomatosis

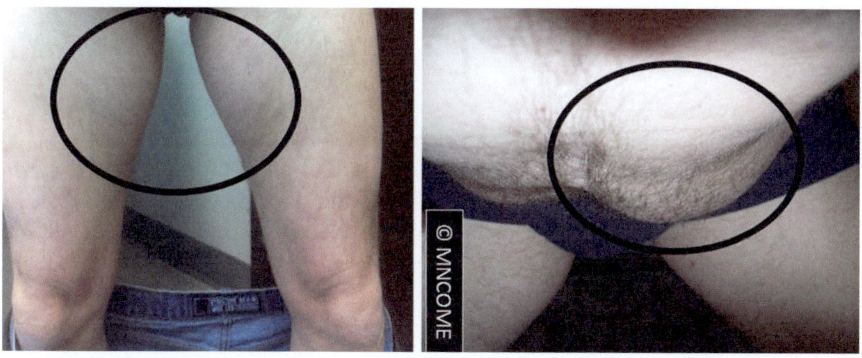

Fig. 6.7 Lipohypertrophy

Finally, edema is common in patients with obesity. It may be due to venous insufficiency of the lower extremities, increased intra-abdominal pressure decreasing venous return to the heart, portal hypertension from the development of a cirrhotic liver in the setting of progressive steatohepatitis, or heart failure itself. Lipedema may occur, and this must be distinguished from pitting edema. Lipedema is the accumulation of fat mass around the lower limbs (Fig. 6.8). There are several stages of lipedema. Weight loss may not help lipedema that is long standing, but it does help early stages.

Collectively, these distinct disorders represent distinct manifestations of adiposopathy. For individuals with these regional fat distribution syndromes, improving

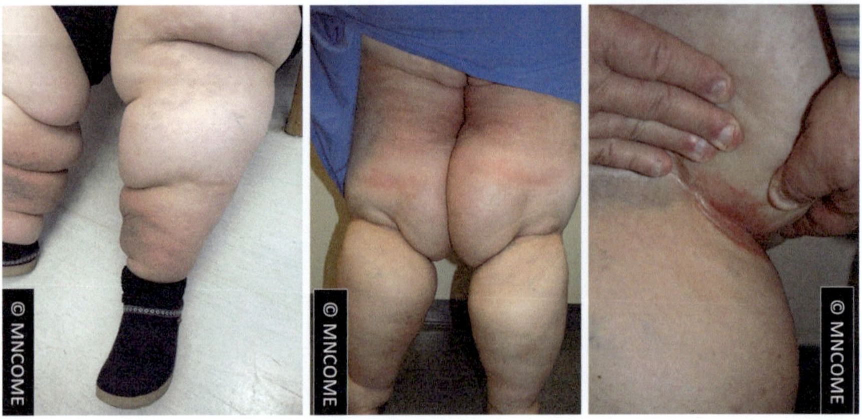

Fig. 6.8 Lipoedema

quality of life involves removal of symptomatic adipose tissue deposits. Liposuction or excision remains the main treatment. An important parallel goal is to treat the underlying overweight or obesity as a chronic disease with the goals to reduce overall fat mass, to prevent reaccumulation of abnormal fat deposits, and to return adipose tissue function to normal.

6.7 Conclusion

Adipose tissue becomes diseased as it experiences changes in structure and function due to the accumulation of fat mass. Adipose tissue is at the crossroads of metabolism, and adiposopathy contributes to the generation of other metabolic diseases. Bariatric endocrinology recognizes that adipose tissue is an endocrine organ and makes the treatment of adiposopathy a primary treatment target. Recognized disorders of regional fat distribution need to be addressed in individual patients, so the bariatric endocrinologist must be fluent with them.

Reading List

Bays HE. Adiposopathy is "sick fat" a cardiovascular disease? J Am Coll Cardiol. 2011; 57(25):2461–73. Epub 2011/06/18.

Bays HE, Gonzalez-Campoy JM. Adiposopathy. In: Friedberg E, Castrillon DH, Galindo RL, Wharton K, editors. New-opathies. Hackensack: World Scientific; 2012. p. 105–68.

Bays H, Rodbard HW, Schorr AB, Gonzalez-Campoy JM. Adiposopathy: treating pathogenic adipose tissue to reduce cardiovascular disease risk. Curr Treat Options Cardiovasc Med. 2007;9(4):259–71. Epub 2007/09/01.

Bays HE, Gonzalez-Campoy JM, Henry RR, Bergman DA, Kitabchi AE, Schorr AB, et al. Is adiposopathy (sick fat) an endocrine disease? Int J Clin Pract. 2008;62(10):1474–83. Epub 2008/08/07.

Bluher M. Adipose tissue dysfunction contributes to obesity related metabolic diseases. Best Pract Res Clin Endocrinol Metab. 2013;27(2):163–77. Epub 2013/06/05.

Bozec, A., Hannemann, N. Mechanism of Regulation of Adipocyte Numbers in Adult Organisms Through Differentiation and Apoptosis Homeostasis. J. Vis. Exp. (112), e53822, https://doi.org/10.3791/53822 (2016).

Buechler C, Krautbauer S, Eisinger K. Adipose tissue fibrosis. World J Diabetes. 2015;6(4):548–53. Epub 2015/05/20.

Choe SS, Huh JY, Hwang IJ, Kim JI, Kim JB. Adipose tissue remodeling: its role in energy metabolism and metabolic disorders. Front Endocrinol. 2016;7:30. Epub 2016/05/06.

Chong PS, Vucic S, Hedley-Whyte ET, Dreyer M, Cros D. Multiple symmetric lipomatosis (Madelung's disease) caused by the MERRF (A8344G) mutation: a report of two cases and review of the literature. J Clin Neuromuscul Dis. 2003;5(1):1–7. Epub 2003/09/01.

Cohen PG. Abdominal obesity and intra-abdominal pressure: a new paradigm for the pathogenesis of the hypogonadal-obesity-BPH-LUTS connection. Horm Mol Biol Clin Invest. 2012;11(1):317–20. Epub 2012/10/01.

De Pergola G, Silvestris F. Obesity as a major risk factor for cancer. J Obes. 2013;2013:291546. Epub 2013/09/28.

Dercum FX. Three cases of a hitherto unclassified affection resembling in its grosser aspects obesity, but associated with special nervous symptoms—adiposis dolorosa. Am J Med Sci. 1892;104(6):521–85.

Farb MG, Gokce N. Visceral adiposopathy: a vascular perspective. Horm Mol Biol Clin Invest. 2015;21(2):125–36. Epub 2015/03/18.

Farb MG, Ganley-Leal L, Mott M, Liang Y, Ercan B, Widlansky ME, et al. Arteriolar function in visceral adipose tissue is impaired in human obesity. Arterioscler Thromb Vasc Biol. 2012;32(2):467–73. Epub 2011/11/19.

Findlay GH, Duvenage M. Acquired symmetrical lipomatosis of the hands—a distal form of the Madelung-Launois-Bensaude syndrome. Clin Exp Dermatol. 1989;14(1):58–9. Epub 1989/01/01.

Garcia-Fuentes E, Santiago-Fernandez C, Gutierrez-Repiso C, Mayas MD, Oliva-Olivera W, Coin-Araguez L, et al. Hypoxia is associated with a lower expression of genes involved in lipogenesis in visceral adipose tissue. J Transl Med. 2015;13:373. Epub 2015/12/02.

Gonzalez-Campoy JM, Richardson B, Richardson C, Gonzalez-Cameron D, Ebrahim A, Strobel P, et al. Bariatric endocrinology: principles of medical practice. Int J Endocrinol. 2014;2014:917813. Epub 2014/06/06.

Goossens GH, Blaak EE. Adipose tissue oxygen tension: implications for chronic metabolic and inflammatory diseases. Curr Opin Clin Nutr Metab Care. 2012;15(6):539–46. Epub 2012/10/06.

Greene ML, Glueck CJ, Fujimoto WY, Seegmiller JE. Benign symmetric lipomatosis (Launois-Bensaude adenolipomatosis) with gout and hyperlipoproteinemia. Am J Med. 1970;48(2):239–46. Epub 1970/02/01.

Heilbronn LK, Campbell LV. Adipose tissue macrophages, low grade inflammation and insulin resistance in human obesity. Curr Pharm Des. 2008;14(12):1225–30. Epub 2008/05/14.

Hodson L. Adipose tissue oxygenation: effects on metabolic function. Adipocytes. 2014;3(1):75–80. Epub 2014/02/28.

Hosogai N, Fukuhara A, Oshima K, Miyata Y, Tanaka S, Segawa K, et al. Adipose tissue hypoxia in obesity and its impact on adipocytokine dysregulation. Diabetes. 2007;56(4):901–11. Epub 2007/03/31.

Klopstock T, Naumann M, Seibel P, Shalke B, Reiners K, Reichmann H. Mitochondrial DNA mutations in multiple symmetric lipomatosis. Mol Cell Biochem. 1997;174(1–2):271–5. Epub 1997/10/06.

Landini L, Honka MJ, Ferrannini E, Nuutila P. Adipose tissue oxygenation in obesity: a matter of cardiovascular risk? Curr Pharm Des. 2015;22(1):68–76. Epub 2015/11/12.

Leung NW, Gaer J, Beggs D, Kark AE, Holloway B, Peters TJ. Multiple symmetric lipomatosis (Launois-Bensaude syndrome): effect of oral salbutamol. Clin Endocrinol. 1987;27(5):601–6. Epub 1987/11/01.
Neels JG, Olefsky JM. Inflamed fat: what starts the fire? J Clin Invest. 2006;116(1):33–5. Epub 2006/01/06.
Noh E. An unusual complication of morbid obesity: epidural lipomatosis. Am J Emerg Med. 2015;33(5):742 e3–4. Epub 2015/01/27.
Plotnicov NA, Babayev TA, Lamberg MA, Altonen M, Syrjanen SM. Madelung's disease (benign symmetric lipomatosis). Oral Surg Oral Med Oral Pathol. 1988;66(2):171–5. Epub 1988/08/01.
Prantl L, Schreml J, Gehmert S, Klein S, Bai X, Zeitler K, et al. Transcription profile in sporadic multiple symmetric lipomatosis reveals differential expression at the level of adipose tissue-derived stem cells. Plast Reconstr Surg. 2016;137(4):1181–90. Epub 2016/03/29.
Rasmussen JC, Herbst KL, Aldrich MB, Darne CD, Tan IC, Zhu B, et al. An abnormal lymphatic phenotype is associated with subcutaneous adipose tissue deposits in Dercum's disease. Obesity (Silver Spring). 2014;22(10):2186–92. Epub 2014/07/22.
Requena L, Hasson A, Arias D, Martin L, Barat A. Acquired symmetric lipomatosis of the soles. A plantar form of the Madelung-Launois-Bensaude syndrome. J Am Acad Dermatol. 1992;26(5 Pt 2):860–2. Epub 1992/05/01.
Schuler FA 3rd, Graham JK, Horton CE. Benign symmetrical lipomatosis (Madelung's disease). Case report. Plast Reconstr Surg. 1976;57(5):662–5. Epub 1976/05/01.
Sreekantaiah C, Leong SP, Karakousis CP, McGee DL, Rappaport WD, Villar HV, et al. Cytogenetic profile of 109 lipomas. Cancer Res. 1991;51(1):422–33. Epub 1991/01/01.
Subash M, Aziz A, O'Doherty M, Olver JM. Lipomatosis of the orbits: possibly a form of Madelung's disease. Eye (Lond). 2012;26(6):894–5. Epub 2012/04/14.
Ulusoy OL, Kafadar C, Ozturk E, Mutlu A, Sirvanci M. Idiopathic thoracic epidural lipomatosis presenting with back pain. Spine J. 2016;16(8):e487–8. Epub 2016/01/24.
Weber FP. Diffuse Symmetrical Lipomatosis. Proc R Soc Med. 1912;5(Clin Sect):142. Epub 1912/01/01.
Wood IS, de Heredia FP, Wang B, Trayhurn P. Cellular hypoxia and adipose tissue dysfunction in obesity. Proc Nutr Soc. 2009;68(4):370–7. Epub 2009/08/25.
Ye J. Emerging role of adipose tissue hypoxia in obesity and insulin resistance. Int J Obes. 2009;33(1):54–66. Epub 2008/12/04.
Yin J, Gao Z, He Q, Zhou D, Guo Z, Ye J. Role of hypoxia in obesity-induced disorders of glucose and lipid metabolism in adipose tissue. Am J Physiol Endocrinol Metab. 2009;296(2):E333–42. Epub 2008/12/11.
Zachar V, Duroux M, Emmersen J, Rasmussen JG, Pennisi CP, Yang S, et al. Hypoxia and adipose-derived stem cell-based tissue regeneration and engineering. Expert Opin Biol Ther. 2011;11(6):775–86. Epub 2011/03/19.
Zhang X, Lam KS, Ye H, Chung SK, Zhou M, Wang Y, et al. Adipose tissue-specific inhibition of hypoxia-inducible factor 1{alpha} induces obesity and glucose intolerance by impeding energy expenditure in mice. J Biol Chem. 2010;285(43):32869–77. Epub 2010/08/19.

Chapter 7
Clinical Definition of Overweight and Obesity

W. Timothy Garvey

Pearls of Wisdom

- BMI inter-relates height and weight and is not a direct measure of adiposity. It is useful in screening patients but must be interpreted when used to diagnose overweight or obesity in the context of a physical exam that confirms increased adipose tissue mass.
- BMI does indicate the degree to which adiposity or the development of adiposopathy adversely impact health, as manifest by weight-related complications.
- Best practices require a careful evaluation for the presence and severity of weight-related complications in all patients presenting with overweight and obesity.
- Key weight-related complications can be identified during an initial patient evaluation consisting of physical examination, history, clinical laboratory testing, and an obesity-focused review of systems.
- In bariatric endocrinology an optimal diagnostic framework incorporates an anthropometric measure of increased adiposity (i.e., BMI) together with an assessment of the presence and severity of weight-related complications (including adiposopathy).

W. Timothy Garvey
Department of Nutrition Sciences, The University of Alabama at Birmingham, University of Alabama Hospital, Birmingham, AL, USA

The Birmingham VA Medical Center, Birmingham, AL, USA
e-mail: garveyt@uab.edu

J. M. Gonzalez-Campoy et al. (eds.), *Bariatric Endocrinology*,
https://doi.org/10.1007/978-3-319-95655-8_7

7.1 Introduction

Body mass index (BMI) is widely used in the screening, diagnosis, and classification of overweight and obesity. The World Health Organization (WHO) criteria shown in Table 7.1 are widely accepted, with BMI 25–29.9 kg/m^2 indicative of overweight and BMI $\geq$ 30 kg/m^2 indicative of obesity, designated as class I (BMI = 30–34.9 kg/m^2), class II (35–39.9 kg/m^2), or severe class III ($\geq$40 kg/m^2). BMI is an anthropometric measurement that inter-relates height and weight (kg/m^2) and does not provide a direct measure of adipose tissue mass. Furthermore, BMI does not indicate the degree to which excess adiposity can lead to adiposopathy, or adversely affects the health of individual patients. The risk, presence, and severity of multiple weight-related complications vary markedly among patients at any given BMI level. It is the presence and severity of complications that indicate whether any degree of excess adiposity has caused adiposopathy and is adversely affecting the health of individual patients. While the likelihood of weight-related complications generally increases as a function of progressive obesity, there can be a poor correlation between BMI and the emergence of complications. Patients with overweight or obesity need not have weight-related complications and can be free of disease-related morbidity and mortality. For these reasons, the diagnostic evaluation of obesity extends beyond BMI and requires a careful clinical assessment for weight-related complications. This is consistent with the genetic model for chronic disease where the interaction between susceptibility genes and the environment produces the disease, and additional and perhaps overlapping subsets of genes interacting with the environment determine the severity of the disease and the emergence and severity of complications.

This chapter will discuss the advantages and limitations of BMI when used in the diagnosis of overweight or obesity. While BMI can suffice as a screening tool for obesity, the need for clinical interpretation is required in the use of BMI as a mea-

Table 7.1 Classification of overweight and obesity by BMI and waist circumference

	BMI		Waist	
			Waist circumference and comorbidity risk	
Classification	BMI (kg/m^2)	Comorbidity risk	Men $\leq$40 inches Women $\leq$35 inches	Men >40 inches Women >35 inches
Underweight	<18.5	Low but other problems		
Normal weight	18.5–24.9	Average		
Overweight	25–29.9	Increased	Increased	High
Obesity class I	30–34.9	Moderate	High	Very high
Obesity class II	35–39.9	Severe	Very high	Very high
Obesity class III	$\geq$40	Very severe	Extremely high	Extremely high

Adapted from: World Health Organization (WHO) (1998); used with permission

sure of adiposity for diagnosis of the disease. In addition, the careful clinical assessment of the risk, presence, and severity of weight-related complications will be emphasized as an integral component of best practices in obesity management. As will be discussed, this assessment can be accomplished with a "new patient" history, physical examination, and laboratory testing in addition to an obesity-focused review of systems (ROS). Thus, the optimal diagnostic framework has two components: the assessment of adipose tissue mass and the impact of excess adiposity on health as manifest by disease complications. This diagnostic framework is clinically actionable since it provides an indication of disease severity and can help guide clinical decisions regarding the modality and intensity of therapy.

7.2 The Anthropometric Component of the Diagnosis of Obesity

7.2.1 BMI and the Assessment of Adipose Tissue Mass

Adolphe Quetelet first proposed the Quetelet Index, body mass (kg)/height (m^2), as a measure of obesity in 1859. He was a Belgian astronomer and mathematician who developed an interest in quantifying individual variation in human traits and behaviors, a discipline he termed "social physics." In 1972, the Quetelet Index was renamed the BMI by Ancel Keys, a polymath, nutritionist, epidemiologist, and inventor, after "validating" BMI against skin fold thickness in his Seven Countries Study, which established a relationship between serum cholesterol and heart disease and the first endorsement of the "Mediterranean Diet." Other approaches used to assess obesity include the Ponderal Index (weight/height^3) first proposed by Ridolpho Livi in 1898 but popularized by F. Rohrer in 1921 as the Corpulence Index and applied to newborns (weight/crown-to-heel-length^3). The rationale for the Ponderal Index was that a cubic function was more appropriate for an obesity measurement that essentially represents a volume. Another approach is the relative body weight using actuarial tables of the Metropolitan Life Insurance Company to assess relative weight for a given height after adjusting for a small, medium, or large frame. Relative body weight has the disadvantage of not providing an absolute value of body mass and uses actuarial standards from 1959 that do not reflect the average increments in average body weight that have occurred over the past three decades.

The WHO adopted BMI for the clinical classification of obesity in 1998. The WHO promulgated the widespread application of BMI in epidemiology and medicine (Table 7.1). The National Institutes of Health adopted BMI as the measure for obesity classification and interventional recommendations soon thereafter, as delineated in Table 7.2. Subsequently, BMI cut-offs have predominated in the diagnosis of obesity and in the clinical classification of the severity of obesity. BMI is widely employed in epidemiological and physiological scientific investigations, guidelines for obesity management advocated by multiple health care organizations, by the

Table 7.2 NHLBI obesity treatment guidelines

Treatment	BMI category (kg/m²) 25–26.9	27–29.9	30–34.9	35–39.9	≥40
Diet, physical activity, and behavior	Appropriate NHLBI guidelines	+	+	+	+
Pharmacotherapy	No	With comorbidities	+	+	+
Surgery[a]	No	No	No[a]	With comorbidities	+

Adopted from: Summary of recommendations in the clinical guidelines on the identification, evaluation, and treatment of overweight and obesity in adults. National Institutes of Health/National Heart, Lung and Blood Institute; 1998. http://www.nhlbi.nih.gov/guidelines/obesity/ob_gdlns.pdf
No = not indicated, + = clinically indicated for consideration
[a]US Food and Drug Administration (FDA)-approved gastric banding surgery for patients with BMI of at least 30 kg/m² and one weight-related medical condition (February 2011)

FDA in setting indications for weight loss medications, and in the clinical evaluation of patients as the basis for the diagnosis of obesity. In children and adolescents, obesity is defined as ≥ 95% percentile of BMI, as a function of age and gender, using the Centers for Disease Control growth charts.

The use of BMI in screening and diagnosis of obesity has advantages and disadvantages. Height and weight are easily measured, and BMI generally correlates with adipose tissue mass in population studies. It is useful for the initial screening to detect excess body fat, and higher BMI levels are associated with increased risk of complications of obesity. There is a large body of evidence correlating higher BMI with diabetes, gestational diabetes, and atherosclerotic cardiovascular disease (CVD), including stroke and recurrent coronary events in those with coronary artery disease. BMI confers increasing risk of coronary artery disease beyond 25 kg/m² in both genders. Mortality generally correlates with increasing BMI above 25 kg/m². The mortality correlation carries varying degrees of consistency among different populations and is partly explained by a correlation between BMI and certain types of cancer. In the general population and in patients with type 2 diabetes mellitus (T2DM), there is a J-shaped curve relating BMI with mortality. In those individuals who have never smoked cigarettes, BMI values >30 kg/m² are consistently associated with higher mortality. In these individuals, the increased risk of mortality is not as clearly defined for the BMI range 25–30 kg/m². The increases in metabolic diseases and CVD are conferred more directly by other risk factors that may be associated with obesity. The impact of BMI is diminished when these risk factors are accounted for in multivariate analyses.

BMI cut-offs for identifying excess adiposity and risk of metabolic and cardiac diseases are lower for some Asian-Pacific populations and should be taken into account when screening. Based upon the evidence that lower BMI values are correlated with the risk of T2DM, the American Diabetes Association recommends that screening for diabetes should be considered for all Asian American adults who present with a BMI of ≥23 kg/m². The body of evidence addressing this issue, including meta-analyses performed by the Working Group on Obesity in China, suggests that using a BMI cut-off of ≥23 kg/m^2 would be the optimal single criterion for screening all Asian ethnicities.

Regarding the limitations of BMI, it is important to consider that BMI is an anthropometric measure that inter-relates the height and weight of individuals. The weight measurement used in the calculation incorporates lean mass, fat mass, bone mass, and fluid status; all of these body components contribute to weight. Therefore, BMI is only an indirect measure for the estimation of total body fat mass. Lean mass and body water can vary independently from fat mass, and, for this reason, BMI alone cannot identify excess adiposity and establish a diagnosis of overweight or obesity in all instances. BMI may have poor inter-individual consistency for estimating body fat percentage and distribution. BMI will overestimate adiposity in athletes with high muscle mass and low percent body fat and underestimate adiposity in elderly patients with sarcopenia. The degree of adiposity is also overestimated in patients with edema. The imprecision of BMI as a measure of adiposity weakens the association of BMI with health risks and impairs its utilization as a risk factor. For example, BMI inadequately predicts the risk of metabolic and vascular diseases in those with sarcopenic obesity. Waist circumference is a more accurate predictor than BMI of the high mortality rates that characterize these patients. Along these same lines, low lean mass index predicts mortality in the elderly better than BMI.

The limitations in BMI as a measure of adiposity have important clinical ramifications. While BMI can be used to screen for the presence of obesity, it cannot by itself be used to diagnose overweight or obesity. For diagnosis, the BMI measurement must be clinically interpreted based on medical history and physical examination of the patient. It will be important to ascertain whether the patient has edema or sarcopenia, or is an athlete with high muscle mass, or other conditions listed in Table 7.3. Clinical judgment must then be used to identify those with a low BMI but with excess adiposity, as well as those with high BMI but normal or low percent body fat.

Additional approaches are available that primarily estimate body fat mass as shown in Table 7.4. Some methods involve high-cost equipment. Others are more feasibly conducted in the research arena, such as magnetic resonance imaging, three-dimensional photonic scanning, and total body water dilution techniques. Other measures can be applied in patient care venues. There are several commercially available bioelectric impedance plethysmography devices that are inexpensive and which can estimate body fat. Bioelectric impedance analyses are dependent on the state of hydration of the patient and become less accurate at high degrees of adiposity. Other methods entail more expensive equipment but provide measures that are more highly correlated with results using underwater weighting as the "gold standard." These include air displacement plethysmography and dual-energy X-ray absorptiometry (DXA). DXA has the advantages of providing measures of bone mass and density, lean mass, and fat mass in addition to regional fat distribution (i.e., limbs versus trunk). DXA can quantify intra-abdominal fat by subtracting subcutaneous fat estimates from total trunk adipose. Body fat percentage cut-off points for obesity have been proposed by the WHO to be 25% and 35% for men and women, respectively. One measurement available from a DXA scan is the fat mass

Table 7.3 Limitations of BMI in the screening and diagnosis of obesity

1. BMI inter-relates height and weight but does not directly measure adiposity
2. When applied as an index of adiposity, BMI requires interpretation based on individual clinical assessment with attention to the following: Muscularity Volume status – edema and dehydration Sarcopenia Age Gender Pregnancy Third space fluid accumulation (e.g., ascites) Large tumors (e.g., uterine leiomyosarcomas) Lipodystrophy Loss of muscle mass due to denervation or intrinsic myopathy
3. BMI does not indicate location or distribution of fat Intracellular Extracellular but within the tissue (e.g., "marbling") Peri-organ (mesenteric, pericardial, and perinephric) Subcutaneous versus intra-abdominal Adipose tissue depots (omentum and gluteal) Brown fat versus white fat
4. BMI does not indicate the degree to which excess adiposity is adversely affecting the health of the patient.

Table 7.4 Methods for quantifying adipose tissue mass

Feature measured	Advantages	Method	Limitations
Total body water Extracellular and intracellular fluid spaces	Ease of use Low cost Speed (fast)	Bioelectrical impedance analysis (BIA)	Population specific Poor accuracy in individuals
Total and regional body fat Total and regional lean mass	Ease of use Low radiation exposure Accurate	Dual-energy X-ray absorptiometry (DXA)	Biased for body size, sex, and fatness High equipment cost Specially trained personnel
Total body water Extracellular fluid	Ease of use OK for all ages	Dilution techniques	Inaccurate in disease High equipment cost Labor-intensive analysis
Total body volume Total body fat	Relatively good accuracy Speed (fast)	Air displacement plethysmography	Less accurate in disease High equipment cost
Total and regional body volume	OK for very obese Ease of use	3D photonic scanning	Limited availability
Total body water Total body fat	Ease of use Safety Speed (fast)	Quantitative magnetic resonance imaging	High equipment cost Limited availability
Total and regional adipose tissue Skeletal muscle	Highly accurate and reproducible	Magnetic resonance imaging (MRI)	Costly

index, which is calculated as total body fat mass (kg) divided by height (m^2). The fat mass index is analogous to the BMI but incorporates only fat mass as the weight measure instead of total body weight.

7.2.2 *Waist Circumference and the Importance of Intra-abdominal Fat Mass*

Beyond the assessment of BMI, the next consideration is the distribution of body fat. Accumulation of excess fat in different fat depots can have significant implications for disease risk. The accumulation of visceral adipose tissue, which surrounds organs in the intra-abdominal compartment, is central to the pathophysiology of metabolic and vascular diseases. Central to the disease process is insulin resistance, which progresses to dysmetabolic syndrome, prediabetes, and finally to T2DM, CVD, or both, in individual patients. Also integral to disease pathogenesis is adiposopathy, with inflammation and dysregulated secretion of adipocytokines in visceral adipose tissue, which leads to the development of the dysmetabolic syndrome trait complex. On the other hand, a relative distribution of fat to the periphery (i.e., upper and lower extremities and hips) generally occurs in the subcutaneous space. Subcutaneous adipose tissue accumulation carries a lower risk of metabolic or vascular disease, when adjusting for BMI and age.

Waist circumference estimates visceral adipose tissue and is the simplest anthropometric measurement of abdominal adiposity in clinical settings. Waist circumference consistently and strongly predicts components of dysmetabolic syndrome, T2DM, CVD risk factors, and CVD events in cross-sectional studies and prospective cohorts. The predictive value of waist circumference for CVD and all-cause mortality is generally independent of and stronger than BMI and is even evident in lean individuals with BMI < 25 kg/m^2. As shown in Table 7.1, adding waist circumference to BMI more precisely categorizes metabolic and vascular risk in patients with overweight or obesity. Waist circumference should be measured when screening for obesity and obesity-related comorbidities. This is best done in a private setting using a tension-controlled tape measure placed around the waist just above the anterior superior iliac spine, on a plane horizontal to the floor. Threshold values that are indicative of increased risk of diabetes and CVD are delineated in Table 7.5, as recommended in a joint statement from multiple professional organizations attempting to harmonize criteria for the dysmetabolic syndrome.

Three salient points are important concerning the interpretation of waist circumference measurements. First, waist circumference cut-off points for predicting metabolic and vascular diseases exhibit ethnic variation, including a consistently lower threshold in South Asian, Southeast Asian, and East Asian adults. Therefore, population-specific cut-off values should be used as established by epidemiological studies in regional cohorts (Table 7.5). Second, waist circumference measurements are most discriminative of greater chronic disease risk in individuals with BMI ≤ 35 kg/m^2. When the BMI exceeds 35 kg/m^2, most patients will exceed the

Table 7.5 Waist circumference thresholds for abdominal obesity

Population	Organization	Men	Women
Europid	IDF	≥94 cm ≥37 inches	≥80 cm ≥31 inches
Caucasian	WHO	≥94 cm (↑ risk) ≥37 inches ≥102 cm (↑↑ risk ≥40 inches	≥80 cm (↑ risk) ≥31 inches ≥88 cm (↑↑ risk) ≥35 inches
United states	AHA/NHLBI (ATPIII)	≥102 cm ≥40 inches	≥88 cm ≥35 inches
Canada	Health Canada	≥102 cm ≥40 inches	≥88 cm ≥35 inches
European	European Cardiovascular Societies	≥102 cm ≥40 inches	≥88 cm ≥35 inches
Asian (including Japanese)	IDF	≥90 cm ≥35 inches	≥80 cm ≥31 inches
Asian	WHO	≥90 cm ≥35 inches	≥80 cm ≥31 inches
Japanese	Japanese Obesity Society	≥85 cm ≥33 inches	≥90 cm ≥35 inches
China	Cooperative Task Force	≥85 cm ≥33 inches	≥80 cm ≥31 inches
Middle East, Mediterranean	IDF	≥94 cm ≥37 inches	≥80 cm ≥31 inches
Sub-Saharan African	IDF	≥94 cm ≥37 inches	≥80 cm ≥31 inches
Ethnic Central and South American	IDF	≥90 cm ≥35 inches	≥80 cm ≥31 inches

Adapted from: Alberti et al. (2009)
IDF International Diabetes Federation, *WHO* World Health Organization, *AHA* American Heart Association, *NHLBI* National Heart, Lung, and Blood Institute, *ATPIII* Adult Treatment Panel III

waist circumference cut-off value, whether or not they have insulin resistance or have manifestations of metabolic disease. Finally, it is important to understand that risks conferred by waist circumference are continuous despite the use of categorical cut-off values. Thus, at any given BMI (above and below a BMI of 35 kg/m^2), risks of T2DM and CVD increase progressively, with additional increments in waist circumference.

The waist circumference encompasses subcutaneous adipose tissue, trunk musculature, and abdominal organs, and, therefore, it represents only an estimation of intra-abdominal fat. Intra-abdominal fat can be estimated in the analyses of DXA scans by subtracting subcutaneous fat (from fat mass estimates in the lateral flanks) from total abdominal fat. Intra-abdominal fat can be quantified by magnetic resonance imaging or transverse CAT scan, although these measures are primarily relegated to research studies.

It is unclear whether waist circumference or waist-to-height ratio (WHtR) is a better predictor of T2DM and CVD risks. However, WHtR has better discriminatory power for CVD risk variables than BMI. A WHtR cut-off value of 0.5 is optimal for identifying those with a higher CVD risk across different genders and ethnicities.

7.3 The Clinical Component of the Diagnosis of Obesity

7.3.1 Relationship Between BMI and Weight-Related Complications

As an anthropometric measurement, BMI alone does not indicate the impact of adiposity on the health of individual patients. Since BMI alone is not a sufficient indicator of health status in overweight and obesity, all patients should be clinically evaluated for weight-related complications. While the likelihood of weight-related complications generally increases as a function of progressive obesity, there can be a poor correlation between BMI and the emergence of complications. Patients with overweight or obesity need not have weight-related complications and be free of disease-related morbidity and mortality. The variable associations between BMI and weight-related complications are exemplified below for several key complications that can adversely affect the health of patients with overweight or obesity. While it is clear that elevated BMI per se does not ensure that specific complications are present, the important consideration is that weight loss will ameliorate or prevent many weight-related complications, thus justifying a careful evaluation for their presence.

7.3.1.1 Diabetes Risk, Dysmetabolic Syndrome, and Prediabetes

Obesity is a major risk factor for the development of dysmetabolic syndrome and prediabetes (impaired fasting glucose (IFG) or impaired glucose tolerance (IGT)). Obesity is also a risk for progression to overt T2DM and CVD. However, many individuals with metabolic disease with progression to T2DM and/or CVD are lean. In addition, a significant proportion of individuals with obesity are insulin sensitive, do not exhibit dysmetabolic syndrome traits, and have been referred to as "metabolically healthy obese." While obesity can exacerbate insulin resistance, insulin sensitivity largely varies independent of BMI, and the risks of T2DM and CVD are largely conferred by the presence of metabolic traits associated with adiposopathy and insulin resistance (e.g., increased waist circumference, high triglycerides, low HDL-c, elevated blood pressure, and abnormal glucose tolerance) rather than BMI per se. Therefore, overweight or obesity as assessed by BMI are neither sufficient nor necessary as a pathogenic factor in the development of adiposopathy, insulin resistance, dysmetabolic syndrome, and prediabetes.

It is for this reason that the cardiometabolic risk staging was developed as a quantitative clinical tool that stratifies risks for T2DM and CVD in patients with overweight and obesity. CMDS assigns patients to one of five risk categories using parameters readily available to the clinician, including waist circumference, systolic and diastolic blood pressures, fasting blood glucose, triglycerides, and HDL-C, as well as the 2-h oral glucose tolerance test (OGTT) glucose value. As shown in Fig. 7.1, with advancement from stage 0 to stage 4, there are significant increments in risk and adjusted hazard ratios for diabetes. This is validated by using the Coronary Artery Risk Development in Young Adults (CARDIA) study national cohort. There is also an increased risk and hazard ratios for both all-cause and CVD-related mortality in the National Health and Nutrition Examination Survey (NHANES) cohort. The CMDS staging system is a strong predictor of risk for diabetes, CVD, and all-cause mortality independent of BMI.

More recently, a weighted CMDS system was developed that assigns different weights in the form of integer values to the various risk factors based on their relative contribution to T2DM risk. The range of the sum of integer values for all risk factors was set at 0–100 providing an overall score that was validated to be

Stage	Criteria	Specifications
0	No risk factors	Metabolically healthy obese
1	1 or 2 risk factors	Waist, blood pressure, triglycerides, HDL -c
2	Metabolic syndrome OR prediabetes	Only one of the following: metabolic syndrome or IFG or IGT
3	Metabolic syndrome plus prediabetes	Two or more of the following: metabolic syndrome, IFG, IGT
4	T2DM and/or CVD	End stage cardiometabolic disease

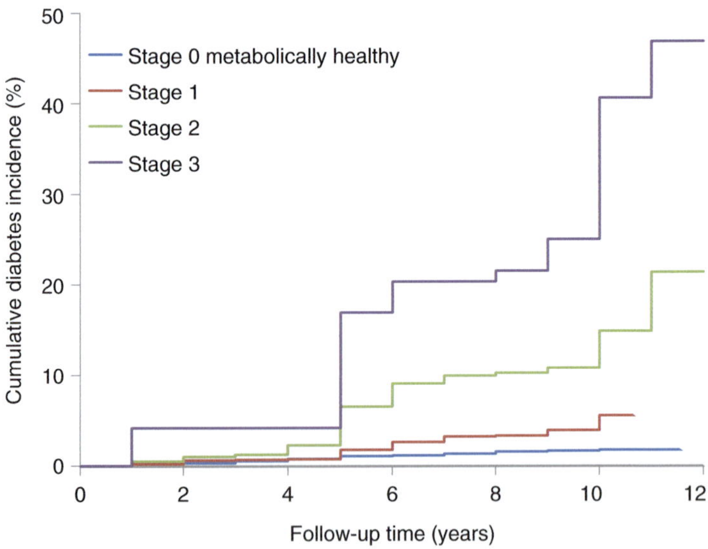

Fig. 7.1 Cardiometabolic disease staging with validation using data from the National CARDIA Study Cohort. (Adapted from: Guo et al. 2014; used with permission)

proportional to the risk of future diabetes. The relative contribution of various traits to diabetes risk varied as a function of gender and race allowing for greater precision of risk quantification in individual patients. This risk engine provides the clinician with the ability to target more aggressive weight loss therapy to those patients at the greatest risk of future T2DM and CVD.

7.3.1.2 T2DM

The proportion of adults who had normal weight at the time of incident diabetes ranged from 9% to 21% (overall 12%) across a substantial number of large cohort studies (ARIC, CARDIA, CHS, Framingham, and MESA). In the Behavior Risk Factor Surveillance System, the prevalence of diabetes is 4.1% in individuals with normal weight, 7.3% in individuals with overweight, 14.9% in class 2 obesity, and 25.6% in class 3 obesity. Thus, the clear majority of individuals with obesity do not have diabetes. While BMI is a strong risk factor for T2DM, the data indicate that BMI is a poor indicator of the presence or absence of diabetes.

7.3.1.3 Hypertension

In the serial NHANES III cross-sectional surveys from 1988 to 1994, there is a strong association between elevated BMI and hypertension. Hypertension is present in 23% of patients with a normal weight, 34–39% in patients with overweight, 48–49% in patients with class 1 obesity, 55–65% in patients with class 2 obesity, and 63–64% in patients with class 3 obesity. Thus, not all patients with overweight or obesity have hypertension. Hypertension has other risk factors independent of obesity, including age, ethnicity/race, sedentary lifestyle, cigarette smoking, high sodium intake, heavy alcohol use, stress, family history, insulin resistance, dysmetabolic syndrome, and genetic factors.

7.3.1.4 CVD Events and CVD Mortality

BMI is associated with an increased risk of CVD events, principally through its association with other risk factors. The independent risk of CVD events conferred by BMI is negated or minimized in multivariate analyses.

7.3.1.5 Nonalcoholic Fatty Liver Disease/Nonalcoholic Steatohepatitis

Seventy percent of patients with obesity have nonalcoholic fatty liver disease (NAFLD), whereas 30% do not. Only 15–20% of patients with obesity have nonalcoholic steatohepatitis (NASH). While the factors that predict which patients with NAFLD will progress to NASH and cirrhosis have not been elucidated, factors other than generalized obesity, such as insulin resistance and the dysmetabolic syndrome, appear to predominate as major contributors to NAFLD and NASH.

7.3.1.6 Female Infertility and Polycystic Ovary Syndrome (PCOS)

The prevalence rates of PCOS in women who have normal weight, overweight, or class 1 obesity were 9.8%, 9.9%, and 9.0%, respectively, with rates rising to 12.4% when the BMI is >35 kg/m^2. Thus, the majority of women who have overweight or obesity do not experience infertility or PCOS, and these problems also afflict women with a normal weight. Central adiposity and dysmetabolic syndrome are risk factors associated with PCOS independent of BMI.

7.3.1.7 Obstructive Sleep Apnea (OSA)

OSA affects ~70% of patients with obesity, and prevalence rates rise progressively as the BMI exceeds 29 kg/m^2. Clearly, not all patients with obesity have OSA. Insulin resistance, abdominal obesity, enlarged neck circumference, and T2DM are also risk factors for OSA.

7.3.1.8 Osteoarthritis

Increasing BMI is associated with progressive increments in the odds ratio for osteoarthritis of the knee in patients with severe obesity when compared with normal-weight individuals. However, osteoarthritis can afflict both individuals who are lean or who have obesity, and not all patients with overweight or obesity have osteoarthritis. Other independent risk factors for osteoarthritis include age, work history, knee trauma, participation in certain sports, and adiposopathy with elevated adipocytokines.

7.3.1.9 Urinary Stress Incontinence

BMI increases risk for stress urinary incontinence, although the majority of women who have overweight or obesity do not experience incontinence, and this disorder affects individuals with normal weight as well. Other factors in addition to BMI constitute independent risk factors for urinary incontinence, including age, waist circumference, parity, previous hysterectomy, dysmetabolic syndrome, and depression.

7.3.1.10 Gastroesophageal Reflux Disease

While there is an association with elevated BMI, GERD is common in both individuals who are lean and those with obesity. Odds ratios attributable to obesity are somewhat modest in the range of 1.22–2.8. The pathophysiology involves abnormal functioning of the lower esophageal sphincter, and other risk factors include positive family history, cigarette smoking, hiatal hernia, delayed gastric emptying, *Helicobacter pylori* infection, and alcohol consumption.

In summary, it is clear that the presence of overweight or obesity by BMI is not a good predictor of any weight-related complications. Best practices for obesity management will always necessitate a careful evaluation for the presence or absence of adiposopathy and weight-related complications.

7.3.2 Clinical Evaluation of Patients for Weight-Related Complications

The identification of weight-related complications and the staging of the severity of these complications are important for two reasons in patients with overweight or obesity. First, the presence and severity of weight-related complications will indicate the need for more aggressive therapy to improve the health of individual patients. Second, since these complications can be improved, or reversed by weight loss therapy, the evaluation will establish therapeutic targets for weight loss and the integration of these goals as desired outcomes into the therapeutic plan. For example, if a patient is diagnosed to have the dysmetabolic syndrome or prediabetes and the goal of therapy is to prevent progression to T2DM, then 10% body weight loss is a rational goal, since this represents a threshold for maximal diabetes prevention. Similarly, weight loss of 10% or greater is required to predictably decrease the apnea–hypopnea index in patients with OSA. On the other hand, if the patient has T2DM and the goal of weight loss is to improve glycemia, dyslipidemia, and hypertension, there does not appear to be a threshold of weight loss for maximal clinical benefit. For example, the Look AHEAD study demonstrated that reductions in HbA1c, blood pressure, and triglycerides and increments in HDL-c were progressive as weight loss increased from 5% to >15% body weight in patients with T2DM.

From this perspective, the goals of weight loss therapy are to improve the health of patients with overweight or obesity by treating and preventing weight-related complications. This is consistent with the "complications-centric" approach to obesity management as advocated by the American Association of Clinical Endocrinologists (AACE). In these guidelines, it is not so much the baseline BMI that is important in establishing the indications for the modality and aggressiveness of weight loss therapy but the presence and severity of weight-related complications, as illustrated by the algorithm in Fig. 7.2. This is a medical model for obesity care wherein weight loss therapy is employed to treat or prevent weight-related complications as the endpoint of therapy. This stands in contrast to a "BMI-centric" approach, such as advocated by the National Heart, Lung and Blood Institute (NHLBI) (Table 7.2), where the baseline BMI largely sets the indications for utilization of treatment modalities and where a set decrease in weight or BMI is the endpoint of therapy.

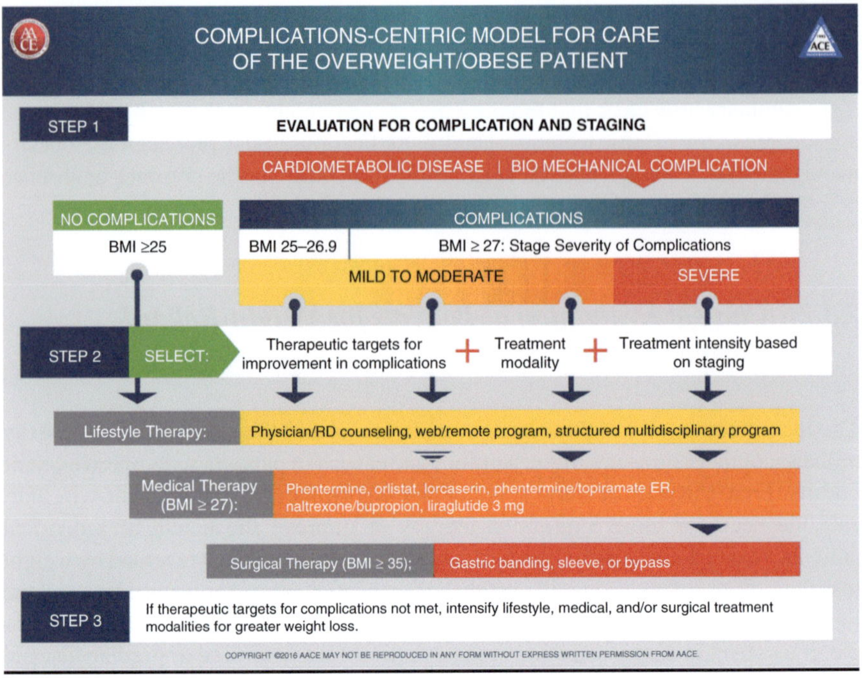

Fig. 7.2 AACE algorithm for obesity management. (Reprinted with permission from American Association of Clinical Endocrinologists © 2018. Endocr Pract. 2018;24:90–120)

The identification of complications does not involve an extensive or extraordinary degree of testing but can be ascertained in the course of an initial patient evaluation consisting of medical history, review of systems (ROS), physical examination, and laboratory studies. In the initial evaluation, the clinician will need to pay particular attention to the relevant aspects of the history and examination and conduct an obesity-focused ROS assessing potential symptomatology of weight-related complications. Clinical data that are important to obtain in the initial evaluation are listed in Table 7.6 for the physical examination, ROS, and clinical laboratory testing. These data can be used to identify the key complications that can be treated or prevented by weight loss. In many cases, the information gathered in the initial examination is sufficient for the diagnosis of certain weight-related complications. For other complications, the initial information augments the degree of suspicion, and additional testing consistent with standards of care is then necessary to confirm the diagnosis and for staging the severity of the complication. Depending on the expertise of the clinician, referral may be indicated for further evaluation and treatment of specific complications. The complications that can be prevented or treated by weight loss therapy are listed in Table 7.7 together with the basis for screening or diagnosis using clinical data obtained at the initial patient evaluation and the follow-up tests that are potentially helpful in confirming certain diagnoses and staging their severity.

Table 7.6 Key clinical data to be obtained at the initial evaluation of patients with overweight or obesity

Initial evaluation	System	Findings	Relevant complication[a]
Physical examination	Anthropometrics	Weight, BMI, waist circumference	Anthropometric component of the diagnosis of obesity, Dysmetabolic syndrome (waist)
		Neck circumference	Obstructive sleep apnea
	Vital signs	Blood pressure	Hypertension, Dysmetabolic syndrome
	General	Mobility and physical ability	Disability secondary to excess weight
	Skin	Acanthosis nigricans	Insulin resistance
		Hirsutism	Polycystic ovary syndrome
	Pulmonary	Wheezing, prolonged expiratory phase	Asthma
	Extremities	Edema	Interpretation of BMI, Edema-forming state
	Joints	Swelling, tenderness, crepitance, decreased range of motion	Osteoarthritis
	Liver	Enlarged, firm	Nonalcoholic fatty liver disease
	Muscle	Increased muscularity	Interpretation of BMI
		Weakness	Sarcopenia
	Endocrine	Thyroid, findings consistent with hypo/hyperthyroidism	Hypo/hyperthyroidism
		Stigmata of hypercortisolism	Cushing's disease
Medication history		Medications predisposing to weight gain	Iatrogenic obesity
Review of systems (obesity focused)	Metabolic	Symptoms of hyperglycemia	Diabetes
	Cardiovascular	For example, chest pain, syncope, palpitations, orthopnea, dyspnea, transient ischemic attacks, stoke history/symptoms, claudication	Cardiovascular disease
	Menstruation	Menstrual history, fertility	Polycystic ovary disease
	Pulmonary	Shortness of breath, wheezing, allergy	Asthma
		Snoring, daytime fatigue, restless sleep	Obstructive sleep apnea
	Gastrointestinal	Heartburn, indigestion	GERD
	Urinary	Leaking, wetting, stress versus urge symptoms	Urinary incontinence
	Skeletal	Joint pain, limited functionality, and range of motion	Osteoarthritis
	Functional capacity	Activities of daily living, weakness	Disability, Sarcopenia
	Psychological complications/ disease	Depression, binge eating, stigmatization	Depression, Binge eating syndrome

(continued)

Table 7.6 (continued)

Initial evaluation	System	Findings	Relevant complication[a]
Clinical laboratory	Fasting glucose, HbA1c, 2-h OGTT glucose	Prediabetes: Fasting 100–125 mg/dl (IFG); 2-h 140–199 mg/dl (IGT); HbA1c 5.7–6.4%	Prediabetes, Dysmetabolic syndrome (IFG), Diabetes
	Total cholesterol, triglycerides, HDL-c, LDL-c, non-HDL-c	Triglycerides ≥ 150 mg/dl; HDL-c < 40 mg/dl men, <50 women; LDL-c ≥100 mg/dl; non-HDL-c ≥ 130 mg/dl	Dyslipidemia, Dysmetabolic syndrome (HDL-c and triglycerides), LDL-c target for CVD risk reduction
	Transaminases (AST, ALT), liver function tests	Transaminase levels above normal	Nonalcoholic fatty liver disease

Notes: The table illustrates key aspects in the evaluation but should not be considered all inclusive
[a]The diagnosis of each "Relevant Complication" may be complete based on findings in the initial evaluation, while other potential complications will be suspected and will require further testing for diagnosis or staging (see Table 7.7)

In this context, an "Advanced Framework for a New Diagnosis of Obesity" emerged from multidisciplinary discussions at the AACE/ACE Consensus Conference on Obesity held in Washington, DC, in March 2014. The consensus was that the diagnosis of obesity based solely on BMI was not medically meaningful or actionable and that this represented an impediment to concerted action to fight obesity among health care professionals, regulators, payers, and employers. BMI may not reflect the impact of weight gain on the health or well-being of the individual, and its significance varies as a function of different ethnicities and body types. An improved medically relevant diagnosis would consist of the continued use of BMI (together with other anthropometrics such as waist circumference) and an assessment of the presence and severity of obesity-related complications. Furthermore, strategy regarding prevention and treatment of obesity should conform to the three classic phases of chronic disease prevention: primary, to prevent the disease in the first place; secondary prevention, once the disease has appeared but before the emergence of complications; and tertiary prevention, after complications develop. Therefore, the new obesity diagnostic algorithm (Table 7.8) incorporates two components: (*1*) an assessment of body mass, including validated ethnicity-adjusted anthropometrics to identify individuals with increased adipose tissue placing them at risk and (*2*) the presence and severity of weight-related complications as shown in Table 7.8. The approach emphasizes risk stratification and complications staging in order to target more aggressive interventions to those patients who will most benefit from weight loss therapy. Each complication is evaluated for severity and impact on the patient's health using complication-specific criteria: stage 0 (no complication is present), stage 1 (complication is mild to moderate), or stage 2 (complication is severe).

Table 7.7 Screening and diagnoses of weight-related complications in patients with overweight/obesity

Weight-related complication	Basis for screening and/or diagnosis	Secondary testing when needed to confirm diagnosis, stage severity, or guide therapy
Prediabetes	Fasting glucose, HbA1c	If fasting glucose is 100–125 mg/dl, a repeat elevated fasting glucose completes diagnosis of IFG; however, 2-h OGTT glucose should also be performed to exclude diabetes and IGT. Fasting and 2-h OGTT glucose should be performed if initial fasting glucose is normal and HbA1c is elevated, or in high-risk patients based on family history or dysmetabolic syndrome
Dysmetabolic syndrome	Waist circumference, blood pressure, fasting glucose, triglycerides, HDL-c	Initial evaluation completes diagnosis
Type 2 diabetes	Fasting glucose, HbA1c, ROS	Overtly elevated (i.e., ≥200 mg/dl) or a repeat fasting glucose ≥126 mg/dl completes diagnosis. If fasting glucose and/or HbA1c is consistent with prediabetes, 2-h OGTT should be performed to test for diabetes. HbA1c should be performed to help guide therapy
Hypertension	Blood pressure	Repeat elevated blood pressure measurements complete diagnosis; home blood pressure or ambulatory blood pressure monitoring may help complete testing
Dyslipidemia	Lipid panel (total cholesterol, HDL-c, triglycerides, LDL-c, non-HDL-c)	Lipid panel completes diagnosis; lipoprotein subclasses, apoB-100 may further define risk
NAFLD/NASH	Physical exam, LFTs	Imaging (e.g., ultrasound, MRI, elastography) and/or liver biopsy needed to complete diagnosis
PCOS	Physical exam, ROS	Hormonal testing (e.g., androgen levels LH/FSH) needed to complete diagnosis
Obstructive sleep apnea	Physical exam, neck circumference, ROS	Polysomnography needed to complete diagnosis
Osteoarthritis	Physical exam, ROS	Radiographic imaging may be needed to complete diagnosis
Urinary stress incontinence	Physical exam, ROS	Urine culture and urodynamic testing may be needed to complete diagnosis
GERD	Physical exam, ROS	Endoscopy and esophageal motility study may be needed to complete diagnosis
Disability	Physical exam, ROS	Functional testing may be helpful
Asthma/ respiratory disease	Physical exam, ROS	Chest X-ray and respirometry studies may be needed to complete diagnosis
Depression/ stigmatization	Physical exam, ROS	Psychological testing and evaluation may be needed to complete diagnosis

(continued)

Table 7.7 (continued)

Weight-related complication	Basis for screening and/or diagnosis	Secondary testing when needed to confirm diagnosis, stage severity, or guide therapy
Obesity secondary to hormonal disorder	Physical exam, ROS	TSH for suspected hypothyroidism; serum/urine cortisol for hypercortisolism, if clinical findings or symptoms are present
Iatrogenic obesity (e.g., secondary to medications)	Review current medications and medication history	Follow-up following withdrawal of offending medication and/or substitution with a weight-neutral alternative may be needed to complete diagnosis
Genetic syndrome	Physical exam, ROS, family history	If clinical findings are suggestive, genetic testing of the patient and perhaps family members may be needed to complete diagnosis

Table 7.8 Two-component diagnostic framework for overweight/obesity consistent with the phases of chronic disease prevention

Diagnosis	Anthropometric component	Clinical component[a]	Phases of prevention/ treatment
Normal	BMI < 25 kg/m^2		Primary
Overweight stage 0	BMI 25–29.9 kg/m^2	No obesity-related complications	Secondary
Obesity stage 0	BMI ≥ 30 kg/m^2	No obesity-related complications	
Obesity stage 1	BMI ≥ 25 kg/m^2	Presence of one or more mild-to-moderate obesity-related complications	Tertiary
Obesity stage 2	BMI ≥ 25 kg/m^2	Presence of one or more severe obesity-related complications	

Adapted from Garvey et al. (2014a)
[a]Staging of complications as mild-to-moderate (Stage 1) or severe (Stage 2) is based on complication-specific criteria

Interventions for primary prevention might include public education or modifications in the built environment to prevent overweight or obesity. Secondary prevention strategies are designed to prevent further weight gain and/or promote weight loss in patients with overweight or obesity and to prevent the emergence of complications. Once complications develop, it is evident that the excess adiposity is adversely affecting the health of the patient, and a more intensive approach to management is indicated. Tertiary prevention/treatment is then required to treat the complications by achieving sufficient weight loss to ameliorate them. Thus, the diagnostic framework that combines a measure of adiposity and an assessment of the presence and severity of weight-related complications is actionable. This diagnostic framework indicates disease severity and aids in therapeutic decisions. It renders a diagnosis that dictates what to treat and why.

7.4 Conclusion

The diagnosis of overweight or obesity based solely on BMI is insufficient for two major reasons. First, overweight and obesity represent a continuum of excess adiposity, and BMI is not a direct measure of adipose tissue mass. Thus, while BMI can be used as a parameter for screening, an evaluation is necessary to interpret the BMI measurement for diagnostic purposes and assure that elevated values reflect fat mass and not excess muscularity, edema, pregnancy, large tumors, third-space fluid collection, etc. Furthermore, BMI does not indicate distribution of fat in different adipose tissue depots. On the other hand, waist circumference is useful in identifying relative accumulation in the intra-abdominal depot, which is an element of adiposopathy, and is central to the development of metabolic and vascular complications. Second, BMI does not indicate the degree to which adiposity adversely impacts health since the presence and severity of adiposopathy and weight-related complications varies tremendously among individual patients at any given BMI value. In bariatric endocrinology, best practices require a careful evaluation for the presence and severity of weight-related complications (including adiposopathy) in all patients presenting with overweight and obesity. Key weight-related complications can be identified during an initial patient evaluation consisting of history, an obesity-focused review of systems, physical examination, and clinical laboratory testing. An optimal diagnostic framework incorporates an anthropometric measure of increased adiposity (i.e., BMI) together with an assessment of the presence and severity of weight-related complications, which provides both an indication of disease severity and the intensity of weight loss therapy required to improve health.

Reading List

Abdullah A, Peeters A, de Courten M, Stoelwinder J. The magnitude of association between overweight and obesity and the risk of diabetes: a meta-analysis of prospective cohort studies. Diabetes Res Clin Pract. 2010;89(3):309–19.

Alberti KG, Eckel RH, Grundy SM, et al. Harmonizing the metabolic syndrome: a joint interim statement of the International Diabetes Federation task force on epidemiology and prevention; National Heart, Lung, and Blood Institute; American Heart Association; World Heart Federation; International Atherosclerosis Society; and International Association for the Study of Obesity. Circulation. 2009;120(16):1640–5.

Ashwell M, Gunn P, Gibson S. Waist-to-height ratio is a better screening tool than waist circumference and BMI for adult cardiometabolic risk factors: systematic review and meta-analysis. Obes Rev. 2012;13(3):275–86.

Barak N, Ehrenpreis ED, Harrison JR, Sitrin MD. Gastro-oesophageal reflux disease in obesity: pathophysiological and therapeutic considerations. Obes Rev. 2002;3(1):9–15.

Browning LM, Hsieh SD, Ashwell M. A systematic review of waist-to-height ratio as a screening tool for the prediction of cardiovascular disease and diabetes: 05 could be a suitable global boundary value. Nutr Res Rev. 2010;23(2):247–69.

Bugianesi E, Leone N, et al. Expanding the natural history of non-alcoholic steatohepatitis: from cryptogenic cirrhosis to hepatocellular carcinoma. Gastroenterology. 2002;123:134–40.

Carnethon MR, De Chavez PJD, Biggs ML, et al. Association of weight status with mortality in adults with incident diabetes. JAMA. 2012;308(6):581–90.

Cefalu WT, Bray GA, Home PD, Garvey WT, Klein S, Pi-Sunyer FX, Hu FB, Raz I, Van Gaal L, Wolfe BM, Ryan DH. Advances in the science, treatment, and prevention of the disease of obesity: reflections from a diabetes care editors' expert forum. Diabetes Care. 2015;38(8):1567–82.

Cerhan JR, Moore SC, Jacobs EJ, Kitahara CM, Rosenberg PS, Adami HO, Ebbert JO, English DR, Gapstur SM, Giles GG, Horn-Ross PL, Park Y, Patel AV, Robien K, Weiderpass E, Willett WC, Wolk A, Zeleniuch-Jacquotte A, Hartge P, Bernstein L, Berrington de Gonzalez A. A pooled analysis of waist circumference and mortality in 650,000 adults. Mayo Clin Proc. 2014;89(3):335–45.

Chang SH, Beason TS, Hunleth JM, Colditz GA. A systematic review of body fat distribution and mortality in older people. Maturitas. 2012;72(3):175–91.

Coughlin SR, Mawdsley L, Mugarza JA, et al. Obstructive sleep apnoea is independently associated with an increased prevalence of metabolic syndrome. Eur Heart J. 2004;25:735e41.

Daniel S, Soleymani T, Garvey WT. A complications-based clinical staging of obesity to guide treatment modality and intensity. Curr Opin Endocrinol Diabetes Obes. 2013;20(5):377–88.

Davis MA, Ettinger WH, Neuhaus JM. Obesity and osteoarthritis of the knee: evidence from the National Health and Nutrition Examination Survey (NHANES I). Semin Arthritis Rheum. 1990;20:34–41.

de Koning L, Merchant AT, Pogue J, Anand SS. Waist circumference and waist-to-hip ratio as predictors of cardiovascular events: meta-regression analysis of prospective studies. Eur Heart J. 2007;28(7):850–6.

Després J-P, Lemieux I. Abdominal obesity and metabolic syndrome. Nature. 2006;444:881–7.

Eckel RH, Grundy SM, Zimmet PZ. The metabolic syndrome. Lancet. 2005;365:1415–28.

Eknoyan G. Adolphe Quetelet (1796–1874)-the average man and indices of obesity. Nephrol Dial Transplant. 2008;23(1):47–51.

Flegal KM, Kit BK, Orpana H, Graubard BI. Association of all-cause mortality with overweight and obesity using standard body mass index categories: a systematic review and meta-analysis. JAMA. 2013;309(1):71–82.

Frankenfield DC, Rowe WA, Cooney RN, Smith JS, Becker D. Limits of body mass index to detect obesity and predict body composition. Nutrition. 2001;17(1):26–30.

Garber AJ, Abrahamson MJ, Barzilay JI, Blonde L, Bloomgarden ZT, Bush MA, Dagogo-Jack S, Davidson MB, Einhorn D, Garber JR, Garvey WT, Grunberger G, Handelsman Y, Hirsch IB, Jellinger PS, McGill JB, Mechanick JI, Rosenblit PD, Umpierrez GE. Consensus statement by the American association of clinical endocrinologists and American college of endocrinology on the comprehensive type 2 diabetes management algorithm—2015 executive summary. Endocr Pract. 2015;21(12):1403–14.

Garvey WT. New tools for weight-loss therapy enable a more robust medical model for obesity treatment: rationale for a complications-centric approach. Endocr Pract. 2013;19(5):864–74.

Garvey WT, Garber AJ, Mechanick JI, Bray GA, Dagogo-Jack S, Einhorn D, Grunberger G, Handelsman Y, Hennekens CH, Hurley DL, McGill J, Palumbo P, Umpierrez G, on Behalf of the AACE Obesity Scientific Committee. American Association of Clinical Endocrinologists and American College of Endocrinology position statement on the 2014 advanced framework for a new diagnosis of obesity as a chronic disease. Endocr Pract. 2014a;20(9):977–89.

Garvey WT, Garber AJ, Mechanick JI, et al. American Association of Clinical Endocrinologists and American College of Endocrinology consensus conference on obesity: building an evidence base for comprehensive action. Endocr Pract. 2014b;20(9):956–76.

Garvey WT, Ryan DH, Henry R, Bohannon NJ, Toplak H, Schwiers M, et al. Prevention of type 2 diabetes in subjects with prediabetes and metabolic syndrome treated with phentermine and topiramate extended release. Diabetes Care. 2014c;37:912–21.

Gomez-Ambrosi J, Silva C, Galofre JC, et al. Body mass index classification misses subjects with increased cardiometabolic risk factors related to elevated adiposity. Int J Obes. 2012;36(2):286–94.

Guh DP, Zhang W, Bansback N, et al. The incidence of co-morbidities related to obesity and overweight: a systematic review and meta-analysis. BMC Public Health. 2009;9(1):88.

Guo F, Garvey WT. Development of a weighted cardiometabolic disease staging (CMDS) system for the prediction of future diabetes. J Clin Endocrinol Metab. 2015;100(10):3871–7.

Guo F, Moellering DR, Garvey WT. The progression of cardiometabolic disease: validation of a new cardiometabolic disease staging system applicable to obesity. Obesity. 2014;22:110–8.

Hamman RF, Wing RR, Edelstein SL, et al. Effect of weight loss with lifestyle intervention on risk of diabetes. Diabetes Care. 2006;29:2102–7.

He W, Li Q, Yang M, Jiao J, et al. Lower BMI cutoffs to define overweight and obesity in China. Obesity. 2015;23(3):684–91.

Heymsfield SB, Peterson CM, Thomas DM, et al. Scaling of adult body weight to height across sex and race/ethnic groups: relevance to BMI. Am J Clin Nutr. 2014;100(6):1455–61.

Hsu WC, Araneta MRG, Kanaya AM, et al. BMI cut points to identify at-risk Asian Americans for type 2 diabetes screening. Diabetes Care. 2015;38:150–8.

Hunskaar S. A systematic review of overweight and obesity as risk factors and targets for clinical intervention for urinary incontienence in women. Neurourol Urodyn. 2008;27:749–57.

Jacobs EJ, Newton CC, Wang Y, et al. Waist circumference and all-cause mortality in a large US cohort. Arch Intern Med. 2010;170(15):1293–301.

Katzmarzyk PT, Craig CL, Bouchard C. Adiposity, adipose tissue distribution and mortality rates in the Canada fitness survey follow-up study. Int J Obes Relat Metab Disord: J Int Assoc Study Obes. 2002;26(8):1054–9.

Katzmarzyk PT, Bray GA, Greenway FL, et al. Ethnic-specific BMI and waist circumference thresholds. Obesity. 2011;19(6):1272–8.

Kaul S, Rothny MP, Peters DM, Wacker WK, Davis CE, Shapitro MD, Ergun DL. Dual-energy X-ray absorptiometry for quantification of visceral fat. Obesity. 2012;20(6):1313–8.

Kendler DL, Borges JL, Fielding RA, et al. The official positions of the international society for clinical densitometry: indications of use and reporting of DXA for body composition. J Clin Densitom. 2013;16(4):496–507.

Keys A, Fidanza F, Karvonen MJ, Kimura N, Taylor HL. Indices of relative weight and obesity. Int J Epidemiol. 2014;43(3):655–65.

Kodama S, Horikawa C, Fujihara K, et al. Comparisons of the strength of associations with future type 2 diabetes risk among anthropometric obesity indicators, including waist-to-height ratio: a meta-analysis. Am J Epidemiol. 2012;176(11):959–69.

Lago F, Dieguez C, Gomez-Reino J, Gualillo O. The emerging role of adipokines as mediators of inflammation and immune responses. Cytokine Growth Factor Rev. 2007;18:313–25.

Lee CMY, Huxley RR, Wildman RP, Woodward M. Indices of abdominal obesity are better discriminators of cardiovascular risk factors than BMI: a meta-analysis. J Clin Epidemiol. 2008;61(7):646–53.

Locke AE, Kahali B, Berndt SI, Justice AE, Pers TH, et al. Genetic studies of body mass index yield new insights for obesity biology. Nature. 2015;518(7538):197–206.

Mariotti S, Capocaccia R, Farchi G, Menotti A, Verdecchia A, Keys A. Differences in the incidence rate of coronary heart disease between north and south European cohorts of the Seven Countries Study as partially explained by risk factors. Eur Heart J. 1982;3(5):481–7.

McGee DL, Diverse Populations Collaboration. Body mass index and mortality: a meta-analysis based on person-level data from twenty-six observational studies. Ann Epidemiol. 2005;15(2):87–97.

Mechanick JI, Garber AJ, Handelsman Y, Garvey WT. American Association of Clinical Endocrinologists' position statement on obesity and obesity medicine. Endocr Pract. 2012;18(5):642–8.

Meigs JB, Wilson PW, Fox CS, et al. Body mass index, metabolic syndrome, and risk of type 2 diabetes or cardiovascular disease. J Clin Endocrinol Metab. 2006;91:2906–12.

Melville JL, Katon W, Kristin Delaney K, Newton K. Urinary incontinence in US women: a population-based study. JAMA Intern Med. 2005;165(5):537–42.

Mokdad AH, Ford ES, Bowman BA, Dietz WH, Vinicor F, Bales VS, Marks JS. Prevalence of obesity, diabetes, and obesity-related health risk factors, 2001. JAMA. 2003;289(1):76–9.

Mongraw-Chaffin ML, Peters SA, Huxley RR, Woodward M. The sex-specific association between BMI and coronary heart disease: a systematic review and meta-analysis of 95 cohorts with 1.2 million participants. Lancet Diabetes Endocrinol. 2015;3(6):437–49.
Murphy RA, Reinders I, Garcia ME, et al. Adipose tissue, muscle, and function: potential mediators of associations between body weight and mortality in older adults with type 2 diabetes. Diabetes Care. 2014;37(12):3213–9.
Must A, Spadano J, Coakley EH, Field AE, Colditz G, Dietz WH. The disease burden associated with overweight and obesity. JAMA. 1999;282:1523–9.
National Heart, Lung, and Blood Institute. Clinical guidelines on the identification, evaluation, and treatment of overweight and obesity in adults: the evidence report. Bethesda: National Institutes of Health; 1998. Accessed at www.nhlbi.nih.gov/guidelines/obesity/ob_gdlns.pdf.
Prentice AM, Jebb SA. Beyond body mass index. Obes Rev. 2001;2(3):141–7.
Romero-Corral A, Somers VK, Sierra-Johnson J, et al. Accuracy of body mass index in diagnosing obesity in the adult general population. Int J Obes. 2008;32(6):959–66.
Ruhl CE, Everhart JE. Overweight, but not high dietary fat intake, increases risk of gastroesophageal reflux disease hospitalization: the NHANES I Epidemiologic Followup Study. First National Health and Nutrition Examination Survey. Ann Epidemiol. 1999;9:424–35.
Stavig GR, Leonard AR, Igra A, Felten P. Indices of relative body weight and ideal weight charts. J Chronic Dis. 1984;37(4):255–62.
Tobias DK, Pan A, Jackson CL, et al. Body-mass index and mortality among adults with incident type 2 diabetes. N Engl J Med. 2014;370(3):233–44.
Torloni MR, Betran AP, Horta BL, et al. Prepregnancy BMI and the risk of gestational diabetes: a systematic review of the literature with meta-analysis. Obes Rev. 2009;10(2):194–203.
Tuomilehto H, Seppa J, Uusitupa M. Obesity and obstructive sleep apnea—clinical significance of weight loss. Sleep Med Rev. 2013;17:321–9.
van Dis I, Kromhout D, Geleijnse JM, Boer JM, Verschuren WM. Body mass index and waist circumference predict both 10-year nonfatal and fatal cardiovascular disease risk: study conducted in 20,000 Dutch men and women aged 20–65 years. Eur J Cardiovasc Prev Rehabil. 2009;16(6):729–34.
Van Gaal LF, Mentens IL, De Block CE. Mechanisms linking obesity with cardiovascular disease. Nature. 2006;444:875–80.
Wannamethee SG, Shaper AG, Lennon L, Whincup PH. Decreased muscle mass and increased central adiposity are independently related to mortality in older men. Am J Clin Nutr. 2007;86(5):1339–46.
Whitlock G, Lewington S, Sherliker P, et al. Prospective Studies Collaboration: Body-mass index and cause-specific mortality in 900 000 adults: collaborative analyses of 57 prospective studies. Lancet. 2009;373(9669):1083–96.
WHO (World Health Organization). Physical status: the use and interpretation of anthropometry: report of a WHO expert committee. World Health Organ Tech Rep Ser. 1995;854:1–452.
WHO EC. Appropriate body-mass index for Asian populations and its implications for policy and intervention strategies. Lancet. 2004;363(9403):157.
Wildman RP, Muntner P, Reynolds K, et al. The obese without cardiometabolic risk factor clustering and the normal weight with cardiometabolic risk factor clustering: prevalence and correlates of 2 phenotypes among the US population (NHANES 1999–2004). Arch Intern Med. 2008;1(68):1617–24.
Wing RR, Lang W, Wadden TA, et al., The Look AHEAD Research Group. Benefits of modest weight loss in improving cardiovascular risk factors in overweight and obese individuals with type 2 diabetes. Diabetes Care. 2011;34:1481–6.
World Health Organization (WHO). Report of a WHO consultation on obesity. Obesity: preventing and managing the global epidemic. Geneva: WHO; 1998. Available at: http://whqlibdoc.who.int/hq/1998/WHO_NUT_NCD_98.1_(p1–158).pdf.
Wormser D, Kaptoge S, Di Angelantonio E, et al., the Emerging Risk Factors Collaboration. Separate and combined associations of body-mass index and abdominal adiposity with cardiovascular disease: collaborative analysis of 58 prospective studies. Lancet. 2011;377(9771):1085–95.

Yildiz BO, Knochenhauer ES, Azziz R. Impact of obesity on the risk for polycystic ovary syndrome. J Clin Endocrinol Metab. 2008;93(1):162–8.

Young T, Peppard PE, Gottlieb DJ. Epidemiology of obstructive sleep apnea. A population health perspective. Am J Respir Crit Care Med. 2002;165:1217–39.

Yusuf S, Hawken S, Ounpuu S, et al. Obesity and the risk of myocardial infarction in 27,000 participants from 52 countries: a case-control study. Lancet. 2005;366(9497):1640–9.

Zeb I, Katz R, Nasir K. Relation of nonalcoholic fatty liver disease to the metabolic syndrome: the multi-ethnic study of atherosclerosis. J Cardiovasc Comput Tomogr. 2013;7:311–8.

Zhou BF, Cooperative Meta-Analysis Group of the Working Group on Obesity in China. Predictive values of body mass index and waist circumference for risk factors of certain related diseases in Chinese adults—study on optimal cut-off points of body mass index and waist circumference in Chinese adults. Biomed Environ Sci. 2002;15(1):83–96.

Zhu Q, Shen F, Ye T, Zhou Q, Deng H, Gu X. Waist-to-height ratio is an appropriate index for identifying cardiometabolic risk in Chinese individuals with normal body mass index and waist circumference. J Diabetes. 2014;6(6):527–34.

Chapter 8
Evaluation and Management of the Patient with Obesity or Overweight

Israel Hartman

Pearls of Wisdom

- Overweight and obesity should be treated with the same model of chronic disease management used for other endocrine and metabolic diseases.
- The treatment of overweight and obesity must address the social and medical stigmas. Patients with overweight and obesity require special accommodations within the clinic that are essential to success.
- The desired goal is not merely weight loss but a return of normal metabolism and adipocyte function.
- Realistic goals specific to each patient will better ensure success and deter relapse.

8.1 Introduction

An effective bariatric endocrinology practice is designed to address the unique neuro-endocrinological considerations of its patients in addition to practical and structural needs required to best facilitate their treatment and ensure the financial success of the clinic itself. The ideal clinic requires the right infrastructure and properly trained staff. An individual encounter should be tailored to mainstream the care of patients with obesity or overweight. The encounter itself necessitates its own nuanced approach with a special focus being given to the patient's medical and pharmacological history, and regular risk re-stratification, including laboratory testing.

I. Hartman, MD FACE
University of Texas Southwestern Medical School, Department of Endocrinology, Dallas, TX, USA
e-mail: drhartman@israelhartmanmd.com

J. M. Gonzalez-Campoy et al. (eds.), *Bariatric Endocrinology*,
https://doi.org/10.1007/978-3-319-95655-8_8

Much like the treatment of diabetes and other endocrine diseases, behavior modification is an essential component not only in the treatment of patients with obesity but also in gauging the success of the course of treatment. A bariatric clinic should offer nutritional and physical activity education for the patient and family and develop realistic, goal-based plans.

It is important to recognize that, as with other chronic endocrine conditions, regular follow-up appointments are essential to assure adherence with the plan of treatment and for ultimate success in the management of the patient with obesity or overweight. Several studies have demonstrated that after initial evaluation, patients with obesity or overweight that were asked to follow-up every month with a dedicated nurse, in order to be weighed and discuss treatment, yielded higher rates of success and adherence to the regimen. Developing long-term strategies for treatment with regular re-evaluation and re-stratification will break from historically short-sighted approaches treating overweight, obesity, and adiposopathy.

8.2 Infrastructure: Clinic, Equipment, and Staff Training

In a study of patients with a body mass index (BMI) greater than 55 kg/m^2, 68% of those surveyed reported delay in seeking professional treatment to manage their obesity. The reasons for this delay included past instances of disrespectful treatment, feelings of embarrassment, or inadequate accommodations. An adequate clinic setting in order to promote success in the treatment of obesity or overweight is of paramount importance. A welcoming, sensitive, front desk and nursing staff is integral to maintaining a positive atmosphere. Since many patients with obesity or overweight experience psychological issues often exacerbated by the social stigma surrounding obesity, it is important that all staff members are trained to use "patient-first" language.

In a clinic-based study, 53% of the patients reported inappropriate comments from their doctors about their weight, and doctors were the second most common source of stigma (69%), following family (72%). Stigma and bias refer to negative attitudes that affect our interpersonal interactions and activities in a detrimental way. Stigma may come in several forms, including verbal types of bias (ridicule, teasing, insults, stereotypes, and derogatory names), physical stigma (touching, grabbing, or other aggressive behavior), or other barriers and obstacles due to weight such as medical equipment that is too small or unsafe for patients with obesity or overweight. It is necessary to make patients comfortable as a preliminary step to proper treatment. Strategies should be implemented in the clinical setting in order to reduce weight stigma and improve attitudes within the clinical setting.

The concept of obesity as an illness extends into how the terms "overweight" and "obesity" are used in the clinical setting. These terms should not be used as adjectives and instead referred to only as medical conditions that the patients are being treated for. Thus, “obese patient” would be replaced with “patient with obesity.” The staff should be conscious not to suggest any judgment in their language, gestures, even when the patient is not present, as these may be perceived as disrespectful of the patient’s condition. These initial interactions are an important component of the patient encounter and can help shape it in a positive manner. The same sensitivity applies to the nursing staff’s training in the morphometric assessment of patients, as the habitus of patients with obesity or overweight might present certain difficulties during examination. This will ensure not only consistent measurements but also the comfort of the patient. Staff should be well trained to measure a blood pressure cuff, how to obtain a proper height measurement for the calculation of the BMI, and how to adequately measure waist and hip circumferences.

Due to the size and weight of patients with obesity or overweight, a bariatric endocrinology clinic will need to offer an accommodating workspace ideally suited for the needs of both patient and staff. Wide door frames, hallways, and examination rooms will accommodate severe corpulence and steel-reinforced furniture designed to handle large weights is ideal for waiting and examination rooms. Building entry points need to be designed with comfortable ramps featuring handrails. Doors for examination rooms are recommended to be 3 feet 6 inches wide and the recommended opening size for patient rooms and procedure areas is 4 feet. Paired doors or sliding doors can be used as an alternative. Ample sized, weight-tested wheelchairs should be available to transport patients by the front door. In areas where oversize wheelchairs are to be used, a 72-inch turning radius is recommended, in lieu of the 60-inch radius generally required by the American with Disabilities Act (ADA). In general, it is recommended that 10–20% of general seating in the waiting areas should be specified in bariatric sizes, due to the fact that patients with obesity often times will be accompanied by family members who will require similar types of accommodations.

Bathroom doors and facilities should be equally accommodating to the patient with overweight or obesity. Vitreous China toilets have a maximum capacity of about 300 pounds. The most common solution on the market today is floor-mounted stainless steel toilets. Both toilets and sinks should be floor mounted, and the center line for toilets should be 24 inches versus 18 inches on the center line for a standard toilet. Bathrooms should also be equipped with weight-tested bars or handles on the walls to assist patients and reduce the risk of injury.

A large-sized platform scale (able to accommodate up to 800 pounds) is necessary, as the standard models are unable to handle the weight of many patients. Hydraulic examination tables will also assist patients who have limited mobility as a result of their excess mass, rising from normal sitting level to a height ideal for the examiner. Many other items of standard clinical equipment are not able to accommodate patients with severe obesity. A dedicated bariatric clinic should have examination gowns, blood pressure cuffs, and measuring tapes in extra-large sizes. These fittings along with a thoroughly trained staff will ensure an atmosphere conducive to a comfortable patient encounter. Since many of those with obesity or overweight qualify as having a disability under the ADA, it is important to review the other recommendations outlined in its guidelines. The ADA guide is available from the US Department of Justice.

Contingency plans for emergencies should be in place and well rehearsed. An often-unrecognized need when treating patients with severe obesity is the safety of the health-care professionals who care for them. The National Safety Council reports that the health-care worker is 41% more likely than the average worker to need time off because of serious occupational injuries. An estimated 12% of nurses annually leave their profession due to back injuries. Thus, proper training of the health-care workers on how to prevent this type of injuries when assisting patients around the clinic is essential. OSHA injury prevention guidelines should be reviewed for this purpose. Training in how to physically assist patients with overweight or obesity (such as boosting and lifting) will help prevent any serious injuries to the staff while avoiding discomfort for the patient. In the instance of a medical emergency, an alarm system should be used to notify staff so that multiple staff members can be on hand to assist any patient with excess body weight. Incorporation of this training into evacuation procedures is also important. Staff should be familiar with the necessary procedures to lift a patient weighing over 400 pounds onto a gurney, if needed during an evacuation or medical emergency.

These accommodations are recommended for an ideal clinic that treats patients with obesity or overweight. While financial or structural considerations might limit a clinic's ability to follow all of these recommendations, the patient's safety and comfort should be the priority.

8.3 Team Approach to Obesity

Continuing to use the treatment model of chronic endocrine diseases, the team approach is integral to effective long-term lifestyle modification. Access to a variety of educational materials will greatly benefit patients and meet individual needs. Printed and electronic educational materials can greatly enhance patient education in the clinic. Web-based materials can provide patients access to ongoing education between visits. Providing these materials will also aid in recruiting and engaging relatives in the treatment plan. Both at home and at work, the involvement of individuals to support patient behavior change is desirable. Support from others ensures that patients adhere to treatment plans. Other tools such as pedometers or web/mobile applications can allow the patient or family members to track progress on a regular basis. Interactive tools can also provide motivational support to the patient. Monitoring, logging, and objectively measuring progress help achieve short-term, specific goals. In order to achieve long-term goals, it is essential to establish short-term objectives, as not to disenfranchise the patient. Setting goals for activity or weight loss will help the patient adhere to the long-term treatment plan.

Access to a specially designed health-care team is also essential. An ideally staffed clinic might include both well-trained front desk and nursing staff but also nutritionists/dieticians, mental health professionals, behavior counselors, physical therapists, rehabilitation consultants, and sleep and pain specialists. This will allow the clinic to address the multifaceted needs of each patient. A team approach is ideal to effectively treat and manage the many complications caused by obesity or overweight, which, when present, can prevent attainment of treatment goals. Many third-party providers do not cover dietician or nutritionist visits unless bundled with that of a physician. Thus, the team-based model of a bariatric clinic is also ideal for financial success. Providing access to other specialists such as bariatric surgeons and cardiologists in a multispecialty practice helps to meet the overhead of the team.

Group meetings for patients have also been shown to be beneficial. These group meetings can be held in the clinic. Alternatively, patients can be referred to commercial weight loss programs, which have been shown to be successful in conjunction with lifestyle modifications overseen by a medical professional. Commercial weight loss programs can be an alternative for endocrinology clinics with staff or financial limitations, where an in-clinic dietician or other specialist is not feasible. Support groups and group classes have been shown to help engage patients and inspire adherence and dedication to the treatment plan. In-office classes, referral to physical activity education, or health-centric cooking courses can help educate patients to make better choices in their daily lives.

It is important that the team approach encompasses not only trained professionals but also the patient's family as well. A patient with an invested family network will better adhere to treatment recommendations and have improved outcomes. Awareness of ethnic, cultural, religious, educational, and social differences among patients is also important in discussing meal plan guidelines, as these may provide additional obstacles or advantages to each treatment plan.

8.4 Patient Encounter

Patient encounter provides opportunities for risk stratification (including an obesity-focused review of the medical history), building patient satisfaction and trust, validation of charges, and documentation of all work.

The obesity-focused history will cover any major life events that might have coincided with weight gain. Past events such as changes in career or marital status, medications, pregnancies, and lifestyle are all important to document. Additionally, current habits determine an individual patient's energy balance. A patient's medication history will provide opportunities for intervention. There are medications that are well known to cause weight gain. A general strategy is to avoid them and substitute with alternatives that are associated with weight loss (Table 8.1).

Table 8.1 Medications that promote weight gain or help maintain or lose weight

Promote weight gain
Pyschiatric/Neuro
Antipsychotics
Antidepressants
Lithium
Steroid hormones
Prednisone
Estrogens, progestins
Diabetic agents
Sulfonylureas,
Thiazolidinediones,
Insulin
Beta-adrenergic blockers
Antihistamines
Antiepileptics
Help maintain or lose weight
Pyschiatric/Neuro
Ziprasidone
Celexa
Bupropion
Topiramate
Diabetic agents
Metformin, GLP-1 agonists,
Pramlintide, α-glucosidase
Inhibitors, SGLT-2 blockers
ACE inhibitors

A detailed history should also include documentation of current food intake, physical activity levels, and sleeping habits. A psychological assessment for mood disorders is important, as this may contribute to obesity or overweight, or complicate treatment.

Patient assessment should also look for complications of obesity and overweight because many become obstacles to effective weight loss. Sleep apnea, restrictive lung disease, fatigue, osteoarthritis, degenerative disc disease, angina pectoris, peripheral vascular disease, insulin resistance, and hypogonadism are examples of complications of obesity that become obstacles to effective weight loss. These, along with other complications, should be targeted not only to develop a course of treatment but also for billing purposes.

The physical examination of the patient encounter will encompass both standard measurements of height and weight, and if possible, the percentage of body fat. The patient's BMI should be calculated, and the waist circumference (WC) should be measured, since they are the major factors in stratifying health risk in patients with obesity or overweight. The World Health Organization has defined obesity starting at a BMI of 25 kg/m^2 for a Caucasian population, or 23 kg/m^2 for an Asian popula-

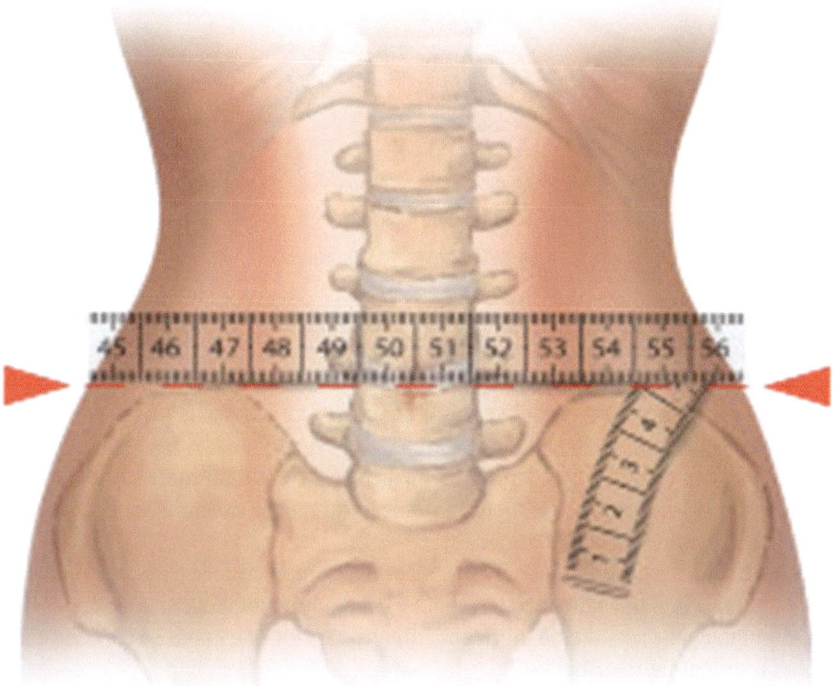

Fig. 8.1 A proper technique for measuring waist circumference. Locate the superior iliac crests and the lower rib margins and place the measuring tape around the abdomen above iliac crests, keeping the loop of the tape parallel to the floor. Ensure the measuring tape is snug but not compressing the skin. (Adapted from: Allison DB, Downey M, Atkinson RL, Billington CJ, Bray GA, Eckel RH, et al. Obesity as a disease: a white paper on evidence and arguments commissioned by the Council of the Obesity Society. Obesity (Silver Spring). 2008;16(6):1161–77. Epub 2008/05/10; used with permission)

tion. While not all patients with obesity or overweight, as defined by BMI criteria, have metabolic diseases or excess adipose tissue, and conversely not all that have metabolic dysfunction have obesity or overweight, the correlation between the two is strong enough that it is clinically appropriate for diagnosis. Distribution of adipose tissue and measures of body composition add another dimension to the assessment of individual patients. Measuring WC is a strong tool for gauging the volume of intra-abdominal or visceral adipose tissue. Those with a WC above 40 inches are at a higher risk of both metabolic diseases, as well as cardiac disease. Figure 8.1 describes the proper way to measure WC, and Table 8.2 shows the accepted variations in WC by ethnic group.

Table 8.2 Ethnic variations in waist circumference risk thresholds

Ethnic/regional origin	Men, in (cm)	Women, in (cm)
Europid	≥37 (94)	≥31 (80)
Caucasian	≥37 (94)	≥31 (80)
North American, European	≥40 (102)	≥35 (88)
Asian	≥35 (90)	≥31 (80)
Middle Eastern, Mediterranean	≥37 (94)	≥31 (80)
Sub-Saharan African	≥37 (94)	≥31 (80)
Central and South American	≥37 (94)	≥31 (80)

Abbreviation: *cm* centimeters

A focused cardiovascular examination includes systolic and diastolic blood pressure readings (SBP/DBP), an electrocardiogram (ECG), as well as screening for dyspnea. Depending on clinical judgment, a full cardiovascular evaluation should be undertaken before a recommendation of increased activity is given to a patient. Since some pharmacological agents used to treat obesity and overweight have been associated with valvular heart disease in the past (fenfluramine and dexfenfluramine), a physical examination focused on heart sounds is essential before prescription of any weight loss medication.

The physical examination will reveal other complications of obesity or overweight, including musculoskeletal changes, edema, lymphedema, venous stasis, and skin changes (acanthosis nigricans, hirsutism, skin tags, and striae) and disorders of regional fat distribution.

Further assessment of body composition can also be useful in diagnosing obesity and overweight. Though many third-party payers do not cover the measurements, they are useful in diagnosis and may provide an additional source of income to the practice if found to be sustainable. Methods such as bioelectrical impedance analysis (BIA), dual-energy X-ray absorptiometry (DEXA), and magnetic resonance imaging (MRI) can all be used to document body composition. Each method has different advantages and limitations that define its effectiveness as a diagnostic tool, and its financial feasibility.

The fat mass index (FMI) is a more precise way of evaluating fat mass. This requires that fat mass be measured, as can be done with DEXA. The patient's FMI is defined as the fat mass in kilograms divided by the height in meters squared.

Laboratory testing should be conducted to stratify health risk. Laboratories are needed to document if there are causes of weight gain or an inability to lose weight, such as insulin resistance, thyroid disorders, and Cushing's syndrome. For primary and secondary laboratory tests, see Table 8.3. Laboratory tests should all be ordered using diagnostic codes other than for obesity or overweight to avoid lack of coverage. Appropriate diagnoses for each test are included in Table 8.3.

Testing of the patient's leptin-to-adiponectin ratio defines adipose tissue health. Leptin levels increase with increasing fat mass. Adiponectin levels drop with adipose tissue dysfunction. Trending the ratio documents the state of adipose tissue health for an individual over time. A ratio of leptin to adiponectin that increases over

Table 8.3 Minimal laboratory evaluation of a patient with overweight or obesity

Laboratory test	Diagnoses/symptoms
Primary tests	
Complete metabolic panel	Fatigue, kidney failure, fatty liver, diabetes mellitus
Complete blood count	Anemia, fatigue, dyspnea
Hemoglobin A1c	Prediabetes, diabetes mellitus, hyperglycemia
Lipid panel	Dyslipidemia, hypothyroidism, diabetes mellitus, hypertension
Secondary tests	
Overnight oximetry	Anemia, fatigue, dyspnea, hypersomnia, loud snoring
Thyroid-stimulating hormone	Fatigue, dyslipidemia, goiter
Testosterone(males)	Loss of libido, fatigue, anemia, erectile dysfunction

time signals progressive adipose tissue dysfunction (adiposopathy) and is a strong predictor of worsening metabolism. On the other hand a ratio of leptin to adiponectin that decreases over time signals improvement in adipose tissue function. Commercial assays for these two adipose tissue hormones are available from national reference laboratories.

8.5 Defining Success

The primary goal of treatment for patients with obesity or overweight is not weight loss on a scale. Rather, clinical endocrinology focuses on returning derangements of metabolism to normal, and this must now include adipose tissue dysfunction. Effective behavior modification is required for success in the long-term management of patients. The desired result is for the patient to achieve a negative energy balance.

Achieving a lean body weight is often an unrealistic goal in the management of overweight and obesity. A reduction of weight of 5–10% will reduce health risk drastically. This 5–10% reduction in body weight should be a desired goal for the ensuing 6–12 months of treatment. At any point in time, this goal of treatment should be reapplied to encourage ongoing weight loss. Most patients will not return to a lean BMI; hence, after any weight loss, the priority will be in the maintenance of the achieved lower weight. It is important to continue to set long-term realistic goals and to encourage decreased caloric intake and a higher amount of physical activity. This emphasis should replace the traditional adage of "diet and exercise" which suggests short-term measures and more immediate results.

Lifestyle changes will be easier to implement, and when stressed repeatedly, more likely to be integrated into the patient's daily habits if they are realistic, achievable, sustainable, and incremental over time. For example, it is best to recommend small amounts of physical activity repeatedly over the day, as opposed to one instance of prolonged physical activity. The use of stairs instead of an escalator or elevator, and parking further from entrances, each increases physical activity without the stigma of "exercise." Similarly, a decrease in caloric intake can be implemented as a decrease in calorie-dense foods and not necessarily the volume or frequency of meals. There are several clinical strategies that can be implemented to restrict caloric intake by making the patient more aware of serving sizes and eating habits. Small changes such as reducing the size of the physical plate, avoiding buffets or self-service tables, and prereducing restaurant portions in to-go containers can greatly reduce intake without drastically changing the patient's lifestyle.

Since these modifications won't result in immediate or drastic results, it is important that patients understand the concept of obesity as a chronic illness. Overweight, obesity, and adiposopathy do not have short-term solutions. Their treatment should be framed in this context so that patients do not become disillusioned and adhere to their treatment plan in the long term. Once the desired weight loss has been achieved, a program of weight maintenance will need to be implemented. Success in both achieving weight loss and maintaining lower weight should be individualized to the patient. Since the rate of recidivism is high in the treatment for obesity and overweight, it is important to incorporate certain components of behavior therapy, such as relapse prevention, which will prepare the patient to expect setbacks and view them as temporary. It is also important to highlight the patient's success and not to chastise mistakes. This approach can be effective in treating even severe obesity and can produce significant results over long periods of time.

8.6 Financial Management of a Bariatric Endocrinology Clinic

As obesity and overweight rates have risen in the United States, coverage for bariatric care has often been deemed too expensive for employers to offer to their employees and has been excluded for coverage in order to reduce health-care premiums. Until recently, this approach has also been reflected in most federal and state-funded coverage plans including Medicare. As a result, office visits, medical nutrition therapy, and pharmacotherapy for overweight and obesity have been excluded from coverage by most health plans.

In 2013, obesity and overweight were recognized by the American Medical Association as a disease continuum. Shifting of health-care resources from treatment to prevention, chiefly through the implementation of provisions of the Affordable Care Act (ACA), has set a precedent for the work of dedicated bariatric clinics to soon be covered through the International Classification of Diseases (ICD) codes for obesity and overweight. Until then, it is imperative that a clinic bill for medical care of the many complications of obesity. As of the publication of this textbook, third-party payer coverage of the billing codes for obesity or overweight is inconsistent, but there is consistent coverage for major complications. Billing codes for obesity and overweight should still be used in regard to billing.

It is important for a clinic to know what the local market will bear. The team-based approach is the most beneficial for treatment; however, many third-party payers may not cover the costs of specialists. Laboratory testing as well as other screenings can be costly and, due to gaps in coverage, may ultimately be the patient's financial responsibility; therefore, being able to gauge the makeup of the practice patient base is vital to success. A successful patient encounter is one that will foremost be beneficial to the patient and also be financially successful for the practice. Ideally, medical care for overweight, obesity, and adiposopathy would not be subsidized by the clinic. Thus, it is important that each encounter meets the overhead of the practice.

8.7 Conclusion

Overweight, obesity, and adiposopathy are chronic illnesses for which there is no cure. The goal of treatment will always be maintenance of a healthy lifestyle and the return of adipose tissue to proper function. Meeting these goals will result in a loss of excess fat mass. The models of care used for other chronic endocrine diseases should be applied to the treatment of overweight, obesity, and adiposopathy. The proper clinic and staff play a pivotal role in helping patients achieve long-term success. Bariatric endocrinology practices will be crucial in changing the prevailing attitudes of health-care professionals about patients with obesity.

Reading List

Alberti KG, Eckel RH, Grundy SM, Zimmet PZ, Cleeman JI, Donato KA, et al. Harmonizing the metabolic syndrome: a joint interim statement of the International Diabetes Federation Task Force on Epidemiology and Prevention; National Heart, Lung, and Blood Institute; American Heart Association; World Heart Federation; International Atherosclerosis Society; and International Association for the Study of Obesity. Circulation. 2009;120(16):1640–5. Epub 2009/10/07.

Collingnon A. Strategies for accommodation obese patients in a acute care setting. AAH J [Internet]. 2008 [Cited 2015 June 1]. Available from http://www.aia.org/practicing/groups/kc/AIAS076325.

de Koning L, Merchant AT, Pogue J, Anand SS. Waist circumference and waist-to-hip ratio as predictors of cardiovascular events: meta-regression analysis of prospective studies. Eur Heart J. 2007;28:850–6.

Gudzune KA, Doshi RS, Mehta AK, Chaudhry ZW, Jacobs DK, Vakil RM, et al. Efficacy of commercial weight-loss programs: an updated systematic review. Ann Intern Med. 2015;162:501–12. https://doi.org/10.7326/M14–2238.

Latner JD, Stunkard AJ. Getting worse: the stigmatization of obese children. Obes Res. 2003;11:452–6.

Neumark-Sztainer D, Story M, Faibisch L. Perceived stigmatization among overweight African-American and Caucasian adolescent girls. J Adolesc Health. 1998;23:264–70.

Neumark-Sztainer D, Story M, Harris T. Beliefs and attitudes about obesity among teachers and school health care providers working with adolescents. J Nutr Educ. 1999;31:3–9.

Puhl R, Brownell KD. Bias, discrimination, and obesity. Obes Res. 2001;9:788–805.
Puhl R, Brownell KD. Psychosocial origins of obesity stigma: toward changing a powerful and pervasive bias. Obes Rev. 2003;4:213–27.
Roehling MV. Weight-based discrimination in employment: psychological and legal aspects. Pers Psychol. 1999;52:969–1017.
Schwartz MB, O'Neal H, Brownell KD, Blair S, Billington C. Weight bias among health professionals specializing in obesity. Obes Res. 2003;11:1033–9.
Shaw K, O'Rourke P, Del Mar C, Kenardy J. Psychological interventions for overweight or obesity. Cochrane Database of Syst Rev. 2005;(2): CD003818.
Use of Workers' Compensation Data for Occupational Safetey and Health. Proceedings from June 2012 workshop. DHHS (NIOSH) publication no. 2013–147. Cincinnati.
Vazquez G, Duval S, Jacobs DR Jr, Silventoinen K. Comparison of body mass index, waist circumference, and waist/hip ratio in predicting incident diabetes: a meta-analysis. Epidemiol Rev. 2007;29:115–28.
Vega GL, Grundy SM. Metabolic risk susceptibility in men is partially related to adiponectin/leptin ratio. J Obes. 2013;2013:409679. https://doi.org/10.1155/2013/409679.
Wignall D. Design as a critical tool in bariatric patient care. J Diabetes Sci Technol. 2008; 2(2):263–7.
Williams DS. Bariatr Nurs Surg Patient Care. 2008;3(1):39–40. https://doi.org/10.1089/bar.2008.9993.

Chapter 9
Primary Causes of Adipose Tissue Weight Gain

Yi-Hao Yu and Jila Kaberi-Otarod

Pearls of Wisdom

- A large percentage of the human population is predisposed to obesity. Individuals who are susceptible to obesity have a permissive genetic background for excessive caloric intake and/or relatively reduced energy expenditure; obesity develops when these individuals are persistently exposed to an obesogenic environment.
- Monogenic obesity is relatively rare and is caused by single gene defects. It is usually characterized by severe and early-onset obesity. It is highly responsive to treatment, however, if correction of the defect is clinically attainable.
- Syndromic obesity is rare and may be caused by a single gene defect or defects of multiple functionally unrelated genes as a result of a gross genetic defect, such as chromosomal deletion, rearrangement, and/or imprinting. Obesity usually occurs early in life as one of the multiple phenotypic manifestations characteristic of the syndromes.
- The common forms of obesity may involve tens and even hundreds of gene variants in a susceptible individual, and the mode of disease transmission (genetic inheritance) varies due to the polygenic nature of the disease as well as the dependency of the disease manifestation on the environmental factors (lifestyles).

Y.-H. Yu (✉)
Greenwich Hospital and Endocrinology Associates of Greenwich, Northeast Medical Group, Yale-New Haven Health, Greenwich, CT, USA

Weight Loss and Diabetes Center, Department of Endocrinology, Stamford, CT, USA
e-mail: yihao.yu@greenwichhospital.org

J. Kaberi-Otarod
Geisinger System – North East, Department of Nutrition and Weight Management, Scranton, PA, USA

J. M. Gonzalez-Campoy et al. (eds.), *Bariatric Endocrinology*,
https://doi.org/10.1007/978-3-319-95655-8_9

- The common forms of obesity may be categorized into two major types: Metabolic obesity, characterized by an elevated body weight set point, and hedonic obesity, caused by sustained hedonic overeating that overrides the metabolic signals for energy abundance. Treatment modalities should be tailored to address the specific etiologies.

9.1 Introduction

Determining the etiology of obesity is as important in clinical practice as it is for understanding obesity out of academic interest. Treatment strategies that prove to be most effective are the ones that take into account the underlying causes of the disorders to be treated. Like diabetes mellitus, which is defined by elevated blood glucose level inclusive of all of its causes, obesity is the ultimate manifestation of excessive body fat (or body weight as a convenient but at times inaccurate surrogate), irrespective of its etiology. Also like diabetes, obesity is a disorder that actually has various underlying causes. Understanding and defining these causes are still a work in progress, but recognizing the specific types of obesity we already know is important and sometimes necessary to a treating clinician. Distinguishing between primary and secondary obesity, for example, is a job a clinician must make first. While primary obesity is managed by employing the usual weight loss treatment modalities, secondary obesity must be treated by addressing its primary etiologies, such as Cushing's syndrome, hypothyroidism, or other abnormalities, leading to the manifestation of obesity. Symptomatic treatment using a usual antiobesity regimen is rarely effective if the underlying abnormality is not corrected in these situations.

This chapter deals with the primary etiologies of obesity, which are diverse. The next chapter deals with secondary causes of obesity.

9.2 Metabolic Versus Hedonic Etiology

Primary causes of obesity are diverse, multifactorial, and may involve numerous biochemical and neuroendocrine pathways. We are at a relatively early stage of understanding, defining, and characterizing them. However, primary causes of obesity may be categorized into two distinct types, metabolic disorders and hedonic disorders (Fig. 9.1). There is overlap between the two types of disorders, as the neuroendocrine networks of the hedonic and metabolic systems in the brain cross-talk with each other. Additionally, an individual with obesity may also harbor a disorder in both the hedonic and the metabolic systems. The key is to determine the cause(s) of obesity or weight gain at the time of therapeutic intervention to make the therapy more effective.

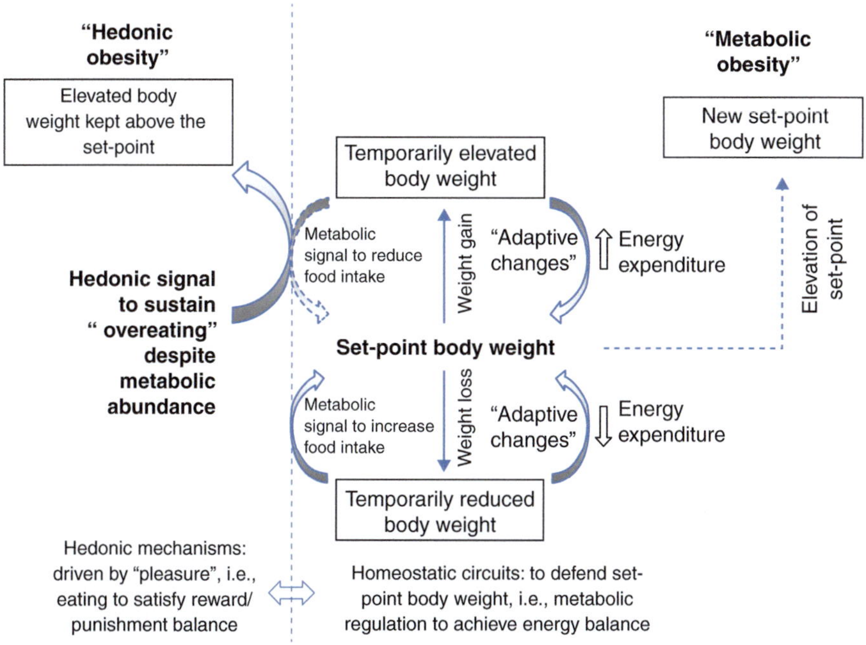

Fig. 9.1 Metabolic and hedonic obesity as related to their respective mechanisms of weight gain. The homeostatic weight regulatory system located primarily in the hypothalamus and the brainstem accounts for weight regulation around a body weight set point. Deviation of body weight from this set point elicits compensatory changes in food intake (cumulative over a long time period) and energy expenditure, in opposite directions, in order to restore the previous set point body weight. Obesity characterized by an elevated body weight set point, which is metabolically defended just as a normal set point body weight is defended, is termed "metabolic obesity." Hedonic eating is governed by the reward system to satisfy the need of pleasure and is nonhomeostatic with regard to energy balance. Dysfunction of the reward system may lead to hedonic overeating in susceptible individuals despite that the metabolic signals indicate energy abundance, leading to sustained weight gain above the metabolic set point weight; this form of obesity is termed "hedonic obesity"

9.2.1 Metabolic Obesity

Metabolic obesity is caused by elevation of body weight set point. Body weight set point defines the steady state body weight of an adult individual. Usually, body weight of an adult is fairly constant over a long period of time (years to decades), if the individual is not undergoing a significant physiological (e.g., menopause) or pathological (e.g., developing Cushing's syndrome) change. Any individual's body weight may fluctuate on a regular basis, as it may be influenced by variations in food consumption and energy expenditure; the caloric ins and outs may not always balance out at any given moment if measured by hours, days, or weeks. However, the weight changes are not random; body weight oscillates around a set point. Any significant deviation of body weight from the set point triggers compensatory metabolic responses that affect caloric intake and energy expenditure, which in turn restore the set point body weight. This type of body weight regulation is unconscious and controlled by the "metabolic brain," primarily composed of specific nuclei in the hypothalamus, the brainstem, and other specific brain structures. When an individual loses 5, 10, or 20 pounds of body weight due to an acute illness (e.g., a bad flu with anorexia or an acute kidney infection requiring hospitalization), the individual will readily gain back the weight after the illness is resolved. Conversely, if an individual gains 5–10 pounds during a vacation or a holiday season, his or her weight usually falls back to its previous level after the individual resumes his or her "normal" life. Of course, each individual has a unique body weight set point, just like the individual's height, blood pressure, or some other phenotypical or physiological characteristics. The individual's body weight set point is in part determined by the individual's genetics (which is generally believed to be of 40–80% heritability, but 20–90% have been reported by various studies). The rest of the influences on body weight set point are attributed to developmental and environmental factors.

An individual's set point may be raised even in adulthood due to certain genetic-environmental interactions. A large body of evidence suggests that our obesogenic environment in the past few decades, particularly high-fat, high-sugar, and caloric-dense foods, has triggered the expression of a higher body weight set point in genetically susceptible individuals. It is believed that persistent exposure to high-fat and high-sugar foods can cause functional and structural changes in the neural circuits in the brain that control energy intake and expenditure, leading to resetting of the body weight set point. Leptin, or the *ob* gene product, an adipocyte-derived humoral signal that informs the brain of the energy reserve status, is an intrinsic part of the brain homeostatic energy balance circuitry that defines the body weight set point. A meal plan composed of high-fat and high-sugar foods impairs leptin signaling, and the acquired leptin resistance is one way of resetting the set point to a higher level. Additionally, loss of synaptic connectivity in hypothalamic POMC (pro-opiomelanocortin)/CART (cocaine- and amphetamine-regulated transcript) neurons, a critical set of neurons that is part of the energy balance circuitry, has also been implicated as a cause of elevated body weight set point and, hence, metabolic obesity. This change is also environment triggered, due to diet-induced inflammation, reactive gliosis, and/or aging of hypothalamic neurons.

9.2.2 Hedonic Obesity

Hedonic obesity is caused by a disorder of the hedonic regulation system, the "cognitive and emotional brain" that controls the reward and pleasure derived from ingesting palatable foods. This hedonic system is composed of a set of brain structures that is distinct from the metabolic brain. It is known as the cortico-limbic neural network. The core components of this system are the signaling pathways for "liking" (the level of pleasure or reward) and "wanting" (the motivation or drive to consume food). Like the metabolic brain, the signaling activities controlling these processes are subconscious. Implicit "liking" is believed to be mediated by μ (mu)-opioid receptor and CB1 cannabinoid receptor signaling networks, centered in the nucleus accumbens (NAc) of the ventral striatum and ventral pallidum. Implicit "wanting" is chiefly encoded in the mesolimbic dopaminergic neurons that project from ventral tegmental area (VTA) to NAc. The liking and wanting are also modulated by multiple other neuronal pathways. These include metabolic signals from the "metabolic brain" reflecting the energy balance status. They also include neuronal processes involving emotion, stress, and even arousal, irrespective of energy balance. The hedonic system integrates some of the basic midbrain, hindbrain, and hypothalamic functions with more complex cortical functions involving conscious and volitional aspects of the brain that are essential for meeting the reward balance, as in, for example, the cortical function of procurement of food. The NAc of the basal forebrain and the VTA of the midbrain, two major sites where liking and wanting are processed and interpreted, have connections to multiple brain areas, including the hippocampus, amygdala, gustatory and orbitofrontal cortex, hypothalamus, and other brainstem structures. These connections are believed to play an important role in coordinating the conscious and unconscious components related to hedonic eating.

Derangements of the hedonic system may be explained by the two prevailing hypotheses related to food evaluation and rewards. The "gluttony hypothesis" emphasizes a positive correlation between the amount of dopaminergic signaling in an individual and the pleasure derived from the sensory experience of ingestion. The "reward deficiency hypothesis" suggests that a deficiency in dopaminergic signaling is the cause of overindulgence in food; such overindulgence is a compensatory reaction to the difficulty in achieving pleasure. Impairments of the reward system may stem from sustained exposure to processed, calorically dense foods. Chronic consumption of these foods can lead to elevated dopamine release and transporter expression, as well as downregulation of dopamine D1 and D2 receptor expression in the NAc and dorsal striatum. The changes in the dopamine reward pathway can be demonstrated in "food addicts," and these changes, particularly the downregulation of dopamine receptors, are similar to those seen in drug addiction. These changes in the dopaminergic pathway lead to sustained overconsumption of foods and calories because of the need to achieve and maintain the level of reward/pleasure in a flawed hedonic system. The hedonic demands are sufficiently powerful to override metabolic signals that would otherwise keep energy balance in check. Hedonic obesity develops when the body weight is raised significantly above the usual set point body weight despite the metabolic signals that already indicate energy surplus.

Patients with hedonic obesity likely have an underlying eating disorder or even "food addiction," although the latter is not a prerequisite. Also frequently seen in these patients are psychiatric co-morbidities, such as depression, anxiety, chronic stress, and sleep deprivation. Hedonic obesity may often be identified on these clinical grounds in association with the finding of constant hedonic hunger present in these individuals. However, a subjective physiological characteristic is an increased resting and/or total energy expenditure per unit of body weight or "metabolic weight," compared to people without obesity, or people with metabolic obesity.

Behavioral and lifestyle modifications, including traditional behavior therapy and possibly pharmacotherapy, would be the primary treatment modalities for treating hedonic obesity. On the other hand, metabolic modifications that are aimed at lowering the body weight set point would be necessary to effectively treat metabolic obesity. This is a fertile ground for future pharmacological exploration. The available data from studies of bariatric surgery suggest that, in general, bariatric surgery has the potential to modify hedonic pathways and alter body weight set point, and therefore, this surgery may be suitable for treating both hedonic and metabolic obesity.

9.3 Genetic Influence

9.3.1 Monogenic Obesity and Syndromic Obesity

People with monogenic obesity have an identifiable underlying genetic trait (defect) as the cause of obesity. Monogenic forms of obesity are relatively rare. Affected individuals usually develop obesity early in life, and the degree of obesity is usually more severe. However, monogenic obesity is also highly responsive to treatment, if correction of the defect is clinically attainable. Families with monogenic obesity have been reported in the literature, and the genetic defects reported so far include several genes in the leptin-melanocortin pathways, including leptin, leptin receptor, POMC, MC4R (melanocortin 4 receptor), and prohormone convertase 1 (PCSK1) and Src homology 2B adaptor protein 1 (SH2B1). For details of the pathways, see Chap. 4 and the relevant references listed in this chapter.

Patients with leptin deficiency and leptin receptor deficiency were identified shortly after the positional cloning of the leptin and leptin receptor genes in 1994 and 1995, respectively. The defects in these genes are responsible for the phenotype of extreme obesity of the respective mouse strains, *ob/ob* and *db/db*. Patients homozygous for loss-of-function mutations of LEP (leptin) or LEPR (leptin receptor) genes are characterized by normal birthweight. But they rapidly gain weight (predominantly fat) shortly after birth due to hyperphagia and altered energy partition in favor of fat deposition. Although early linear growth and cognitive development are usually normal, these patients have severely impaired pubertal development due to hypogonadotropic hypogonadism and hypothalamic hypothyroidism. As an indicator of the size of body's energy store, leptin serves as a permissive factor for normal pubertal development, reproduction, and immunity. Normal functions of the hypothalamic gonadotropin-releasing hormone (GnRH) neurons and thyrotropin-releasing hormone (TRH) neurons require leptin signaling. Ironically, in the case of leptin and leptin receptor deficiency, the lack of leptin signaling makes a false representation of extreme energy deficit, despite the massive obesity. Administration of recombinant leptin to children with congenital leptin deficiency reverses the hyperphagia and obesity with a preferential loss of fat mass (Fig. 9.2). There is also normalization of thyroid function and resumption of pubertal development in leptin-treated children.

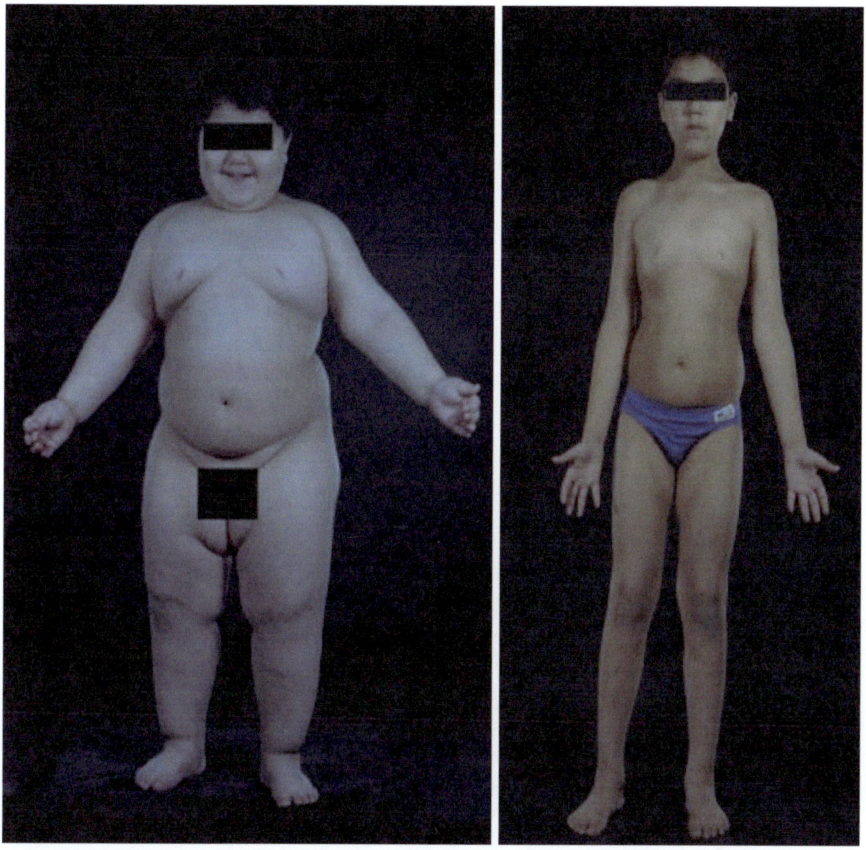

Fig. 9.2 Congenital leptin deficiency. A 3-year-old boy with congenital leptin deficiency weighing 42-kg began treatment with recombinant leptin (left). At age 7 years, he weighed 32 kg (right). (Adapted from Farooqi and O'Rahilly (2014)

POMC deficiency is another intriguing form of monogenic obesity. POMC is a propeptide and undergoes post-translational cleavage to produce multiple active hormones. In the pituitary gland, POMC is cleaved to produce adrenocorticotropic hormone (ACTH), melanotropins, and endorphins, among several other cleavage products. One of the melanotropins, alpha-melanocyte-stimulating hormone (alpha-MSH), binds to the melanocortin receptor of melanocytes in the skin, MC1R, to stimulate the production of black/brown pigment (eumelanin). Alpha-MSH also plays an important role in controlling food intake and energy expenditure through its action on two of the melanocortin receptors in the hypothalamus, MC3R and MC4R. Understandably, congenital POMC deficiency produces a phenotype of hypocortisolism (typically presenting with neonatal hypoglycemia and cholestatic jaundice), early onset of obesity, and red hair and pale skin (Fig. 9.3). While the classical triad of the phenotype of POMC deficiency is well appreciated, a note of caution is also needed, as not all POMC-deficient patients have red hair. More

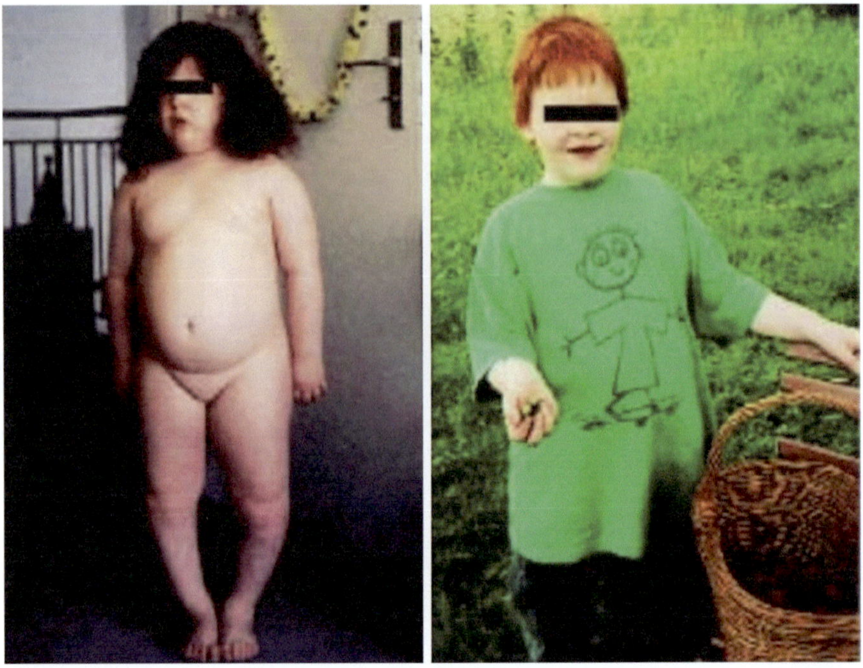

Fig. 9.3 Congenital pro-opiomelanocortin deficiency. Pro-opiomelanocortin deficiency produces a phenotypic triad of red hair (due to melanocyte-stimulating hormone deficiency), hypocortisolism (due to adrenocorticotropic hormone deficiency), and childhood obesity which begins shortly after birth (due to a lack of second-order neuron melanocortin receptor stimulation in the hypothalamus). The girl on the left was found to be a compound heterozygote for two mutations in exon 3 (G7013 T, C7133Δ) which interfere with the appropriate synthesis of ACTH and alpha-MSH. The boy on the right was homozygous for a mutation in exon 2 (C3804A) which abolishes POMC translation. (Adapted from Krude et al. (1998)

recently, non-red-haired POMC-deficient patients have also been described. They display two of the phenotypic triad, early onset of obesity, and adrenal insufficiency, but they have dark hair. It is believed that in some non-Caucasian ethnic groups, eumelanin may also be produced independently of alpha-MSH.

Single gene defects in LEP, LEPR and POMC, MC4R, PCSK1, and SH2B1 as a cause of monogenic obesity are summarized in Table 9.1.

It should be noted that heterozygous carriers of the LEP, LEPR, POMC, and PCSK1 gene mutations do not exhibit the severe obesity phenotype of their homozygous counterparts. In contrast, haploinsufficiency in MC4R can lead to severe obesity. Additionally, MC4R gene defect variants are very common, with a population prevalence of >0.05%. The prevalence sampled among children with obesity is up to 1–6% and that among adults with obesity is 0.5–1%. Human loss-of-function mutations have been described in heterozygous carriers with severe early-onset obesity.

Syndromic obesity is due to a genetic defect that causes obesity in association with a distinct set of other phenotypic characteristics and/or functional deficits recognized

Table 9.1 Examples of monogenic obesity

Gene	Defect	Characteristics
LEP	Congenital leptin deficiency	Severe hyperphagia and morbid obesity Responds well to treatment with recombinant leptin
LEPR	Leptin receptor deficiency	Very similar phenotype as in LEP Presently, no specific treatment is available that targets the defect
POMC	Pro-opiomelanocortin deficiency	Hyperphagia and obesity (loss of melanocortin signaling at MC4R) Pale skin and red hair (loss of melanocortin signaling at MC1R) Adrenal crisis (ACTH deficiency) Selective MC4R agonists are being developed and expected to be effective
MC4R	Defect in melanocortin 4 receptor	Hyperphagia and obesity, as well as increased lean mass (big-boned) No specific treatment available yet, but selective MC4R agonist being developed may be effective, particularly for the heterozygotic defect
PCSK1	Prohormone convertase 1 deficiency	Obesity and hypocortisolism (impaired processing of POMC) Postprandial hypoglycemia (related to processing defect of proinsulin and hypocortisolism) Hypogonadotropic hypogonadism and small bowel dysfunction (impaired processing of gonadal and gut prohormones, respectively) No specific treatment available presently
SH2B1	Src homology 2B adaptor protein 1 deficiency	Hyperphagia and obesity, insulin resistance, reduced adult height, and behavioral abnormalities including social isolation and aggression No specific treatment available that targets the defect

Note: Heterozygous forms of MC4R (melanocortin 4 receptor), LEP (leptin), LEPR (leptin receptor), and POMC (pro-opiomelanocortin) exhibit a less severe and nonfully penetrant form of obesity. MC4R mutations are the most common, with a population prevalence of at least 0.05%, a prevalence of 0.5–1% among adults with obesity, and a prevalence of1–6% among children with obesity

as a syndrome. Syndromic obesity may be due to a single gene defect or defects in multiple genes as occurring in chromosomal deletion/rearrangement. Summarized in Table 9.2 are several well-recognized syndromic obesity disorders.

9.3.2 Common Forms of Obesity: Polygenic Attributes

The common forms of obesity are of polygenic origin. Through unbiased genome-wide association studies (GWAS), 97 loci containing about 405 genes (most of these are conceivably not BMI-associated genes) have been identified to contribute to obesity. More BMI-associated loci may be identified in the future, but they likely confer less risk than those already identified. Many of the genes contained in the

Table 9.2 Examples of syndromic obesity

Syndrome	Phenotype	Genetic defect
Prader-Willi syndrome (PWS) Rare but most common syndromal cause of human obesity: 1/50,000	Extreme hyperphagia and early central obesity accompanied by muscular hypotonia, short stature, small hands and feet, hypogonadotropic hypogonadism, and significant cognitive deficits	Loss of expression of imprinted paternal genes on 15q11–13, mostly (75%) because of deletions on paternal chromosome Candidate genes include the dectin (NDN) gene, small nuclear ribonucleoprotein polypeptide N (SNRPN) gene, the ring zinc finger 127-polypeptide gene, the MAGE-like gene, and the Prader-Willi critical region 1 gene The precise mechanisms by which the candidate genes lead to obesity remains unclear Ghrelin, the "hunger gene" product, which was found to be 4.5-fold elevated in PWS than in non-PWS obesity, has been implicated in the pathogenesis of hyperphagia in PWS
Bardet-Biedl syndrome (BBS) Rare autosomal recessive obesity syndrome: <1/100,000	Central obesity (in 75% of patients) associated with mental retardation, dysphormic extremities, retinal dystrophy or pigmentary retinopathy, hypogonadism, and structural abnormalities of the kidney	Heterogeneous disorder involving mutations of BBS genes that have been mapped to at least eight loci: BBS1 (11q13), BBS2 (16q21), BBS3 (3p13-p12), BBS4 (15q22.3-q23), BBS5, BBS6 (20q12), BBS7 (4q27), and BBS8 (14q32.11) BBS genes are believed to involve in the genesis of cilia and flagella, and the obesity phenotype is speculated to be due to defected cilia functions of the hypothalamic neurons BBS8 localizes to centrosomes and basal bodies and interacts with a protein involved in ciliogenesis, pericentriolar material 1 protein (PCM1), and BBS4 is an adaptor to recruit PCM1 Defects in BBS4 cause abnormal cytokinesis and apoptosis Specific mutations in BBS6 also cause McKusick-Kaufman syndrome
Alstrom syndrome Very rare autosomal recessive obesity syndrome	Early onset of obesity associated with retinal dystrophy, neurosensory deafness, and diabetes Subsets of affected individuals may present with dilated cardiomyopathy, hepatic dysfunction, hypothyroidism, male hypogonadism, developmental delay, and short stature	Mutations in a single gene, ALMS1, a cilia-related gene associated with the primary cilia function (a sensory function of most cell types) are responsible defects

Carpenter syndrome Very rare autosomal recessive obesity syndrome	Obesity associated with characteristic craniofacial malformations (e.g., a tower-shaped skull or pointed head), additional digits or fused fingers or toes (syndactyly), and variable mental retardation. It is also called acrocephalopolysyndactyly type II	Mutations in a single gene RAB23, encoding a protein, which is a member of the RAB family of small guanosine triphosphatases at the primary cilium
Borjeson-Forssman-Lehmann syndrome Very rare X-linked obesity syndrome	Obesity with gynecomastia and large ears Affected individuals have moderate-to-severe mental retardation, epilepsy, and hypogonadism	Mutations in the widely expressed zinc finger gene, plant homeodomain (PHD)-like finger, PHF6, has been linked to this syndrome. PHF6 is localized in the cell nucleus and nucleolus and plays a role in transcription regulation, but the mechanism for obesity has not been worked out
Cohen syndrome Very rare autosomal recessive obesity syndrome	Obesity associated with microcephaly with characteristic facial features, progressive retinochoroidal dystrophy, and mental retardation	Mutations in the VPS13B (COH1) gene encoding a Golgi matrix protein, widely expressed in the brain. The exact mechanism unknown
Albright's hereditary osteodystrophy (AHO) Very rare autosomal dominant obesity syndrome	Obesity with short stature, round face, and skeletal defects including typical brachydactyly and ectopic soft tissue ossification (AHO phenotype) Maternal transmission leads to AHO phenotype plus resistance to parathyroid hormone in target tissues (pseudohypoparathyroidism type 1A); paternal transmission leads only to AHD phenotype without resistance to parathyroid hormone (pseudopseudohypoparathyroidism)	Mutations in a single gene encoding the alpha subunits of the stimulatory G protein (Gsa), GNAS1 are responsible for this syndrome. GNAS1 is imprinted in a tissue-specific manner It is expressed primarily from the maternal allele in certain tissues and biallelically expressed in most other tissues Hormone (multiple) resistance occurs only when Gsa mutations are inherited maternally
WAGR syndrome One of the best-studied contiguous gene syndromes	A subset of WAGR syndrome shows severe early-onset obesity The affected individuals are predisposed to developing Wilms tumor, aniridia, genitourinary anomalies (gonadoblastoma), and (mental) retardation	Chromosomal deletions at 11p13, which encompasses many genes including the PAX6 ocular development gene and the Wilms' tumor gene, WT1 Haplodeficiency of BDNF (brain-derived neurotrophic factor) is believed to be responsible for hyperphagia and obesity in affected individuals

BMI-associated genetic loci are highly expressed in the central nervous system (CNS). The majority of the tissues enriched with these genes are located in the CNS structures implicated in the regulation of energy metabolism, such as the hypothalamus, the pituitary gland, the limbic system, and the hippocampus. These data provide independent support for both metabolic and hedonic causes of obesity as described above in Sect. 9.2. Pathway analyses suggest the involvement of several well-known CNS pathways as well as biochemical and cellular processes linked to energy metabolism. These include regulation of hormones relevant to weight control such as insulin and glucagon-like peptide 1 (GLP-1), and cellular signaling via mitogen-activated protein (MAP) kinase and mammalian target of rapamycin (mTOR); the latter is known as a cellular nutrient sensor. Many novel pathways have also been implicated. Interestingly, the novel pathways seem to highlight the role of synaptic function and long-term potentiation, that is, signaling via the neurotransmitters glutamate, dopamine, norepinephrine, serotonin, and gamma-aminobutyric acid (GABA). These synaptic functions are associated with a wide spectrum of CNS roles in memory, learning, cognition, emotion, physical activity, and coordination. Energy metabolism is thus regulated via the reward system as well as the metabolic circuitry. Finally, analyses of the enriched gene set also suggest the involvement of the process of chromatin organization and modification, which may provide a link between obesity and epigenetic modifications (see Sect. 9.4.2 below).

9.4 Environmental Influences

9.4.1 Obesogenic Environment

The prevalence of obesity has reached an epidemic level. This is a recent phenomenon in the long human history. We are still bearing witness to the rising obesity rate. In the United States, for example, the obesity prevalence was about 22% in the late 1980s. It increased to 30% in the late 1990s, and by the late 2000s, it reached to 35%. The human gene pool has not changed significantly during this time. Our genetic makeup predisposes us to efficiently store excess energy as body fat. The ability to store energy effectively is due to the "thrifty genes" that we have inherited over the long human evolutionary history. For the most part in human history, food shortage and famine were the "norm," and acquiring food required physical labor. The thrifty genes conferred tremendous evolutionary advantages in these settings. However, this evolutionary pressure has changed with the development and maturation of agriculture, the modern industrialization in many parts of the world, and particularly with the rise in the food industry in the past few decades. Foods become abundant and easily attainable, and physical activity is much less demanded in association with modernization of transportation and the increase in deskwork jobs. Processed foods are energy dense and can be manufactured cheaply in large quantities. The flavor of these foods is ever improving to tailor to human's taste for fat and sugar. There is evidence that where "healthy" and "natural" foods cannot be priced reasonably as compared to the high-energy processed foods, obesity is more prevalent. The fact that the prevalence of obesity is greater in people with a lower socioeconomic status perhaps speaks to the fact that obesity is no longer a condition of the rich people, as was the case before the era of the processed food industry.

Much work and innovations are needed to reverse the current obesogenic environment. We need to improve the micro- and macro-environments of our homes, our close social circles, and our large surroundings. However, it is a matter of debate whether regulations of the agriculture and food industries are necessary and appropriate to prevent cheap processed foods from stuffing the shelves of our grocery stores and the pantries of our homes. It also remains controversial whether it has to take measures such as urban and city redesigning and planning (streets, schools, and shopping spaces, etc.) in order to promote healthy eating and more physical activity. Surely we will remain ineffective in combating the current obesity epidemic, until we can correct the environment that promotes obesity.

9.4.2 Developmental Factors and Epigenetic Alteration

From the GWAS studies, it has been estimated that over 20% of BMI variability may be explained by common genetic differences in the 100 or so genetic loci already identified. This number is smaller than the empirically estimated 40–80% BMI variability due to genetic influences expected from earlier non-GWAS studies. This gap may be explained by the following: (1) overestimation of genetic and/or underestimation of environmental influences, (2) the possibility that there are hundreds or thousands more genes that are participants in energy metabolism, the influence of each of these genes being too small to be detected by the current GWAS studies but in aggregate conferring a significant fraction of the genetic risk for obesity, and (3) underappreciated gene-gene and gene-environment interactions.

The body weight of a parent is a powerful determinant of the body weight of an offspring. In addition to the shared genes (genetic transmission) and the shared environment (eating habits and other similar lifestyle factors), epigenetic transmission may also play a role. This type of transmission is through gene-environment interactions that alter the expression of susceptible genes via DNA methylation and/or histone modification in selective DNA segments, without altering the DNA sequences. Understanding the epigenetic mechanisms of obesity development is of particular interest because developmental programming of obesity is potentially an avoidable event. Unlike the genetic transmission of DNA codes, epigenetic transmission is preventable. Prevention requires that we know what environmental factors turn on the epigenetic modifications, and at which developmental stage, which may even include preconception stages represented by the yet unfertilized maternal or paternal gametes. If we can modify the environment during pregnancy and/or early life, we may succeed in preventing obesity later in life.

Developmental studies in humans are complex but have yielded much information regarding potential environmental factors that predict obesity later in life, particularly with regard to maternal nutrition and the birth weight of the children. Many mechanistic insights into epigenetic alterations come from animal studies. A recent study in the fruit fly *Drosophila melanogaster* illustrated nicely how epigenetic mechanisms work. A gene product, Su(vart), has been shown to participate in epigenetic changes (i.e., altering chromatin conformation and gene expression) in response to a high-sugar diet fed to the offspring. This happened only if the male flies were fed the same diet 2 days before mating, during which time epigenetic changes can occur in the sperm. The gene product Su(vart) is conserved in humans. Microarray studies in paired human monozygotic twins suggest that obesity versus lean phenotypes in the paired twins are also associated with differentially expressed levels of this protein.

9.5 Conclusion

Obesity is characterized by excessive adipose tissue (and body) weight, which frequently leads to serious metabolic derangements. Excessive adiposity is caused by net caloric storage resulting from excess caloric intake relative to the body's energy expenditure over a long period of time. The primary etiology of human obesity is linked to both genetic predisposition and obesogenic environments. Monogenic and syndromic obesities are predominantly genetic in etiology and are usually characterized by severe and early-onset obesity. On the other hand, the common forms of obesity vary in severity and result from interaction of an obesogenic environment and multiple obesity-prone gene variants in susceptible individuals. Dozens (possibly hundreds) of gene variants are at play, producing a permissive condition for obesity to develop when environmental conditions are met. This makes the common forms of obesity extremely difficult to treat. A treatment modality targeting a few selective genetic deficits may not solve the problem of excessive weight gain. The complex polygenic nature of the common forms of obesity may be better appreciated by considering that there are numerous biochemical pathways involved in the regulation of energy metabolism and that each of these may be affected by genetic, epigenetic, and environmental factors. The sum of these effects, likely inconsequential individually, may translate into significant alterations in the body's metabolic circuitry of energy balance and/or the hedonic neuro-circuitry, resulting in metabolic obesity and/or hedonic obesity, respectively. The classification into metabolic obesity and hedonic obesity is important, and it may allow more tailored treatments to be developed for the two specific disorders. These treatment modalities may include pharmacological, behavioral, and surgical interventions and their appropriate combinations. In addition, environmental modifications at the societal level will likely be necessary in order to curtail the continued rise of obesity rate worldwide.

Reading List

Ahima RS, Saper CB, Flier JS, Elmquist JK. Leptin regulation of neuroendocrine systems. Front Neuroendocrinol. 2000;21(3):263–307.

Allen PJ, Batra P, Geiger BM, Wommack T, Gilhooly C, Pothos EN. Rationale and consequences of reclassifying obesity as an addictive disorder: neurobiology, food environment and social policy perspectives. Physiol Behav. 2012;107(1):126–37.

Barsh GS, Farooqi IS, O'Rahilly S. Genetics of body-weight regulation. Nature. 2000;404(6778):644–51.

Bell CG, Walley AJ, Froguel P. The genetics of human obesity. Nat Rev Genet. 2005;6(3):221–34.

Berridge KC, Robinson TE, Aldridge JW. Dissecting components of reward: 'liking', 'wanting', and learning. Curr Opin Pharmacol. 2009;9(1):65–73.

Berthoud HR. Metabolic and hedonic drives in the neural control of appetite: who is the boss? Curr Opin Neurobiol. 2011;21(6):888–96.

Berthoud HR, Morrison C. The brain, appetite, and obesity. Annu Rev Psychol. 2008;59:55–92.

Clement K, Dubern B, Mencarelli M, Czernichow P, Ito S, Wakamatsu K, et al. Unexpected endocrine features and normal pigmentation in a young adult patient carrying a novel homozygous mutation in the POMC gene. J Clin Endocrinol Metab. 2008;93(12):4955–62.

Cummins S, Macintyre S. Food environments and obesity—neighbourhood or nation? Int J Epidemiol. 2006;35(1):100–4.

Doche ME, Bochukova EG, Su HW, Pearce LR, Keogh JM, Henning E, et al. Human SH2B1 mutations are associated with maladaptive behaviors and obesity. J Clin Invest. 2012;122(12):4732–6.

Elmquist JK, Coppari R, Balthasar N, Ichinose M, Lowell BB. Identifying hypothalamic pathways controlling food intake, body weight, and glucose homeostasis. J Comp Neurol. 2005;493(1):63–71.

Farooqi IS, O'Rahilly S. Monogenic obesity in humans. Annu Rev Med. 2005;56:443–58.

Farooqi IS, O'Rahilly S. 20 years of leptin: human disorders of leptin action. J Endocrinol. 2014;223(1):T63–70.

Farooqi IS, Jebb SA, Langmack G, Lawrence E, Cheetham CH, Prentice AM, et al. Effects of recombinant leptin therapy in a child with congenital leptin deficiency. N Engl J Med. 1999;341(12):879–84.

Farooqi IS, Drop S, Clements A, Keogh JM, Biernacka J, Lowenbein S, et al. Heterozygosity for a POMC-null mutation and increased obesity risk in humans. Diabetes. 2006;55(9):2549–53.

Flier JS. Clinical review 94: what's in a name? In search of leptin's physiologic role. J Clin Endocrinol Metab. 1998;83(5):1407–13.

Garvey W, Mechanick JI, Einhorn D. The American Association of Clinical Endocrinologists and the American College of Endocrinology: 2014 advanced framework for a new diagnosis of obesity as a chronic disease 2014. Available from: https://www.aace.com/files/2014-advanced-framework-for-a-new-diagnosis-of-obesity-as-a-chronic-disease.pdf.

Govaerts C, Srinivasan S, Shapiro A, Zhang S, Picard F, Clement K, et al. Obesity-associated mutations in the melanocortin 4 receptor provide novel insights into its function. Peptides. 2005;26(10):1909–19.

Grill HJ, Hayes MR. Hindbrain neurons as an essential hub in the neuroanatomically distributed control of energy balance. Cell Metab. 2012;16(3):296–309.

Harris RB. Role of set-point theory in regulation of body weight. FASEB J. 1990;4(15):3310–8.

Hebebrand J, Hinney A, Knoll N, Volckmar AL, Scherag A. Molecular genetic aspects of weight regulation. Dtsch Arztebl Int. 2013;110(19):338–44.

Horvath TL, Sarman B, Garcia-Caceres C, Enriori PJ, Sotonyi P, Shanabrough M, et al. Synaptic input organization of the melanocortin system predicts diet-induced hypothalamic reactive gliosis and obesity. Proc Natl Acad Sci U S A. 2010;107(33):14875–80.

Ifland JR, Preuss HG, Marcus MT, Rourke KM, Taylor WC, Burau K, et al. Refined food addiction: a classic substance use disorder. Med Hypotheses. 2009;72(5):518–26.

Johannsen DL, Knuth ND, Huizenga R, Rood JC, Ravussin E, Hall KD. Metabolic slowing with massive weight loss despite preservation of fat-free mass. J Clin Endocrinol Metab. 2012;97(7):2489–96.

Krude H, Biebermann H, Luck W, Horn R, Brabant G, Gruters A. Severe early-onset obesity, adrenal insufficiency and red hair pigmentation caused by POMC mutations in humans. Nat Genet. 1998;19(2):155–7.

Lake A, Townshend T. Obesogenic environments: exploring the built and food environments. J R Soc Promot Heal. 2006;126(6):262–7.

Leibel RL. Is obesity due to a heritable difference in 'set point' for adiposity? West J Med. 1990;153(4):429–31.

Leibel RL. Molecular physiology of weight regulation in mice and humans. Int J Obes. 2008;32(Suppl 7):S98–108.
Leibel RL, Rosenbaum M, Hirsch J. Changes in energy expenditure resulting from altered body weight. N Engl J Med. 1995;332(10):621–8.
Locke AE, Kahali B, Berndt SI, Justice AE, Pers TH, Day FR, et al. Genetic studies of body mass index yield new insights for obesity biology. Nature. 2015;518(7538):197–206.
Maes HH, Neale MC, Eaves LJ. Genetic and environmental factors in relative body weight and human adiposity. Behav Genet. 1997;27(4):325–51.
McNay DE, Speakman JR. High fat diet causes rebound weight gain. Mol Metab. 2012;2(2):103–8.
McNay DE, Briancon N, Kokoeva MV, Maratos-Flier E, Flier JS. Remodeling of the arcuate nucleus energy-balance circuit is inhibited in obese mice. J Clin Invest. 2012;122(1):142–52.
Mendiratta MS, Yang Y, Balazs AE, Willis AS, Eng CM, Karaviti LP, et al. Early onset obesity and adrenal insufficiency associated with a homozygous POMC mutation. Int J Pediatr Endocrinol. 2011;2011(1):5.
Morton GJ, Cummings DE, Baskin DG, Barsh GS, Schwartz MW. Central nervous system control of food intake and body weight. Nature. 2006;443(7109):289–95.
Ng SF, Lin RC, Laybutt DR, Barres R, Owens JA, Morris MJ. Chronic high-fat diet in fathers programs beta-cell dysfunction in female rat offspring. Nature. 2010;467(7318):963–6.
Ost A, Lempradl A, Casas E, Weigert M, Tiko T, Deniz M, et al. Paternal diet defines offspring chromatin state and intergenerational obesity. Cell. 2014;159(6):1352–64.
Ozanne SE. Epigenetic signatures of obesity. N Engl J Med. 2015;372(10):973–4.
Poston L. Maternal obesity, gestational weight gain and diet as determinants of offspring long term health. Best Pract Res Clin Endocrinol Metab. 2012;26(5):627–39.
Ravussin Y, Gutman R, Diano S, Shanabrough M, Borok E, Sarman B, et al. Effects of chronic weight perturbation on energy homeostasis and brain structure in mice. Am J Physiol Regul Integr Comp Physiol. 2011;300(6):R1352–62.
Rosenbaum M, Hirsch J, Gallagher DA, Leibel RL. Long-term persistence of adaptive thermogenesis in subjects who have maintained a reduced body weight. Am J Clin Nutr. 2008;88(4):906–12.
Sabin MA, Werther GA, Kiess W. Genetics of obesity and overgrowth syndromes. Best Pract Res Clin Endocrinol Metab. 2011;25(1):207–20.
Sesack SR, Grace AA. Cortico-Basal Ganglia reward network: microcircuitry. Neuropsychopharmacology. 2010;35(1):27–47.
Speliotes EK, Willer CJ, Berndt SI, Monda KL, Thorleifsson G, Jackson AU, et al. Association analyses of 249,796 individuals reveal 18 new loci associated with body mass index. Nat Genet. 2010;42(11):937–48.
Thaler JP, Yi CX, Schur EA, Guyenet SJ, Hwang BH, Dietrich MO, et al. Obesity is associated with hypothalamic injury in rodents and humans. J Clin Invest. 2012;122(1):153–62.
Volkow ND, Wang GJ, Tomasi D, Baler RD. Obesity and addiction: neurobiological overlaps. Obes Rev. 2013;14(1):2–18.
Waalen J. The genetics of human obesity. Transl Res. 2014;164(4):293–301.
Walley AJ, Asher JE, Froguel P. The genetic contribution to non-syndromic human obesity. Nat Rev Genet. 2009;10(7):431–42.
Wells JC. The evolution of human fatness and susceptibility to obesity: an ethological approach. Biol Rev Camb Philos Soc. 2006;81(2):183–205.
York D, Bouchard C. How obesity develops: insights from the new biology. Endocrine. 2000;13(2):143–54.
Yu YH, Vasselli JR, Zhang Y, Mechanick JI, Korner J, Peterli R. Metabolic vs. hedonic obesity: a conceptual distinction and its clinical implications. Obes Rev. 2015;16(3):234–47.
Zhang Y, Proenca R, Maffei M, Barone M, Leopold L, Friedman JM. Positional cloning of the mouse obese gene and its human homologue. Nature. 1994;372(6505):425–32.

Chapter 10
Secondary Causes of Adipose Tissue Weight Gain

Daniel L. Hurley

Pearls of Wisdom

- There is a strong relationship between total energy expenditure, resting energy expenditure, and fat-free mass. The differences in fat-free mass account for a large percentage of total energy expenditure variance among individuals.
- Hypothalamic obesity is rare in humans and is usually due to injury, surgery, tumor, or infiltrative disease.
- Patients with hypothyroidism may have a modest increase in weight due to slowing of metabolic activity, and marked weight gain is uncommon. Conversely, severe obesity may be accompanied by subclinical biochemical hypothyroidism, manifested by mild thyroid-stimulating hormone elevation that corrects with weight loss.
- An increased body mass index in the second and third decades in life, but not later, is more frequently associated with oligo/amenorrhea and polycystic ovarian syndrome in women.
- Obesity, diabetes, and depression often coexist. When assessing causes of weight gain, it is important to review the patient's medication list, as a number of commonly prescribed drugs can cause weight gain, including oral diabetes agents, insulin, steroid hormones (including progesterone), antidepressants, and other mood-altering drugs.

D. L. Hurley
Mayo Graduate School of Medicine, Mayo Clinic, Division of Endocrinology, Diabetes, Metabolism, and Nutrition, Rochester, MN, USA
e-mail: hurley.daniel@mayo.edu

J. M. Gonzalez-Campoy et al. (eds.), *Bariatric Endocrinology*,
https://doi.org/10.1007/978-3-319-95655-8_10

10.1 Introduction

An increase in excess body weight stems from multiple factors, including socioeconomic and environmental triggers that contribute to an unhealthy lifestyle of increased consumption of calorie-dense foods and decreased work-related and free-time activity. However, it is also apparent that there is a strong genetic component in the development of obesity. Genetic factors have been reported to explain a large component of body mass index (BMI) variability in family studies, including twin studies (50–90% of BMI variance), adoption studies (20–60% of BMI variance), and parent–offspring and sibling correlations (20–80% of BMI variance). Wardle and colleagues carried out twin analyses of BMI and waist circumference (WC) in 5092 twin pairs aged 8–11. Quantitative genetic model-fitting confirmed 77% heritability for both BMI and WC. Bivariate genetic analyses showed that, although the genetic influence on WC was 60% common to BMI, there was also a significant independent genetic effect. A very modest shared-environment effect was present for both BMI and WC, and the remaining environmental variance was unshared. Longitudinal studies have identified both parental obesity and childhood obesity as strong predictors of obesity in adulthood. The influence of having one parent with obesity throughout an individual's childhood and adolescence increases that person's risk of obesity in adulthood by 2.2–3.2-fold, with a substantially higher risk if both parents have obesity. In addition, a child who develops obesity at the age of 10–14 years of age has a 22-fold increased risk of obesity in adulthood.

Genome-wide association studies have provided new insights into the genetic factors that contribute to the development of obesity. While the connection between a particular single nucleotide polymorphism (SNP) and adiposity is not always clear, an increasing number of mutated genes can be traced to obesity phenotypes. Leptin deficiency is characterized by hyperphagia and severe obesity, and mutations in the leptin pathway and receptor gene may account for 3–4% of severe, early-onset obesity. Mutations in pro-opiomelanocortin have been described, characterized by a lack of central appetite signaling and hyperphagia. Affected individuals may have hypoglycemia, hypogonadotropic hypogonadism, and adrenal insufficiency. The melanocortin-3 and melanocortin-4 receptors are key in feeding behaviors and mutations of these receptors are found in up to 3% of severe, early-onset obesity in children. Polymorphisms of the "fat mass and obesity-associated" (FTO) gene are associated with adiposity and have been associated with weight regain after lifestyle intervention in children and adults with and without type 2 diabetes mellitus (T2DM). Obesity risk alleles were characterized in 3899 adults with T2DM and overweight or obesity who lost 3% or more of the entry weight after one year, from the Look AHEAD (Action for Health in Diabetes) study, a randomized trial to assess the effects of intensive lifestyle intervention and diabetes support and education. Although SNPs were not associated with weight loss, the FTO gene predicted weight regain in the diabetes support and education group, suggesting variations in the FTO gene may be important in weight regain.

The genetic influence on excess adiposity may occur in two ways. First, genes may serve as the primary factors in the development of obesity. Second, environmental factors may interact upon susceptibility genes that play a role in weight gain. There are major variations in the susceptibility to weight gain among individuals under similar external influences (decreased physical activity and increased calorie intake), depending on the genetic background. Metabolic risk factors for weight gain are reported to include low metabolic rate, increased carbohydrate oxidation, insulin resistance, and low sympathetic activity. Low energy expenditure is one factor that may promote weight gain. Approximately 70% of total energy expenditure (TEE) is utilized for the metabolic basal or resting energy expenditure (REE) needs. These include the REE involved in maintaining body temperature, cellular integrity and ion gradients, cardiac and respiratory muscle function, gastrointestinal motility and secretion, and storage and mobilization of metabolic fuels. Another 10% of TEE is dissipated through the thermic effects of food digestion, and the remaining energy expenditure is from activities of daily living and exercise. There is a strong relationship between TEE, REE, and fat-free mass (FFM), and differences in FFM account for a large percentage of TEE variance among individuals. Piaggi and colleagues studied energy metabolism in 612 healthy adult men and women (mean values for age 29.5 years, BMI 33.0 kg/m^2, and percent body fat 30.9%) with follow-up of 292 subjects after a mean 6.7 years. TEE and REE were measured by indirect calorimetry in a 24-h respiratory chamber, and body composition was assessed by either underwater weighing or dual-energy X-ray absorptiometry (DEXA). The 24-h TEE was inversely related to the rate of weight change ($p = 0.007$) and change in FFM ($p = 0.012$), such that 100 kcal below the expected 24-h TEE corresponded to 0.2 kg/year weight gain, of which 0.1 kg/year was fat mass. Thus, measures of REE and substrate oxidation were predictors of long-term weight change, indicating a small but potentially significant role for a reduced REE in weight gain over an individual's lifetime.

Significant weight loss and loss of FFM may slow the REE. Thus, an important goal during weight loss is to maximize the loss of fat while preserving metabolically active FFM. Johannsen and colleagues studied whether restriction of caloric intake and vigorous physical activity would preserve FFM and maintain REE during weight loss in 16 patients with severe obesity (BMI 49.4 ± 9.4 kg/m^2 and body fat 49 ± 5%). There were measurements of body composition by DEXA, REE by indirect calorimetry, and TEE by double-labeled water. Subjects lost greater than one-third (38 + 9%) of their body weight at 30 weeks, to include 17% from FFM and 83% from fat. Although energy expenditure from physical activity increased significantly, the REE declined out of proportion to the decrease in body mass, demonstrating a substantial metabolic adaptation, with a decline of 504 ± 171 kcal/day ($p < 0.01$). Physical activity did not prevent a significant decline in REE during rapid weight loss, suggesting that patients may be predisposed to weight regain if physical activity and/or caloric restriction are not maintained. The Health, Aging, and Body Composition Study followed body composition change in 147 adults (54% women, 38% African–American) over a weight-cycling period (defined as ≥3% weight loss with weight regain within ±3% of baseline over 2 years) compared to gender- and race-matched weight-stable subjects. More lean mass was lost during the weight-loss period than was gained during the weight-regain period, especially in men, although not statistically significant when compared to the weight-stable group.

With this background of the genetic influence on body adiposity, and the importance of TEE variability during weight change, this chapter will review the potential endocrine causes of excess body fat, and the role of medications in promoting weight gain.

10.2 Endocrine Causes of Weight Gain

10.2.1 Hypothalamus–Pituitary–Adrenal (HPA) Axis

Hypothalamic obesity is a rare syndrome in humans. In animals, injury to the ventromedial or paraventricular region of the hypothalamus regularly results in obesity. These brain regions are responsible for sensing hunger and satiety, and hyperphagia occurs when the hypothalamus is damaged. Causes of hypothalamic obesity are listed in Table 10.1. Craniopharyngiomas are the most common intracranial tumors of nonglial origin in the pediatric population, and hypothalamic involvement is a major risk factor for obesity in these children. In 90 children with a diagnosis of craniopharyngioma, early reductions in growth rates and late increases in BMI standard deviation (SD) scores were seen. In 48 children with hypothalamic involvement, BMI SD scores were higher at diagnosis and annual follow-up ($p < 0.001$ for both) compared to 42 patients without hypothalamic involvement (Fig. 10.1). Both hypothalamic tumor involvement and BMI SD scores had relevant and independent

Table 10.1 Etiologies of hypothalamic obesity

Single gene mutations	Leptin, leptin receptor, CART, POMC, prohormone convertase-1, MC4R, BDNF (TrkB), single-minded 1(SIM-1)
Genetic syndromes	Prader–Willi syndrome, Bardet–Biedl syndrome
Tumors	Craniopharyngioma, angiosarcoma, cholesteatoma, chordoma, colloid cysts, endothelioma, ependymoma, epidermoid, epithelioma, ganglioneuroma, germinoma, glioma, hamartoma, Langerhans cell, leukemia, meningioma, pituitary macroadenoma, pinealoma, teratoma, metastases
Inflammatory or infiltrative disease	Sarcoidosis, tuberculosis, arachnoiditis, histiocytosis X, encephalitis
Injury	Head trauma, neurosurgery, radiotherapy, aneurysm
Medications	Antidepressants, mood stabilizers, antipsychotics

Adapted from Bereket A, Kiess W, Lustig RH, et al. Hypothalamic obesity in children. Obes Rev. 2012;13:780–98; used with permission

BDNF (TrkB) brain-derived neurotrophic factor (tyrosine kinase B), *CART* cocaine- and amphetamine-related transcript, *MC4R* melanocortin 4 receptor, *POMC* pro-opiomelanocortin

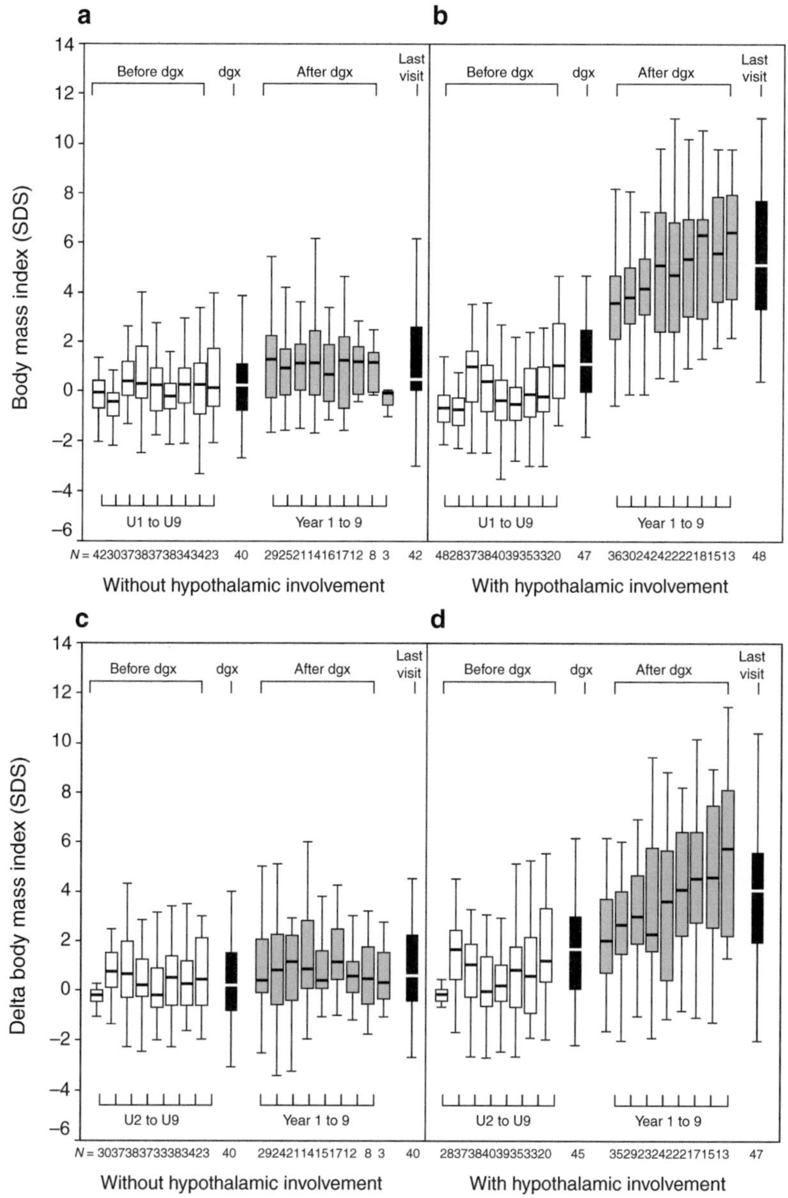

Fig. 10.1 Body mass index (expressed as standard deviation scores, SDS) before, at (mean age 8 years), and after diagnosis of craniopharyngioma and hypothalamic involvement to last visit ($n = 90$, 50 girls and 40 boys). Ages: U1, birth; U2, third to tenth day of life; U3, third to fourth week; U4, third to fourth month; U5, sixth to seventh month; U6, 10th to 12th month; U7, 21st to 24th month; U8, years 3.5 to 4; and U9, year 5. Data were retrospectively analyzed based on medical records, and results are shown as box plots for patients who presented without (**a**, **c**) or with (**b**, **d**) hypothalamic involvement by craniopharyngioma. (Adapted from Müller et al. 2004; used with permission)

impacts on the development of childhood obesity ($p < 0.001$ for both). In a report of 42 adults treated with surgery and/or radiotherapy for hypothalamic tumors, 52% had obesity at 5-year follow-up compared to 24% at baseline.

Growth hormone (GH) is known to increase lean body mass and reduce fat mass. Long-term GH treatment provides beneficial weight change for children who have either underweight or obesity, independent of the indication for GH therapy. However, GH replacement has also been associated with variable changes in adiposity in children. Changes in BMI SD scores between starting GH treatment and attaining near-adult height were analyzed in 2643 children with idiopathic GH deficiency, 281 children small for gestational age, 142 children with Prader–Willi syndrome, and 1661 girls with Turner syndrome identified from an international growth database. Children with obesity had decreased BMI SD scores, while children with underweight had increased BMI SD scores following GH therapy. Of interest, normal-weight children had an unexpected increase in BMI SD scores during GH treatment. Adult GH deficiency is associated with an increase in abdominal and visceral fat and a decrease in lean body mass. GH replacement in adults has been shown to have significant favorable effects on body composition compared to controls, to include increased FFM and decreased fat mass.

There is dysregulation of cortisol in the setting of excess adiposity. Obesity is associated with changes in adrenal function, which include an increase in adrenal medullary catecholamine output, changes in adipose tissue glucocorticoid (GC) metabolism, and enhanced adipocyte mineralocorticoid receptor activity. It is unknown whether these changes are in part responsible for the increase in adiposity and related metabolic dysfunction, or an adaptive response to obesity instead. GC secretion not only depends on the HPA circadian rhythm but also the intracellular regulation of cortisol by 11-beta-hydroxysteroid dehydrogenase (11ß-HSD). The enzyme 11ß-HSD-1 catalyzes the conversion of the inactive cortisone to active cortisol and thus amplifies GC tissue action in the liver, muscle, and fat. Excess adipose tissue 11ß-HSD-1 activity may be an important component of increased GC receptor activation. In contrast, 11ß-HSD-2 inactivates cortisol into inactive cortisone metabolites, thereby reducing the activation of the GC receptor. This balance of local cortisol activation and inactivation may play an essential role in metabolic disorders that are related to obesity. In addition, cortisol-binding globulin concentrations are often significantly reduced in obesity, resulting in higher free levels of cortisol. Patients with obesity and dysmetabolic syndrome have reportedly higher visceral adipose tissue expression of 11ß-HSD-1, higher adipose tissue expression of the GC receptor, and increased HPA axis activity compared to patients with obesity but without dysmetabolic syndrome. Of interest, weight loss after bariatric surgery has been shown to result in decreased levels of circulating cortisol and lower adipose tissue 11ß-HSD-1 expression, when compared to control subjects with normal weight.

Physiologic stressors can stimulate the HPA axis, which in turn can activate the mesolimbic dopaminergic system, a brain network strongly related to reward. Individuals with a high BMI show a stronger association between chronic stress and weight gain than those with a low BMI who experience similar degrees of stress. Several studies have examined the association of high-fat, high-sugar meal plans and activity of the HPA axis. Consistent with this notion, stress-related eating is significantly associated with obesity in women. Restrained eating refers to the voluntary cognitive effort to restrict food intake typically for the purpose of controlled weight loss or weight maintenance. High cognitive restraint is associated with increased cortisol concentrations. In addition, both epidemiological and experimental data support the association between sleep deprivation and disrupted physiological rhythms as being a possible risk for developing obesity. It is estimated that approximately one-third of adults in the United States sleep less than 6 h per night. Although studies suggest that restricting sleep may lead to weight gain via increased food consumption, methodologies have been inconsistent and the data, to include effects on energy expenditure, are mixed.

Approximately 5–20% of adrenal incidentalomas present with subclinical cortisol hypersecretion. This disorder has been described as subclinical Cushing's syndrome (CS), characterized by the absence of a clinical Cushing's phenotype and subtle alterations of the HPA axis due to adrenal autonomy, although there is lack of consensus as to the biochemical diagnostic criteria. Zografos and colleagues reported on 21 studies of adrenal incidentalomas and reported an increased prevalence of obesity ($n = 11$ studies, prevalence 25–78%), impaired glucose tolerance or T2DM ($n = 11$, 25–69%), T2DM only ($n = 7$, 16–33%), arterial hypertension ($n = 18$, 45–100%), and dyslipidemia ($n = 7$, 9–71%) irrespectively of adrenal function but being possibly higher in patients with subclinical CS. Rossi and colleagues prospectively studied the clinical and hormonal features of 50 consecutive patients with incidentally discovered adrenal adenomas. All subjects had hormone assays at regular intervals to assess the function of the HPA axis for a median period of 38 months, with comparison to 107 age- and gender-matched controls. For all patients with incidentalomas, T2DM was present in 24%, dyslipidemia in 28%, and BMI >25 kg/m^2 in 36% with significantly higher serum cortisol ($p < 0.001$), lower adrenocorticotropic hormone (ACTH) concentrations ($p < 0.05$), and impaired dexamethasone cortisol suppression ($p < 0.001$). Criteria for subclinical CS were met by 12 (24%) patients, with a BMI >25 kg/m^2 in 50%, T2DM in 42%, and dyslipidemia in 50%. It is noteworthy that obesity, hypertension, T2DM, and dyslipidemia are not specific to cortisol excess and are highly prevalent in the general population. This is especially so beyond the sixth decade of life, when adrenal incidentalomas are more frequent. Nevertheless, improvement in T2DM and insulin sensitivity has been reported after adrenalectomy in patients with adrenal incidentalomas, with or without subclinical CS. Rossi et al. documented that adrenal hormonal features improved in all patients undergoing adrenalectomy but appeared unchanged in patients not treated by surgery during a follow-up period ranging from 9 to 73 months. These findings suggest that subclinical hypercortisolism may contribute to increased adiposity, adiposopathy, and metabolic abnormalities.

The first evidence that cortisol levels were related to obesity and metabolic disease was derived from clinical observations of CS with associated central body obesity, glucose intolerance, and hypertension. The effect of GCs in CS can be explained by the induction of 11ß-HSD-1 and enhanced lipogenic capacity in visceral adipose tissue. GCs increase de novo lipid production in hepatocytes through increased expression of fatty acid synthase. GCs also promote conversion of preadipocytes to mature adipocytes and have an acute antilipolytic effect on adipocytes. However, the long-term effects of GCs on adipose tissue lipolysis remain unknown, and there is controversy as to whether these mechanisms contribute to fat hypertrophy in adiposopathy.

CS due to bilateral adrenocortical hyperplasia can be classified as ACTH-independent macronodular adrenocortical disease (>1 cm) that is more frequent in older adults, and micronodular disease (<1 cm), more frequent in children and young adults. The cyclic adenosine monophosphate (cAMP) signaling pathway plays a role in bilateral adrenal hyperplasia, either directly due to genetic defects of a central pathway molecule or indirectly via upregulation of ectopically expressed G-protein-coupled receptors in the adrenal cortex. Increased levels of cAMP-dependent protein kinase A (PKA) activity and/or cAMP are increased in adrenocortical lesions, and PKA is known to play an important role in fat metabolism and energy balance. Micronodular adrenal hyperplasia includes a pigmented variant, primary pigmented nodular adrenocortical disease (PPNAD). Mutations of the PRKAR1A gene that codes for the regulatory subunit 1α of PKA (RIα) cause PPNAD. London and colleagues studied CS and non-CS subtypes, both with and without PRKAR1A mutations. PRKAR1A mutations affected cAMP signaling in adipose tissue and were associated with significantly reduced CS-related obesity. BMI and BMI Z-scores were lower in adults with PPNAD and PRKAR1A mutations and in pediatric patients with PPNAD with or without PRKAR1A mutations. PKA activity in adipose tissue differed between CS groups, with higher cAMP levels in patients with PPNAD. Thus, increased cAMP and PKA activity may contribute to increased adiposity and phenotypic differences among CS subtypes.

10.2.2 Thyroid

Many of the actions of thyroid hormone in metabolic regulation involve modulation of other metabolic signaling pathways. Thyroid hormone regulates basal metabolic rate through known targets such as sodium–potassium ATPase, although the overall mechanism is not well established. Thyroid hormone interacts closely with the adrenergic nervous system to generate heat in response to cold exposure, termed adaptive thermogenesis. This process stimulates mitochondrial biogenesis and upregulation of fatty acid oxidation. The conversion of thyroxine (T4) to triiodothyronine (T3), along with the expression of uncoupling protein-1 (UCP1), is required for adaptive thermogenesis in brown adipose tissue, and is stimulated by catecholamines. The UCP1 promoter and the promoter for a rate-limiting enzyme in gluconeogenesis, phosphoenolpyruvate carboxykinase, have a cAMP response element and a thyroid response element in close proximity, and both response elements are required to stimulate gene expression. Thyroid hormone stimulates both lipolysis and lipogenesis and is involved in fatty acid oxidation to mobilize stored triglycerides and generate ATP to meet cellular demands. Regulation of fatty acid oxidation

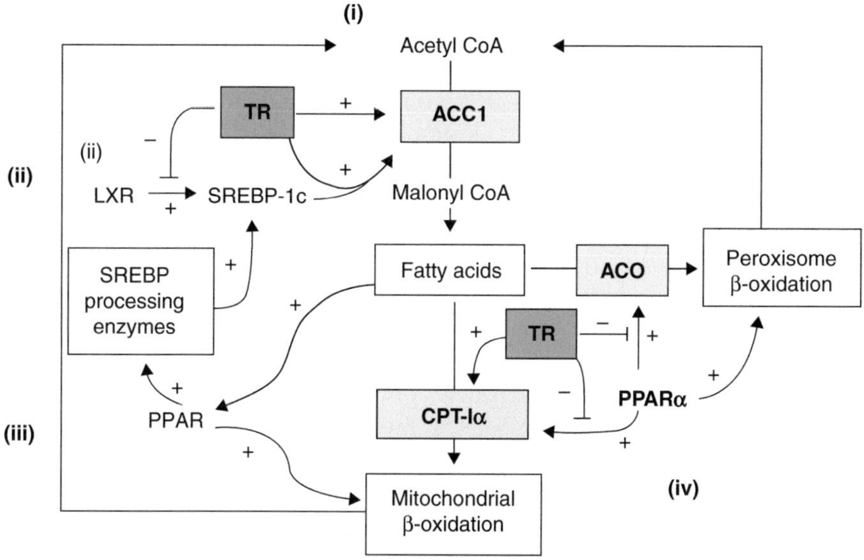

Fig. 10.2 Crosstalk between thyroid hormone signaling and metabolic pathways in fatty acid synthesis and ß-oxidation. (i) Free fatty acid (FAA) synthesis is controlled by acetyl-CoA carboxylase (ACC). Thyroid hormone receptor response element (TR) and sterol regulating element-binding protein (SREBP). (ii) Liver X receptor (LXR) stimulates FFA synthesis by enhancing SREBP-1c gene expression. In the absence of T3, TR competes with LXR. (iii) Peroxisome proliferator-activated receptor (PPAR), an agonist, increases FFA synthesis by enhancing SREBP processing enzymes. (iv) T3 increases FFA oxidation by upregulating palmitoyltransferase (CPT)-Ia. PPARa also stimulates CPT-Ia and acyl–CoA oxidase (ACO), a rate-limiting enzyme. Unliganded TR can block CPT1a and ACO stimulation by PPARa. (Adapted from Liu and Brent 2010; used with permission)

is mainly through key rate-limiting enzymes such as carnitine palmitoyltransferase Iα and acyl-CoA oxidase (Fig. 10.2).

Patients with hypothyroidism may gain weight due to slowing of metabolic activity. Some of this weight gain is fat, but the weight gain is usually modest, and marked weight gain is uncommon. Serum thyroid-stimulating hormone (TSH) levels that are increasing in the normal range or slightly above normal have been associated with a modest increase in body weight. Moreover, there is an inverse correlation between free thyroxine values and BMI, even when free thyroxine levels remain in the normal range. A retrospective analysis of 703 multiethnic children and adolescents found a positive association between TSH concentrations and BMI Z-scores. After adjustment for ethnicity, gender, pubertal stage, and BMI, significant associations remained between TSH levels and hyperglycemia (e.g., impaired fasting glucose and impaired glucose tolerance), and dyslipidemia (e.g., elevated levels of triglycerides, total cholesterol, and LDL-cholesterol). In adults, subclinical hypothyroidism (mean TSH: 6.7 mIU/L) is associated with a slightly higher baseline weight (0.51 kg higher baseline weight per 1 mIU/L higher TSH) in women older than 65 years of age, compared to euthyroid individuals (i.e., TSH 2.2 mIU/L).

However, there is no association observed in men and no weight change over time in women. In contrast, a cross-sectional study in 2037 middle-aged Japanese adults found significant positive associations between the serum TSH and BMI in men only. In a study of 4235 patients with T2DM, patients were divided into two groups based on the thyroid status, those with clinical hypothyroidism on thyroid hormone replacement compared to persons without known thyroid disease. BMI was strongly associated with patients who were found to have hypothyroidism (BMI 32.2 ± 7.4 vs. 29.4 ± 5.7 kg/m^2, $p < 0.0001$) and for patients receiving thyroid hormone therapy for hypothyroidism ($p < 0.0001$; odds ratio [OR] 2.28). Weight change following onset of thyroid hormone therapy was evaluated in a retrospective cohort of 101 adults with newly diagnosed primary hypothyroidism (median TSH ≥18.3 mIU/L, range 10.1–710 mIU/L). The median treatment TSH level was 2.3 mIU/L (range, 0.04–5 mIU/L), and only 52% of patients lost weight, with a mean weight loss of 3.8 ± 4.4 kg. Gender, race, age, initial TSH level, time to normalization of TSH, and initial weight were not associated with changes in weight or BMI after onset of thyroid hormone therapy. Another retrospective analysis compared 245 patients treated with treated hypothyroidism and 162 euthyroid controls. Both groups were similar in height, weight, BMI, and the number of patients with T2DM. The thyroid treated group had more women, Caucasians, and nonsmokers. The average TSH was slightly higher in the treated hypothyroid group compared to controls (median TSH 1.87 vs. 1.55, $p < 0.01$), but there was no significant relationship between TSH and BMI in either group. Thus, it seems unlikely that properly treated hypothyroidism contributes to weight gain.

It has been suggested that abnormalities in thyroid function may be secondary to excess fat mass. However, these changes appear to be functional, since thyroid function becomes normal after weight loss in children and adolescents. In addition, weight loss after bariatric surgery in adults improves or normalizes TSH levels. Chikunguwo and colleagues retrospectively studied thyroid function tests in 86 patients without previous diagnosis of thyroid disorder who underwent gastric bypass or adjustable gastric banding. Before bariatric surgery, 10.5% of subjects had TSH values consistent with subclinical hypothyroidism (defined as elevated TSH with normal free thyroxine). One year after bariatric surgery, all patients experienced significant weight reduction and simultaneous resolution of their subclinical hypothyroidism. The mean BMI change from 49 to 32 kg/m^2 after bariatric surgery was associated with a mean reduction in the TSH level from 4.5 to 1.9 mIU/L. TSH levels correlated positively with BMI ($p < 0.001$) within the BMI range of 30–67 kg/m^2. Of interest, free thyroxine showed no association with BMI and was not significantly influenced by weight loss (Fig. 10.3). Subclinical hypothyroidism is present at the preoperative evaluation for Roux-en-Y gastric bypass in 43% of 503 patients. One year after bariatric surgery, the mean BMI declined from 47 ± 8 kg/m^2 to 33 ± 6 kg/m^2 ($p < 0.001$) and was associated with significant decreases in both TSH (5.8 ± 2.0 to 2.8 ± 1.3 mIU/L, $p < 0.001$) and free thyroxine (15.2 ± 2.1 to 13.9 ± 2.3 pmol/L, $p < 0.001$). Subclinical hypothyroidism resolved in 87% of patients, and this high rate of spontaneous recovery suggests that follow-up alone is sufficient in the majority of patients undergoing bariatric surgery with mild TSH elevations.

10.2.3 Ovaries

Polycystic ovary syndrome (PCOS) is a common endocrine disorder. PCOS affects 6–18% of premenopausal women. Approximately one-half of women with PCOS are reported to have obesity, with increased abdominal and visceral fat. The factors responsible for this association are not fully understood. Excess adiposity is associated with insulin resistance and compensatory hyperinsulinemia and leads to decreased sex hormone-binding globulin synthesis in the liver, and excessive androgen production in the ovaries. These changes lead to a hyperandrogenic state when compared to women of normal weight. There is a significant association between weight gain in early adulthood and symptoms or diagnosis of PCOS. Ollila and colleagues evaluated women with both oligo/amenorrhea and hirsutism at age 31 (n = 126), or diagnosed with PCOS by age 46 (n = 181), as compared to women without PCOS (n = 1577). An increased BMI between the ages of 14 and 31, but not later, was more frequent in all groups of women with isolated oligo/amenorrhea (p = 0.006), oligo/amenorrhea plus hirsutism, (p = 0.001), and PCOS (p = 0.001).

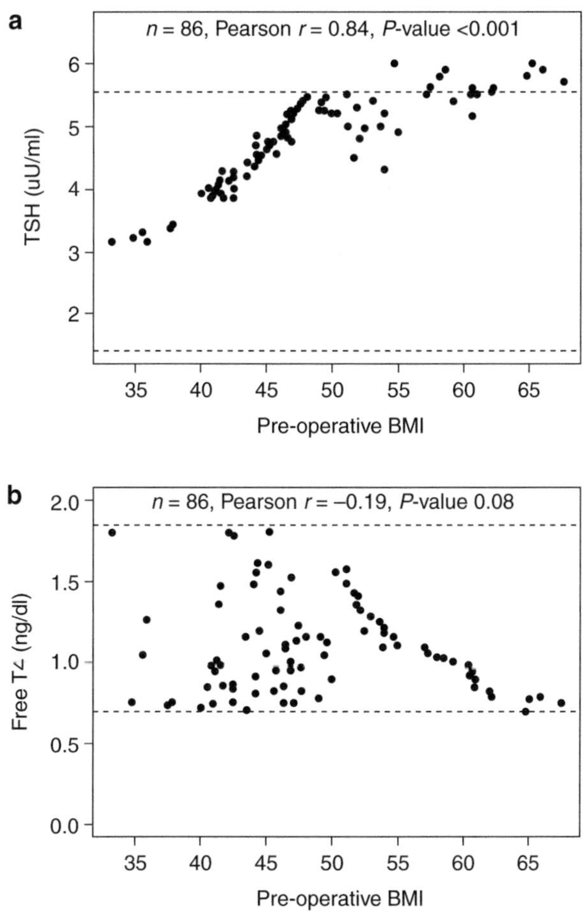

Fig. 10.3 Influence of obesity and surgical weight loss on thyroid hormone levels. Left: Correlation between preoperative BMI and preoperative (**a**) serum TSH and (**b**) free T4 levels. Right: Correlation between BMI 6 months after bariatric surgery and (**a**) serum TSH and (**b**) free T4 levels. Dotted lines represent lower and upper limits of normal range for thyroid hormone concentrations. (Adapted from Chikunguwo et al. 2007; used with permission)

Fig. 3 (continued)

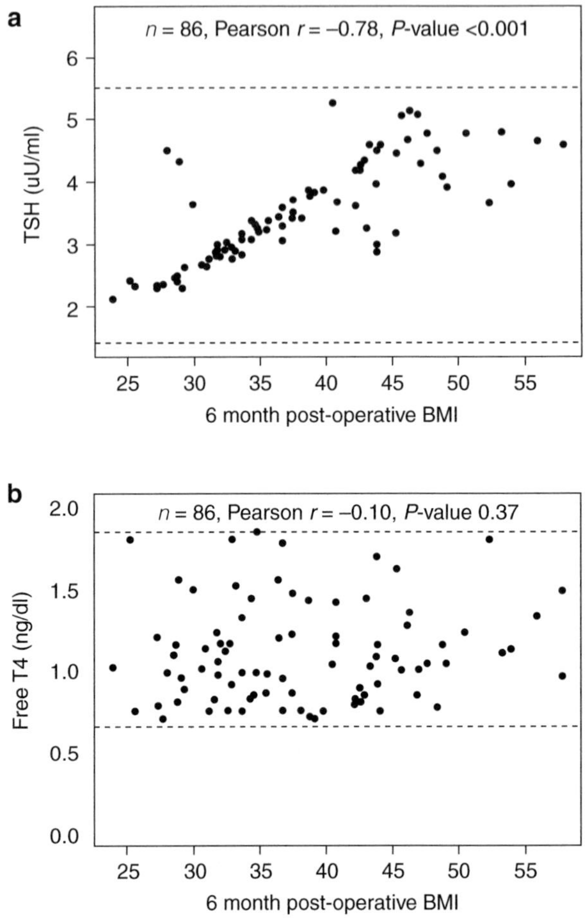

PCOS was significantly associated with increased BMI and higher concentrations of androgens, insulin, and triglycerides.

Cytochrome P450c17α is a key enzyme in the biosynthesis of ovarian androgens and has both 17α-hydroxylase and 17,20-lyase activity. In ovarian theca cells, P450c17α converts progesterone to 17α-hydroxyprogesterone via 17α-hydroxylase, and then converts 17α-hydroxyprogesterone to androstenedione by 17,20-lyase activity. Weight loss using a hypocaloric meal plan in women with PCOS reduces plasma testosterone and glucose-stimulated insulin levels and improves hirsutism. A decline in the waist-to-hip ratio correlates positively with decreases in glucose-stimulated insulin levels and inversely with the decreases in plasma 17-beta-estradiol. Metformin therapy, 500 mg three times a day in women with PCOS, as compared to placebo, significantly reduces the levels of serum insulin, 17α-hydroxyprogesterone, luteinizing hormone, sex hormone-binding globulin, and testosterone, all independent of BMI, although the waist-to-hip ratio decreases with metformin administration ($p = 0.02$). Glintborg and colleagues studied body composition in 90 patients with PCOS randomized to 1 year of metformin (2 g/day), metformin plus oral contraception (150 mg desogestrel +30 mcg ethinyl estradiol), or oral contraception alone. Treatment with metformin alone or in combination with oral contraception was associated with greater declines in body weight and regional fat mass compared to oral contraception alone. Testosterone levels were comparable between groups.

10.3 Medication-Related Weight Gain: Commonly Used Drugs for Common Diseases

When assessing causes of weight gain, it is important to review the patient's medication list as a number of medications can cause weight gain, including oral diabetes agents, insulin, antidepressants and other mood-altering drugs, antiepileptic drugs, and hormones (Tables 10.2 and 10.3).

Table 10.2 The potential effects of diabetes therapeutic agents on weight change

Drug class	Drug agent(s)	Weight change
Amylin analogs	*Pramlintide*	↓↓
Biguanides	*Metformin*	↓
GLP-1 receptor agonists	*Albiglutide, dulaglutide, exenatide, liraglutide*	↓↓
SGLT-2 inhibitors	*Canagliflozin, dapagliflozin, empagliflozin*	↓
α-Glucosidase inhibitors	*Acarbose, miglitol*	↔
Bile acid sequestrants	*Colesevelam*	↔
DPP-4 inhibitors	*Alogliptin, linagliptin, saxagliptin, sitagliptin*	↔
Dopamine-2 agonists	*Bromocriptine*	↔
Glinides	*Nateglinide, repaglinide*	↑
Sulfonylureas	*Glimepiride, glipizide, glyburide*	↑↑
Insulins	*Aspart, detemir, glargine, glulisine, lispro, NPH, regular*	↑↑
Thiazolidinediones	*Pioglitazone, rosiglitazone*	↑↑

Table 10.3 The potential effects of CNS psychoactive agents on weight change

Drug class	Related to weight gain	Related to weight neutrality or loss
Antidepressants	*Mirtazapine, TCAs, SSRIs (paroxetine)*	*Bupropion, venlafaxine, SSRIs (fluoxetine, sertraline)*
Antipsychotics	*Clozapine, olanzapine, quetiapine, risperidone, thioridazine*	*Aripiprazole, ziprasidone*
Antiepileptics	*Gabapentin, valporate*	*Lamotrigine, topiramate, zonisamide*
Others	*Lithium*	

CNS central nervous system, *SSRIs* selective serotonin reuptake inhibitors, *TCAs* tricyclic antidepressants (i.e., amitriptyline, clomipramine, doxepin, imipramine)

10.3.1 Diabetes-Related Drugs

The risk of developing T2DM and hypertension increases with increasing BMI and WC. BMI and WC are each independently and strongly associated with T2DM, with WC being a stronger risk factor in women than in men. Many patients with obesity have prediabetes or T2DM, and vice versa, and may be treated for metabolic complications with drugs that are weight promoting. Beta-blockers and alpha-blockers prescribed as antihypertensive agents may cause weight gain. Lee and colleagues found that among patients taking beta-blockers and matched to controls, meal-induced thermogenesis, fat oxidation rate, and weekly activity were lower by 50% ($p < 0.01$), 32% ($p = 0.04$), and 30% ($p < 0.01$), respectively. The adjusted mean body weight was significantly higher in these patients who attended either a diabetes clinic (9.2 ± 1.2 kg, $p = 0.0002$) or hypertension clinic (17.2 ± 3.2 kg, $p = 0.004$), compared to patients attending these clinics and not treated with beta-blockers. Weight-neutral agents to control blood pressure would include angiotensin-converting enzyme inhibitors, angiotensin receptor blockers, and calcium channel blockers, although more robust studies of the effect of antihypertension drugs on weight change are needed. In addition, there is a high rate of depression in patients with obesity and T2DM, and many psychoactive agents commonly prescribed to improve mood in these patients may promote weight gain. Thus, all patients with prediabetes, T2DM, or obesity should have their medication list carefully reviewed for drugs that can cause weight gain.

Insulin administration is associated with weight gain, for both conventional and intensive insulin therapy. Patients receiving insulin gain approximately 1–3 kg more weight than those receiving other diabetes agents. In the Diabetes Control and Complications Trial, a mean increase in weight of 5.1 kg was seen in the intensive treatment group, versus 2.4 kg in the conventional treatment group. Sulfonylureas and thiazolidinediones are associated with weight gain, whereas metformin use in the Diabetes Prevention Program resulted in a significant 2-kg weight loss in patients with impaired glucose tolerance. Other oral diabetes agents are weight neutral or associated with a small decline in weight (i.e., dipeptidyl peptidase-4 inhibitors, alpha-glucosidase inhibitors, and sodium glucose transport-2 inhibitors). Injectable glucagon-like peptide-1 (GLP-1) receptor agonists used in the treatment of T2DM have been shown to provide improved glycemic control, blood pressure reduction, and weight loss. Patients with T2DM and overweight or obesity should receive instruction in healthy eating patterns and regular physical activity. They should also be treated with diabetes medications that are safe, effective, and weight neutral, or associated with weight loss.

10.3.2 Antidepressants

The Netherlands Study of Depression and Anxiety evaluated data from 2542 adults with major depressive disorder over 6 years of observation, compared to healthy controls. A current, but not remitted, major depressive disorder was significantly associated with both weight gain and weight loss. Antidepressant use was significantly associated with weight gain both for selective serotonin reuptake inhibitors (OR 1.26, 95% CI, 1.05–1.52) as well as for other antidepressants (OR 1.36, 95% CI, 1.00–1.84) ($p < 0.05$ for both). Compared to patients who lost weight, those who gained weight had lower initial BMI, were younger, had more anxiety disorders, and had poorer quality of mood and reduced appetite as depressive symptoms. Overweight or obesity was found in 72% of a cohort of 127 adult ambulatory patients with depression, studied by Correia and colleagues. A longer duration of depression was associated with significantly higher BMI values and greater fat mass ($p < 0.003$). Weight gain during the observed time of depression was reported in 87% of patients. Antidepressants and benzodiazepines were prescribed in 75% and 72% of patients, respectively, and both were associated with significant weight gain. The tricyclic antidepressants amitriptyline, clomipramine, doxepin, and imipramine are all associated with significant weight gain. In contrast, not all SSRIs have been associated with weight gain. In a randomized study of 284 patients with depression receiving one of three SSRIs (fluoxetine, sertraline, or paroxetine), a significant increase in weight occurred only in the paroxetine group, while no significant weight change was observed in patients taking sertraline or fluoxetine.

10.3.3 Antipsychotics

Both "conventional" first-generation antipsychotics (i.e., thioridazine) and "atypical" second-generation antipsychotics (Table 10.3) can cause significant weight gain, reportedly between 0.8 and 4.4 kg. Antagonism of histamine H1 receptors has been identified as the main cause of second-generation antipsychotic-induced obesity, but the molecular mechanisms are unclear. Blocking hypothalamic H1 receptors by second-generation antipsychotics activates AMP-activated protein kinase (AMPK). During short-term second-generation antipsychotic treatment, hypothalamic H1 receptor antagonism may activate the AMPK-carnitine palmitoyltransferase 1 signaling to rapidly increase caloric intake. During long-term treatment, hypothalamic H1 receptor antagonism can reduce thermogenesis and thus may contribute to fat accumulation by decreasing lipolysis and increasing lipogenesis. Central opioidergic neurotransmission may be implicated in the development of olanzapine metabolic disturbances. Of interest, the addition of naltrexone or placebo to olanzapine in a randomized, double-blind pilot study did not result in BMI differences between groups. However, subjects taking naltrexone plus olanzapine had a significant decrease in fat, increase in FFM, and a trend toward improvement in homeostatic model assessment of insulin resistance, compared to controls. In another randomized, double-blinded, placebo-controlled trial, melatonin was found to be effective in attenuating adverse metabolic effects of second-generation antipsychotics in patients with bipolar disorder but not with schizophrenia. Significant beneficial outcomes with melatonin were seen on fat mass and diastolic blood pressure, compared to placebo. Second-generation antipsychotics also seem to induce a hypometabolic state. Adolescents taking olanzapine, quetiapine, or risperidone monotherapy were analyzed using anthropometric measurements, bioelectrical impedance analysis, and indirect calorimetry to measure REE. Patients gained 10.8 ± 6.2 kg (60% as fat mass) and increased WC by 11.1 ± 5.0 cm after only 1 year of treatment. The REE/kg body mass ratio decreased ($p = 0.027$), and the REE/percentage FFM ratio increased ($p = 0.007$) during treatment. This could explain, at least in part, the changes in weight and body composition observed in these patients. Taken together, these findings support a centrally mediated imbalance during use of mood-altering drugs that can lead to changes in weight and body composition, as well as adiposopathy and adverse metabolic clinical outcomes.

10.3.4 Antiepileptics

The antiepileptic drugs valproic acid and carbamazepine are also used in the management of bipolar disorder and are associated with weight gain. Gabapentin is commonly used for treatment of neuropathic pain and can also cause weight gain, whereas topiramate and zonisamide do not promote weight gain. Shapiro and colleagues reported on 47 adolescent patients with an average BMI of 30.2 kg/m^2 who were first prescribed topiramate or zonisamide and subsequently had the addition of at least one mood-altering drug. Of these patients, topiramate was initially prescribed in 91% of adolescents due to its safety profile, and 92% were later prescribed an antipsychotic (e.g., aripiprazole, quetiapine, or risperidone). Anticonvulsant dosage was associated with an average decline in BMI of 3.2–6.1 kg/m^2 for every 6 months of treatment in patients with a baseline BMI ≥25 kg/m^2, and weight reduction was not statistically different between patients taking topiramate or zonisamide.

10.3.5 Gonadal hormones

Many progestin-only contraceptives are long acting and cost effective in preventing pregnancy, but concerns about weight gain can deter initiation, or cause early discontinuation of their use. In a review of contraceptive use studies, weight change for women taking progestin-only contraceptives generally did not differ significantly from their comparison contraceptive group, with a mean weight gain <2 kg for most studies of 1-year duration. However, three studies showed significant differences for progestin-only contraceptives compared to women not using a hormonal method of contraception. Three-year weight gain is greater with depot medroxyprogesterone acetate (DMPA) use compared to women using a nonhormonal IUD. DMPA users also have significantly greater percent increases in body fat and a decrease in lean body mass. There is a 1 year greater increase in weight with DMPA use, compared to women using an IUD contraceptive, with the weight increase due to an increase in fat mass. In contrast, women who used DMPA postpartum do not differ from women choosing bilateral partial salpingectomy sterilization in either weight or percent body fat at 1-year follow-up. About half the women using DMPA return to their prepregnancy weight. However, the other half of DMPA users gain weight, with a higher prepregnancy BMI associated with postpartum weight gain.

Serum testosterone level decreases in men by 0.4–2% per year after the third decade of life. In addition to increasing age, obesity has been associated with decreased serum testosterone. There is evidence that low testosterone levels promote fat accumulation, suggesting a bidirectional relationship between adiposity and testosterone. A total of 3369 community-dwelling men aged 40–79 years were evaluated as part of the European Male Aging Study and categorized as eugonadal (n = 1909), incident secondary hypogonadal (n = 140), or persistent secondary hypogonadal (n = 123). Incident secondary hypogonadism is predicted by a BMI of ≥30 kg/m^2 (OR 2.86, $p < 0.0001$), weight gain (OR 1.79, $p = 0.011$), and increased WC (OR 1.73 for WC 94–102 cm, $p = 0.026$ and 2.64 for WC ≥102 cm, $p < 0.0001$). Late-onset hypogonadism occurs in middle-aged and elderly men and is defined by hypogonadal symptoms in the presence of low testosterone levels. In the European Male Aging Study, 63 men (2.1%) were classified as having moderate or severe late-onset hypogonadism. Only men with severe late-onset hypogonadism showed significant associations with WC, insulin resistance, and dysmetabolic syndrome, although men with low testosterone levels only had lesser magnitudes of association for the same end points. Androgen deprivation therapy is employed in men with locally advanced, recurrent, and metastatic prostate cancer and has been prospectively shown to cause decreased lean muscle mass, increased fat mass, weight gain, increased cholesterol and triglycerides, and insulin resistance. Mean increases in body weight and WC after 1 year of androgen-deprivation therapy have been reported as 2.9% and 3.0%, respectively. Visceral and subcutaneous fat (measured by computerized tomography) both increase by >20%, although the increase in subcutaneous fat is significantly greater than that measured in visceral fat. Studies in men taking androgen-deprivation therapy are needed. Physical activity is associated with significantly improved health and disease-specific quality of life in men taking androgen-deprivation therapy. However, physical activity does not have a beneficial effect on weight, WC, lean mass, fat mass, blood pressure, or lipids.

10.4 Conclusion

Patients inquire about, and physicians and other health-care providers often screen for, endocrine-related disorders as a cause of weight gain in persons who have overweight or obesity. Endocrine disorders may be associated with modest weight gain, as seen in subclinical hypothyroidism or subclinical hypercortisolism, but they rarely are the sole culprit for marked or continued weight gain. Cushing's syndrome is rare and has an unmistakable phenotype. Hypothyroidism is common but rarely results in significant weight gain, even in patients with profound hypothyroidism. These endocrine disorders, Cushing's syndrome and myxedema, are usually quickly diagnosed and properly treated. The more difficult scenario is the patient with T2DM who has overweight or obesity and may have anxiety and depression. Polypharmacy is common in these patients, and they may be taking drugs for diabetes, depression, anxiety, and pain that promote weight gain. Behavioral change is critical to the prevention and treatment of patients who have overweight or obesity. However, a focus solely on modifying individual behaviors for healthy eating and increased physical activity may have had limited success if physicians and healthcare providers are not aware of the genetic variability between individuals in energy metabolism and the effect that commonly prescribed medications can have on weight change.

Reading List

Anderson RJ, Freedland KE, Clouse RE, et al. The prevalence of comorbid depression in adults with diabetes: a meta-analysis. Diabetes Care. 2001;24(6):1069–78.

Anderson DA, Shapiro JR, Lundgren JD, et al. Self-reported dietary restraint is associated with elevated levels of salivary cortisol. Appetite. 2002;38(1):13–7.

Aziz KM. Association between hypothyroidism, body mass index, systolic blood pressure and proteinuria in diabetic patients: does treated hypothyroid with thyroxine replacement therapy prevent nephropathy/chronic renal disease? Curr Diabetes Rev. 2015;12:297. [Epub ahead of print].

Baudrand R, Vaidya A. Cortisol dysregulation in obesity-related metabolic disorders. Curr Opin Endocrinol Diabetes Obes. 2015;22(3):143–9.

Baudrand R, Carvajal CA, Riquelme A, et al. Overexpression of 11beta-hydroxysteroid dehydrogenase type 1 in hepatic and visceral adipose tissue is associated with metabolic disorders in morbidly obese patients. Obes Surg. 2010;20(1):77–83.

Bieler BM, Gaughan J, Khan M, et al. Lack of an association between BMI and TSH in treated hypothyroid patients and euthyroid controls. Endocr Pract. 2015;22:555. [Epub ahead of print].

Binnerts A, Deurenberg P, Swart GR, et al. Body composition in growth hormone-deficient adults. Am J Clin Nutr. 1992;55(5):918–23.

Block JP, He Y, Zaslavsky AM, et al. Psychosocial stress and change in weight among US adults. Am J Epidemiol. 2009;170(2):181–92.

Chikunguwo S, Brethauer S, Nirujogi V, et al. Influence of obesity and surgical weight loss on thyroid hormone levels. Surg Obes Relat Dis. 2007;3(6):631–5.

Chiodini I, Morelli V, Salcuni AS, et al. Beneficial metabolic effects of prompt surgical treatment in patients with an adrenal incidentaloma causing biochemical hypercortisolism. J Clin Endocrinol Metab. 2010;95(6):2736–45.

Constantinopoulos P, Michalaki M, Kottorou A, et al. Cortisol in tissue and systemic level as a contributing factor to the development of metabolic syndrome in severely obese patients. Eur J Endocrinol. 2015;172(1):69–78.

Correia J, Ravasco P. Weight changes in Portuguese patients with depression: which factors are involved? Nutr J. 2014;13(1):117.

Crocker MK, Yanovski JA. Pediatric obesity: etiology and treatment. Endocrinol Metab Clin N Am. 2009;38(3):525–48.

Cuerda C, Merchan-Naranjo J, Velasco C, et al. Influence of resting energy expenditure on weight gain in adolescents taking second-generation antipsychotics. Clin Nutr. 2011;30(5):616–23.

Dal'Ava N, Bahamondes L, Bahamondes MV, et al. Body weight and body composition of depot medroxyprogesterone acetate users. Contraception. 2014;90(2):182–7.

Daousi C, Dunn AJ, Foy PM, et al. Endocrine and neuroanatomic features associated with weight gain and obesity in adult patients with hypothalamic damage. Am J Med. 2005;118(1):45–50.

De Boer H, Blok GJ, Voerman HJ, et al. Body composition in adult growth hormone-deficient men, assessed by anthropometry and bioimpedance analysis. J Clin Endocrinol Metab. 1992;75(3):833–7.

DeUgarte CM, Bartolucci AA, Azziz R. Prevalence of insulin resistance in the polycystic ovary syndrome using the homeostasis model assessment. Fertil Steril. 2005;83(5):1454–60.

Domecq JP, Prutsky G, Leppin A, et al. Clinical review: drugs commonly associated with weight change: a systematic review and meta-analysis. J Clin Endocrinol Metab. 2015;100(2):363–70.

Drab SR. Glucagon-like peptide-1 receptor agonists for type 2 diabetes: a clinical update of safety and efficacy. Curr Diabetes Rev. 2015;12:403. [Epub ahead of print].

Farooqi S. Insights from the genetics of severe childhood obesity. Horm Res. 2007;68(Suppl 5):5–7.

Farooqi IS, Wangensteen T, Collins S, et al. Clinical and molecular genetic spectrum of congenital deficiency of the leptin receptor. N Engl J Med. 2007;356(3):237–47.

Fava M, Judge R, Hoog SL, et al. Fluoxetine versus sertraline and paroxetine in major depressive disorder: changes in weight with long-term treatment. J Clin Psychiatry. 2000;61(11):863–7.

Fox CS, Pencina MJ, D'Agostino RB, et al. Relations of thyroid function to body weight: cross-sectional and longitudinal observations in a community-based sample. Arch Intern Med. 2008;168(6):587–92.

Gambineri A, Pelusi C, Vicennati V, et al. Obesity and the polycystic ovary syndrome. Int J Obes Relat Metab Disord. 2002;26(7):883–96.

Garber AJ, Abrahamson MJ, Barzilay JI, et al. American Association of Clinical Endocrinologists' comprehensive diabetes management algorithm 2013 consensus statement—executive summary. Endocr Pract. 2013;19(3):536–57.

Garin MC, Arnold AM, Lee JS, et al. Subclinical hypothyroidism, weight change, and body composition in the elderly: the Cardiovascular Health Study. J Clin Endocrinol Metab. 2014;99(4):1220–6.

Gibson-Smith D, Bot M, Milaneschi Y, et al. Major depressive disorder, antidepressant use, and subsequent 2-year weight change patterns in the Netherlands Study of Depression and Anxiety. J Clin Psychiatry. 2015;77:e144. [Epub ahead of print].

Glintborg D, Altinok ML, Mumm H, et al. Body composition is improved during 12 months' treatment with metformin alone or combined with oral contraceptives compared with treatment with oral contraceptives in polycystic ovary syndrome. J Clin Endocrinol Metab. 2014;99(7):2584–91.

Goncalves P, Araujo JR, Martel F. Antipsychotics-induced metabolic alterations: focus on adipose tissue and molecular mechanisms. Eur Neuropsychopharmacol. 2015;25(1):1–16.

He M, Deng C, Huang XF. The role of hypothalamic H1 receptor antagonism in antipsychotic-induced weight gain. CNS Drugs. 2013;27(6):423–34.

Heymsfield SB, Harp JB, Reitman ML, et al. Why do obese patients not lose more weight when treated with low-calorie diets? A mechanistic perspective. Am J Clin Nutr. 2007;85(2):346–54.

Hochberg I, Hochberg Z. Expanding the definition of hypothalamic obesity. Obes Rev. 2010;11(10):709–21.

InterAct Consortium, Langenberg C, Sharp SJ, Schulze MB, et al. Long-term risk of incident type 2 diabetes and measures of overall and regional obesity: the EPIC-InterAct case-cohort study. PLoS Med. 2012;9(6):e1001230.

Janssen IM, Homan J, Schijns W, et al. Subclinical hypothyroidism and its relation to obesity in patients before and after Roux-en-Y gastric bypass. Surg Obes Relat Dis. 2015;11(6):1257–63.

Johannsen DL, Knuth ND, Huizenga R, et al. Metabolic slowing with massive weight loss despite preservation of fat-free mass. J Clin Endocrinol Metab. 2012;97(7):2489–96.

Kargi AY, Iacobellis G. Adipose tissue and adrenal glands: novel pathophysiological mechanisms and clinical applications. Int J Endocrinol. 2014;2014:614074.

Knowler WC, Barrett-Connor E, Fowler SE, et al. Reduction in the incidence of type 2 diabetes with lifestyle intervention or metformin. N Engl J Med. 2002;346(6):393–403.
Knudsen N, Laurberg P, Rasmussen LB, et al. Small differences in thyroid function may be important for body mass index and the occurrence of obesity in the population. J Clin Endocrinol Metab. 2005;90(7):4019–24.
Laitinen J, Taponen S, Martikainen H, et al. Body size from birth to adulthood as a predictor of self-reported polycystic ovary syndrome symptoms. Int J Obes Relat Metab Disord. 2003;27(6):710–5.
Larger E. Weight gain and insulin treatment. Diabetes Metab. 2005;31(4 Pt 2):4S51–6.
Lasserre AM, Glaus J, Vandeleur CL, et al. Depression with atypical features and increase in obesity, body mass index, waist circumference, and fat mass: a prospective, population-based study. JAMA Psychiat. 2014;71(8):880–8.
Lee JS, Visser M, Tylavsky FA, et al. Weight loss and regain and effects on body composition: the Health, Aging, and Body Composition Study. J Gerontol A Biol Sci Med Sci. 2010;65((1):78–83.
Lee P, Kengne AP, Greenfield JR, et al. Metabolic sequelae of beta-blocker therapy: weighing in on the obesity epidemic? Int J Obes. 2011;35(11):1395–403.
Lee SY, Braverman LE, Pearce EN. Changes in body weight after treatment of primary hypothyroidism with levothyroxine. Endocr Pract. 2014;20(11):1122–8.
Leslie WS, Hankey CR, Lean ME. Weight gain as an adverse effect of some commonly prescribed drugs: a systematic review. QJM. 2007;100(7):395–404.
Liu YY, Brent GA. Thyroid hormone crosstalk with nuclear receptor signaling in metabolic regulation. Trends Endocrinol Metab. 2010;21(3):166–73.
London E, Rothenbuhler A, Lodish M, et al. Differences in adiposity in Cushing syndrome caused by PRKAR1A mutations: clues for the role of cyclic AMP signaling in obesity and diagnostic implications. J Clin Endocrinol Metab. 2014;99(2):E303–10.
Loos RJF. Genetic determinants of common obesity and their value in prediction. Best Pract Res Clin Endocrinol Metab. 2012;26(2):211–26.
Lopez LM, Edelman A, Chen M, et al. Progestin-only contraceptives: effects on weight. Cochrane Database Syst Rev. 2013;7:CD008815.
Luppino FS, de Wit LM, Bouvy PF, et al. Overweight, obesity, and depression: a systematic review and meta-analysis of longitudinal studies. Arch Gen Psychiatry. 2010;67(3):220–9.
Maes HH, Neale MC, Eaves LJ. Genetic and environmental factors in relative body weight and human obesity. Behav Genet. 1997;27(4):325–51.
Manji N, Boelaert K, Sheppard MC, et al. Lack of association between serum TSH or free T4 and body mass index in euthyroid subjects. Clin Endocrinol. 2006;64(2):125–8.
March WA, Moore VM, Willson KJ, et al. The prevalence of polycystic ovary syndrome in a community sample assessed under contrasting diagnostic criteria. Hum Reprod. 2010;25(2):544–51.
Marras V, Casini MR, Pilia S, et al. Thyroid function in obese children and adolescents. Horm Res Paediatr. 2010;73(3):193–7.
Matsuo T, Nakata Y, Hotta K, et al. The FTO genotype as a useful predictor of body weight maintenance: initial data from a 5-year follow-up study. Metabolism. 2014;63(7):912–7.
McCaffery JM, Papandonatos GD, Huggins GS, et al., Genetic Subgroup of Look AHEAD; Look AHEAD Research Group. FTO predicts weight regain in the Look AHEAD clinical trial. Int J Obes. 2013;37(12):1545–52.
McLean JA, Barr SI, Prior JC. Cognitive dietary restraint is associated with higher urinary cortisol excretion in healthy premenopausal women. Am J Clin Nutr. 2001;73(1):7–12.
Methlie P, Dankel S, Myhra T, et al. Changes in adipose glucocorticoid metabolism before and after bariatric surgery assessed by direct hormone measurements. Obesity. 2013;21(12):2495–503.
Mitsuzuka K, Kyan A, Sato T, et al. Influence of 1 year of androgen deprivation therapy on lipid and glucose metabolism and fat accumulation in Japanese patients with prostate cancer. Prostate Cancer Prostatic Dis. 2015; https://doi.org/10.1038/pcan.2015.50. [Epub ahead of print].
Morton NM, Seckl JR. 11beta-hydroxysteroid dehydrogenase type 1 and obesity. Front Horm Res. 2008;36:146–64.

Müller HL, Emser A, Faldum A, et al. Longitudinal study on growth and body mass index before and after diagnosis of childhood craniopharyngioma. J Clin Endocrinol Metab. 2004;89(7):3298–305.

Nestler JE, Jakubowicz DJ. Decreases in ovarian cytochrome P450c17 alpha activity and serum free testosterone after reduction of insulin secretion in polycystic ovary syndrome. N Engl J Med. 1996;335(9):617–23.

Nyirati M, Habash DL, Shaffer LE. Weight and body fat changes in postpartum depot-medroxyprogesterone acetate users. Contraception. 2013;88(1):169–76.

Ollila MM, Piltonen T, Puukka K, et al. Weight gain and dyslipidemia in early adulthood associate with polycystic ovary syndrome: prospective cohort study. J Clin Endocrinol Metab. 2015;101:739:jc20153543. [Epub ahead of print].

Pasquali R, Antenucci D, Casimirri F, et al. Clinical and hormonal characteristics of obese amenorrheic hyperandrogenic women before and after weight loss. J Clin Endocrinol Metab. 1989;68(1):173–9.

Peckett AJ, Wright DC, Riddell MC. The effects of glucocorticoids on adipose tissue lipid metabolism. Metabolism. 2011;60(11):1500–10.

Pereira CD, Azevedo I, Monteiro R, et al. 11beta-Hydroxysteroid dehydrogenase type 1: relevance of its modulation in the pathophysiology of obesity, the metabolic syndrome and type 2 diabetes mellitus. Diabetes Obes Metab. 2012;14(10):869–81.

Piaggi P, Thearle MS, Bogardus C, et al. Lower energy expenditure predicts long-term increases in weight and fat mass. J Clin Endocrinol Metab. 2013;98(4):E703–7.

Prasad-Reddy L, Isaacs D. A clinical review of GLP-1 receptor agonists: efficacy and safety in diabetes and beyond. Drugs Context. 2015;4:212283.

Radhakishun NN, van Vliet M, von Rosenstiel IA, et al. Increasing thyroid-stimulating hormone is associated with impaired glucose metabolism in euthyroid obese children and adolescents. J Pediatr Endocrinol Metab. 2013;26(5–6):531–7.

Rastrelli G, Carter EL, Ahern T, et al. Development of and recovery from secondary hypogonadism in aging men: prospective results from the EMAS. J Clin Endocrinol Metab. 2015;100(8):3172–82.

Reinehr T, Lindberg A, Koltowska-Haggstrom M, et al. Is growth hormone treatment in children associated with weight gain?—longitudinal analysis of KIGS data. Clin Endocrinol. 2014a;81(5):721–6.

Reinehr T, Wolters B, Roth CL, et al. FTO gene: association to weight regain after lifestyle intervention in overweight children. Horm Res Pediatr. 2014b;81(6):391–6.

Reiter RJ, Tan DX, Korkmaz A, et al. Obesity and metabolic syndrome: association with chronodisruption, sleep deprivation, and melatonin suppression. Ann Med. 2012;44(6):564–77.

Rodríguez-Arnao J, Jabbar A, Fulcher K, et al. Effects of growth hormone replacement on physical performance and body composition in GH deficient adults. Clin Endocrinol. 1999;51(1):53–60.

Romo-Nava F, Alvarez-Icaza Gonzalez D, Fresan-Orellana A, et al. Melatonin attenuates antipsychotic metabolic effects: an eight-week randomized, double-blind, parallel-group, placebo-controlled clinical trial. Bipolar Disord. 2014;16(4):410–21.

Rosén T, Bosaeus I, Tölli J, et al. Increased body fat mass and decreased extracellular fluid volume in adults with growth hormone deficiency. Clin Endocrinol. 1993;38(1):63–71.

Rossi R, Tauchmanova L, Luciano A, et al. Subclinical Cushing's syndrome in patients with adrenal incidentaloma: clinical and biochemical features. J Clin Endocrinol Metab. 2000;85(4):1440–8.

Saad F, Aversa A, Isidori AM, et al. Testosterone as potential effective therapy in treatment of obesity in men with testosterone deficiency: a review. Curr Diabetes Rev. 2012;8(2):131–43.

Sakurai M, Nakamura K, Miura K, et al. Association between a serum thyroid-stimulating hormone concentration within the normal range and indices of obesity in Japanese men and women. Intern Med. 2014;53(7):669–74.

Saylor PJ, Smith MR. Adverse effects of androgen deprivation therapy: defining the problem and promoting health among men with prostate cancer. J Natl Compr Cancer Netw. 2010;8(2):211–23.

Shah PK, Mudaliar S, Chang AR, et al. Effects of intensive insulin therapy alone and in combination with pioglitazone on body weight, composition, distribution and liver fat content in patients with type 2 diabetes. Diabetes Obes Metab. 2011;13(6):505–10.
Shapiro M, Reid A, Olsen B, et al. Topiramate, zonisamide and weight loss in children and adolescents prescribed psychiatric medications: a medical record review. Int J Psychiatry Med. 2016;51(1):56–68.
Skelton JA, Irby MB, Grzywacz J, et al. Etiologies of obesity in children: nature and nurture. Pediatr Clin N Am. 2011;58(6):1333–54.
Spencer SJ, Tilbrook A. The glucocorticoid contribution to obesity. Stress. 2011;14(3):233–46.
St-Onge MP. The role of sleep duration in the regulation of energy balance: effects on energy intakes and expenditure. J Clin Sleep Med. 2013;9(1):73–80.
Tajar A, Huhtaniemi IT, O'Neill TW, et al. Characteristics of androgen deficiency in late-onset hypogonadism: results from the European Male Aging Study (EMAS). J Clin Endocrinol Metab. 2012;97(5):1508–16.
Taveira TH, Wu WC, Tschibelu E, et al. The effect of naltrexone on body fat mass in olanzapine-treated schizophrenic or schizoaffective patients: a randomized double-blind placebo-controlled pilot study. J Psychopharmacol. 2014;28(4):395–400.
Teede HJ, Joham AE, Paul E, et al. Longitudinal weight gain in women identified with polycystic ovary syndrome: results of an observational study in young women. Obesity. 2013;21(8):1526–32.
Teleni L, Chan RJ, Chan A, et al. Exercise improves quality of life in androgen deprivation therapy-treated prostate cancer: systematic review of randomised controlled trials. Endocr Relat Cancer. 2016;23(2):101–12.
The DCCT Research Group. Weight gain associated with intensive therapy in the diabetes control and complications trial. Diabetes Care. 1988;11(17):567–73.
Trasande L, Cronk C, Durkin M, et al. Environment and obesity in the National Children's Study. Environ Health Perspect. 2009;117(2):159–66.
Travison TG, Araujo AB, Kupelian V, et al. The relative contributions of aging, health, and lifestyle factors to serum testosterone decline in men. J Clin Endocrinol Metab. 2007;92(2):549–55.
Varughese AG, Nimkevych O, Uwaifo GI. Hypercortisolism in obesity-associated hypertension. Curr Hypertens Rep. 2014;16(7):443.
Vidarsdottir S, de Leeuw van Weenen JE, Frolich M, et al. Effects of olanzapine and haloperidol on the metabolic status of healthy men. J Clin Endocrinol Metab. 2010;95(1):118–25.
Wardle J, Carnell S, Haworth CM, et al. Evidence for a strong genetic influence on childhood adiposity despite the force of the obesogenic environment. Am J Clin Nutr. 2008;87(2):398–404.
Whitaker RC, Wright JA, Pepe MS, et al. Predicting obesity in young adulthood from childhood and parental obesity. N Engl J Med. 1997;337(13):869–73.
Willett WC, Dietz WH, Colditz GA. Guidelines for healthy weight. N Engl J Med. 1999;341(6):427–34.
Woods C, Corrigan M, Gathercole L, et al. Tissue specific regulation of glucocorticoids in severe obesity and the response to significant weight loss following bariatric surgery (BARICORT). J Clin Endocrinol Metab. 2015;100(4):1434–44.
Wu FC, Tajar A, Pye SR, et al. Hypothalamic-pituitary-testicular axis disruptions in older men are differentially linked to age and modifiable risk factors: the European Male Aging Study. J Clin Endocrinol Metab. 2008;93(7):2737–45.
Yau YHC, Potenza MN. Stress and eating behaviors. Minerva Endocrinol. 2013;38(3):255–67.
Zografos GN, Perysinakis I, Vassilatou E. Subclinical Cushing's syndrome: current concepts and trends. Hormones. 2014;13(3):323–37.

Chapter 11
Physical Manifestations of Obesity

Jeffrey Sicat

Pearls of Wisdom

- Obesity and sleep apnea have a bidirectional relationship in that obesity can cause and worsen sleep apnea, and conversely sleep apnea can contribute to and worsen obesity.
- Untreated, undiagnosed sleep apnea, and reduced sleep duration cause insulin resistance, worsening diabetes control, reduced leptin levels, increased ghrelin, increased cortisol, increased sympathetic activity, and increased appetite and cravings for sweets and salts.
- Diagnosis and treatment of sleep disorders may improve multiple cardiometabolic parameters including improved glycemic control, insulin sensitivity, and appetite regulation.
- Obesity increases the risk of osteoarthritis, knee replacement, postoperative complications, and need for repeat joint replacement surgery, and weight reduction of 10% can dramatically improve each of these factors.
- Hepatobiliary disease is highly associated with obesity, including an increased risk of cholesterol gallstones. Rapid weight loss via both very low-calorie meal plan and bariatric surgery acutely increases the risk of gallstones, and this risk may be attenuated by ursodeoxycholic acid or a daily meal including at least 10 grams of dietary fat.

J. Sicat
Virginia Weight and Wellness, Glen Allen, VA, USA

J. M. Gonzalez-Campoy et al. (eds.), *Bariatric Endocrinology*,
https://doi.org/10.1007/978-3-319-95655-8_11

11.1 Introduction

The progressive shift toward obesity over the last 30 years has resulted in a tremendous and widespread impact on metabolic, psychiatric, and physical complications of obesity. This chapter specifically discusses the physical manifestations of obesity. While obesity impacts multiple organ systems (Table 11.1), this chapter focuses specifically on the respiratory, musculoskeletal, and gastrointestinal systems, with particular focus on the interplay of obesity and sleep disorders, knee osteoarthritis (OA), and gallstone disease.

11.2 Obesity and Sleep Disorders Have a Bidirectional Effect

Obesity is the most significant risk factor for obstructive sleep apnea (OSA). OSA is the most common type of sleep-disordered breathing and is characterized by recurrent episodes of upper airway obstruction and/or collapse, causing reduced airflow or complete cessation of airflow during sleep. Episodes commonly manifest as loud snoring, gasping, and choking, causing acute reductions of oxygenation. These can occur as often as 1–2 episodes per minute, with up to hundreds of episodes through the night, resulting in recurrent arousals and preventing progression to deep restorative sleep.

Table 11.1 Overview of physical manifestations of obesity by organ system

Cardiovascular	Congestive heart failure	Deep venous thrombosis
Pulmonary/ respiratory	*Sleep apnea* Obesity hypoventilation syndrome	Restrictive lung disease Dyspnea
Neurologic	Cerebrovascular accident Compressive neuropathies	Carpal tunnel syndrome Papilledema
Gastrointestinal	Gastroesophageal reflux disease *Gallstones*	Hernias
Genitourinary	Urinary incontinence Cystocele Uterine prolapse	Sexual dysfunction (including inability to penetrate, inability to use some sexual positions, genital overcrowding, orgasmic dysfunction, and erectile dysfunction)
Musculoskeletal	*Osteoarthritis* Lumbago—back pain (originating from degenerative disc disease and degenerative joint disease)	Gout Immobility
Dermatologic	Cellulitis Cutaneous candidiasis Edema Lymphedema	Acanthosis nigricans Hirsutism Venous stasis and ulcers Skin tags
Reproductive	Pregnancy-related complications	

Risk factors for OSA include a neck circumference >16″ in women and >17″ in men, male gender, increasing age, alcohol use, sedative use, and supine sleeping position. Endocrine conditions associated with OSA include obesity, adiposopathy, hypothyroidism, postmenopausal status, and acromegaly. The risk in men is doubled compared to women (approximately 30% in men and 15% in women). Postmenopausal women have a more than fourfold increased risk, compared to premenopausal women. This risk for postmenopausal women increases until the age of 65 and then reaches a plateau. Approximately 25% of adults with a body mass index (BMI) between 25 and 28 kilograms (kg)/meter $(m)^2$ have at least mild OSA. OSA is present in up to 45% of patients with stage 3 or higher obesity. Similarly, obesity is the biggest risk factor for OSA. Approximately 70% of patients with OSA have obesity. The prevalence of OSA in stage 3 or higher obesity is nearly double that seen in normal-weight adults.

Obesity potentiates OSA due to excess soft tissue and fat deposition in the mouth, throat, upper airway, and peripharyngeal regions. This extra soft tissue may result in a smaller airway lumen as well as increased external pressure on the airway. The net effect of these changes is an increased collapsibility of the upper airway leading to apnea. An increasing neck circumference correlates with increasing severity of OSA. Apnea episodes occur during sleep due to decreased airway muscle tone during sleep, as well as the pull of gravity while in the supine position.

11.2.1 OSA and Reduced Sleep Duration Can Cause Obesity and Insulin Resistance

While obesity is the most significant risk factor for OSA, there is a bidirectional effect. OSA and reduced sleep duration contribute to the development of obesity and type 2 diabetes mellitus (T2DM).

Over the last 40 years, self-reported sleep duration has declined by 1.5–2 h in the United States. A poll by the National Sleep Foundation in 2009 demonstrated that American adults sleep an average of 6 h 30 min on weekdays and 7 h 12 min on weekends, whereas the average duration of sleep was 8.5 h in 1960.

There is an increased risk of developing T2DM over 3 years, depending on the severity of nocturnal hypoxia (mild hypoxia episode odds ratio [OR] = 1.26; moderate-to-severe hypoxia OR = 1.69), even after adjustments for BMI, gender, and other risk factors.

OSA severity may be categorized based on the apnea-hypopnea index (AHI), which is calculated based on the number of apnea events divided by the number of hours of sleep. Normal is an AHI < 5 apnea episodes per hour; mild OSA is an AHI 5–14; moderate OSA is an AHI 15–29, and severe OSA is an AHI ≥ 30.

The Wisconsin Sleep Study (*n* = 1387) demonstrated a twofold increase in the incidence of T2DM in patients with an AHI > 15 compared to those with an AHI < 5 (OR = 2.3), even after adjustments for BMI and other risk factors. The Sleep Heart

Study ($n = 6441$) also showed that patients with overweight or obesity with sleep-disordered breathing had significantly higher rates of impaired fasting glucose (IFG), impaired glucose tolerance (IGT), and T2DM even after adjusting for BMI. Even those with sleep-disordered breathing and normal bodyweight had a 2.5 greater prevalence of T2DM compared to patients with normal breathing patterns.

11.2.2 Why Does OSA Increase the Risk of T2DM?

OSA may increase glucose intolerance through several mechanisms. Intermittent hypoxemia has been shown to stimulate the sympathetic nervous system. The resulting elevation in catecholamines may directly cause insulin resistance. Fragmented sleep, as seen in OSA, increases cortisol levels, which can also lead to insulin resistance. Stamatakis et al. demonstrated a 25% reduction in insulin sensitivity after just 2 days of sleep fragmentation. Lastly, reduced sleep duration has been shown to stimulate orexigenic hormones, such as ghrelin, leading to further weight gain and insulin resistance.

11.2.3 Increasing Severity of OSA Is Associated with Worsening Glucose Control

OSA is highly prevalent in patients with T2DM. Tasali et al. screened 60 consecutive patients with T2DM for sleep apnea, demonstrating that 77% had sleep apnea. Increasing severity of sleep apnea was associated with worsening glucose control. The presence of mild, moderate, or severe OSA increased mean-adjusted hemoglobin A1c (A1c) values by 1.49%, 1.93%, and 3.69%, respectively.

11.2.4 OSA Treatment and T2DM Improvement

Continuous positive airway pressure (CPAP) therapy in patients with T2DM with OSA can improve glucose control. Nighttime glucose levels improve following initiation of CPAP therapy. Pallayova showed that even after one night of initiating CPAP therapy, there are significant improvements in overnight glucose control as well as reduced glucose variability. Dawson et al. demonstrated that after 5 weeks of CPAP, mean overnight glucose levels improved from 121 milligrams/deciliter (mg/dL) to 102 mg/dL. Babu et al. evaluated patients with diabetes before and after 3 months of CPAP therapy and showed an A1c reduction of 0.6% (in patients with a baseline A1c > 7%) as well as significant improvements in postprandial glucose after all three meals (191 mg/dL pre-therapy and 130 mg/dL post 3 months of CPAP therapy).

While several controlled studies have shown a benefit of CPAP on glucose metabolism and insulin sensitivity, others have not shown improvement in A1c or insulin sensitivity. However, the average nighttime use of CPAP treatment was less than 5 h per night in the studies demonstrating a lack of benefit, with some studies averaging as low as 3 h of CPAP use per night.

11.2.5 Weight Loss Through Very Low-Calorie Meal Plan (VLCMP), Pharmacologics, or Surgery May Improve OSA

Currently, the standard of care for OSA is treatment with CPAP. Unfortunately, when factoring in patient acceptance and adherence to CPAP, the success rates of CPAP can be as low as 50%.

OSA in patients with overweight or obesity can improve with significant weight loss, whether achieved through lifestyle modification, medication, or bariatric surgery. Longitudinal studies have demonstrated that a 1% decrease in body weight decreases the AHI by approximate 3%.

11.2.5.1 VLCMP Weight Loss

Johansson et al. treated patients with obesity and moderate-to-severe OSA with a VLCMP for 9 weeks, followed by a weight maintenance program, resulting in 27 pounds (lbs) or 10% weight loss at 1 year. This weight loss significantly reduced apnea episodes, with 48% of patients no longer requiring CPAP. Further analysis demonstrated that a 10-kg weight loss was associated with an average decrease of 5 events/h on the AHI score. Tuomilehto et al. treated patients with mild OSA. They demonstrated that with a 10% reduction in body weight at 1 year, 63% of patients were cured from OSA (defined as AHI < 5 events/hour).

11.2.5.2 Pharmacological Weight Loss

Treatment for 28 weeks with extended-release phentermine/topiramate in patients with obesity and OSA demonstrated significant weight reduction compared to placebo (10.2% vs. 4.3%). It also resulted in a greater reduction of apnea events per hour compared to placebo (−31.5 events/h vs. −16.6 events/h). From baseline to week 28, patients in the phentermine/topiramate group reduced their mean AHI from 44 to 14 events/h (68% reduction).

11.2.5.3 Surgical Weight Loss

Out of 597 consecutive patients about to undergo bariatric surgery, 48% had OSA (19% severe OSA, 11% moderate OSA, and 18% mild OSA). At a median of 11 months postbariatric surgery, the mean BMI was reduced from 56 to 38 kg/m^2 and the number of patients using CPAP or bilevel positive airway pressure reduced from 81 to 31 patients postoperatively.

11.2.6 Reduced Sleep Duration Is Associated with Obesity

Short sleep duration is associated with obesity, independent of BMI. Cappuccio et al. performed a meta-analysis of 45 cross-sectional studies (including 604,509 adults and 30,002 children) and showed a relationship between short sleep (<5 h per night in adults and <10 h per night in children) and obesity, with an OR of 1.55 in adults and 1.89 in children. In adults, every 1 h of reduced sleep duration was associated with an increase in BMI of 0.35 kg/m^2.

11.2.7 Reduced Sleep Duration Changes Neuroendocrine Hormones (Reduced Leptin and Increased Ghrelin)

Spiegal et al. published the first detailed lab study on the effect of recurrent partial sleep deprivation on hormonal and metabolic variables involved in appetite regulation. Young healthy men underwent six consecutive nights of sleep deprivation (4 h sleep/night), followed by seven nights of sleep recovery (12 h of sleep/night). At the end of 6 days of sleep deprivation, leptin levels were reduced 19% compared to baseline, with a 40% decrease in glucose tolerance consistent with a state of glucose intolerance and a significant reduction in acute insulin response to glucose. The postbreakfast homeostatic model assessment of insulin resistance was significantly elevated (+56%) after the sleep-deprived state compared to the fully rested state. Thus, insulin resistance develops even with short-term sleep deprivation.

A small, shorter, follow-up study (n = 12) was performed involving 2 days of sleep restriction (4 h) compared to 2 days of full sleep (10 h). Results after brief sleep restriction showed a significant reduction in leptin (−18%) and significant increases in ghrelin (+28%), hunger, appetite (+23%), and appetite specifically for high carbohydrate.

Larger population-based studies, including the Wisconsin Sleep Cohort Study (n = 1024) and the Quebec Family Study (n = 740) demonstrated identical reductions in leptin and identical increases in ghrelin. These observations help explain the propensity for increased appetite and energy intake in patients with a reduced sleep duration (5 h).

11.2.8 Sleep Loss Increases Adrenocorticotropic Hormone (ACTH) and Cortisol and Dampens Evening Reduction of Cortisol

Sleep loss, whether partial or total sleep deprivation (from insomnia or recurrent sleep deprivation), results in elevated evening cortisol levels. Guyon et al. demonstrated that two nights of sleep restriction (from 10 h to 4 h) was associated with a

19% increase in overall ACTH levels, a 21% increase in total cortisol levels, and the usual physiological evening circadian cortisol decline was attenuated by 21%. Evening total and free cortisol levels were increased by 30% and 200%, respectively, in the sleep-deprived versus normal sleep groups. An increase in appetite was correlated with the increase in total cortisol.

11.2.9 Reduced Sleep Duration Can Affect Body Composition Changes During Weight Loss

Nedeltcheva et al. reported a 2-week study of sleep restriction compared to normal sleep time (5.5 vs. 8.5 h/night) while on a hypocaloric meal plan. Subjects in both groups lost a similar amount of total body weight (3 kg), but sleep-restricted subjects lost 60% more lean body mass and 55% less fat mass. These findings suggest that adequate sleep may play a key role in preserving lean body mass during periods of caloric restriction, whereas sleep deprivation may lead to loss of lean body mass during weight loss.

11.2.10 Effect of Sleep Restriction on Energy Expenditure

Sleep disturbance or nighttime wakefulness is associated with lower daytime physical activity. Gupta et al. found that for each 1-h decrease in sleep, obesity increased by 80% and physical activity was reduced by 3%. Ortega et al. found that short sleep duration was associated with morning tiredness, less physical activity, and excessive TV watching. In addition, sleep restriction in humans reduces leptin levels, and rodent studies have shown that reduction of leptin may reduce energy expenditure by reducing physical activity and core body temperature.

11.2.11 Effect of Circadian Disruption

Continuous disruption of circadian rhythms, as seen in shift workers, has been associated with body weight gain, T2DM, and cardiovascular disease. In ten subjects who underwent a forced desynchrony protocol, short-term circadian misalignment increased postprandial glucose, insulin, and blood pressure, decreased 24-h leptin levels, and inverted the cortisol profile (increased cortisol at the end of the wake episode and beginning of the sleep episode). Pan et al. followed >170,000 nurses in the Nurses' Health Study and found that healthcare workers working night shifts for the highest duration had the greatest risk of developing obesity, excess weight gain, and diabetes (Fig. 11.1).

A summary of the impact of sleep deprivation on endocrine metabolic factors is given in Fig. 11.2.

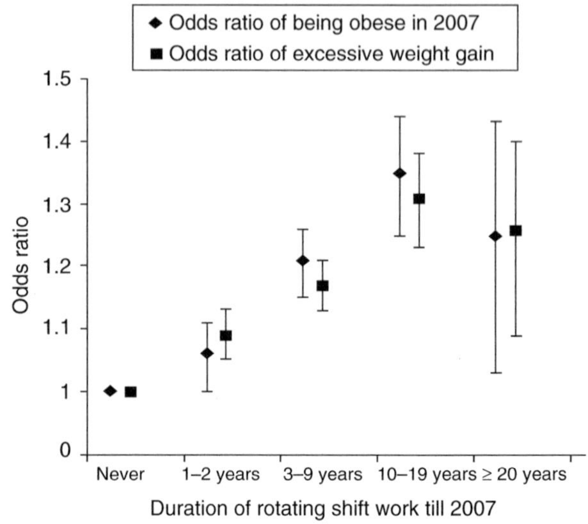

Fig. 11.1 Duration of rotating night shift work and the risk of obesity and excess weight gain in the Nurses' Health Study II. Increased duration of rotating night shift work was associated with an increased odds ratio of being obese in 2007 as well as excessive weight gain from 1989 to 2007. Excess weight gain was defined as an increase of more than 5% body weight above the baseline bodyweight from 1989. (From: Pan et al. 2011; used with permission)

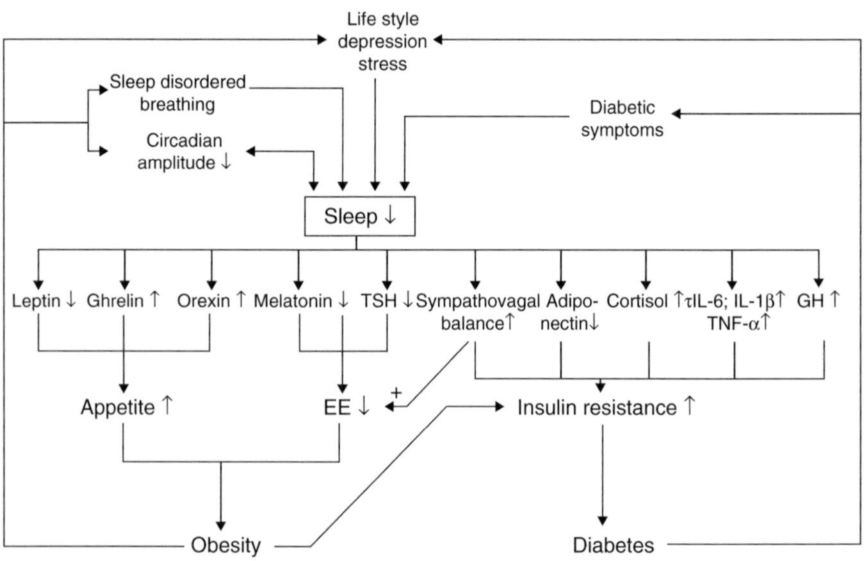

Fig. 11.2 Reduced sleep duration and sleep-disordered breathing may cause endocrine/metabolic disruptions leading to obesity and diabetes. Reduced sleep duration and quality may increase the risk of obesity and diabetes via multiple hormonal and physiological changes causing an increase in appetite, a decrease in energy expenditure (EE), and an increase in insulin resistance (Abbreviations: EE energy expenditure, GH growth hormone, IL-1ß interleukin-1 beta, IL-6 interleukin 6, TNF-α tumor necrosis factor alpha, TSH thyroid-stimulating hormone). (From: Lucassen et al. 2012; used with permission)

11.2.12 Increasing Sleep Time May Reduce Appetite

Limited data suggest that increasing sleep time may reduce appetite. Tasali et al. prospectively studied young adults with overweight, with baseline habitual sleep duration <6.5 h. Subjects' sleep time was increased to 8.5 h for 2 weeks. On average, participants obtained 1.6 h of extra sleep (5.6 vs. 7.1 h) and reported less sleepiness and higher energy levels. Increasing sleep time led to a 14% decrease in overall appetite and a 62% decrease in the desire for sweet and salty foods.

11.2.13 Sleep Summary

In summary, obesity and sleep disorders have a bidirectional impact. Obesity is the most significant risk factor for OSA, and OSA is a significant risk factor for T2DM. Sleep disorders and reduced sleep can cause an increase in insulin resistance, cortisol, sympathetic catecholamines, and orexigenic hormones, as well as a decrease in energy expenditure and physical activity. Treatment of OSA and increase in sleep duration can significantly improve glucose control, insulin resistance, and hunger and may promote weight loss. Bariatric endocrinology subspecialists should be highly attuned to this bidirectional relationship and be aggressive in diagnosing and treating sleep disorders, especially in patients with treatment-resistant diabetes and/or obesity.

11.3 Musculoskeletal Section

Obesity is the strongest modifiable risk factor for the development of osteoarthritis (OA). In the first National Health and Nutrition Examination Survey study, women with a BMI > 30 kg/m^2 compared to BMI < 30 kg/m^2 had fourfold increased risk of OA and men had a fivefold increased risk. Excess body weight increases the amount of force across a joint, which may cause cartilage breakdown eventually leading to OA. Approximately 719,000 knee replacements are performed yearly in the US. Three to six times one's bodyweight is exerted across the knee while walking, and thus, an increase of 10 lbs in body weight may increase the mechanical forces on the knee by 60 lbs. Patients in the Framingham Heart Study Cohort (mean age: 37 years), who had overweight or obesity, demonstrated a higher rate of development of knee OA at an average age of 73 versus normal-weight subjects. Obesity is not only associated with OA of the knees but also OA of the hands. This observation suggests that obesity causes not only biomechanical effects on joints but also joint destruction from circulating systemic proinflammatory cytokines in OA. Specifically, elevated levels of the inflammatory cytokine IL-6 have been implicated in the pathogenesis of OA.

Felson et al. found that in patients who had overweight or obesity, 10 lbs of weight gain increased the risk of knee OA by 40%, while 10 lbs of weight loss reduced the risk of knee OA. Based on estimates from the Framingham OA data, if men and women with a BMI > 30 kg/m^2 were able to reduce enough weight to achieve a BMI < 30 kg/m^2, it is estimated that the incidence of symptomatic knee OA would be reduced by 21% in men and by 33% in women.

Messier et al. prospectively studied patients with obesity and knee OA ($n = 453$) to evaluate the impact of ≥10% bodyweight loss. Knee compressive forces, IL-6 levels, and pain scores were significantly reduced by 10%, 15%, and 45%, respectively, with the greatest reductions seen in patients who lost the most weight. Niklas et al. showed that weight loss through dietary interventions reduced inflammatory cytokine IL-6 levels, whereas exercise (without weight loss) did not affect IL-6 levels.

While previous data were inconsistent regarding the impact of obesity on post-knee surgery complications, more recent data suggest a graded effect on complications based on the severity of obesity. A meta-analysis of 20 studies reviewing the impact of obesity on postoperative knee arthroplasty complications showed patients with a BMI > 30 kg/m^2, compared to <30 kg/m^2, had increased infection rates (OR = 1.9), deep infections requiring surgical debridement (OR = 2.38), and an increased need for surgical revisions (OR = 1.3).

A recent analysis of more than 1.6 million Medicare patients undergoing total knee replacement between 2005 and 2011 showed increasing BMI levels (BMI < 30 kg/m^2, BMI 30–39 kg/m^2, BMI 40–49 kg/m^2, and BMI >50 kg/m^2) were associated with increased risks of local complications (postoperative infection and postoperative stiffness requiring manipulation under anesthesia) and systemic complications (deep venous thromboses, pulmonary emboli, myocardial infarctions, cerebrovascular accidents, urinary tract infections, pneumonia, and renal failure). Patients with a BMI of >50 kg/m^2 had about double the rates of complications than patients with a BMI of 40–49 kg/m^2, triple that of patients with a BMI of 30–39 kg/m^2, and quadruple that of patients with a BMI < 30 kg/m^2.

It is thought that patients with obesity and severe OA cannot lose weight due to reduced mobility and increased joint pain. Postoperatively, both of these factors improve and should facilitate weight loss. Thus, many people assume that weight loss improves after knee replacement surgery by increasing one's ability to be more active. In fact, most patients with obesity do not lose weight after knee replacement surgery.

Donovan et al. showed that in the year after knee arthroplasty, while patients had increased mobility and less pain, there was no significant change in body weight. Zeni et al. showed that in the 2 years after total knee arthroplasty (TKA), 66% of patients gained weight with an average weight gain of 14 lbs.

Amin et al. prospectively followed up patients with a BMI > 40 kg/m^2 who were matched with patients with a BMI < 30 kg/m^2 after knee replacement. They found that at less than 4 years postoperatively, patients with a BMI > 40 kg/m^2 had increased complications and increased need for repeat knee replacement compared to patients who did not have obesity (25.8% vs. 0%).

11.3.1 Musculoskeletal Summary

In summary, excess body weight is the most significant risk factor for OA of the knee with mechanical compressive forces on the knee amplified up to 600% for every pound of weight gain. Ten percent bodyweight loss has been associated with almost a 50% reduction in knee pain. Obesity is associated with increased need for knee replacement surgery, increased perioperative complications, and increased need for repeat joint revision surgery. While most patients report improved mobility and pain control after knee replacement surgery, most patients do not lose weight postoperatively. A BMI > 40 kg/m^2 is associated with a higher need for repeat joint replacement surgery. Thus, weight loss should be an important focus both prior to and after joint replacement surgery to improve outcomes and reduce the need for repeat surgery.

11.4 Gastrointestinal Section: Focus on Gallstones

Obesity is commonly associated with several hepatobiliary diseases including gallstones, pancreatitis, and hepatic steatosis. This section focuses on gallstone disease, as more than 700,000 cholecystectomies are performed yearly in the USA. Nongenetic risk factors for gallbladder disease include female gender, estrogen, pregnancy, increasing age, smoking, fibrates, dyslipidemia, metabolic syndrome, obesity, and rapid weight loss through either meal planning or surgery.

11.4.1 Obesity Is a Significant Risk Factor for Gallstones

The Nurses' Health Study showed that during 8 years of follow-up, there was a linear correlation between BMI and risk for cholecystectomy. The risk of cholecystectomy was increased eightfold in women with a BMI $\geq$ 45 kg/m^2 compared to those with a BMI < 25 kg/m^2. Women with a BMI $\geq$ 30 kg/m^2 and BMI $\geq$ 45 kg/m^2 had an approximately 1% and 2% incidence per year for cholecystectomy, respectively.

11.4.2 Why Does Obesity Increase the Risk of Gallstones?

More than 80% of gallstones are in the form of cholesterol gallstones, which are composed of conglomerates of cholesterol monohydrate crystals, mucin gel, calcium bilirubinate, and proteins which grow and accumulate in the gallbladder. Cholesterol gallstones result from: (1) cholesterol supersaturation of bile, (2) presence of a kinetic defect that allows for the nucleation and growth of cholesterol crystals, and (3) gallbladder hypomotility and thus bile stasis.

Cholesterol gallstones are commonly seen in patients with excess body weight since obesity increases the activity of 3-hydroxy-3-methyl-glutaryl-CoA reductase (HMG-CoA reductase), the rate-limiting step in cholesterol synthesis, thus increasing cholesterol synthesis. This causes a higher rate of biliary cholesterol secretion resulting in highly supersaturated gallbladder bile. Weight loss reduces bile cholesterol saturation, thus reducing the risk of stone formation. Weight regain causes a return to the more supersaturated bile, thus returning to baseline the risk of stone formation.

11.4.3 Rapid Weight Loss Can Increase the Formation of Stones (VLCD and Surgical)

Rapid weight loss, whether achieved through a VLCD or bariatric surgery, is associated with an increased risk of gallstones. Pooled data from multiple rapid weight loss studies showed that 12% of VLCD (500–800 calories/daily) patients developed gallstones within 26 weeks and 37% of bariatric surgery patients developed gallstones within 18 months. For this reason, some bariatric surgery centers recommend routine cholecystectomy during the bariatric surgery procedure.

Shiffman et al. showed that in women on a 520-calorie/day VLMP, a higher rate of monthly weight loss was associated with an increased risk of gallstones (10–15 lbs/month = 32% risk of gallstone formation, >15–20 lbs/month = 65%, and >20 lbs/month = 100% risk of gallstone formation).

11.4.4 Why Does Rapid Weight Loss Increase the Risk of Gallstones?

At baseline, patients with obesity have increased cholesterol supersaturation of bile. During the process of caloric restriction, gallbladder hypomotility and reduced gallbladder emptying may occur, contributing to stone growth. Gallbladder hypomotility and reduced emptying occur when patients consume a low-calorie meal plan and may be seen, especially when a meal plan contains <10 grams of fat per day.

A higher fat intake during a VLCMP reduces the risk of gallstones. Gephard et al. induced 22% bodyweight loss using either 520 cal/day (<2 g fat/day) versus 900 cal/day (30 g fat/day) and gallstones developed in 66% and 0% of patients, respectively. Festi et al. similarly demonstrated that treating patients with a VLCMP using similar caloric intake (535–577 cal/day) but different fat intake resulted in a higher rate of gallstone formation over 3 months in patients receiving 3 grams of fat versus 12 grams of fat (55% vs. 0%) daily.

11.4.5 Medical Treatments to Reduce Gallstones During VLCMP and Bariatric Surgery

Ursodeoxycholic acid (UDCA) (Actigall®) is a prescription bile salt that reduces cholesterol secretion into bile and also improves biliary cholesterol solubility. Shiffman et al. prospectively studied 1004 patients with obesity undergoing a 16-week, 520-calorie/day VLCMP. Escalating doses of UDCA significantly reduced the development of gallstones in a dose-dependent manner (placebo = 28%, 300 mg/day = 8%, 600 mg/day = 3%, and 1200 mg/day = 2%). The recommended dose of UDCA is 600 mg/day.

Sugerman et al. prospectively studied 233 patients undergoing gastric bypass and also found UDCA to be effective in preventing gallstones 6 months after surgery. In placebo, and 300 mg and 600 mg of UDCA doses, gallstones formed in 32%, 13%, and 2% of patients, respectively. A total of 600 mg is an effective daily dose of UDCA for the prevention of gallstones during rapid weight loss after gastric bypass.

Similar benefits were found using UDCA in patients with gastric sleeve and gastric band. Miller et al. prospectively treated patients with gastric sleeve or gastric band for 6 months with UDCA or placebo and found the risk of gallstone formation was reduced (3% and 22%, respectively), as well as the need for cholecystectomy (4.7% and 12%, respectively) at 1 year.

11.4.6 Gastrointestinal Summary

In summary, as obesity increases across our population, so does the risk of hepatobiliary disease, gallstones, subsequent cholecystectomies, and interventional biliary procedures for stone management. Obesity upregulates the activity of HMG-CoA reductase, which increases biliary cholesterol excretion and saturation in bile. Therefore, obesity increases the risk of cholesterol gallstones (the most common type of stones). Reduction of body weight is associated with lower gallstone risk. However, rapid weight loss, as seen with VLCMP or bariatric surgery, can significantly increase the risk of stone formation due to biliary stasis. The risk of biliary stone formation during rapid weight loss may be reduced with pharmacologic agents such as UDCA (to improve dissolution of stones) and through the ingestion of fat (>10 g) at one daily meal during VLCMP (by reducing biliary stasis).

Reading List

Amin AK, Clayton RA, Patton JT, Gaston M, Cook RE, Brenkel IJ. Total knee replacement in morbidly obese patients. Results of a prospective matched study. J Bone Joint Surg Br. 2006;88(10):1321–6.

Aronsohn RS, Whitmore H, Van Cauter E, Tasali E. Impact of untreated obstructive sleep apnea on glucose control in type 2 diabetes. Am J Respir Crit Care Med. 2010;181:507–13.

Babu AR, Herdegen J, Fogelfeld L, Shott S, Mazzone T. Type 2 diabetes, glycemic control, and continuous positive airway pressure in obstructive sleep apnea. Arch Intern Med. 2005;165:447–52.
Bennion LJ, Grundy SM. Risk factors for the development of cholelithiasis in man (second of two parts). N Engl J Med. 1978;299(22):1221–7.
Bixler EO, Vgontzas AN, Ten Have T, Tyson K, Kales A. Effects of age on sleep apnea in men: prevalence and severity. Am J Respir Crit Care Med. 1998;157(1):144–8.
Bixler EO, Vgontzas AN, Lin HM, et al. Prevalence of sleep disordered breathing in women: effects of gender. Am J Respir Crit Care Med. 2001;163(3 Pt 1):608–13.
Bonfrate L, Wang DQ, Garruti G, Portincasa P. Obesity and the risk and prognosis of gallstone disease and pancreatitis. Best Pract Res Clin Gastroenterol. 2014;28(4):623–35.
Cappuccio FP, Taggart FM, Kandala NB, et al. Meta-analysis of short sleep duration and obesity in children and adults. Sleep. 2008;31:619–26.
Centers for Disease Control and Prevention: FastStats inpatient surgery data for the U.S. [Internet]. 2010 [cited 2015 May 24]. Available from: http://www.cdc.gov/nchs/fastats/inpatient-surgery.htm.
Chaput JP, Despres JP, Bouchard C, Tremblay A. Short sleep duration is associated with reduced leptin levels and increased adiposity: results from the Quebec family study. Obesity. 2007;15:253–61.
Crispim CA, Waterhouse J, Dâmaso AR, et al. Hormonal appetite control is altered by shift work: a preliminary study. Metabolism. 2011;60:1726–35.
Davies RJ, Stradling JR. The relationship between neck circumference, radiographic pharyngeal anatomy, and the obstructive sleep apnoea syndrome. Eur Respir J. 1990;3:509–14.
Dawson A, Abel SL, Loving RT, Dailey G, Shadan FF, Cronin JW, et al. CPAP therapy of obstructive sleep apnea in type 2 diabetics improves glycemic control during sleep. J Clin Sleep Med. 2008;4:538–42.
Donovan J, Dingwall I, McChesney S. Weight change 1 year following total knee or hip arthroplasty. ANZ J Surg. 2006;76:222–5.
Everhart JE. Contributions of obesity and weight loss to gallstone disease. Ann Intern Med. 1993;119:1029–35.
Felson DT. Weight and osteoarthritis. J Rheumatol. 1995;43:7–9.
Felson DT, Anderson JI, Naimark A, Walker AM, Meenan RF. Obesity and knee osteoarthritis. Ann Intern Med. 1988;109:18–24.
Felson DT, Zhang Y, Hannan MT, et al. Risk factors for incident radiographic knee osteoarthritis in the elderly: the Framingham Study. Arthritis Rheum. 1997;40:728–33.
Festi D, Colecchia A, Orsini M, et al. Gallbladder motility and gallstone formation in obese patients following very low calorie diets: use it (fat) to lose it (well). Int J Obes Relat Metab Disord. 1998;22:592–600.
Gebhard RL, Prigge WF, Ansel HJ, et al. The role of gallbladder emptying in gallstone formation during diet-induced rapid weight loss. Hepatology. 1996;24:544–8.
Gupta NK, Mueller WH, Chan W, Meininger JC. Is obesity associated with poor sleep quality in adolescents? Am J Hum Biol. 2002;14:762–8.
Guyon A, Balbo M, Morselli LL, Tasali E, Leproult R, L'Hermite-Balériaux M, et al. Adverse effects of two nights of sleep restriction on the hypothalamic-pituitary-adrenal axis in healthy men. J Clin Endocrinol Metab. 2014;99:2861–8.
Haines KL, Nelson LG, Gonzalez R, Torrella T, Martin T, Kandil A, et al. Objective evidence that bariatric surgery improves obesity-related obstructive sleep apnea. Surgery. 2007;141:354–8.
Johansson K, Hemmingsson E, Harlid R, et al. Longer term effects of very low energy diet on obstructive sleep apnoea in cohort derived from randomised controlled trial: prospective observational follow-up study. BMJ. 2011;342:d3017.
Kakkar RK, Berry RB. Positive airway pressure treatment for obstructive sleep apnea. Chest. 2007;132:1057–72.
Kerkhoffs GM, Servien E, Dunn W, et al. The influence of obesity on the complication rate and outcome of total knee arthroplasty: a meta-analysis and systematic literature review. J Bone Joint Surg Am. 2012;94(20):1839–44.

Kripke DF, Simons RN, Garfinkel L, Hammond EC. Short and long sleep and sleeping pills. Is increased mortality associated? Arch Gen Psychiatry. 1979;36:103–16.

Lam JC, Lam B, Yao TJ, Lai AY, Ooi CG, Tam S, et al. A randomised controlled trial of nasal continuous positive airway pressure on insulin sensitivity in obstructive sleep apnoea. Eur Respir J. 2010;35:138–45.

Lucassen EA, Rother KI, Cizza G. Interacting epidemics? Sleep curtailment, insulin resistance, and obesity. Ann N Y Acad Sci. 2012;1264:110–34.

Messier SP, Mihalko SL, Legault C, Miller GD, Nicklas BJ, DeVita P, et al. Effects of intensive diet and exercise on knee joint loads, inflammation, and clinical outcomes among overweight and obese adults with knee osteoarthritis: the IDEA randomized clinical trial. JAMA. 2013;310:1263.

Miller K, Hell E, Lang B, Lengauer E. Gallstone formation prophylaxis after gastric restrictive procedures for weight loss a randomized double-blind placebo-controlled trial. Ann Surg. 2003;238:697–702.

Morikawa Y, Nakagawa H, Miura K. Shift work and the risk of diabetes mellitus among Japanese male factory workers. Scand J Work Environ Health. 2005;31:179–83.

Muraki I, Tanigawa T, Yamagishi K, Sakurai S, Ohira T, Imano H, et al. Nocturnal intermittent hypoxia and the development of type 2 diabetes: the Circulatory Risk in Communities Study (CIRCS). Diabetologia. 2010;53:481–8.

Narkiewicz K, van de Borne PJ, Montano N, Dyken ME, Phillips BG, Somers VK. Contribution of tonic chemoreflex activation to sympathetic activity and blood pressure in patients with obstructive sleep apnea. Circulation. 1998;97:943–5.

National Sleep Foundation 2012 Bedroom Poll [Internet]. 2015 [cited 2015 Nov 20]. Available from: https://sleepfoundation.org/sites/default/files/bedroompoll/NSF_Bedroom_Poll_Report.pdf.

Nedeltcheva AV, Kilkus JM, Imperial J, Schoeller DA, Penev PD. Insufficient sleep undermines dietary efforts to reduce adiposity. Ann Intern Med. 2010;153:435–41.

Nicklas BJ, Ambrosius W, Messier SP, et al. Diet-induced weight loss, exercise, and chronic inflammation in older, obese adults: a randomized controlled clinical trial. Am J Clin Nutr. 2004;79(4):544–51.

Ortega FB, Chillón P, Ruiz JR, et al. Sleep patterns in Spanish adolescents: associations with TV watching and leisure-time physical activity. Eur J Appl Physiol. 2010;110:563–73.

Pallayova M, Donic V, Tomori Z. Beneficial effects of severe sleep apnea therapy on nocturnal glucose control in persons with type 2 diabetes mellitus. Diabetes Res Clin Pract. 2008;81(1):e8–e11.

Pan A, Schernhammer ES, Sun Q, Hu FB. Rotating night shift work and risk of type 2 diabetes: two prospective cohort studies in women. PLoS Med. 2011;8(12):e1001141. https://www.ncbi.nlm.nih.gov/pubmed/?term=Pan+A%2C+Schernhammer+ES%2C+Sun+Q%2C+Hu+FB.+Rotating+night+shift+work+and+risk+of+type+2+diabetes%3A+two+prospective+cohort+studies+in+women.+PLoS+Med.+2011%3B8(12)%3Ae1001141.

Reichmuth KJ, Austin D, Skatrud JB, Young T. Association of sleep apnea and type II diabetes: a population-based study. Am J Respir Crit Care Med. 2005;172:1590–5.

Romero-Corral A, Caples S, Lopez-Jimenez F, Somers V. Interactions between obesity and obstructive sleep apnea implications for treatment. Chest. 2010;137(3):711–9.

Scheer FA, Hilton MF, Mantzoros CS, Shea SA. Adverse metabolic and cardiovascular consequences of circadian misalignment. Proc Natl Acad Sci U S A. 2009;106:4453–8.

Seicean S, Kirchner HL, Gottlieb DJ, et al. Sleep-disordered breathing and impaired glucose metabolism in normal-weight and overweight/obese individuals: the Sleep Heart Health Study. Diabetes Care. 2008;31:1001–6.

Shiffman ML, Kaplan GD, Brinkman-Kaplan V, et al. Prophylaxis against gallstone formation with ursodeoxycholic acid in patients participating in a very-low-calorie diet program. Ann Intern Med. 1995;122:899–905.

Spiegel K, Leproult R, Van Cauter E. Impact of sleep debt on metabolic and endocrine function. Lancet. 1999;354:1435–9.

Spiegel K, Tasali E, Penev P, Van Cauter E. Sleep curtailment in healthy young men is associated with decreased leptin levels, elevated ghrelin levels and increased hunger and appetite. Ann Intern Med. 2004;141:846–50.

Stamatakis K, Punjabi NM. Effects of sleep fragmentation on glucose metabolism in normal subjects. Chest. 2010;137(1):95–101.

Stampfer MJ, Maclure KM, Colditz GA, Manson JE, Willett WC. Risk of symptomatic gallstones in women with severe obesity. Am J Clin Nutr. 1992;55:652–8.

Sugerman HJ, Brewer WH, Shiffman ML, et al. A multicenter, placebo controlled, randomized, double-blind, prospective trial of prophylactic ursodiol for the prevention of gallstone formation following gastric bypass-induced rapid weight loss. Am J Surg. 1995;169:91–6.

Taheri S, Lin L, Austin D, Young T, Mignot E. Short sleep duration is associated with reduced leptin, elevated ghrelin, and increased body mass index (BMI). PLoS Med. 2004 Dec;1(3):e62:210–7.

Tasali E, et al. The effects of extended bedtimes on sleep duration and food desire in overweight young adults: a home-based intervention. Appetite. 2014;80:220–4.

Tuomilehto HP, Seppa JM, Partinen MM, et al. Lifestyle intervention with weight reduction: first-line treatment in mild obstructive sleep apnea. Am J Respir Crit Care Med. 2009;179:320–7.

van de Wall E, Leshan R, Xu AW, Balthasar N, Coppari R, Liu SM, et al. Collective and individual functions of leptin receptor modulated neurons controlling metabolism and ingestion. Endocrinology. 2007;149:1773–85.

Van Drongelen A, Boot CRL, Merkus SL, Smid T, van der Beek AJ. The effects of shift work on body weight change—a systematic review of longitudinal studies. Scand J Work Environ Health. 2011;37:263–75.

Weinstock TG, Wang X, Rueschman M, Ismail-Beigi F, Aylor J, Babineau DC, et al. A controlled trial of CPAP therapy on metabolic control in individuals with impaired glucose tolerance and sleep apnea. Sleep. 2012;35:617–25.

Werner BC, Evans CL, Carothers JT, Browne JA. Primary total knee arthroplasty in super-obese patients: dramatically higher postoperative complication rates even compared to revision surgery. Arthroplasty. 2015;30(5):849–53.

West SD, Nicoll DJ, Wallace TM, Matthews DR, Stradling JR. Effect of CPAP on insulin resistance and HbA1c in men with obstructive sleep apnoea and type 2 diabetes. Thorax. 2007;62:969–74.

Winslow DH, Bowden CH, DiDonato KP McCullough PA. A randomized, double-blind, placebo-controlled study of an oral, extended-release formulation of phentermine/topiramate for the treatment of obstructive sleep apnea in obese adults. Sleep. 2012;35(11):1529–39.

Young T, Palta M, Dempsey J, Skatrud J, Weber S, Badr S. The occurrence of sleep-disordered breathing among middle aged adults. N Engl J Med. 1993;328(17):1230–5.

Young T, Shahar E, Nieto FJ, et al. Sleep Heart Health Study Research Group. Predictors of sleep-disordered breathing in community-dwelling adults: the Sleep Heart Health Study. Arch Intern Med. 2002;162(8):893–900.

Young T, Peppard P, Gottlieb DJ. Epidemiology of obstructive sleep apnea a population health perspective. Am J Respir Crit Care Med. 2002;165:1217–39.

Zeni JA, Snyder-Mackler L. Most patients gain weight in the 2 years after total knee arthroplasty: comparison to a healthy control group. Osteoarthr Cartil. 2010;18(4):510–4.

Chapter 12
Evaluation and Treatment of Atherogenic Dyslipidemia

J. Michael Gonzalez-Campoy and Caroline M. Houston

Pearls of Wisdom

- Adipose tissue is the largest storage organ for lipids in the human body. Adiposopathy leads to an inability of adipose tissue to process circulating fats, with the development of dyslipidemia.
- Any patient with dyslipidemia should be evaluated for overweight, obesity, and adiposopathy, and if present, treatment should be instituted. Conversely, any patient with overweight, obesity, or adiposopathy should have an evaluation for dyslipidemia, and if present, it should be treated.
- Dyslipidemia is one of the multiple risk factors for cardiovascular disease. Therefore, cardiovascular risk assessment should include the use of new risk equations derived from a more contemporary and diverse population, and initiation of treatment for dyslipidemia should be based on each patient's overall risk.
- The first line of treatment for dyslipidemia should be with the highest intensity of a statin that will reduce cardiovascular risk while minimizing the risk of side effects.
- Substitution therapy with newer lipid-lowering therapies should be implemented for patients who are intolerant of statins, and combination therapy should be used when a statin alone cannot sufficiently lower the risk of cardiovascular disease.

J. M. Gonzalez-Campoy (✉)
Minnesota Center for Obesity, Metabolism and Endocrinology, PA (MNCOME), Eagan, MN, USA
e-mail: drmike@mncome.com

C. M. Houston
The Brody School of Medicine at East Carolina University, Division of Endocrinology, Diabetes, and Metabolism, Greenville, NC, USA

J. M. Gonzalez-Campoy et al. (eds.), *Bariatric Endocrinology*,
https://doi.org/10.1007/978-3-319-95655-8_12

12.1 Introduction

Adipose tissue is the largest reservoir of energy in the human body. The energy reserves in adipose tissue are in the form of fats collected in the fat vacuoles of adipocytes and are not for immediate use. Rather, complex molecules have to be broken down in adipocytes, and the byproducts then have to be shuttled to other tissues. To the extent that adipose tissue is able to regulate the storage of energy and its distribution in times of need, the concentrations of lipoproteins and free fatty acids in the blood remain normal. Adipose tissue dysfunction results in derangements of the blood lipids. Clinically, chronic exposure to abnormal lipoprotein levels results in progression of atherosclerosis, with eventual organ damage from ischemia. This chapter will outline the adipose tissue handling of lipids, the derangements that develop with adiposopathy, the clinical impact of these derangements, and treatment options.

12.2 Role of Adipose Tissue in Lipid Metabolism

12.2.1 Adipose Tissue Contributions to Lipid Homeostasis

Triglycerides (TGs) are the largest component of adipocytes. TGs (e.g., triacylglycerides) are composed of three fatty acid chains of variable lengths attached to a three-carbon glycerol structural backbone. Each fatty acid chain has a variable number of single and double bonds along its length. Hormone-sensitive lipase (HSL) is the main intracellular enzyme that catalyzes the hydrolysis of TG esters in adipocytes. Hydrolysis of a TG yields a diglyceride. The diglyceride is rapidly cleaved to a monoglyceride by diglyceride lipase. The one remaining fatty acid is in turn cleaved by monoglyceride lipase. This process allows each adipocyte to release stored energy to meet the body's needs (free fatty acids' (FFAs') outflow).

HSL is the major intra-adipocyte lipolytic enzyme affected by hormones and is upregulated by catecholamines (i.e., beta-adrenergic stimulation) and cortisol. HSL is downregulated by insulin. Through this mechanism, increased sympathetic nervous system activity and increased cortisol secretion are catabolic, while hyperinsulinemia is anabolic, with regard to TG storage in adipocytes.

FFAs are the major secretory product of adipose tissue. Circulating FFA may be saturated or unsaturated. The fatty acids most easily released from adipose tissue by HSL are shorter (16–20 carbons) and more unsaturated. The circulating levels of FFA are determined by:

- The fed state (digestion of fats results in the absorption of TG from the intestine).
- The storage capacity of adipose tissue (saturated storage prevents accretion of TG by adipocytes).
- The degree to which other body organs store FFA as TG.
- The degree to which body organs metabolize FFA.

Lipoprotein lipase (LPL) is an enzyme produced by adipocytes and released into the extracellular space. LPL then diffuses to nearby capillaries, where it attaches to large, branched proteins bound to the inner capillary surface, including heparan sulfate proteoglycans. LPL is inactive until it becomes bound to its cofactor, apolipoprotein (apo) CII. Apo CII is attached to very low-density lipoproteins (VLDL) when they are secreted from the liver. Chylomicrons do not initially have apo CII, but receive it (and apo E) from circulating high-density lipoproteins (HDL). In exchange, the chylomicron transfers its apoprotein A1 to the HDL. When the apo CII on a TG-rich lipoprotein contacts LPL on the inner surface of capillaries in adipose tissue, it becomes activated. LPL hydrolyzes the TG in the lipoprotein into FFA and monoglyceride. The lipoprotein and attached enzyme can detach from the capillary wall and circulate, but the hydrolysis continues as long as the enzyme remains attached. Human adipocytes rely upon LPL to hydrolyze circulating TG into FFA. FFAs are transported into the adipocytes and are used for lipogenesis (FFA inflow). In the fed state, LPL interacts with chylomicrons and other TG-rich lipoproteins. In the fasting state, LPL mainly interacts with VLDL and other TG-rich lipoproteins.

In the fed state, plasma glucose levels rise. This causes the beta-cells of the pancreatic islets of Langerhans to secrete insulin. The blood supply of adipose tissue during the fed states provides higher glucose and insulin levels compared to the fasting state. Insulin receptor activation in adipocytes during the fed state:

- Promotes the incorporation of glucose transporter (GLUT) 4 into the adipocyte cell membrane, leading to glucose absorption by adipocytes.
- Stimulates extracellular LPL, leading to adipocyte uptake of FFA and resulting in the formation of intra-adipocyte triacylglycerols.
- Downregulates HSL, which breaks down intra-adipocyte triacylglycerols into fatty acids and glycerol, promoting storage in fat vacuoles.

Thus, glucose is indispensable to normal adipocyte function and lipogenesis, both directly and indirectly through insulin stimulation. The active influx of glucose into adipocytes in the fed state leads to the generation of intra-adipocyte glycerol 3-phosphate. Glycerol originates from glucose or pyruvate, which means that adipocytes must have access to glucose in order to store fatty acids as TG. Glycerol is phosphorylated by glycerol kinase and is then acylated to fatty acid-CoA by glycerol-3-phosphate acyltransferase (GPAT), to form lysophosphatidic acid. Lysophosphatidic acid is acylated to another fatty acid-CoA by acylglycerophosphate acyltransferase (AGPAT), to form phosphatidic acid. Phosphatidic acid is dephosphorylated by phosphatidic acid phosphorylase (PAP) to form diacylglycerol and is then acylated to a final fatty acid-CoA by diacylglycerol acyltransferase (DGAT), to form triacylglycerol. By these mechanisms, glycerol is esterified to intra-adipocyte FFA, to form and store intra-adipocyte TG. Largely because of nutrient-induced increases in insulin levels which downregulate HSL and upregulate LPL, FFA are dramatically decreased (by ~70% or more) after meals. This helps create and "trap" circulating FFA into adipocytes.

In the fasting state plasma glucose levels decrease to normal. This causes cessation of beta-cell stimulation in the pancreatic islets of Langerhans, with a drop in insulin levels. The blood supply of adipose tissue in the fasting state provides lower levels of glucose and insulin compared to the fed state. With fasting insulin levels, adipocytes lack the stimulation of LPL or downregulation of HSL by insulin. Adipocytes may respond to catecholamine and atrial natriuretic peptide stimulation of HSL, which then promotes lipolysis in the fasting state. Growth hormone and cortisol contribute to lipolysis during prolonged physical activity. All of this leads to increased FFA release from adipocytes, increased circulating FFA, increased FFA available to the muscle for beta-oxidation (FFAs are a primary source of energy in the muscle), and increased FFA uptake in the liver (used for hepatic beta-oxidation, ketogenesis, lipogenesis, and gluconeogenesis).

12.2.2 Adiposopathy and Lipotoxicity

With the development of adiposopathy (as occurs with insufficient adipogenesis and impaired adipocyte function), there is inadequate storage of excessive FFA in adipose tissue. Excess FFAs are shunted to other body tissues, such as the liver, muscle, and pancreas. This leads to the deposition of FFAs in these tissues, leading to pathophysiological effects, often termed "lipotoxicity."

Lipotoxicity causes dysfunction of body organs. The dysfunction is induced by the adverse effects of excessive free fatty acids and their products (e.g., ceramides and diacylglycerols). Lipotoxicity causes hepatic and muscle insulin resistance, decreased insulin secretion from the pancreas leading to pancreatic endocrine insufficiency, and dysfunction of other body organs (the heart, vasculature, kidney, etc.). Lipotoxicity helps explain why patients with diabetes mellitus (DM) have increased circulating fasting and postprandial free fatty acid levels compared to those without it. Insulin therapy can rapidly reduce very high TG blood levels in patients with hyperglycemia and poorly controlled DM. Increasing LPL activity is a major mechanism of action by which fibrates and omega-3 fatty acids lower TG levels.

Excess carbohydrate ingestion also leads to the storage of lipids in the liver (hepatosteatosis). Conversely, decreased carbohydrate intake (especially decreased simple sugars or carbohydrates high in glycemic index) may reduce hepatosteatosis. Prolonged fasting (greater than 7 days) may markedly increase circulating FFA, increase hepatosteatosis, increase ketosis, potentially result in a transient rise in TG and total cholesterol (TC), and worsen insulin sensitivity (even as glucose blood levels are reduced).

Lipogenesis is not exclusive to adipose tissue. Although lipogenesis is often thought to be virtually absent in the muscle, the liver has the enzymes for it. If glycogen stores are replete, additional ingested carbohydrates are converted into glucose 6-phosphate, which then generates acetyl-CoA through the glycolytic process in hepatocytes. Acetyl-CoA is used by hepatocytes to form fatty acids that combine with glycerol to form hepatic TG (hepatic lipogenesis).

Increased FFA delivery to the liver increases hepatic secretion of TG-enriched VLDL. This is clinically manifested by elevated fasting TG levels. Once in the circulation, VLDL particles generated by the liver undergo enzymatic exchanges with other lipoprotein particles such as HDL and low-density lipoproteins (LDL), via cholesteryl ester transfer protein (CETP). The resulting TG-rich lipoprotein particles are subjected to various lipases. The HDL particles become smaller and are more apt to undergo metabolism and excretion by the kidney, resulting in low HDL cholesterol levels. When TG-rich LDL particles interact with lipases, they may also become smaller and denser. The VLDL particles may undergo further lipolysis, resulting in VLDL remnants, which are also atherogenic.

Thus, adiposopathy causes:

- Hypertriglyceridemia
- Low HDL cholesterol (HDL-C)
- Small, dense LDL cholesterol (LDL-C)
- VLDL remnants

These lipid changes from adiposopathy are distinct from other atherogenic dyslipidemias such as isolated severe hypercholesterolemia, which is often the result of genetic disorders.

12.2.3 Adiposopathy and Cardiovascular (CV) Risk

Irrespective of the CV risk conveyed by elevated LDL-C plasma levels, the dyslipidemia of adiposopathy predicts the majority of the increased risk of CV disease in patients with overweight or obesity. Each component of atherogenic dyslipidemia predicts CV disease, but low HDL-C is the best predictor. There is an inverse relationship between HDL-C levels and the incidence of CV disease. Even if LDL-C levels are lowered below 70 milligrams (mg)/deciliter (dL), low HDL-C conveys increased risk of CV disease. Therefore, HDL-C has an atheroprotective effect. HDL-C is responsible for reverse cholesterol transport—shuttling of cholesterol from peripheral tissue (including adipose tissue) to the liver. Cholesterol may then be excreted in the feces. In addition, HDL-C inhibits thrombosis, oxidation, and inflammation.

Hypertriglyceridemia independently predicts CV disease. Hypertriglyceridemia almost invariably accompanies a low HDL-C. The predictive power of hypertriglyceridemia for CV disease persists after adjusting for HDL-C levels. In a meta-analysis of 21 population-based prospective studies involving a total of 65,863 men and 11,089 women, an 89 mg/dL rise in plasma TG led to a 32% increase in coronary artery disease in men (relative risk or RR, 5 1.30; 95% confidence interval or CI, 1.25–1.35) and a 76% increase in women (RR, 51.69; 95% CI, 1.45–1.97). This increased risk was independent of TC, LDL-C, HDL-C, BMI, blood pressure, or diabetes. The goal of treatment is therefore to return TG levels to less than 150 mg/dL. Patients with high (200–499 mg/dL) or very high (≥500 mg/dL) TG levels should have the non-HDL-C calculated:

(non-HDL Cholesterol) = Total cholesterol – (HDL – cholesterol)

Both TC and HDL-C may be directly measured regardless of the fed state. Non-HDL-C assists in the risk stratification of these patients and includes all atherogenic particles, including LDL-C, intermediate-density lipoproteins, VLDL-C, VLDL remnants, chylomicron remnants, and lipoprotein (a) (Lp(a)). Non-HDL-C is also useful for patients with diabetes, and/or established arteriosclerotic CV disease.

For all patients, TG levels should be part of routine lipid screening, which requires a fasting lipid panel. Moderate elevations of the TG (≥150 mg/dL) may identify individuals with adiposopathy and insulin resistance. TG levels ≥200 mg/dL help identify individuals at substantially increased risk for CV disease.

Apo B is present in each potentially atherogenic particle. The apo B level in the circulation directly reflects the number of circulating atherogenic particles. As is the case with non-HDL-C, apo B does not require that a patient be fasting for it to be accurately measured. Apo B is useful to assess residual risk for CV disease once the LDL-C and non-HDL-C are treated to goal.

In 2001, the National Cholesterol Education Program, Adult Treatment Panel III, included high TG and low HDL-C as two of five elements defining the metabolic syndrome. High blood pressure, high blood sugar, and high waist circumference were the other three elements. When the international classification of diseases included a billing code for this cluster of CV risk factors, it was for "*dysmetabolic syndrome*." The inclusion of waist circumference strongly tied adipose tissue intra-abdominal mass to CV risk and adiposopathy as a key element. There have been refinements to the clustering of findings that make up dysmetabolic syndrome, to include insulin resistance and waist circumference thresholds for various populations. Indeed, insulin resistance is now known to precede the clinical onset of the dyslipidemia of adiposopathy.

In the broadest definition of lipid disorders, one may think of a high LDL-C as one category of dyslipidemia and of hypertriglyceridemia with a low HDL-C as a second category of dyslipidemia. Awareness of secondary causes for these two broad categories of dyslipidemia is important and can be addressed through the history, physical examination, and laboratory testing (Table 12.1). Elevated LDL-C has been the major target to modify the risk for CV disease. Thus, most guidelines have focused on intervention when the plasma levels of LDL-C are high. More recently, the non-HDL-C has become a treatment target as well, since it is strongly and directly linked to the risk for CV disease.

12.2.4 Adipocytokines and Dyslipidemia

The role of adipocytokines in lipid metabolism is still being defined. Leptin, produced by adipocytes, has both central and peripheral effects on lipids. Central administration of leptin in laboratory animals increases the resting metabolic rate,

Table 12.1 Secondary causes of dyslipidemia

Dyslipidemia phenotype	Secondary cause
Elevated LDL-C	Hypothyroidism Nephrotic syndrome Dysgammaglobulinemia Systemic lupus erythematosus Multiple myeloma Progestin treatment Anabolic steroid treatment Cholestatic diseases of the liver (due to abnormal lipoproteins) Protease inhibitors for the treatment of HIV infection
Hypertriglyceridemia and/or low HDL-C	Chronic renal failure Type 2 diabetes mellitus Adiposopathy, overweight, and obesity Excessive alcohol intake Hypothyroidism Antihypertensive medications Thiazide diuretics β-adrenergic blocking agents Corticosteroid therapy (or severe stress that increases endogenous corticosteroids) Orally administered estrogens including oral contraceptives Pregnancy Protease inhibitors for the treatment of HIV infection

results in lower TG content in tissues, and lowers circulating TG. On the other hand, the peripheral administration of leptin stimulates lipolysis of TG.

Adiponectin levels are reduced in obesity, insulin resistance, diabetes, and dyslipidemia. Adiponectin has anti-atherothrombotic effects, so the reduced levels in metabolic diseases contribute to vascular events in these patients. Adiponectin levels are inversely related to plasma TG and positively correlated with HDL-c levels in humans. The positive correlation between HDL-C and adiponectin levels is independent of BMI and insulin resistance. The mechanisms whereby a low HDL-C may lead to adiponectin deficiency, or conversely, adiponectin deficiency may lead to a low HDL-C, are not yet defined. However, in adiponectin-deficient mice, adiponectin administration improves glycemia and dyslipidemia. With adiponectin administration, there is increased lipid oxidation and reduced vascular thickening.

Resistin gene expression is suppressed by thiazolidinediones. Therefore, resistin plays a role in insulin resistance and obesity. Resistin levels are elevated in obesity in rodents, but human data are not congruent.

12.3 Bariatric Endocrinology and Dyslipidemia

In the National Health and Nutritional Examination Surveys, using the 1999–2002 database, there is a relationship between BMI and the prevalence of metabolic diseases. The classification of metabolic diseases is based on the following definitions: (1) DM = diagnosed and previously undiagnosed type 1 or type 2 DM; (2) hypertension = administration of antihypertensive medication or systolic blood pressure ≥ 140 millimeters of mercury (mmHg) or diastolic blood pressure ≥ 90 mmHg; and (3) dyslipidemia = any of the following: TC ≥ 240 mg/dL, TG ≥ 200 mg/dL, LDL-C ≥ 160 mg/dL, or HDL-C < 40 mg/dL. For patients with a BMI ≥ 40 kg/m^2, the incidences of dyslipidemia, hypertension, and DM were 62.5%, 44%, and 16.4%, respectively. Therefore, at a BMI ≥ 40 kg/m^2, 37.5% of patients do not have dyslipidemia, 56% of patients do not have hypertension, and 83.6% of patients do not have DM. Clearly, fat mass alone does not predict metabolic diseases.

The concept that adiposopathy has to develop for metabolic diseases to follow underscores the need to have a diagnostic paradigm that is not based on fat mass alone. For the bariatric endocrinologist, metabolic derangements are a reflection of adipose tissue dysfunction. Therefore, a primary goal of treatment is to reverse adiposopathy, which in turn translates into improvement in metabolic parameters. This incorporates all clinical tools available for the treatment of each metabolic disorder but also aggressively reducing fat mass with all available means.

In the 1940s, CV events were diagnosed and treated. There was no insight as to the causes of CV events. With the inception of the Framingham Heart Study in 1948 began the quest for identifying these causes. In 1957, high blood pressure and high plasma TC were highly correlated to CV events. In 1961, the term "risk factor" was introduced into the literature to focus attention on modifiable clinical conditions, which, when treated, might decrease the likelihood of a vascular event. In 1962, tobacco use was associated with CV disease. Over time, many additional risk factors for CV disease have been identified. Although some are not modifiable, where possible, treatment of these risk factors became the primary prevention of CV disease (Table 12.2). Preventing subsequent vascular events became the secondary prevention. The identification of CV risk is now aided by risks calculators that are offered by various organizations. This helps stratify the magnitude of CV risk.

Then the question became, what are risk factors for the risk factors of CV disease? How can we prevent CV risk factors to begin with? The medical community came up with new definitions which included insulin resistance, dysmetabolic syndrome, prediabetes, impaired fasting glucose, glucose intolerance, and prehypertension. Intervention here became the new norm, and it became the primary prevention of CV disease. Traditional risk factor modification became the secondary prevention, and preventing subsequent vascular events once one had occurred now became the tertiary prevention (Fig. 12.1). Thus, treating overweight or obesity, and modifying adiposopathy, become the primary prevention target for the bariatric endocrinologist. Prevention of overweight, obesity, and adiposopathy to begin with, shifts everything, making prevention of subsequent vascular events the quaternary prevention.

Terminology has changed over time. The pharmaceutical company Sanofi Aventis developed rimonabant for the treatment of obesity. Sanofi Aventis coined the term "cardiometabolic risk" to create a platform to launch and sell rimonabant for the treatment of obesity. The product never came to market because of reports of suicides in clinical trials. But the term remains and has become pervasive. Metabolic

Table 12.2 Cardiovascular risk factors

Nonmodifiable risk factors	Modifiable risk factors
Advancing age	Elevated total cholesterol
Family history of cardiovascular disease	Elevated LDL-C
Family history of dyslipidemia	Elevated small, dense LDL-C
Chronic kidney disease	Elevated low-density lipoprotein particle concentration
Male gender (vs. females before the menopause)	Elevated non-HDL-C
African ancestry	Elevated triglycerides
Asian ancestry	Elevated triglyceride-rich remnants
Poverty (a life full of stress, social isolation, anxiety, depression, and an inability to break out of poverty)	Low HDL-C
Apo E4 isoform	Elevated Apo B
History of pre-eclampsia or eclampsia	Elevated lipoprotein (a)
	Hyperglycemic states (prediabetes and diabetes)
	Hypertension/high salt intake
	Tobacco use
	Increased intra-abdominal fat
	Polycystic ovary syndrome
	Elevated clotting factors/hypercoagulable states
	Inflammatory milieu (i.e., C-reactive protein elevation)
	Elevated homocysteine levels
	Elevated uric acid
	Sedentary lifestyle/physical inactivity
	Excess alcohol ingestion
	Unhealthy meal plan
	Excess stress

Abbreviations: *HDL-C* high-density lipoprotein cholesterol, *LDL-C* low-density lipoprotein cholesterol, *Apo* apolipoprotein

risk develops from the accrual of fat mass and the development of adiposopathy. Vascular events come much later. Although popularized by some, and commercialized by many, the term "cardiometabolic" is best avoided.

12.4 Guidelines for the Management of Dyslipidemia

LDL levels are directly and linearly related to the risk of having a vascular event. The definition of an LDL-C threshold for starting lipid-lowering treatment, however, has shifted over time. In 1988, the first Adult Treatment Panel chose an LDL-C level of 160 mg/dL as a threshold for intervention. This was a value above which the

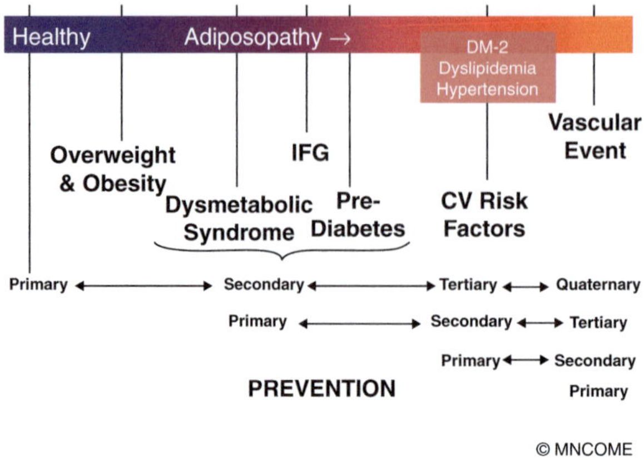

Fig. 12.1 *Development and prevention of cardiovascular disease.* Awaiting for a vascular event to happen makes prevention of any subsequent events the *primary prevention.* Interventions to modify known cardiovascular risk factors make prevention of any subsequent events *secondary prevention.* Interventions to modify the risk factors of the known cardiovascular risk factors make prevention of any subsequent events *tertiary prevention.* Early intervention to preserve a healthy lifestyle and prevent the development of overweight, obesity, and adiposopathy makes prevention of any subsequent events *quaternary prevention.* Abbreviations: IFG impaired fasting glucose, DM-2 type 2 diabetes mellitus, CV cardiovascular, MNCOME Minnesota Center for Obesity, Metabolism and Endocrinology, PA

risk of CV disease increased "steeply" given the data available at the time. This threshold also corresponded to "approximately the 75th percentile for the adult US population."

The American College of Cardiology (ACC) and the American Heart Association (AHA) published their recommendations in 2013. The work on these recommendations was started by the National Heart, Lung, and Blood Institute in 2008 and was then turned over to ACC–AHA. In these guidelines, there are four categories for starting treatment:

- Adults with atherosclerotic CV disease
- Adults with diabetes aged 40–75 years with LDL-C levels between 70 and 189 mg/dL
- Adults with LDL-C levels of 190 mg/dL or higher
- Adults aged 40–75 years of age who have LDL levels between 70 and 189 mg/dL and 7.5% or greater 10-year risk of atherosclerotic CV disease

There has been debate about the appropriate treatment targets for dyslipidemia. The methodology used by the ACC–AHA, and the questions asked, led to the conclusion of the committee that there was no scientific evidence to support specific treatment goals for either LDL-C or HDL-C. All trials of various statins available for review compared drug to placebo, and did not have a specific LDL treatment target. The committee recommended follow-up measurements of LDL-C solely for the assessment of adherence to treatment, comparing each patient to their baseline. No LDL targets were provided.

The ACC–AHA recommendations ran counter to those of other major organizations, including the American Association of Clinical Endocrinologists' (AACE) Guidelines for Management of Dyslipidemia and Prevention of Atherosclerosis (March and April 2012), the European Atherosclerosis Society consensus statement on treating familial hypercholesterolemia (August 2013), and the National Lipid Association Recommendations for Patient-Centered Management of Dyslipidemia (September 2014), all of which maintained specific LDL-C targets in the management of dyslipidemia.

Published data subsequent to the ACC-AHA review warranted the change, since new evidence does suggest that the lower the LDL-C, the lower the risk of vascular events. In IMPROVE-IT (IMProved Reduction of Outcomes: Vytorin Efficacy International Trial), published in 2015, among individuals with recent acute coronary syndrome, the addition of ezetimibe to moderate-intensity statin therapy reduced the incidence of CV mortality, major CV events, or nonfatal stroke, when compared to statin therapy alone. The inclusion criteria included an LDL-C ≥ 50 mg/dL, and the average baseline LDL-C was 94 mg/dL. At the 1-year observation point, the LDL-C was 69.9 mg/dL in the stain group and 53.2% in the statin plus ezetimibe group ($p < 0.001$).

JUPITER (Justification for the Use of Statins in Prevention: an Intervention Trial Evaluating Rosuvastatin) randomized nearly 18,000 patients with normal lipids and elevated highly sensitive C-reactive protein (HS-CRP) to treatment with either rosuvastatin or placebo. Patients were followed to their first CV event. Among patients with normal LDL-C, but elevated HS-CRP, rosuvastatin reduces the incidence of CV events. The LDL-C values, comparing drug versus placebo, at 12 months were 55 versus 110, at 24 months were 54 versus 108, at 36 months were 53 versus 106, and at 48 months were 55 versus 109 mg/dL, respectively.

Proprotein convertase subtilisin/kexin type 9 (PCSK9) inhibitors are the latest addition to the pharmacotherapy for dyslipidemia. Consistently, in their clinical trials, LDL-C levels already under treatment are driven further down. For example, in the FOURIER (Further Cardiovascular Outcomes Research with PCSK9 Inhibition in Subjects with Elevated Risk) trial, the LDL-C was reduced by 59% from a median of 92 to 30 mg/dL in the evolocumab group. This resulted in additional reductions in cardiovascular events compared to placebo.

The latest recommendations issued by the AACE put treatment targets back and are the most appropriate document to guide treatment of patients with overweight, obesity, and adiposopathy, given these new findings (Table 12.3).

12.5 Management of Dyslipidemia

The management of dyslipidemia in patients with overweight, obesity, and adiposopathy starts with lifestyle changes that include increased physical activity (increased caloric expenditure), decreased caloric intake (controlled portions with a high content of nondigestible carbohydrate), and modification of ingested fats. Table 12.4 reviews the effects of ingested fats on the lipid profile.

Table 12.3 ASCVD risk categories and cholesterol treatment goals

Risk category	Risk factors and 10-year risk	Treatment goals		
		LDL-C (mg/dL)	Non-HDL-C (mg/dL)	Apo B (mg/dL)
Extreme risk	Progressive ASCVD including unstable angina in patients after achieving an LDL-C < 70 mg/dL Established clinical ASCVD in patients with DM, CKD 3/4, or HeFH History of premature ASCVD (<55 males, <65 females)	<55	<80	<70
Very high risk	Established or recent hospitalization for ACS, coronary, carotid or peripheral vascular disease, 10-year risk >20% Diabetes or CKD 3/4 with 1 or more risk factor(s) HeFH	<70	<100	<80
High risk	≥2 risk factors and 10-year risk 10–20% Diabetes or CKD 3/4 with no other risk factors	<100	<130	<90
Moderate risk	≤2 risk factors and 10-year risk <10%	<100	<130	<90
Low risk	0 risk factors	<130	<160	Not recommended

Adapted from: Jellinger et al. (2017)
Abbreviations: *Apo* apolipoprotein, *ASCVD* atherosclerotic cardiovascular disease, *CKD* chronic kidney disease, *DM* diabetes mellitus, *HDL-C* high-density lipoprotein cholesterol, *HeFH* heterozygous familial hypercholesterolemia, *LDL-C* low-density lipoprotein cholesterol

It is best to avoid the terms "diet" and "exercise" in counseling patients. Each implies short-lived interventions. Rather, the emphasis should be on life-long, ongoing meal-planning, healthy eating, and good nutrition; and physical activity that is daily, realistic, achievable, sustainable, and incremental over time. The physical activity recommendations for weight management, which are also the ones for lipid management, are included in Chap. 20 of this textbook. A healthy lifestyle is paramount to reverse the metabolic changes of adiposopathy, including dyslipidemia.

12.5.1 Medical Nutrition Therapy

Chapter 19 in this textbook is dedicated to nutritional interventions for weight management and includes a section on nutritional management of lipid disorders. Patient education to achieve effective changes in the meal plan (nutritional intervention) should be implemented early on, and continued. It is best to approach medical nutrition therapy as a team, including registered dieticians in the practice.

Table 12.4 Effect of fat ingestion on serum lipids

Ingested fat	TC	LDL-C	HDL -C	TG	Food Sources
Trans fat	Raises	Raises	Lowers	Raises	Pre-packaged foods Processed foods
Saturated fat	Raises	Raises	Lowers	Raises	Animal fats Cocoa butter (chocolate) Coconut oil Palm oil Hydrogenated vegetable oil
Polyunsaturated fat	Lowers	Lowers	Lowers	Lowers	Safflower oil Corn oil Soyben oil Cottonseed oil Sesame oil Walnuts Flax seed Fish
Monounsaturated fat	Lowers	Lowers	Maintains or Raises	Lowers	Olive oil Peanut oil Canola oil Avocados Nuts Seeds
Omega-3 fatty acids	Lowers	Neutral	Neutral or Raises	Lowers	Fish Oysters

Abbreviations: *TC* Total cholesterol, *LDL* low-density lipoprotein cholesterol, *HDL* high-density lipoprotein cholesterol, *TG* triglycerides
Colors: Bright red = very harmful, bright green = very beneficial, light green = beneficial, light red = harmful

And it is very important to include the family members of the patient in the process of modifying the meal plan.

12.5.2 Pharmacotherapy

The literature on pharmacotherapy for dyslipidemia is vast. It is beyond the scope of this chapter to address all aspects of clinical use of each class of agents. Table 12.5 provides a summary of the lipid-lowering medication classes, their major mechanism of action, and the effects on the lipid profile. The sections below provide an overview of most of these medications. A discussion of pharmacotherapy in patients with concomitant diseases, such as DM, renal failure, or cirrhosis, is not included in the summary below. It is of note that the vast majority of the literature on pharmacotherapy for lipid disorders does not address adiposopathy, overweight, or obesity, other than a tacit acknowledgment of weight gain as a CV risk factor.

Table 12.5 Lipid-lowering medications

Medication class	MOA	LDL-C	TG	HDL-C	Other
Statins (HMGCR inhibitors)	↓ Hepatic cholesterol synthesis (But ↑ intestinal absorption of cholesterol)	↓↓	↓	↑	↓ apo B
Intestinal cholesterol transporter inhibitors	↓ Cholesterol absorption from the intestine (But ↑ cholesterol synthesis in the liver)	↓	↓	↑	↓ apo B
PCSK9 inhibitors	Prevents LDL-C receptor degradation on hepatocytes ↑ LDL-C receptors on hepatocytes	↓↓	↓	↑	↓ Lp(a)
Apo B inhibitors	↓ Formation of apoB-containing lipoproteins	↓↓	↓	↑ or ↔	↓ Lp(a) ↓ apo B
MTTP inhibitors	Inhibit TG transfer to apo B-48 or apo B-100 in intestinal and liver cells, respectively ↓ formation of chylomicrons and VLDL VLDL inhibition leads to LDL inhibition	↓↓	↓↓	↓	↓ apo B
Bile acid sequestrants	↓ Bile acid absorption ↑ Hepatic conversion of cholesterol to bile acids ↑ LDL-C receptors on hepatocytes	↓	↑ or ↔	↑	Improve Glycemia
Fibrates (PPAR α activators)	↑ Activity of lipoprotein lipase ↑ VLDL-C metabolism ↑ Oxidation of FFA in the muscle and adipose tissue ↓ TG synthesis in liver	↓ or ↑	↓↓	↑	↓ apo B
Nicotinic acid (niacin)	↓ Production of VLDL-C ↓ Lipolysis in adipocytes	↑ or ↔	↓↓	↑↑	↓ apo B
Omega-3 fatty acids		↑ or ↔	↓↓	↑ or ↔	↓ apo B

Abbreviations: *apo* apolipoprotein, *FFA* free fatty acids, *HDL-C* high-density lipoprotein cholesterol, *HMGCR* 3-hydroxy-3-methyl-glutaryl-coenzyme A reductase, *LDL-C* low-density lipoprotein cholesterol, *Lp(a)* lipoprotein (a), *MOA* mechanism of action, *PCSK9* proprotein convertase subtilisin/kexin type 9, *PPAR* peroxisome proliferator-activated receptor, *MTTP* microsomal triglyceride transfer protein, *TG* triglycerides, *VLDL-C* very low-density lipoprotein cholesterol

12.5.2.1 Statins

3-Hydroxy-3-methyl-glutaryl-coenzyme A (HMG-CoA) reductase ((HMGCR) is the rate-controlling enzyme which catalyzes the conversion of HMG-CoA to mevalonic acid. This is a necessary step in the synthesis of cholesterol and other isoprenoids. HMGCR inhibitors therefore significantly lower the rate of production of cholesterol. These medications are known as "*statins*." Statins that are approved for use in the USA are discussed in this section.

There are overwhelming data from randomized clinical trials that statins lower the LDL-C and the risk of CV events, compared to placebo. This holds true for both primary and secondary prevention of CV events. In May 2016, the Food and Drug Administration (FDA) approved a generic preparation of rosuvastatin, making it the last patented medication to go generic in this drug category in the United States. Statins are now all generic medications. Because they are safe, effective, and cost effective, statins are the first line of pharmacotherapy for the treatment of dyslipidemia.

Statins are indicated for the treatment of primary hypercholesterolemia, mixed dyslipidemia, and familial hypercholesterolemia. In patients with dyslipidemia but without clinical evidence of vascular disease, they are indicated for the primary prevention of myocardial infarction, to decrease the risk of myocardial revascularization procedures, and to decrease the risk of cardiovascular death. In patients with established cardiovascular disease, statins are indicated for secondary prevention, to decrease the risk of coronary death, myocardial infarction, myocardial revascularization procedures, stroke, transient ischemic attacks, and the progression of CV disease.

Statin therapy may be refined in terms of intensity of treatment. When an LDL-C reduction of over 50% is needed, high doses of atorvastatin or rosuvastatin are needed. Medium (LDL-C reduction of 30–50%) and low (LDL-C reduction of <30%) intensity doses of various statins broaden the therapeutic options (Table 12.6).

Statins are contraindicated in pregnancy and lactation, and with the concomitant administration of potent cytochrome (CY)-P3A4 inhibitors (itraconazole, ketoconazole, protease inhibitors, erythromycin, clarithromycin, telithromycin, and nefazodone) or CY-P2C9 inhibitors (relative contraindication, not dependent on CY-P450 statin metabolism).

Statins are relatively contraindicated in patients older than 70 years, with stages 4 and 5 kidney failure, uncontrolled hypothyroidism, a personal or family history of muscular disorders, a personal history of muscular toxicity with a statin or fibrate, and active alcoholism.

Statins are well tolerated, and the dropout rate in clinical trials as a result of any adverse event was <10%. The statin dropout rates were similar to those of patients taking placebo. Less than 1% were serious adverse events. Skeletal muscle toxicity, hepatotoxicity, hypersensitivity reactions to any statin or the excipients, dyspepsia, sleep disturbance, memory loss, and mood changes are the most common adverse events associated with statin use.

The incidence of muscular adverse events in 180,000 patients who were included in 21 major statin trials, with an average duration of 3 years, was 1.5–3% for

Table 12.6 Statin dosing

Statin	Statin dose (mg)	LDL-C reduction <30% (Low intensity)	30%–50% (Moderate intensity)	>50% (High intensity)
Atorvastatin (Lipitor®)	10		√	
	20		√	
	40			√
	80			√
Fluvastatin (Lescol®)	20	√		
	40	√		
Lovastatin (Mevacor®) (Altocor®, Altoprev®)	20	√		
	40	√		
	40 BID		√	
	XL 80		√	
Pitavastatin (Livalo®)	1	√		
	2		√	
	4		√	
Pravastatin (Pravachol®)	10	√		
	20	√		
	40		√	
	80		√	
Rosuvastatin (Crestor®)	5		√	
	10		√	
	20			√
	40			√
Simvastatin (Zocor®)	10	√		
	20		√	
	40		√	
	80			√[a]

Abbreviations: *BID* twice daily, *mg* milligram, *NA* not applicable, *LDL-C* low-density lipoprotein cholesterol, *XL* extended release

[a]The 80-mg dose of simvastatin should be restricted to patients who have been taking simvastatin 80 mg chronically (e.g., for 12 months or more) without evidence of muscle toxicity. Patients on lower doses of simvastatin should not be titrated to the 80-mg dose

myalgia, 5/100,000 for myopathy with documented creatine kinase elevation, and 1.6/100,000 for rhabdomyolysis. Most of these events occur within the first 3 months of statin therapy. High-dose statin therapy increases the prevalence of muscle complaints to 5.1–18.2% depending on the statin used. Simvastatin high-dose therapy (40–80 mg per day) had the highest prevalence of muscle complaints, so this high dose is to be used with caution, if at all.

In February 2012, the FDA issued a consumer update on statins:

- It acknowledged the possibility of muscular adverse events.
- The FDA recommended that liver enzyme testing be done at the onset of statin therapy, and if symptoms of liver damage develop. Regular monitoring of liver function is no longer recommended for statin therapy.

- New-onset diabetes is associated with statin use, is dose related and is less common with pravastatin and pitavastatin. Patients on statin therapy should have periodic reassessment of their glycemic status. The clinical benefits of statin use are such that their use should be continued, and the hyperglycemia should be addressed as a separate issue.

Statins have effects on adipose tissue:

- They upregulate HSL expression, which enhances lipolysis and decreases lipid accumulation. This in turn prevents adipocyte hypertrophy.
- Intensive statin therapy causes regression of the epicardial fat pad.
- They increase LPL activity, contributing to reductions of VLDL-C and TG.
- They decrease the secretion of inflammatory cytokines from adipose tissue.
- They inhibit leptin expression.
- They improve insulin sensitivity with no changes in body weight or adipose tissue mass.
- They inhibit adipogenesis.

12.5.2.2 Intestinal Cholesterol Transporter Inhibitors

Sterol transporter Niemann-Pick C1-Like 1 (NPC1L1) is involved in the intestinal uptake of cholesterol and phytosterols. Ezetimibe (Zetia®), which is the only agent in this drug category, became available for generic use in the USA as of 2017, and blocks this transporter, reducing the absorption of fat from ingested meals.

Ezetimibe has beneficial effects on all lipid parameters and is synergistic with statins. It is indicated for the reduction of elevated TC, LDL-C, apo B, and non-HDL-C:

- As monotherapy or in combination with a statin in patients with primary (heterozygous familial and nonfamilial) hyperlipidemia
- In combination with fenofibrate in patients with mixed hyperlipidemia

Ezetimibe is also indicated:

- In combination with a statin to lower TC and LDL-C in patients with homozygous FH, as an adjunct to other lipid-lowering treatments (e.g., LDL apheresis), or if such treatments are unavailable
- As monotherapy to lower elevated sitosterol and campesterol levels in patients with homozygous familial sitosterolemia

Ezetimibe is contraindicated in combination with a statin in patients with active liver disease or unexplained, persistent liver enzyme elevations, or known hypersensitivity to the drugs. It is contraindicated for use in nursing mothers or women who are pregnant or may become pregnant.

The incidence of adverse events for ezetimibe was similar to placebo in clinical trials. When used with a statin, it may cause liver enzyme elevation.

12.5.2.3 PCSK9 Inhibitors

PCSK9 binds the LDL-C receptor, resulting in its degradation and leading to a reduction in LDL-C receptor activity. Individuals who have loss of function mutations of the gene encoding for PCSK9 get a phenotype of low LDL-C and a reduction in CV risk. PCSK9 inhibitors are monoclonal antibodies directed against PCSK9. They are available for subcutaneous injection every 2–4 weeks. The loss of PCSK9 activity results in higher LDL-C receptor activity, which reduces LDL-C levels in the circulation within days.

There are two PCSK9 inhibitors in the market as of 2017, and others under development. Alirocumab (Praluent®—Sanofi) and evolocumab (Repatha®—Amgen) entered clinical trials in 2009 for a wide variety of lipid disorders and on a variety of background therapies. In addition to lowering the LDL-C, they raise the HDL-C and lower the TG. An additional effect has been a consistent reduction in LP(a) of 25–30%.

PCSK9 inhibitors are approved for use in adults with heterozygous familial hypercholesterolemia (FH), or clinical atherosclerotic CV disease, not treated to goal on maximally tolerated statin therapy. Evolocumab is approved for homozygous FH patients ages 13 or older.

Three-year data with PCSK9 inhibitors show that they are safe. A few injection site reactions have been reported, but like other injectable proteins, there are no issues with the subcutaneous delivery. No serious adverse events have been reported in the more than 40,000 patients who have been treated with PCSK9 inhibitors. The manufacturers and FDA regulators had concerns about the patients who achieved very low LDL-C levels (<25 or <15 mg/dL), but there are no differences in adverse events compared to those with higher LDL-C, or those treated with placebo or standard of care.

12.5.2.4 Apo-B Synthesis Inhibitors

Mipomersen (Kynamro®) is an oligonucleotide inhibitor of apo B-100 synthesis. Apo B is the principal apolipoprotein of LDL and its metabolic precursor, VLDL. Mipomersen crosses the hepatocyte and nuclear membranes, and in the nucleus, it inhibits the synthesis of apo-B by sequence-specific binding to its messenger ribonucleic acid (mRNA). Sequence-specific binding to apo-B mRNA results in the degradation of the mRNA through enzyme-mediated pathways, or disruption of mRNA function through binding alone.

Mipomersen thus prevents translation to form apo-B, decreased formation of apo B-containing lipoproteins, including LDL-C (40–50% reduction). Mipomersen also decreases Lp(a) concentrations.

Mipomersen is approved by the FDA only as an orphan drug and is indicated as an adjunct to lipid-lowering medications to reduce LDL-C, apo B, TC, and non HDL-C in patients with homozygous FH. Mipomersen minimizes the need for apheresis in these patients.

Mipomersen is contraindicated in patients with moderate or severe hepatic impairment (Child–Pugh category B or C), as well as in patients with active liver disease or persistent elevated serum transaminase levels.

Side effects of mipomersen include injection site reactions in 88.5% of patients, influenza-like symptoms in half the patients, and nausea in 11% of patients. Hepatic steatosis with elevated liver enzymes was documented in up to a third of the patients. The FDA has restricted mipomersen and made it available only through a risk evaluation and mitigation strategy (REMS). Prescribers and pharmacies need additional certification to prescribe and dispense the medication.

12.5.2.5 Microsomal Triglyceride Transfer Protein (MTTP) Inhibitors

MTTP catalyzes the transport of triglyceride, cholesterol ester, and phospholipid across phospholipid surfaces. Lomitapide (Juxtapid®) directly binds and inhibits MTTP, which resides in the lumen of the endoplasmic reticulum. By doing so, lomitapide inhibits TG transfer to apo B-48 or apo B-100 in intestinal and liver cells, respectively, which decrease the formation of chylomicrons and VLDL. The inhibition of the synthesis of VLDL leads to reduced levels of plasma LDL-C and other apo B-containing lipoproteins.

Lomitapide is indicated as an adjunct to other lipid-lowering treatments, including LDL apheresis where available, to reduce LDL-C, TC, apo B, and non-HDL-C in patients with homozygous FH. Lomitapide dosing needs to be titrated up. The initial dose is 5 mg once daily. The dose is then titrated up based on acceptable safety and tolerability to 10 mg daily after at least 2 weeks. Further titrations up on the dose are then done at a minimum of 4-week intervals, to 20 mg, 40 mg, and up to the maximum recommended dose of 60 mg daily.

The safety and effectiveness of lomitapide have not been established in patients with hypercholesterolemia who do not have homozygous FH. The effect of lomitapide on cardiovascular morbidity and mortality has not been determined.

In clinical trials, lomitapide caused increased stool frequency, hepatic steatosis, and serum transaminase levels. Because of the risk of hepatotoxicity, lomitapide is available only through the Juxtapid REMS Program. Before treatment, measurements of liver enzymes, alkaline phosphatase, and total bilirubin need to be documented. A negative pregnancy test needs to be done for all females of reproductive potential. Also, before treatment, a low-fat meal plan supplying <20% of energy from fat must be implemented. Due to reduced absorption of fat-soluble vitamins and fatty acids, daily vitamin E, linoleic acid, alpha-linolenic acid, eicosapentaenoic acid, and docosahexaenoic acid supplements should be dosed.

12.5.2.6 Bile Acid Sequestrants

Bile acid sequestrants available for use in the USA include cholestyramine (Questran®, Prevalite®), colestipol (Colestid®, Flavored Colestid®), and colesevelam (Welchol®). They are indicated to lower the TC and LDL-C.

Bile acid sequestrants bind bile acids in the intestine and increase the excretion of bile acids in the stool. This reduces the amount of bile acids returning to the liver. The liver is then forced to produce more bile acids to replace the bile acids lost in the stool. In order to produce more bile acids, the liver converts more cholesterol into bile acids, which lowers the level of cholesterol in the blood.

Bile acid sequestrants achieve modest reductions in LDL-C. Low doses (e.g., 8 gram/day of cholestyramine) can lower LDL cholesterol by 10%–15%. But, even high doses (24 gram/day of cholestyramine) can only lower LDL cholesterol by 25%. Therefore, bile acid sequestrants used alone are not as effective as statins in lowering LDL cholesterol. Bile acid sequestrants are most useful in combination with a statin or niacin. The combination of a statin and bile acid sequestrant can lower LDL-C levels by approximately 50%. The combination of a statin and niacin can reduce LDL-C and elevate HDL-C.

Bile acid sequestrants are not absorbed from the intestinal tract. Their pharmacological effect is all intraenteric. Bile acid sequestrants do not have systemic side effects, and their most common side effects are gastrointestinal.

Bile acid sequestrants can bind to and decrease the absorption (and hence the effectiveness) of other drugs. Warfarin, thyroid hormones, digoxin, and thiazide diuretics, among others, will have decreased absorption if they are co-administered with bile acid sequestrants. It is best if all medications are taken 1 h before or 4–6 h after the administration of a bile acid sequestrant. Bile acid sequestrants reduce the absorption of vitamins A, D, E, and K. Long-term use may thus cause a deficiency of these vitamins.

A beneficial effect of bile acid sequestrants is that they improve glycemia in patients with type 2 DM. Colesevelam now has an indication for the treatment of type 2 DM.

12.5.2.7 Fibrates

Fibric acid derivatives, also known as fibrates, include fenofibrate (Fenoglide®, Lofibra®, Lipofen®, Tricor®, Antara®, Triglide®), gemfibrozil (Lopid®), and fenofibric acid (Trilipix®, Fibricor®). Many of these preparations are generic and affordable.

Fibrates have as their main pharmacological effect a reduction of plasma TG-rich lipoproteins. In patients with elevated LDL-C at the onset of treatment, fibrates generally lower LDL-C by 20–25%. An exception to this is gemfibrozil, which increases LDL-C by 10–15%.

Fibrates are all indicated for treatment of severe hypertriglyceridemia (TG $\geq$ 1000 mg/dL). Fenofibrate and fenofibric acid are indicated to treat dyslipidemia (to decrease TC, LDL-C, triglycerides, and apo B; and to increase HDL-C). Gemfibrozil is the only agent in this class that is indicated for the primary prevention of coronary artery disease, for patients with low HDL-C and high LDL-C and TG.

An additional clinical use for fenofibrate is to lower uric acid levels in patients with gout (off-label use). Therefore, fenofibrate should be included in the treatment of hypertriglyceridemia when patients also have hyperuricemia.

Fibrates are contraindicated in patients with stages 4 and 5 kidney failure, active liver disease, pre-existing gallbladder disease, and known hypersensitivity to the drugs. They should be held for pregnancy and lactation.

Fibrates are well tolerated, and in clinical trials, adverse events were similar to placebo. Gemfibrozil may cause gastrointestinal symptoms in up to 34% of patients when first started. Elevated hepatic transaminases occur in up to 7.5% of patients in those treated with fenofibrate, which return to normal with discontinuation of the drug. Baseline and periodic liver enzyme monitoring is recommended for patients on fenofibrate.

Gemfibrozil is a CY-P2C8 inhibitor and strongly increases the blood levels of its substrates. Among the substrates of CY-P2C8 are the statins, the thiazolidinediones, and repaglinide. Therefore, the risk of muscle toxicity is increased with concomitant use of gemfibrozil and statins. This is not so for fenofibrate or fenofibric acid. Gemfibrozil is best avoided when patients are being treated with any statin.

12.5.3 Other Treatment Options

Medications for weight loss, including pancreatic lipase inhibitors like orlistat, each have a positive impact on the lipid profile. Other interventions for weight loss, leading up to the various bariatric surgeries, all have a positive impact on the lipid profile too. The magnitude of weight loss is the major determinant, and the lipid parameter that most consistently improves is the plasma TG. Modification of secondary causes of hypercholesterolemia, including hyperglycemia, hypercortisolism, and hypothyroidism, improves the lipid profile. Lipoprotein apheresis and partial ileal bypass are interventions reserved for individuals with extreme elevations of the LDL-C. These are subspecialty interventions that require the expertise of a medical center with the resources to make them available.

12.6 Conclusion

Adiposopathy may develop with the accrual of adipose tissue mass. BMI alone is not a good predictor of the emergence of metabolic disorders in association with adiposopathy. Laboratory testing is necessary to identify individuals with dyslipidemia. Atherogenic dyslipidemia is a strong risk factor for premature CV disease. It is imperative to intervene early and to continue the interventions over time. In addition to healthy lifestyle changes, medical nutrition interventions, physical activity counseling, and education to create awareness of risk, there are many treatment options to help patients lose weight. Aggressive management of overweight and obesity are the standard of care now. Beyond this, pharmacotherapy for correction of dyslipidemia is appropriate for most patients. It is now clear that the lower the LDL-C, the lower the risk of CV events. Non-HDL-C and apo-B are now also treatment targets for the prevention of CV disease, since there is residual risk (after LDL-C reductions) that is reflected by these numbers.

Reading list

Abdel-Maksoud MF, Hokanson JE. The complex role of triglycerides in cardiovascular disease. Semin Vasc Med. 2002;2(3):325–33. Epub 2005/10/14.

Adhyaru BB, Jacobson TA. New cholesterol guidelines for the management of atherosclerotic cardiovascular disease risk: a comparison of the 2013 American College of Cardiology/American Heart Association cholesterol guidelines with the 2014 National Lipid Association recommendations for patient-centered management of dyslipidemia. Endocrinol Metab Clin N Am. 2016;45(1):17–37. Epub 2016/02/20.

Aguiar C, Alegria E, Bonadonna RC, Catapano AL, Cosentino F, Elisaf M, et al. A review of the evidence on reducing macrovascular risk in patients with atherogenic dyslipidaemia: a report from an expert consensus meeting on the role of fenofibrate-statin combination therapy. Atheroscler Suppl. 2015;19:1–12. Epub 2015/09/01.

Backes JM, Kostoff MD, Gibson CA, Ruisinger JF. Statin-associated diabetes mellitus: review and clinical guide. South Med J. 2016;109(3):167–73. Epub 2016/03/10.

Bays HE. Adiposopathy is "sick fat" a cardiovascular disease? J Am Coll Cardiol. 2011;57(25):2461–73. Epub 2011/06/18.

Bays H, Rodbard HW, Schorr AB, Gonzalez-Campoy JM. Adiposopathy: treating pathogenic adipose tissue to reduce cardiovascular disease risk. Curr Treat Options Cardiovasc Med. 2007;9(4):259–71. Epub 2007/09/01.

Bays HE, Gonzalez-Campoy JM, Bray GA, Kitabchi AE, Bergman DA, Schorr AB, et al. Pathogenic potential of adipose tissue and metabolic consequences of adipocyte hypertrophy and increased visceral adiposity. Expert Rev Cardiovasc Ther. 2008a;6(3):343–68. Epub 2008/03/11.

Bays HE, Gonzalez-Campoy JM, Henry RR, Bergman DA, Kitabchi AE, Schorr AB, et al. Is adiposopathy (sick fat) an endocrine disease? Int J Clin Pract. 2008b;62(10):1474–83. Epub 2008/08/07.

Bays HE, Toth PP, Kris-Etherton PM, Abate N, Aronne LJ, Brown WV, et al. Obesity, adiposity, and dyslipidemia: a consensus statement from the National Lipid Association. J Clin Lipidol. 2013;7(4):304–83. Epub 2013/07/31.

Cannon CP, Blazing MA, Giugliano RP, McCagg A, White JA, Theroux P, et al. Ezetimibe added to statin therapy after acute coronary syndromes. N Engl J Med. 2015;372(25):2387–97. Epub 2015/06/04.

Chrusciel P, Sahebkar A, Rembek-Wieliczko M, Serban MC, Ursoniu S, Mikhailidis DP, et al. Impact of statin therapy on plasma adiponectin concentrations: a systematic review and meta-analysis of 43 randomized controlled trial arms. Atherosclerosis. 2016;253:194–208. Epub 2016/08/09.

Cleeman JI, Lenfant C. New guidelines for the treatment of high blood cholesterol in adults from the National Cholesterol Education Program. From controversy to consensus. Circulation. 1987;76(4):960–2. Epub 1987/10/01.

De Vera MA, Bhole V, Burns LC, Lacaille D. Impact of statin adherence on cardiovascular disease and mortality outcomes: a systematic review. Br J Clin Pharmacol. 2014;78(4):684–98. Epub 2014/11/05.

Dullaart RP. PCSK9 inhibition to reduce cardiovascular events. N Engl J Med. 2017;376:1790. Epub 2017/03/18.

Endo A. A historical perspective on the discovery of statins. Proc Jpn Acad Ser B Phys Biol Sci. 2010;86(5):484–93. Epub 2010/05/15.

Expert Panel on Detection E, Treatment of High Blood Cholesterol in A. Executive summary of the third report of the National Cholesterol Education Program (NCEP) expert panel on detection, evaluation, and treatment of high blood cholesterol in adults (adult treatment panel III). JAMA. 2001;285(19):2486–97. Epub 2001/05/23.

Farr S, Taher J, Adeli K. Glucagon-like peptide-1 as a key regulator of lipid and lipoprotein metabolism in fasting and postprandial states. Cardiovasc Hematol Disord Drug Targets. 2014;14(2):126–36. Epub 2014/05/08.

Fonseca VA, Handelsman Y, Staels B. Colesevelam lowers glucose and lipid levels in type 2 diabetes: the clinical evidence. Diabetes Obes Metab. 2010;12(5):384–92. Epub 2010/04/27.
Franssen R, Monajemi H, Stroes ES, Kastelein JJ. Obesity and dyslipidemia. Med Clin North Am. 2011;95(5):893–902. Epub 2011/08/23.
Geer EB, Islam J, Buettner C. Mechanisms of glucocorticoid-induced insulin resistance: focus on adipose tissue function and lipid metabolism. Endocrinol Metab Clin N Am. 2014;43(1):75–102. Epub 2014/03/04.
Gonzalez-Campoy JM, St Jeor ST, Castorino K, Ebrahim A, Hurley D, Jovanovic L, et al. Clinical practice guidelines for healthy eating for the prevention and treatment of metabolic and endocrine diseases in adults: cosponsored by the American Association of Clinical Endocrinologists/the American College of Endocrinology and the Obesity Society. Endocr Pract. 2013;19(0):1–82. Epub 2013/10/17.
Gonzalez-Campoy JM, Richardson B, Richardson C, Gonzalez-Cameron D, Ebrahim A, Strobel P, et al. Bariatric endocrinology: principles of medical practice. Int J Endocrinol. 2014;2014:917813. Epub 2014/06/06.
Goodman DS, Hulley SB, Clark LT, Davis CE, Fuster V, JC LR, et al. Report of the National Cholesterol Education Program Expert Panel on detection, evaluation, and treatment of high blood cholesterol in adults. The expert panel. Arch Intern Med. 1988;148(1):36–69. Epub 1988/01/01.
Grundy SM, Bilheimer D, Chait A, Clark LT, Denke M, Havel RJ, et al. Summary of the second report of the National Cholesterol Education Program (NCEP) Expert Panel on detection, evaluation, and treatment of high blood cholesterol in adults (Adult Treatment Panel II). JAMA. 1993;269(23):3015–23. Epub 1993/06/16.
Gulati M, Merz CN. New cholesterol guidelines and primary prevention in women. Trends Cardiovasc Med. 2015;25(2):84–94. Epub 2014/12/03.
Jacobson TA, Ito MK, Maki KC, Orringer CE, Bays HE, Jones PH, et al. National Lipid Association recommendations for patient-centered management of dyslipidemia: part 1—executive summary. J Clin Lipidol. 2014;8(5):473–88. Epub 2014/09/23.
Jacobson TA, Ito MK, Maki KC, Orringer CE, Bays HE, Jones PH, et al. National lipid association recommendations for patient-centered management of dyslipidemia: part 1—full report. J Clin Lipidol. 2015a;9(2):129–69. Epub 2015/04/26.
Jacobson TA, Maki KC, Orringer CE, Jones PH, Kris-Etherton P, Sikand G, et al. National Lipid Association recommendations for patient-centered management of dyslipidemia: part 2. J Clin Lipidol. 2015b;9(6 Suppl):S1–122 e1. Epub 2015/12/25.
Jellinger PS, Smith DA, Mehta AE, Ganda O, Handelsman Y, Rodbard HW, et al. American Association of Clinical Endocrinologists' guidelines for management of dyslipidemia and prevention of atherosclerosis. Endocr Pract. 2012;18(Suppl 1):1–78. Epub 2012/04/24.
Jellinger PS, Handelsman Y, Rosenblit PD, Bloomgarden ZT, Fonseca VA, Garber AJ, et al. American Association of Clinical Endocrinologists and American College of Endocrinology guidelines for management of dyslipidemia and prevention of cardiovascular disease. Endocr Pract. 2017;23(Suppl 2):1–87. Epub 2017/04/25.
Leusink M, Onland-Moret NC, de Bakker PI, de Boer A, Maitland-van der Zee AH. Seventeen years of statin pharmacogenetics: a systematic review. Pharmacogenomics. 2016;17(2):163–80. Epub 2015/12/17.
McGettigan P, Ferner RE. PCSK9 inhibitors for hypercholesterolaemia. BMJ. 2017;356:j188. Epub 2017/01/21.
Mells JE, Anania FA. The role of gastrointestinal hormones in hepatic lipid metabolism. Semin Liver Dis. 2013;33(4):343–57. Epub 2013/11/14.
Nordestgaard BG, Chapman MJ, Humphries SE, Ginsberg HN, Masana L, Descamps OS, et al. Familial hypercholesterolaemia is underdiagnosed and undertreated in the general population: guidance for clinicians to prevent coronary heart disease: consensus statement of the European Atherosclerosis Society. Eur Heart J. 2013;34(45):3478–90a. Epub 2013/08/21.
Orringer CE, Jacobson TA, Saseen JJ, Brown AS, Gotto AM, Ross JL, et al. Update on the use of PCSK9 inhibitors in adults: recommendations from an expert panel of the National Lipid Association. J Clin Lipidol. 2017;11(4):880–90. Epub 2017/05/24.

Ouwens MJ, Nauta J, Ansquer JC, Driessen S. Systematic literature review and meta-analysis of dual therapy with fenofibrate or fenofibric acid and a statin versus a double or equivalent dose of statin monotherapy. Curr Med Res Opin. 2015;31(12):2273–85. Epub 2015/09/24.

Peng W, Qiang F, Peng W, Qian Z, Ke Z, Yi L, et al. Therapeutic efficacy of PCSK9 monoclonal antibodies in statin-nonresponsive patients with hypercholesterolemia and dyslipidemia: a systematic review and meta-analysis. Int J Cardiol. 2016;222:119–29. Epub 2016/08/06.

Ridker PM, Danielson E, Fonseca FA, Genest J, Gotto AM Jr, Kastelein JJ, et al. Rosuvastatin to prevent vascular events in men and women with elevated C-reactive protein. N Engl J Med. 2008;359(21):2195–207. Epub 2008/11/11.

Sabatine MS, Giugliano RP, Keech AC, Honarpour N, Wiviott SD, Murphy SA, et al. Evolocumab and clinical outcomes in patients with cardiovascular disease. N Engl J Med. 2017;376(18):1713–22. Epub 2017/03/18.

Sahebkar A, Catena C, Ray KK, Vallejo-Vaz AJ, Reiner Z, Sechi LA, et al. Impact of statin therapy on plasma levels of plasminogen activator inhibitor-1. A systematic review and meta-analysis of randomised controlled trials. Thromb Haemost. 2016a;116(1):162–71. Epub 2016/03/25.

Sahebkar A, Giua R, Pedone C. Impact of statin therapy on plasma leptin concentrations: a systematic review and meta-analysis of randomized placebo-controlled trials. Br J Clin Pharmacol. 2016b;82(6):1674–84. Epub 2016/08/12.

Sahebkar A, Simental-Mendia LE, Pedone C, Ferretti G, Nachtigal P, Bo S, et al. Statin therapy and plasma free fatty acids: a systematic review and meta-analysis of controlled clinical trials. Br J Clin Pharmacol. 2016c;81(5):807–18. Epub 2015/12/02.

Sattar N. Lipid metabolism. Curr Opin Lipidol. 2013;24(1):101–2. Epub 2013/01/10.

Saxon DR, Eckel RH. Statin intolerance: a literature review and management strategies. Prog Cardiovasc Dis. 2016;59(2):153–64. Epub 2016/08/09.

Shapiro MD, Fazio S. PCSK9 and atherosclerosis—lipids and beyond. J Atheroscler Thromb. 2017;24:462. Epub 2017/03/18.

Shrank WH, Barlow JF, Brennan TA. New therapies in the treatment of high cholesterol: an argument to return to goal-based lipid guidelines. JAMA. 2015;314(14):1443–4. Epub 2015/08/11.

Smith TK, Reynolds TB, Denny PW. Lipid metabolism as a therapeutic target. Biochem Res Int. 2012;2012:158139. Epub 2012/05/09.

Stone NJ, Robinson JG, Lichtenstein AH, Bairey Merz CN, Blum CB, Eckel RH, et al. 2013 ACC/AHA guideline on the treatment of blood cholesterol to reduce atherosclerotic cardiovascular risk in adults: a report of the American College of Cardiology/American Heart Association Task Force on Practice Guidelines. Circulation. 2014;129(25 Suppl 2):S1–45. Epub 2013/11/14.

Chapter 13
Evaluation and Treatment of Insulin Resistance and Hyperglycemic States

Daniel L. Hurley and Farhad Zangeneh

Pearls of Wisdom

- Adipose tissue dysfunction (adiposopathy), includes the accumulation of intra-abdominal fat, which leads to the development of insulin resistance in adipocytes, and the ectopic accumulation of lipids within the liver and muscle cells.
- Body mass index is useful for the initial screening classification of excess adiposity. However, central adiposity is superior in conferring the metabolic risk of developing prediabetes and the dysmetabolic syndrome.
- Younger subjects with prediabetes have a stronger risk of developing type 2 diabetes mellitus than their older counterparts.
- There are strong associations between the accumulation of fat mass leading to overweight or obesity, the development of adiposopathy with inflammation in adipose tissue and insulin resistance, and the arrival of hyperglycemic thresholds to reach the diagnosis of type 2 diabetes mellitus.
- Weight loss enhances insulin sensitivity and improves glycemic control in patients, whether achieved through lifestyle modification, pharmacotherapy, or bariatric surgery.

D. L. Hurley (✉)
Mayo Graduate School of Medicine, Mayo Clinic, Division of Endocrinology, Diabetes, Metabolism, and Nutrition, Rochester, MN, USA
e-mail: hurley.daniel@mayo.edu

F. Zangeneh
Endocrinology, Diabetes and Osteoporosis Clinic, Sterling, VA, USA

J. M. Gonzalez-Campoy et al. (eds.), *Bariatric Endocrinology*,
https://doi.org/10.1007/978-3-319-95655-8_13

13.1 Introduction

Obesity is a chronic disease state that is due to complex interactions among genetic, metabolic, environmental, and socioeconomic factors. Obesity rates have increased over the past few decades, and data from the National Health and Nutrition Examination Surveys show that approximately two-third of adults in the United States have overweight or obesity, and one-third have obesity. Adiposity, the accumulation of fat mass, is often associated with insulin resistance (IR), but not in all individuals. Still, overweight or obesity can worsen IR with progression to the dysmetabolic syndrome, prediabetes, and type 2 diabetes mellitus (T2DM) and thereby increases in the risk for cardiovascular (CV) disease (CVD). The main goal of overweight and obesity management is to improve overall health by reducing body fat and treating weight-related complications. Weight loss enhances insulin sensitivity and improves glycemic control, whether achieved through lifestyle modification, pharmacotherapy, or bariatric surgery. The choice of therapy depends upon both the degree of excess adiposity and the severity of complications related to adiposity and adiposopathy.

13.2 Pathophysiology of Hyperglycemic States

13.2.1 IR

IR may be defined as a subnormal glucose response to either endogenous or exogenous insulin. Exogenous insulin use may lead to the development of insulin antibodies, which is one of the causes of a subnormal glucose response to insulin. With the advent of recombinant human insulin for the treatment of hyperglycemia, anti-insulin antibodies are now a less frequent cause of IR. IR is now commonly encountered in clinical disease states such as overweight or obesity, dysmetabolic syndrome, prediabetes, T2DM, and polycystic ovarian syndrome. There are other causes of IR, some relatively uncommon (Table 13.1).

13.2.2 Hyperglycemia

Overweight and obesity, with the development of adiposopathy, can worsen IR, impair beta cell function, or both, and advance disease progression to the dysmetabolic syndrome, prediabetes, and eventually T2DM. Prediabetes is present when either the fasting plasma glucose (FPG) or the 2-h plasma glucose in an oral glucose tolerance test (OGTT) is above normal, but below the diagnostic threshold for T2DM. The terms "impaired fasting glucose (IFG)" and "impaired glucose tolerance (IGT)," respectively, are used to define these two conditions. Although patients with IFG and IGT both have IR, the site of IR has been shown to differ between these two prediabetes states. In addition to insulin resistance in adipocytes, which contributes

Table 13.1 Clinical conditions associated with IR

Chronic and common states associated with IR	Acute and subacute states causing IR	Uncommon or rare causes of IR
Overweight/obesity/adiposopathy (causal) Dysmetabolic syndrome Gestational diabetes Prediabetes (IFG and IGT) Type 2 diabetes mellitus Polycystic ovarian syndrome	Glucocorticoid excess Infection/inflammation Pregnancy Severe stress (surgery, sepsis, etc.) Uremia	Anti-insulin antibodies Insulin receptor antibodies Insulin receptor mutations (leprechaunism) Lipodystrophy (inherited leptin deficiency; acquired antiretroviral therapy)

FPG fasting plasma glucose = glucose level after >8 h of no caloric intake, *OGTT* oral glucose tolerance test = plasma glucose level 2 h after ingesting 75-g oral glucose in the morning after an overnight fast of >8 h, *IFG* impaired fasting glucose = FPG 100–125 mg/dL, *IGT* impaired glucose tolerance = OGTT 140–199 mg/dL
Type-2 diabetes mellitus = FPG ≥126 mg/dL (twice, barring acute stress), or OGTT ≥200 mg/dL, or symptoms of hyperglycemia (e.g., polyuria, polydipsia, and polyphagia) and a random (casual, nonfasting) plasma glucose ≥200 mg/dL, or A1C ≥6.5%

to hypertriglyceridemia and hyperglycemia, marked muscle IR and mild hepatic IR are present with IGT. On the other hand, IFG has severe IR in the liver and normal or near-normal insulin sensitivity in the muscle. In addition, both IFG and IGT are characterized by a reduction in early-phase insulin secretion, but subjects with IGT also have impaired late-phase insulin secretion. It remains controversial whether IR increases with age, although two studies reported that younger individuals with prediabetes have significantly more IR than their comparative older age cohorts. Considering an age-related deterioration of beta-cell function, a greater impairment in insulin secretion was present in younger versus older subjects with prediabetes. In addition, the younger subjects with IFG were characterized by a higher incidence of the development of T2DM. These disparities highlight that intervention to slow the progression from prediabetes to T2DM should especially target younger adults. The Coronary Artery Risk Development in Young Adults (CARDIA) study, and the Atherosclerosis Risk in Communities cohort study, reported a marked increased risk for T2DM in the presence of dysmetabolic syndrome traits. As previously mentioned, IFG is a component of the dysmetabolic syndrome. Thus, all patients with the dysmetabolic syndrome, to include those with prediabetes, should be informed of their increased risk for both T2DM and CVD. These patients should be counseled on aggressive management of their CVD risk factors.

13.2.3 Adiposopathy and Inflammation

Data from both human studies and animal models suggest strong associations between overweight- or obesity-related IR, chronic inflammation in adipose tissue, and the development of T2DM. Overweight and obesity, and in particular visceral adiposity, are associated with proinflammatory pathways (Fig. 13.1). The change from normal functioning adipose tissue to adiposopathy, with tissue inflammation,

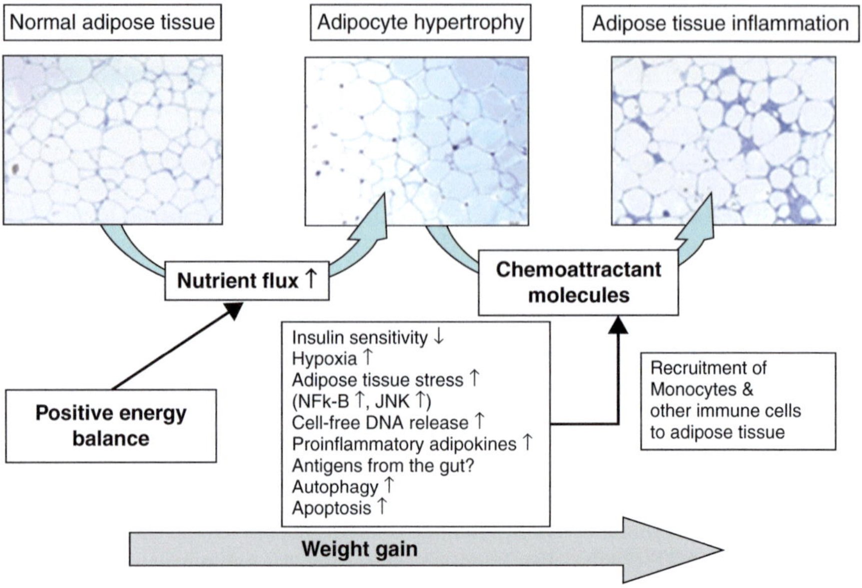

Fig. 13.1 Potential mechanisms for the development of adipose tissue inflammation in adiposopathy. (From Blüher (2016); used with permission)

is likely initiated by adipocyte hypertrophy from chronic lipid accumulation. Increased adipocyte size causes cellular stress with the activation of Jun N-terminal kinase, nuclear factor-κβ, and other stress signaling pathways. Stress signal activation in turn regulates protein phosphorylation and transcriptional events to stimulate fat cells, endothelial cells, and immune cells in adipose tissue. These activated fat cells produce proinflammatory cytokines, endothelial adhesion molecules, and proinflammatory and chemotactic mediators (to include interleukin-6, interleukin 1-beta, tumor necrosis factor-alpha, plasminogen activator inhibitor-1, monocyte chemoattractant protein-1, and colony-stimulating factor-1). Thus, an altered balance between metabolic and inflammatory signaling contributes to the pathophysiology of IR and adiposopathy-related diseases (Fig. 13.2).

13.2.4 Beta-Cells

Pancreatic beta-cell mass is increased with overweight and obesity and decreased with T2DM. In an autopsy study of 124 patients with and without T2DM and matched for obesity, beta-cell mass was significantly decreased regardless of whether they were lean or had obesity. Reduction in beta-cell mass was related to progression of disease and appeared to be related primarily to increased apoptosis. Beta-cell mass was reduced by 63% in subjects with obesity and T2DM compared to those who had obesity without T2DM. The observation that patients with obesity

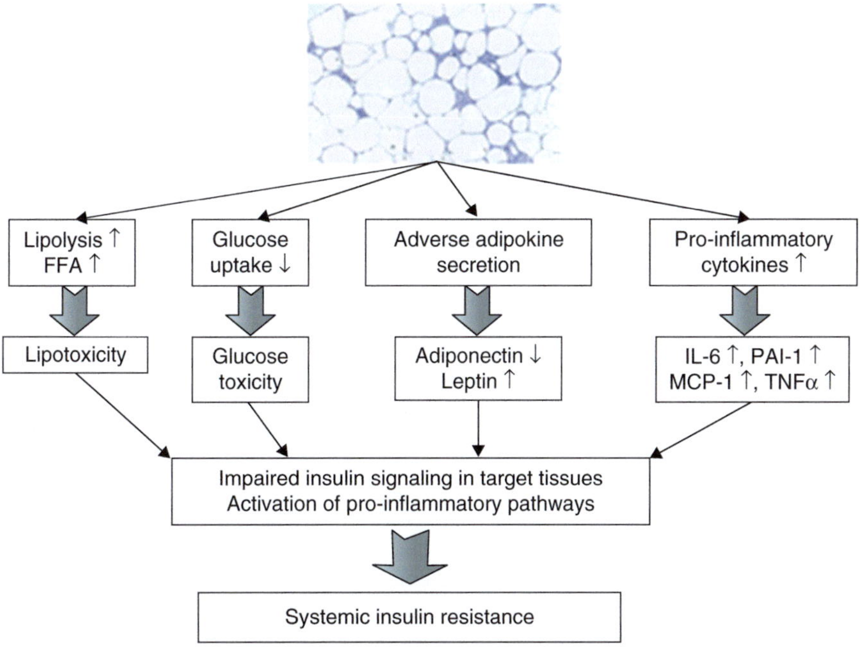

Fig. 13.2 Mechanistic model for the link between adipose tissue inflammation and insulin resistance in adiposopathy. (From Blüher (2016); used with permission)

and IFG had a decrease in beta-cell volume relative to controls provides evidence that beta-cell loss is important in the development of T2DM.

13.2.5 Dysmetabolic Syndrome

IR with impaired glucose metabolism and fatty acid utilization has been linked to vascular endothelial dysfunction, systemic inflammation, dyslipidemia, hypertension (HTN), T2DM, and CVD. IR can be accurately quantified by using the euglycemic insulin clamp technique, whereby insulin-induced glucose uptake is measured while maintaining the blood glucose at a steady concentration using dextrose infusion. In population-based epidemiology studies, simple ratios derived from both FPG and insulin levels have been used (e.g., glucose-to-insulin ratios and homeostasis model assessment of IR [HOMA-IR]). However, these techniques are impractical for clinical use. Common clinical and laboratory features of IR are listed in Table 13.2. The combined presence of hyperglycemia, dyslipidemia, and HTN defines the existence of the dysmetabolic syndrome. This textbook favors this term because it was used when it was added to the *International Classification of Diseases, Ninth edition* (ICD-9). Other names applied to this constellation of findings have included metabolic syndrome, syndrome X, the IR syndrome, the deadly

Table 13.2 Clinical and laboratory features associated with insulin resistance

Clinical features	Adiposity—central/visceral (increased waist circumference) Adiposity—total body (elevated body mass index) Acanthosis nigricans Androgen excess in women (hirsutism, virilization) Oligo- or amenorrhea Infertility
Laboratory tests	Hyperglycemia (elevated FBG and/or A1c, IFG, IGT) Hyperlipidemia (elevated triglyceride and depressed HDL-cholesterol) Hyperandrogenism (elevated serum testosterone, in women) Hyperinsulinemia Hyperleptinemia, hypoadiponectinemia, and elevated leptin to adiponectin ratio

Table 13.3 NCEP ATP III and IDF criteria for diagnosis of the dysmetabolic syndrome

NCEP ATP III	IDF
The presence of any three of the following: Abdominal obesity; WC ≥102 cm (40 in.) in M and ≥ 88 cm (35 in.) in F Serum Tg ≥150 mg/dL (1.7 mmol/L), or drug therapy for elevated Tg Serum HDL-C < 40 mg/dL (1 mmol/L) in M and < 50 mg/dL (1.3 mmol/L) in F, or drug therapy for low HDL-C BP ≥130/85 mmHg, or drug therapy for elevated BP FPG ≥100 mg/dL (5.6 mmol/L), or drug therapy for elevated FPG	Increased WC (with ethnic-specific WC cut-points)[a] plus any two of the following: Tg ≥150 mg/dL (1.7 mmol/L), or therapy for elevated Tg HDL-C <40 mg/dL (1.03 mmol/L) in M or < 50 mg/dL (1.29 mmol/L) in F, or therapy for low HDL-C SBP ≥130, DBP ≥85, or drug therapy for elevated BP FPG ≥100 mg/dL (5.6 mmol/L)[b], or previously diagnosed T2DM

BP blood pressure (S-systolic, D-diastolic), *cm* centimeter, *dL* deciliter, *FPG* fasting plasma glucose, *F* females, *HDL-C* high-density lipoprotein cholesterol, *IDF* International Diabetes Federation, *in* inches, *L* liter, *M* males, *mg* milligrams, *mmHg* millimeters of mercury, *mmol* millimoles, *NCEP ATP III* National Cholesterol Education Program Adult Treatment Panel III, *OGTT* oral glucose tolerance test, *Tg* triglycerides, *T2DM* type 2 diabetes mellitus, *WC* waist circumference

[a]Europid, Middle East, Eastern Mediterranean, and sub-Saharan African M ≥ 94 cm and F ≥ 80 cm. South and Central American, South Asian, Chinese, and Japanese M ≥ 90 cm and F ≥ 80 cm

[b]An OGTT is recommended for patients with an elevated FPG, but not required

quartet, and the obesity-dyslipidemia syndrome. Although the National Cholesterol Education Program (NCEP) Adult Treatment Panel (ATP) III is commonly cited to define the dysmetabolic syndrome, several differing criteria exist and can lead to difficulty in comparing data from human studies (Table 13.3). The National Health and Nutrition Examination Surveys reported a 28% increase in the prevalence of the dysmetabolic syndrome from 1988–1994 to 1999–2000. Contributing factors include an increased prevalence of obesity from 22.5% to 30.5% over the same time period and age-related increments in blood pressure (BP) and FPG. Dyslipidemia associated with IR is characterized by an excess of large, triglyceride-rich, very low-density lipoprotein (VLDL) particles, which are seen as elevated triglyceride and decreased high-density lipoprotein (HDL) cholesterol blood levels. Although the low-density lipoprotein (LDL) cholesterol concentration may not be elevated, the LDL cholesterol is packaged into smaller and denser lipoprotein particles. This results in a higher LDL particle concentration that is more atherogenic for any given level of LDL cholesterol. Elevated triglyceride and low HDL cholesterol concentrations are two of the five diagnostic criteria for the dysmetabolic syndrome and pose an increased risk for CVD. Overweight or obesity and hypertension (HTN) frequently coexist, and it is estimated that 60–70% of elevated BP in adults is attributable to excess body fat, especially increased visceral adiposity with adiposopathy. Cross-sectional and longitudinal studies have reported an association between body weight or body mass index (BMI) and increased risk of HTN as a function of weight gain over time. A meta-analysis of 19 cross-sectional studies compared the performance of BMI against waist circumference (WC) and waist-to-hip ratio (WHR) as indicators of HTN risk. The incremental increases in BP and the additional risk of HTN (defined as SBP/DBP ≥140/90 mmHg) were broadly similar for all measures of adiposity in ethnically diverse populations. However, insulin sensitivity can vary fivefold among individuals, in a manner that is largely independent of BMI, while individuals with IR are at risk of developing prediabetes and/or the dysmetabolic syndrome. Adipocytes with IR develop when there is a redistribution of fat to the intra-abdominal compartment, one of the elements of adiposopathy. IR in intra-abdominal adipose tissue leads to the ectopic accumulation of lipid within liver and muscle cells, another element of adiposopathy. A meta-analysis of 24 cross-sectional and 10 prospective studies, which included 512,809 subjects, documented the value of the waist-to-height ratio (WHtR). WHtR has a stronger association with the dysmetabolic syndrome and T2DM than BMI in cross-sectional studies. WHtR is superior to BMI in detecting CVD and mortality in prospective studies. The usefulness of WHtR appeared to be better in Asian populations. In another meta-analysis of 15 prospective cohort studies, the pooled relative risk (RR) for T2DM was 1.63 for WC, 1.62 for WHtR, 1.55 for BMI, and 1.52 for WHR. Thus, while excess body weight confers metabolic risk, most studies demonstrate that measures of central adiposity are superior to BMI in conferring risk of developing prediabetes or the dysmetabolic syndrome. Therefore, it is best to think in terms of adiposopathy as being the change in adipose tissue that contributes to the genesis of dysmetabolic syndrome, not sheer poundage.

There is a large body of evidence correlating higher BMI values with T2DM and other CV risk factors and atherosclerotic CVD. BMI is useful for the initial screening for the classification of excess weight, as it correlates with individual differences in adiposity and is associated with the risk of comorbidities secondary to excess body fat. However, BMI alone may not identify excess adiposity in all instances due to the variance of lean body mass (muscularity or sarcopenia) and volume status (dehydration or edema/ascites), especially in the overweight (BMI <30 kilogram (kg)/m (meter)^2) and class-1 obesity (BMI 30–34.9 kg/m^2) categories. In addition, despite strong associations, the mechanisms that link adiposity with IR and cardiometabolic disease risk have not been thoroughly established. The convergence of genetic factors that influence beta-cell function, aging, and lifestyle-related behaviors (both cultural and environmental, to include eating habits and level of activity) all play a role. Analyses of the prospective risk for T2DM in the Atherosclerosis Risk in Communities cohort indicated that weight gain in insulin-sensitive persons has no impact on CVD risk, and cumulative rates of incident T2DM remain low.

It is evident that some individuals with excess adiposity do not have dysmetabolic syndrome traits and are called "metabolically healthy obese." We consider them not to have developed adiposopathy, even though they have developed adiposity. Physiological studies have shown that patients with obesity but without dysmetabolic syndrome traits are relatively insulin sensitive, and epidemiologic data indicate a low risk of progression to T2DM and CVD. Thus, while BMI is important, obesity is neither necessary nor sufficient as a predictor of T2DM. By contrast, weight gain in individuals with IR markedly increases the risk of T2DM. Individuals with IR who undergo progressive weight gain have a relatively greater accumulation of fat in visceral adipose tissue. The predictive value of WC is both independent of, and additive to, BMI for both T2DM and CVD risk, up to a BMI of <35 kg/m^2. WC is a strong predictor of both all-cause and CV-related mortality.

13.3 T2DM

13.3.1 Epidemiology

Among adults in the United States, one-third have obesity and > 11% have T2DM. The majority of patients with T2DM have overweight or obesity, and the prevalence of diabetes is estimated to increase to >20% by 2050. The risk of T2DM increases with increasing BMI values in women and men. A meta-analysis of 32 studies conducted in multiple countries between 1985 and 2004 found that the pooled RR for incident T2DM was 1.87 for every standard deviation increase in BMI. Another meta-analysis of 18 prospective cohort studies documented an RR of T2DM of 2.99 and 7.19 for patients who had overweight or obesity, respectively, when compared to persons of normal weight. In addition to baseline BMI, weight gain is also a risk factor for T2DM. A meta-analysis of 15 prospective cohort studies found a pooled RR for incident T2DM was 3.07 and 2.12 for a 5-kg/m^2 increment in BMI occurring earlier versus later in adulthood, respectively.

13.3.2 Approach to the Patient with T2DM

There is a risk continuum for poor clinical outcomes in the progression from normal glucose tolerance to overt T2DM. The American Association of Clinical Endocrinologists (AACE)/American College of Endocrinology (ACE) clinical practice guidelines for obesity outline a complication centric approach to assess and treat patients with increased adiposity. Guidelines are also available for the treatment of patients with T2DM. All patients should have an annual height and weight measured for the calculation of BMI. The BMI and WC should be included as vital signs at every encounter in the bariatric endocrinology practice. If either the BMI or WC is increased, then an assessment of BP, FBG, and lipids is indicated. Epidemiologic evidence shows a continuous relationship between hemoglobin A1c (A1C) and CV and all-cause mortality. The lowest rates of CV and all-cause mortality are at A1C levels <5%. A1C values between 5.5% and 6.4% inclusive should signal consideration for specific glucose testing, especially in patients with overweight or obesity. However, the A1C should be used only as a screening tool for prediabetes or diabetes. Table 13.1 outlines the diagnostic criteria for prediabetes (IFG and IGT) and T2DM. Dysmetabolic syndrome, prediabetes, or T2DM should be aggressively treated.

In addition to lowering glucose, the priority in hyperglycemia management is to minimize the risks of hypoglycemia and weight gain. Intensive lifestyle intervention can improve fitness, glycemic control, and CV risk factors with a relatively modest decline in body weight. Weight loss lowers A1C while also producing significant improvement in BP and lipids, and it can decrease the need for diabetes medications. Weight loss enhances insulin sensitivity and improves glycemic control in patients with T2DM, whether achieved through lifestyle modification, pharmacotherapy, or bariatric surgery. Comprehensive lifestyle modification is generally recommended for all individuals with overweight or obesity, either as the only initial approach to weight loss or in combination with weight-loss medications or bariatric surgery. Lifestyle modification incorporates behavioral therapy, physical activity, and medical nutrition therapy. However, the addition of weight-loss medications consistently results in a greater degree of weight loss than lifestyle alone. Weight-loss medications have been shown to be superior to intensive lifestyle intervention alone in slowing progression from prediabetes to T2DM. Bariatric surgery achieves excellent and superior glycemic control to intensive lifestyle intervention and reduces CV risk factors. Glycemic control improves rapidly after bariatric surgery, even before significant weight loss has occurred, and the majority of patients are able to reduce or even eliminate their dependence on diabetes medications. Although additional studies are needed to demonstrate long-term benefits, bariatric surgery should be considered as a diabetes treatment option in patients with class III obesity (BMI ≥40 kg/m^2), with class II obesity (BMI 35.0–39.9 kg/m^2) when T2DM is inadequately controlled by medical therapy, and with class I obesity (BMI 30.0–34.9 kg/m^2) if hyperglycemia is inadequately controlled despite optimal treatment with either oral and/or injectable diabetes medications.

13.3.3 Pharmacotherapy for T2DM

Complete descriptions of antihyperglycemic agents, their mechanisms of action, and rationale for use can be found in the 2015 AACE and ACE comprehensive diabetes management algorithm consensus statement and clinical practice guidelines, as well in the American Diabetes Association (ADA) standards of medical care in diabetes. Existing pharmacotherapy strategies include stimulating insulin release, adding exogenous insulin, reducing hepatic glucose production, decreasing renal glucose transporter activity, and increasing or mimicking glucagon-like peptide-1 (GLP-1) activity.

As monotherapy progresses to combination therapy for glucose control, there can be an increased risk of hypoglycemia and weight gain. Complex treatment regimens that include hypoglycemia risk require regular glucose monitoring, often several times a day during insulin administration.

Patients with T2DM tend to have slightly more difficulty achieving and maintaining weight loss than those without it. One reason that weight-loss attempts may sometimes be slightly less effective in diabetes is that several medications used to treat diabetes result in weight gain. Clinicians should discuss with their patients the possible weight effects of glucose-lowering medications and consider the use of diabetes medications that promote weight loss or are weight neutral. Sulfonylureas, thiazolidinediones (TZDs), and insulin all cause weight gain. Insulin has the largest weight increase with an average gain of 4.0 kg more than conventional therapy at 10 years in the United Kingdom Prospective Diabetes Study. Metformin and dipeptidyl-peptidase-4 (DPP-4) inhibitors are weight neutral, whereas GLP-1 receptor agonists and sodium glucose transporter-2 (SGLT-2) inhibitors lead to weight loss. Metformin carries a low risk of hypoglycemia, produces durable antihyperglycemic effects, and is also effective when used in combination therapy. Sulfonylureas and glinides increase insulin secretion in a glucose-independent fashion. Sulfonylureas can cause hypoglycemia and may reduce, eliminate, or minimize the weight-loss benefit of drugs such as metformin, GLP-1 receptor agonists, and SGLT2 inhibitors. Although TZDs cause weight gain, they have been shown to improve insulin sensitivity and to preserve or improve beta-cell secretory function in patients with T2DM. The GLP-1 receptor agonists and DPP-4 inhibitors are incretin-based therapies that increase insulin secretion in a glucose-dependent manner. The "incretin effect" is the observation that an oral glucose load produces a greater insulin response than that of an iso-glycemic intravenous glucose infusion. This difference has been attributed to the gastrointestinal peptides GIP (glucose-dependent insulinotropic peptide) and GLP-1 that are secreted by endocrine cells in the epithelium of the small intestine in response to glucose. Glucose appears in the digestive tract following the absorption of ingested carbohydrates and activates a feed-forward mechanism that increases GIP and GLP-1 secretion. GIP and GLP-1 then target the pancreatic beta-cells to secrete more insulin. Like natural incretins, the GLP-1 receptor agonists lower postprandial glucose and can slow gastric emptying, thereby promoting satiety and reducing food intake, which often results in weight loss.

13.3.4 Reductions in mortality by T2DM treatments

Patients with T2DM manifest a two- to threefold greater risk of CV events compared to those without diabetes. CVD is responsible for approximately 80% of overall mortality in people with T2DM. Interventions to lower glycemia are important to blunt this risk.

- Treatment with pioglitazone, one of the TZDs, reduces composite outcome of nonfatal acute myocardial infarction, stroke, and all-cause mortality.

- In a time-to-event analysis, the rate of the first occurrence of death from CV causes, nonfatal myocardial infarction, or nonfatal stroke among 9340 patients with T2DM was lower with liraglutide than with placebo.
- The empagliflozin cardiovascular outcome event trial demonstrated that in patients with T2DM and high CVD risk, empagliflozin reduced the primary major adverse cardiac event endpoint (CV death, nonfatal myocardial infarction, and nonfatal stroke) by 14%. This beneficial effect was driven by a 38% reduction in CV mortality with no significant decrease in nonfatal myocardial infarction or stroke. Although SGLT-2 inhibitors exert multiple metabolic benefits (decreases in A1C, body weight, and BP and an increase in HDL cholesterol), it is unlikely that the reduction in CV mortality can only be explained by empagliflozin's metabolic effects. More likely, hemodynamic effects, specifically reduced BP and decreased extracellular volume, are responsible for the decrease in hospitalization for heart failure and for reduced CV mortality.

13.3.5 Insulin

Insulin is usually initiated when combination therapy with other agents fails to maintain adequate glycemic goals. Insulin is also started when an A1C level is above 9.0%, whether the patient is drug naïve or on treatment. Insulin may be initiated as a basal, basal-bolus, prandial, or premixed regimen. For most patients treated with oral diabetes medication but requiring additional A1C lowering, adding a basal insulin analog regimen is preferred. Hypoglycemia and weight gain are the most common adverse effects of insulin therapy. The combination of basal insulin and GLP-1 receptor agonist therapy has an additive effect to decrease both fasting and postprandial glucose and may limit weight gain and the risk of hypoglycemia compared with basal-bolus insulin regimens. The combined use of DPP-4 inhibitors or SGLT2 inhibitors with insulin is also effective in improving glycemic control with a relatively low risk of hypoglycemia.

13.3.6 Glycemic Targets for T2DM

It is important to note that no randomized controlled trials have established optimal glycemic targets in patients with T2DM. Thus, some professional organizations have recommended a general target A1C level of ≤6.5% while others have recommended <7%. In all patients, safety is paramount, and the potential risks of intensive glycemic control may outweigh its benefits. Less stringent control is appropriate in patients with frequent or severe hypoglycemia, hypoglycemia unawareness, seizure disorder, advanced aged, terminal illness, or active cardiovascular disease.

The challenges associated with improving glycemic control are exemplified by the fact that the ADA target goal for A1c of <7% is not achieved in almost half of patients with T2DM. In patients with obesity and T2DM requiring insulin therapy, choosing the proper insulin regimen (basal, prandial, or biphasic) using appropriate titration and the lowest effective dose would minimize hypoglycemia and weight gain. Combination therapy using metformin, GLP-1 receptor agonists, and/or SGLT-2 inhibitors with insulin should be considered to both mitigate insulin-medicated weight gain and assist in glucose control.

13.4 Conclusion

IR, which develops with adiposopathy, and impaired glucose metabolism have been linked to vascular endothelial dysfunction, systemic inflammation, dyslipidemia, T2DM, and CVD. There is a strong association between overweight and obesity, adiposopathy, and IR. The development of central adiposity leads to adiposopathy and the subsequent development of prediabetes and the dysmetabolic syndrome. In addition, there is a risk continuum for poor clinical outcomes in the progression from normal glucose tolerance to overt T2DM. Thus, the treatment for excess adiposity and adiposopathy should be patient centered and initiated concomitantly to treatment of other obesity-related comorbidities. The priorities in patients with IR and hyperglycemia are to lower the blood glucose but at the same time minimize the risks of hypoglycemia and avoid weight gain.

Lifestyle behavioral change should include structured support for healthy eating with reduced caloric intake and daily physical activity to reduce sedentary lifestyle. However, the addition of weight-loss medications consistently results in a greater degree of weight loss than lifestyle therapy alone. Weight-loss medications have been shown to be superior to intensive lifestyle intervention alone in both decreasing weight and slowing the progression from prediabetes to T2DM. Since obesity-related complications can be significantly improved by weight loss, a multidisciplinary team to help intensify and support therapy should be employed for patients with overweight or obesity. Patients with a BMI of ≥35 kg/m^2 with one or more comorbidities or ≥ 40 kg/m^2 without coexisting medical problem should be considered for referral to an accredited bariatric surgery center.

Reading List

Abdul-Ghani MA, Tripathy D, DeFronzo RA. Contributions of beta-cell dysfunction and insulin resistance to the pathogenesis of impaired glucose tolerance and impaired fasting glucose. Diabetes Care. 2006;29(5):1130–9.

Abdullah A, Peeters A, de Courten M, Stoelwinder J. The magnitude of association between overweight and obesity and the risk of diabetes: a meta-analysis of prospective cohort studies. Diabetes Res Clin Pract. 2010;89(3):309–19.

ADA Standards of Medical Care in Diabetes—2016. Glycemic targets. Diabetes Care. 2016;39(Supplement 1):S39–46.

Alberti KG, Eckel RH, Grundy SM, et al. Harmonizing the metabolic syndrome: a joint interim statement of the International Diabetes Federation task force on epidemiology and prevention; National Heart, Lung, and Blood Institute; American Heart Association; World Heart Federation; International Atherosclerosis Society; and International Association for the Study of Obesity. Circulation. 2009;120(16):1640–5.

Alexander CM, Landsman PB, Teutsch SM, et al. Third National Health and Nutrition Examination Survey (NHANES III), National Cholesterol Education Program (NCEP). NCEP-defined metabolic syndrome, diabetes, and prevalence of coronary heart disease among NHANES III participants age 50 years and older. Diabetes. 2003;52(5):1210–4.

Alexander CM, Landsman PB, Grundy SM. The influence of age and body mass index on the metabolic syndrome and its components. Diabetes Obes Metab. 2008;10(3):246–50.

Ali MK, Bullard KM, Saaddine JB, Cowie CC, Imperatore G, Gregg EW. Achievement of goals in US diabetes care, 1999–2010. N Engl J Med. 2013;368(17):1613–24.

American Diabetes Association. Classification and diagnosis of diabetes. Diabetes Care. 2015;38:S8–S16.

American Diabetes Association Standards of Medical Care in Diabetes—2016. Diabetes Care. 2016a;39(Supplement 1):1–203.

American Diabetes Association Standards of Medical Care in Diabetes—2016. Approaches to glycemic treatment. Diabetes Care. 2016b;39(Suppl 1):S52–9.

Apovian CM, Aronne L, Rubino D, et al. A randomized, phase 3 trial of naltrexone SR/bupropion SR on weight and obesity-related risk factors (COR-II). Obesity (Silver Spring). 2013;21:935–43.

Balkau B, Deanfield JE, Després JP, et al. International Day for the Evaluation of Abdominal Obesity (IDEA): a study of waist circumference, cardiovascular disease, and diabetes mellitus in 168,000 primary care patients in 63 countries. Circulation. 2007;116(17):1942–51.

Bays HE, Chapman RH, Grandy S, SHIELD Investigators' Group. The relationship of body mass index to diabetes mellitus, hypertension and dyslipidaemia: comparison of data from two national surveys. Int J Clin Pract. 2007;61(5):737–47.

Bays HE, Gonzalez-Campoy JM, Henry RR, Bergman DA, Kitabchi AE, Schorr AB, et al. Is adiposopathy (sick fat) an endocrine disease? Int J Clin Pract. 2008;62(10):1474–83. Epub 2008/08/07.

Belalcazar LM, Haffner SM, Lang W, et al. Lifestyle intervention and/or statins for the reduction of C-reactive protein in type 2 diabetes: from the look AHEAD study. Obesity (Silver Spring). 2013;21:944–50.

Blüher M. Adipose tissue inflammation: a cause or consequence of obesity-related insulin resistance? Clin Sci. 2016;130(18):1603–14.

Bolen S, Feldman L, Vassy J, et al. Systematic review: comparative effectiveness and safety of oral medications for type 2 diabetes mellitus [Erratum in *Ann Intern Med* 2007;147:887]. Ann Intern Med. 2007;147:386–99.

Boyle JP, Thompson TJ, Gregg EW, et al. Projection of the year 2050 burden of diabetes in the US adult population: dynamic modeling of incidence, mortality, and prediabetes prevalence. Popul Health Metr. 2010;8:29.

Buse JB, Bergenstal RM, Glass LC, et al. Use of twice daily exenatide in basal insulin-treated patients with type 2 diabetes: a randomized, controlled trial. Ann Intern Med. 2011;154:103–12.

Butler AE, Janson J, Bonner-Weir S, et al. β-cell deficit and increased apoptosis in humans with type 2 diabetes. Diabetes. 2003;52:102–10.

Cerhan JR, Moore SC, Jacobs EJ, et al. A pooled analysis of waist circumference and mortality in 650,000 adults. Mayo Clin Proc. 2014;89(3):335–45.

Chan JM, Rimm EB, Colditz GA, et al. Obesity, fat distribution, and weight gain as risk factors for clinical diabetes in men. Diabetes Care. 1994;17:961–9.

Chen G, Shi L, Cai L, et al. Comparison of insulin resistance and β-cell dysfunction between the young and the elderly in normal glucose tolerance and prediabetes population: a prospective study. Horm Metab Res. 2016; https://doi.org/10.1055/s-0042–111325.

Colditz GA, Willett WC, Rotnitzky A, et al. Weight gain as a risk factor for clinical diabetes mellitus in women. Ann Intern Med. 1995;122:481–6.
de Koning L, Merchant AT, Pogue J, et al. Waist circumference and waist-to-hip ratio as predictors of cardiovascular events: meta-regression analysis of prospective studies. Eur Heart J. 2007;28(7):850–6.
Devries JH, Bain SC, Rodbard HW, et al. Sequential intensification of metformin treatment in type 2 diabetes with liraglutide followed by randomized addition of basal insulin prompted by A1C targets. Diabetes Care. 2012;35:1446–54.
Eckel RH, Kahn SE, Ferrannini E, et al. Obesity and type 2 diabetes: what can be unified and what needs to be individualized? J Clin Endocrinol Metab. 2011;96(6):1654–63.
Ferrannini E, Natali A, Bell P, et al. Insulin resistance and hypersecretion in obesity. European Group for the Study of Insulin Resistance (EGIR). J Clin Invest. 1997;100(5):1166–73.
Flegal KM, Carroll MD, Ogden CL, et al. Prevalence and trends in obesity among US adults, 1999–2000. JAMA. 2002;288(14):1723–7.
Gami AS, Witt BJ, Howard DE, et al. Metabolic syndrome and risk of incident cardiovascular events and death: a systematic review and meta-analysis of longitudinal studies. J Am Coll Cardiol. 2007;49(4):403–14.
Garber AJ. Long-acting glucagon-like peptide 1 receptor agonists: a review of their efficacy and tolerability. Diabetes Care. 2011;34(Suppl 2):S279–84.
Garber AJ, Abrahamson MJ, Barzilay JI, et al. American Association of Clinical Endocrinologists/ American College of Endocrinology' comprehensive diabetes management algorithm 2015. Endocr Pract. 2015;21:438–47.
Garvey WT, Kwon S, Zheng D, et al. Effects of insulin resistance and type 2 diabetes on lipoprotein subclass particle size and concentration determined by nuclear magnetic resonance. Diabetes. 2003;52(2):453–62.
Garvey WT, Ryan DH, Look M, et al. Two-year sustained weight loss and metabolic benefits with controlled release phentermine/topiramate in obese and overweight adults (SEQUEL): a randomized, placebo-controlled, phase 3 extension study. Am J Clin Nutr. 2012;95:297–308.
Garvey WT, Ryan DH, Bohannon NJ, et al. Weight-loss therapy in type 2 diabetes: effects of phentermine and topiramate extended-release. Diabetes Care. 2014a;37:3309–16.
Garvey WT, Ryan DH, Henry R, et al. Prevention of type 2 diabetes in subjects with prediabetes and metabolic syndrome treated with phentermine and topiramate extended release. Diabetes Care. 2014b;37(4):912–21.
Garvey WT, Mechanick JI, Brett EM, et al. American Association of Clinical Endocrinologists and American College of Endocrinology comprehensive clinical practice guidelines for medical care of patients with obesity. Endocr Pract. 2016;22(Suppl 3):1–103.
Gonzalez-Campoy JM. The birth of bariatric endocrinology and the coming of age of obesity medicine. US Endocrinol [Internet]. 2016;12(1):10–1. https://doi.org/10.17925/USE.2016.12.01.10.
Gonzalez-Campoy JM, St Jeor ST, Castorino K, Ebrahim A, Hurley D, Jovanovic L, et al. Clinical practice guidelines for healthy eating for the prevention and treatment of metabolic and endocrine diseases in adults: cosponsored by the American Association of Clinical Endocrinologists/ The American College of Endocrinology and The Obesity Society. Endocr Pract Off J Am Coll Endocrinol Am Assoc Clin Endocrinol. 2013;19(0):1–82. Epub 2013/10/17.
Gonzalez-Campoy JM, Richardson B, Richardson C, Gonzalez-Cameron D, Ebrahim A, Strobel P, et al. Bariatric endocrinology: principles of medical practice. Int J Endocrinol. 2014;2014:917813. Epub 2014/06/06.
Grundy SM, Brewer HB Jr, Cleeman JI, et al. American Heart Association, National Heart, Lung, and Blood Institute. Definition of metabolic syndrome: report of the National Heart, Lung, and Blood Institute/American Heart Association conference on scientific issues related to definition. Circulation. 2004;109(3):433–8.
Guh DP, Zhang W, Bansback N, et al. The incidence of co-morbidities related to obesity and overweight: a systematic review and meta-analysis. BMC Public Health. 2009;9:88.
Guo F, Garvey WT. Development of a weighted cardiometabolic disease staging (CMDS) system for theprediction of future diabetes. J Clin Endocrinol Metab. 2015;100(10):3871–7.

Guo F, Garvey WT. Cardiometabolic disease risk in metabolically healthy and unhealthy obesity: stability of metabolic health status in adults. Obesity (Silver Spring). 2016;24(2):516–25.

Guo F, Moellering DR, Garvey WT. The progression of cardiometabolic disease: validation of a new cardiometabolic disease staging system applicable to obesity. Obesity (Silver Spring). 2014;22(1):110–8.

Handelsman Y, Bloomgarden ZT, Grunberger G, et al. American Association of Clinical Endocrinologists and American College of Endocrinology: clinical practice guidelines for developing a diabetes mellitus comprehensive care plan-2015. Endocr Pract. 2015;21(Suppl 1):1–87.

Herder C, Carstensen M, Ouwens DM. Anti-inflammatory cytokines and risk of type 2 diabetes. Diabetes Obes Metab. 2013;15(Suppl 3):39–50.

Heymsfield SB, Peterson CM, Thomas DM, et al. Scaling of adult body weight to height across sex and race/ethnic groups: relevance to BMI. Am J Clin Nutr. 2014;100(6):1455–61.

Hollander P, Gupta AK, Plodkowski R, et al. Effects of naltrexone sustained-release/bupropion sustained-release combination therapy on body weight and glycemic parameters in overweight and obese patients with type 2 diabetes. Diabetes Care. 2013;36:4022–9.

Hollenbeck C, Reaven GM. Variations in insulin stimulated glucose uptake in healthy individuals with normal glucose tolerance. J Clin Endocrinol Metab. 1987;64(6):1169–73.

Khaw KT, Wareham N, Bingham S, et al. Association of hemoglobin A1c with cardiovascular disease and mortality in adults: the European prospective investigation into cancer in Norfolk. Ann Intern Med. 2004;141:413–20.

Kip KE, Marroquin OC, Kelley DE, et al. Clinical importance of obesity versus the metabolic syndrome in cardiovascular risk in women: a report from the Women's Ischemia Syndrome Evaluation (WISE) study. Circulation. 2004;109(6):706–13.

Kodama S, Horikawa C, Fujihara K, et al. Comparisons of the strength of associations with future type 2 diabetes risk among anthropometric obesity indicators, including waist-to-height ratio: a meta-analysis. Am J Epidemiol. 2012;176(11):959–69.

Kodama S, Horikawa C, Fujihara K, et al. Quantitative relationship between body weight gain in adulthood and incident type 2 diabetes: a meta-analysis. Obes Rev. 2014;15(3):202–14.

Kotchen TA. Obesity-related hypertension: epidemiology, pathophysiology, and clinical management. Am J Hypertens. 2010;23(11):1170–8.

Liao Y, Kwon S, Shaughnessy S, et al. Critical evaluation of adult treatment panel III criteria in identifying insulin resistance with dyslipidemia. Diabetes Care. 2004;27(4):978–83.

Lincoff AM, Wolski K, Nicholls SJ, et al. Pioglitazone and risk of cardiovascular events in patients with type 2 diabetes mellitus: a meta-analysis of randomized trials. JAMA. 2007;298:1180–8.

Look AHEAD Research Group, Wing RR. Long-term effects of a lifestyle intervention on weight and cardiovascular risk factors in individuals with type 2 diabetes mellitus: four-year results of the Look AHEAD trial. Arch Intern Med. 2010;170:1566–75.

Marso SP, Daniels GH, Brown-Frandsen K, et al. LEADER trial. Liraglutide and cardiovascular outcomes in type 2 diabetes. N Engl J Med. 2016;375:311–22.

Meigs JB, Wilson PW, Fox CS, et al. Body mass index, metabolic syndrome, and risk of type 2 diabetes or cardiovascular disease. J Clin Endocrinol Metab. 2006;91(8):2906–12.

Miles JM, Leiter L, Hollander P, et al. Effect of orlistat in overweight and obese patients with type 2 diabetes treated with metformin. Diabetes Care. 2002;25:1123–8.

Misra A, Khurana L. Obesity and the metabolic syndrome in developing countries. J Clin Endocrinol Metab. 2008;93(11 Suppl 1):S9–S30.

Mora S, Szklo M, Otvos JD, et al. LDL particle subclasses, LDL particle size, and carotid atherosclerosis in the Multi-Ethnic Study of Atherosclerosis (MESA). Atherosclerosis. 2007;192(1):211–7.

O'Neil PM, Smith SR, Weissman NJ, et al. Randomized placebo-controlled clinical trial of lorcaserin for weight loss in type 2 diabetes mellitus: the BLOOM-DM study. Obesity (Silver Spring). 2012;20:1426–36.

Obesity in Asia Collaboration. Is central obesity a better discriminator of the risk of hypertension than body mass index in ethnically diverse populations? J Hypertens. 2008;26(2):169–77.

Reaven GM. Insulin resistance: the link between obesity and cardiovascular disease. Med Clin North Am. 2011;95(5):875–92.
Reis JP, Allen N, Gunderson EP, et al. Excess body mass index- and waist circumference-years and incident cardiovascular disease: the CARDIA study. Obesity. 2015;23(4):879–85.
Rubino F, et al. Metabolic surgery in the treatment algorithm for type 2 diabetes: a joint statement by international diabetes organizations. Diabetes Care. 2016;39:861–77.
Savva SC, Lamnisos D, Kafatos AG. Predicting cardiometabolic risk: waist-to-height ratio or BMI. A meta-analysis. Diabetes Metab Syndr Obes. 2013;6:403–19.
Schauer PR, Kashyap SR, Wolski K, et al. Bariatric surgery versus intensive medical therapy in obese patients with diabetes. N Engl J Med. 2012;366:1567–76.
Shah RV, Murthy VL, Abbasi SA, et al. Visceral adiposity and the risk of metabolic syndrome across body mass index: the MESA Study. JACC Cardiovasc Imaging. 2014;7(12):1221–35.
Shoelson SE, Lee J, Goldfine AB. Inflammation and insulin resistance. J Clin Invest. 2006;116:1793–801.
Sjostrom L, Lindroos AK, Peltonen M, et al. Lifestyle, diabetes, and cardiovascular risk factors 10 years after bariatric surgery. N Engl J Med. 2004;351:2683–93.
St-Pierre AC, Cantin B, Dagenais GR, et al. Low-density lipoprotein subfractions and the long-term risk of ischemic heart disease in men: 13-year follow-up data from the Quebec Cardiovascular Study. Arterioscler Thromb Vasc Biol. 2005;25(3):553–9.
The DPP Research Group. Role of insulin secretion and sensitivity in the evolution of type 2 diabetes in the diabetes prevention program. Effect of lifestyle intervention and metformin. J Gerontol. 2006;61:1075–81.
Tobias DK, Pan A, Jackson CL, et al. Body-mass index and mortality among adults with incident type 2 diabetes. N Engl J Med. 2014;370(3):233–44.
Torgerson JS, Hauptman J, Boldrin MN, et al. XENical in the prevention of diabetes in obese subjects (XENDOS) study. Diabetes Care. 2004;27(1):155–61.
Twig G, Afek A, Derazne E, et al. Diabetes risk among overweight and obese metabolically healthy young adults. Diabetes Care. 2014;37(11):2989–95.
van Dis I, Kromhout D, Geleijnse JM, et al. Body mass index and waist circumference predict both 10-year nonfatal and fatal cardiovascular disease risk: study conducted in 20,000 Dutch men and women aged 20–65 years. Eur J Cardiovasc Prev Rehabil. 2009;16(6):729–34.
Vazquez G, Duval S, Jacobs DR, et al. Comparison of body mass index, waist circumference, and waist/hip ratio in predicting incident diabetes: a meta-analysis. Epidemiol Rev. 2007;29:115–28.
Wildman RP, Muntner P, Reynolds K, et al. The obese without cardiometabolic risk factor clustering and the normal weight with cardiometabolic risk factor clustering: prevalence and correlates of 2 phenotypes among the US population (NHANES 1999–2004). Arch Intern Med. 2008;168(15):1617–24.
Wilson PW, D'Agostino RB, Sullivan L, et al. Overweight and obesity as determinants of cardiovascular risk: the Framingham experience. Arch Intern Med. 2002;162(16):1867–72.
Wilson PW, D'Agostino RB, Parise H, et al. Metabolic syndrome as a precursor of cardiovascular disease and type 2 diabetes mellitus. Circulation. 2005;112(20):3066–72.
Wormser D, Kaptoge S, Di Angelantonio E, et al. Emerging Risk Factors Collaboration. Separate and combined associations of body-mass index and abdominal adiposity with cardiovascular disease: collaborative analysis of 58 prospective studies. Lancet. 2011;377(9771):1085–95.
Zhang C, Rexrode KM, van Dam RM, et al. Abdominal obesity and the risk of all-cause, cardiovascular, and cancer mortality: sixteen years of follow-up in US women. Circulation. 2008;117(13):1658–67.
Zinman B, Wanner C, Lachin JM, et al. EMPA-REG OUTCOME Investigators. Empagliflozin, cardiovascular outcomes, and mortality in type 2 diabetes. N Engl J Med. 2015;373:2117–28.

Chapter 14
Evaluation and Treatment of Hypertension

Quang T. Nguyen and Raymond A. Plodkowski

Pearls of Wisdom

- For patients <60 years of age who have overweight or obesity start pharmacotherapy at the blood pressure threshoulds of 140/90 mmHg and continue lifestyle changes.
- Angiotensin converting enzyme inhibitors, angiotensin receptor blockers, or calcium channel blockers are considered first-line agents in the treatment of patients with overweight or obesity, and hypertension. More often, multiple classes are required due to the complex regulatory disturbances seen in this population.
- Treating hypertension in patients with overweight or obesity requires aggressive weight management as part of the therapeutic plan, if not as a primary plan.
- Patients with overweight or obesity, and hypertension, should limit their sodium intake to 2.3–3 g/day, maintain a potassium intake >3.5 g/day, restrict alcohol to <1 oz./day, and engage in physical activity >30 min/day.
- There is a dose-response relationship between the amount of weight loss achieved at up to 3 years by lifestyle intervention and the lowering of blood pressure (5% weight loss, mean reduction in systolic and diastolic BP is 3 mmHg and 2 mmHg, respectively).

Q. T. Nguyen (✉)
Las Vegas Endocrinology, Clinical Education, AZCOM, TUNCOM, Henderson, NV, USA

R. A. Plodkowski
University of California San Diego, Division of Endocrinology and Metabolism, Scripps Clinic, San Diego, CA, USA

J. M. Gonzalez-Campoy et al. (eds.), *Bariatric Endocrinology*,
https://doi.org/10.1007/978-3-319-95655-8_14

- A 5% mean weight loss difference achieved over 4 years by intensive lifestyle intervention in adults with overweight or obesity, and type 2 diabetes, is associated with a lower prevalence of patients who are prescribed antihypertensive medications compared to controls.
- A favorable inverse relationship has been noted between blood pressure and regular physical activity, independent of body weight.

14.1 Introduction with Adipocentric View

Obesity increases the risk for hypertension. The Framingham Heart Study estimated that excess body weight accounted for approximately 26% of cases of hypertension in men and 28% in women and for approximately 23% of cases of coronary heart disease in men and 15% in women. The Swedish Obesity Study reported hypertension being present in approximately 50% of subjects, all of whom had at least a body mass index (BMI) of ≥34 kg/m^2 in men and ≥ 38 kg/m^2 in women. In a report from the Nurses' Health Study, the BMI at age 18 years and at midlife was positively associated with the occurrence of hypertension. Overweight subjects (BMI ≥25 kg/m^2) who gained 5.0–9.9 kg had a relative increased risk of hypertension of 1.7 and 5.2, respectively. This relationship also held true for men in the Health Professionals Follow-up Study where a strong positive association between overall obesity and hypertension and diabetes was observed (Fig. 14.1). Latest data from the American Heart Association (AHA) estimated that at least 75% of the incidence of hypertension in the United States is directly related to obesity. This association was supported by results from the National Health and Nutrition Examination Survey (NHANES) 1999–2004. Researchers from this database observed an increase in the prevalence of hypertension from 18.1% in normal-weight subjects to 52.3% in those with class III (BMI ≥ 40 kg/m^2) obesity. With normal-weight individuals as a reference, individuals with obesity class III had a five (4.8 adjusted odds ratio (OR)) times higher risk of developing hypertension.

The pathophysiology of obesity causing hypertension is not well understood and is likely multifactorial. From a hemodynamic standpoint, obese hypertensive patients are known to have higher cardiac output compared to their lean counterparts. The higher cardiac output is produced predominantly by the increase in stroke volumes via Frank-Starling mechanism (increased preload). As subjects become more deconditioned due to the direct and indirect effects of obesity, heart rate also increases [further] cardiac output, leading to higher blood pressure.

Another proposed mechanism by which obesity raises blood pressure involves the role of excessive central (visceral) obesity leading to peripheral insulin resistance, hyperinsulinemia, endothelial dysfunction, and subsequent activation of the sympathetic nervous system. The pathophysiological link between visceral adiposity and cardiometabolic complications focuses on insulin sensitivity, the sympathetic nervous system, the renin-angiotensin-aldosterone system (RAAS), and the cardiac natriuretic peptide system (CNPS).

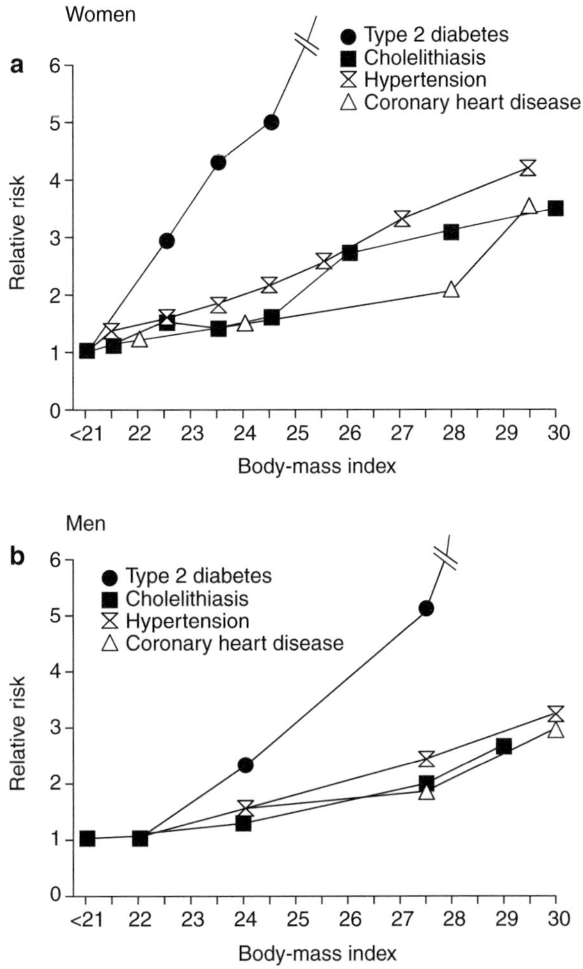

Fig. 14.1 Relation between body mass index up to 30 kg/m^2 and the relative risk of type 2 diabetes, hypertension, coronary heart disease, and cholelithiasis. Panel A shows these relations for women in the Nurses' Health Study, initially 30–55 years of age, who were followed for up to 18 years. Panel B shows the same relations for men in the Health Professionals Follow-up Study, initially 40–65 years of age, who were followed for up to 10 years. (From Willett et al. (1999); used with permission)

Central adipose tissues are metabolically active. In excess, they upregulate (and dysregulate) the renin-angiotensin-aldosterone system causing increased renal sodium reabsorption and subsequent volume expansion. The subsequent increase in angiotensin II level enhances the production of aldosterone in the adrenals as well as contributes to the hypertension due to its vasoconstriction property. Angiotensin II also has tropic effects on adipocytes, thereby ensuring the continued growth of these tissues and maintaining the vicious cycle.

Cardiac natriuretic peptide system is responsible for natriuresis and diuresis, leading to lower plasma volume and lower blood pressure. This system is downregulated in obese patients allowing the renin-angiotensin-aldosterone system to go unchecked leading to higher blood pressure.

Chronic stress, sleep apnea, and physical/mechanical compression of the vasculatures or kidneys by adipose tissues are other mechanisms by which obesity raises blood pressure.

14.2 Epidemiology

The Centers for Disease Control and Prevention estimated that approximately 29% (approximately 70 million) of adults in the United States currently have high blood pressure. Hypertension is the number one diagnosis in the ambulatory setting and is one of the top diagnoses in the nursing home. Data from the Framingham Heart Study suggest that patients who are normotensive at age 55 years have a 90% lifetime risk of developing hypertension. Women are as likely as men to develop high blood pressure during their lifetime. However, for people younger than 45 years old, the condition affects more men than women. For people 65 years old or older, high blood pressure affects more women than men. African Americans develop high blood pressure more often, and at an earlier age, than whites and Hispanics do. More African American women than men have high blood pressure.

Despite the awareness and wide array of treatment options currently available, only 50% individuals with hypertension are currently controlled. About one of five US adults with high blood pressure still do not know that they have hypertension and only seven in ten US adults with high blood pressure are using medications to treat it. More than 360,000 American deaths in 2013 included high blood pressure as a primary or contributing cause, equating to almost 1000 deaths each day. Approximately 10% of the current US total annual drug expenditure is spent on antihypertensive medications. High blood pressure costs the nation $46 billion each year, including cost of health care services, medications to treat high blood pressure, and missed days of work.

Since obesity and hypertension are so closely linked, the number of patients with hypertension is likely to grow as the obesity epidemic worsens.

14.3 Definitions

The definition of "hypertension" has changed over time, and the numeric thresholds vary depending on the specific guidelines and organization. As the body of evidence correlating elevated BP levels with CVD has grown, values defining "normal" BP have declined. The first National Health Examination Survey, conducted from 1960 through 1962, defined hypertension as BP higher than 160/95 mmHg. This threshold was lowered to 140/90 mmHg in 1973 by the National High Blood Pressure Education Program. In 1993, the fifth report of the Joint National Committee (JNC) lowered the definition of normal BP to 130/85 mmHg or below, and in 2003, the seventh report of the JNC (JNC 7) redefined the definition of normal BP to 120/80 mmHg or below (see Table 14.1). The criteria shown in Table 14.1 are based upon the average of two or more properly measured readings at each of two or more office visits after initial screening. The 2014 Evidenced-Based Guidelines for Management of High Blood Pressure in Adults as reported by the panel members appointed to the eighth Joint National Committee (JNC 8) did not address or change the parameters established by JNC 7. As such, the definition of hypertension as

Table 14.1 Blood pressure guidelines

JNC 7 blood pressure classification in adults aged >18 years	
Category	Systolic and diastolic
Normal	<120 and < 80
Prehypertension	120–139 or 80–89
Hypertension, stage 1	140–159 or 90–99
Hypertension, stage 2	≥160 or ≥ 100

From: National Heart, Lung, and Blood Institute; National Institutes of Health; U.S. Department of Health and Human Services, JNC 7 Express

established by JNC 7 is still the most current and accepted definition to guide providers in clinical practice. *The blood pressure goal in obese patients with hypertension is similar to the general population, treating SBP and DBP to targets of < 140/90 mmHg.*

- Normal blood pressure: Systolic <120 mmHg and diastolic <80 mmHg.
- Prehypertension: Systolic 120–139 mmHg or diastolic 80–89 mmHg.
- Hypertension:
  - Stage 1: Systolic 140–159 mmHg or diastolic 90–99 mmHg.
  - Stage 2: Systolic ≥160 mmHg or diastolic ≥100 mmHg.

Isolated systolic hypertension (ISH) (systolic-BP ≥140 mmHg; diastolic BP <90 mmHg) is more common in individuals over 50 years of age, most likely a result of increased arterial stiffness from arteriosclerosis or impairment of nitric oxide-mediated vasodilation. In a hypertension study involving NHANES III survey, isolated hypertension was present in 54% of subjects between the ages of 50 and 59 years and in 87% of hypertensive subjects older than 60 years of age. This is significant because ISH is associated with a two- to four-fold increase in the risk for stroke, myocardial infarction (MI), or cardiovascular (CV) mortality. Under the age of 50 years, diastolic blood pressure is more common and is a better predictor of mortality than systolic blood pressure.

14.4 Overview

14.4.1 Primary Hypertension

Hypertension without known cause or pre-existing renal disease is known as primary or essential hypertension. This form of hypertension is the most common form of hypertension and accounts for 90–95% of adult cases. Arterial blood pressure is determined by the following equation:

$$\text{Blood Pressure}\left(\text{BP}\right) = \text{Cardiac Output}\left(\text{CO}\right) \times \text{Peripheral Resistance}\left(\text{PR}\right).$$

Table 14.2 Risk factors for primary hypertension

Obesity: Excessive blood volume increases cardiac output. Peripheral resistance eventually increases as well, leading to sustained hypertension
Genetic: Hypertension is twice as common in subjects who have one or two hypertensive parents
Age: Hypertension increases with age, especially systolic blood pressure
Race: African Americans develop high blood pressure more often, and at an earlier age, than whites and Hispanics do
Inactivity: Physical inactivity increases the risk for hypertension, and exercise is an effective means of lowering blood pressure
Tobacco use: Second-hand smoke also can increase hypertension risk
Excessive sodium intake: >3000 mg/day increases the risk for hypertension
Alcohol abuse: Excess alcohol intake is associated with the development of hypertension
Diabetes and dyslipidemia: Presence of other cardiovascular risk factors increase risk for hypertension
Depression/personality disorders/traits: Hypertension more common in depression, type A personalities, and other personality traits
Inadequate potassium intake: Insufficient potassium intake may contribute to the development of hypertension
Low/reduced nephron mass: Reduced nephron mass can predispose to hypertension
Hypovitaminosis D: Hypertension is higher with low vitamin D in some population

Any conditions or risk factors that elevate cardiac output or peripheral resistance will cause hypertension. In patients with obesity, the initial defect is due to elevated cardiac output. Over time, peripheral resistance goes up as well, leading to even higher blood pressure. In most patients, increased peripheral resistance eventually will become the primary hemodynamic fault for sustained hypertension. Although the exact cause of primary hypertension is unknown, several risk factors are strongly associated with its development. Table 14.2 lists these risk factors and provides a brief explanation for its pathophysiology.

14.4.2 Secondary Hypertension

Secondary hypertension is hypertension with known causes. This form of hypertension is less common and accounts for approximately 5–10% of adult cases. In many cases, these causes co-exist with risk factors for primary hypertension, requiring a multipronged approach to controlling blood pressure. This is especially true in patients with obesity, who commonly also have metabolic syndrome, diabetes, and dyslipidemia. Table 14.3 lists common causes of secondary hypertension. Renal parenchymal disease is the most common cause of secondary hypertension, followed by renovascular disease, various adrenal disorders, and neurologic disorders. Prescription or over-the-counter drugs also play a role in secondary hypertension. Some of the common culprits used in obese patients

Table 14.3 Major causes of secondary hypertension

Causes		
Renal	Renal parenchymal disease	Acute glomerulonephritis Chronic nephritis Polycystic disease Diabetic nephropathy Hydronephrosis
	Renovascular	Renal artery stenosis Intrarenal vasculitis
	Renin-producing tumors	
	Liddle syndrome	
	Gordon syndrome	
Endocrine	Acromegaly	
	Hypothyroidism	
	Hyperthyroidism	
	Hypercalcemia	Hyperparathyroidism
	Adrenal (cortical)	Cushing syndrome Primary Aldosteronism Congenital adrenal hyperplasia
	Adrenal (medullary)	Pheochromocytoma
	Apparent mineralocorticoid excess	
	Carcinoid	
	Paget disease of the bone	
	Exogenous hormones	Estrogen Glucocorticoids Mineralocorticoids Sympathomimetics Erythropoietin Tyramine-containing foods and monoamine oxidase inhibitors
Coarctation of aorta		
Pregnancy-induced hypertension		
Neurologic disorders	Increase intracranial pressure	
	Sleep apnea	
	Quadriplegia	
	Acute porphyria	
	Familial dysautonomia	
	Guillain-Barre syndrome	
Acute stress	Psychogenic hyperventilation	
	Hypoglycemia	
	Burns	
	Alcohol withdrawal	
	Sickle cell crisis	
	Post resuscitation	
	Perioperative	

(continued)

Table 14.3 (continued)

Causes		
Increased intravascular volume		
Exogenous causes	Alcohol abuse	
	Nicotine	
	Immunosuppressive drugs	
	Heavy metal toxicity	
Increased cardiac output	Aortic valvular insufficiency	
	Arteriovenous fistula, patent ductus	
Rigidity of aorta		

From Zipes et al. (2005); used with permission

include oral contraceptives; glucocorticoids; weight loss medications; stimulants such as methylphenidate, nonsteroidal anti-inflammatory agents, and decongestants. Illicit drugs such as cocaine and methamphetamine will also raise blood pressure.

14.4.3 *Evaluation*

All obese adults over the age of 18 should be screened for elevated blood pressure at least annually. An elevated screening blood pressure should be confirmed using out-of-office measurement and if possible, ambulatory blood pressure monitoring (ABPM) should be utilized.

The evaluation of hypertension involves accurately measuring the patient's blood pressure, performing a focused medical history and physical examination, and obtaining results of routine laboratory studies. The objectives of a thorough evaluation are (1) to assess lifestyle and identify other cardiovascular risk factors or concomitant disorders that may affect prognosis and guide treatment (Tables 14.2 and 14.4); (2) to reveal identifiable causes of high BP (Table 14.3); and (3) to assess the presence or absence of target organ damage and CVD (Table 14.5).

14.4.4 *History and Physical Examination*

This history should search for precipitating causes as well as the duration of hypertension. Since hypertension is a silent disease, many patients may have had undiagnosed hypertension for many years that could accelerate end organ damages.

The physical examination should include an appropriate measurement of BP, with verification in the contralateral arm; examination of the optic fundi; calculation

Table 14.4 Cardiovascular risk factors

Major risk factors
Hypertension*
Cigarette smoking
Obesity* (body mass index ≥30 kg/m²)
Physical inactivity
Dyslipidemia*
Diabetes mellitus*
Microalbuminuria or estimated GFR <60 mL/min
Age (older than 55 for men, 65 for women)
Family history of premature cardiovascular disease (men under age 55 or women under age 65)

*From: National Heart, Lung, and Blood Institute; National Institutes of Health; U.S. Department of Health and Human Services, JNC 7 Express

Table 14.5 Target organ damage

Heart	Left ventricular hypertrophy Angina or prior myocardial infarction Prior coronary revascularization Heart failure
Brain	Stroke Transient ischemic attack
Chronic kidney disease	
Peripheral arterial disease	
Retinopathy	

From: National Heart, Lung, and Blood Institute; National Institutes of Health; U.S. Department of Health and Human Services, JNC 7 Express

of body mass index (BMI) (measurement of waist circumference also may be useful); auscultation for carotid, abdominal, and femoral bruits; palpation of the thyroid gland; thorough examination of the heart and lungs; examination of the abdomen for enlarged kidneys, masses, and abnormal aortic pulsation; palpation of the lower extremities for edema and pulses; and neurological assessment.

Because blood pressures fluctuate considerably throughout the day and are heavily influenced by external and environmental influences, many measurements are often needed. Accurate and proper technique in BP measurement is paramount, especially in the obese population.

14.4.4.1 Accurate (Proper) Blood Pressure Measurement in the Patient with Overweight or Obesity

Many requirements are needed for proper blood pressure measurement, including posture, arm support and position, proper arm selection, and usage of correct cuff and bladder. Improper techniques and equipment usage may lead to overestimation (undercuffing) and underestimation (overcuffing) of the patient's blood pressure. Due to these variables influencing the blood pressure measurement, obese patients usually have a higher rate of inaccurate measurement when compared to nonobese patients mainly due to increased mismatching of the bladder and arm. The regular cuff for adults does not have sufficient length, thus, requiring obese patients to use a larger size cuff.

The shape of the arm also influences the fit of the cuff, with the conical-shaped arm of obese patients being the biggest problem. The shape of the upper arm is usually troncoconical, with the differences in the circumference of proximal and distal being anywhere from 1 to 20 cm, with the average value being 8.7 cm. When the arm circumference near the shoulder is much greater than normal, usually in the case of obesity, a cylindrical cuff does not provide an adequate fit, yielding an inaccurate blood pressure measurement. If a larger size cuff is used, then the distal end of the cuff will remain loose, causing an overestimation of the patient's blood pressure.

Another factor hindering blood pressure measurement in obese patients is the length of the arm. Most obese patients will have a large upper arm circumference along with a short upper arm length. Due to the larger arm circumference, a larger cuff size is needed, but this may also result in the cuff being too long and passing the elbow. With this paradoxical circumstance, it may be difficult to select the proper cuff size for an accurate blood pressure measurement. Because of these problems, alternative methods are required for blood pressure measurement in obese patients.

In patients with overweight or obesity, it may be necessary to use special cuffs that can accommodate those with "irregular" arm dimensions. Another solution is to use automated devices with special software that can yield an accurate blood pressure measurement even with incorrect cuffing. These devices can adjust the cuff accordingly to the patient's arm, thus, providing a proper cuffing.

Another method of measuring blood pressure in patients with "irregular" arm size is to circumvent the arm itself. With the creation of oscillometric automated BP measurement, wrist blood pressure measurement has become more popular and is readily available for consumer use. In normal-weight individuals, arm cuff is still recommended over wrist devices, but for obese patients, wrist BP measurement may be more suitable than arm cuff due to the problems discussed above.

Table 14.6 summarizes the steps to properly measure blood pressure in patients with overweight or obesity.

14.4.5 Laboratory Tests and Other Diagnostic Procedures

Laboratory tests recommended before initiating therapy include an electrocardiogram (EKG); urinalysis; blood glucose and hematocrit; serum potassium, creatinine (or the corresponding estimated glomerular filtration rate [GFR]), and calcium and a lipid profile that includes high-density lipoprotein cholesterol and low-density lipoprotein cholesterol and triglycerides. Optional tests include the measurement of urinary albumin excretion or albumin-to-creatinine ratio. More extensive testing for identifiable causes is not indicated generally unless BP control is not achieved. Table 14.7 summarizes the recommended laboratory tests and diagnostic procedures. Table 14.8 summarizes features of inappropriate hypertension when secondary causes of hypertension should be entertained. Table 14.9 lists the recommended workup for the common form of secondary hypertension.

Table 14.6 Guideline for measuring blood pressure of patients with overweight or obesity

Blood pressure should be measured after the patient has emptied their bladder and has been seated for 5 min, with their back supported and legs resting on the ground (not crossed)
A longer and wider cuff is required for sufficient compression of brachial artery due to the patient's arm size
The center of the bladder should be placed over the brachial artery pulse
Even if the arm length is insufficient despite larger arm circumference, a very long cuff is still preferred due to difficulty of fitting a standard cuff around the arm
If the arm circumference is larger than 50 cm, then a thigh cuff may be used in place of the arm cuff
If neither thigh nor arm cuff fits, then a forearm cuff may be used. The forearm should be raised to the heart level while searching for radial pulse
Korotkoff sounds could be used for detecting systolic pressure by using a Doppler probe or other oscillometric device over the radial artery. This method usually results in an overestimation of diastolic pressure but will give a good estimation for systolic pressure

Adapted from Pickering et al. (2005); used with permission

Table 14.7 Suggested initial evaluation of patients with overweight or obesity, and hypertension

History and physical examination
Urinalysis—Evaluating microalbuminuria
Chemical profile, including creatinine, blood glucose, potassium, uric acids, and lipids. A hemoglobin A1c is an option in patients with history of hyperglycemia
Electrocardiogram

Table 14.8 Features indicative of secondary hypertension

Age less than 30 years in nonobese, nonblack patients with a negative family history of hypertension and no other risk factors (e.g., obesity) for hypertension
Sudden-onset, intermittent, or labile blood pressure
Resistant to appropriate therapy
Associate with abnormal clinical and laboratory findings; cardiomegaly, left ventricular hypertrophy (LVH), funduscopic findings of grade 2 or above, abdominal bruit, variable features of tremor, tachycardia, sweating
Level of blood pressure > 180/110 mmHg
Proven age of onset before puberty

Table 14.9 Tests for common causes of secondary hypertension

	Diagnosis procedures	
Diagnosis	Initial	Confirming
Renovascular disease	Duplex sonography	CT angiogram, MRI, MRA, aortogram
Coarctation	Blood pressure in legs	Echocardiogram, aortogram
Chronic renal disease	Urinalysis, serum creatinine, renal ultrasound	Renal biopsy
Pheochromocytoma	Plasma free metanephrines, timed urine collection for metanephrines, urine collection (24-h specimen) for free catecholamines and metanephrines	CT scanning, MRI of the adrenal glands, MIBG scintigraphy
Primary hyperaldosteronism	Aldosterone/plasma renin activity ratio	Saline suppression test, CT scan or MRI of adrenals, adrenal venous sampling (AVS)
Cushing's syndrome	24-h free cortisol excretion, overnight dexamethasone suppression, late-night serum/salivary cortisol	Adrenal CT scan, pituitary MRI, petrosal sinus sampling for ACTH, high-dose dexamethasone suppression
Thyroid disease	Serum thyroid function tests	Thyroid antibodies, thyroid uptake, and scan +/− ultrasound
Hyperparathyroidism	Serum calcium, phosphorus, and parathyroid levels	Parathyroid scan, neck ultrasound, CT scan of the neck

14.5 Hypertension Management

The cornerstone to hypertension management is meal planning and lifestyle changes. These changes will promote weight loss that will help to bring blood pressure to goals. In addition there should be a reduction of sodium intake and moderation of alcohol intake to maximize improvement in blood pressure levels.

Initial management of hypertension should include a healthy diet, weight control, and regular physical activity. In some cases, this may decrease or eliminate the need for medication. Ongoing weight management, dietary changes, and physical activity also have the potential for minimizing chronic medications and multidrug therapy.

In the setting of overweight and obesity, it is important to consider sodium intake as well as weight loss in patients with hypertension. The Dietary Approaches to Stop Hypertension (DASH-Sodium) trial showed low sodium intake decreased blood pressure in patients with high-to-normal blood pressure or stage 1 hypertension. Individuals with high-to-normal blood pressure or stage 1 hypertension should reduce sodium intake to 3 g or less per day.

Alcohol consumption levels should also be considered. Patients who drink alcohol daily tend to have higher blood pressure levels than people who do not drink daily. Patients who drink daily had systolic blood pressure levels 6.6 mmHg higher and diastolic BP levels 4.7 mmHg higher than once daily drinkers.

The Look AHEAD study gave insights into the effects of weight loss on hypertension. In overweight or obese adults with elevated cardiovascular disease risk including type 2 diabetes and hypertension, there is a dose-response relationship between the amount of weight loss achieved for up to 3 years with diet and lifestyle changes alone or combined with orlistat. The study showed that at weight losses less than 5%, reductions in blood pressure were mild and variable. However, at a 5% weight loss, a weighted mean reduction in systolic and diastolic blood pressures of approximately 3 and 2 mmHg was seen, respectively. This trial also showed that a 5% weight loss achieved by intensive lifestyle intervention in overweight and obese adults with type 2 diabetes is associated with a lower prevalence of patients who are prescribed medications compared with controls.

The Report from the Panel Members Appointed to the Eighth Joint National Committee (JNC8) gave guidance regarding initial therapy. In the general nonblack population, including those with diabetes, initial antihypertensive treatment should include a thiazide-type diuretic, a calcium channel blocker (CCB), angiotensin-converting enzyme inhibitor (ACEI), or angiotensin receptor blocker (ARB). In the general black population, including those with diabetes, initial antihypertension treatment should include a thiazide-type diuretics, CCB, ACEI, or ARB.

14.5.1 ACE Inhibitors

There have been studies that investigated a possible link between obesity and the renin-angiotensin system (RAS). Data have clearly demonstrated the presence of a fully functional RAS in animal and human adipose tissue. Evidence from genetically manipulated animals or from experiments in which the RAS was blocked suggests that the activity of the RAS is directly related to the accumulation of body fat. In a rodent study, melanocortin-4 receptor-deficient female rates were used because functional loss of melanocortin receptor MCR4 activity leads to hyperphagia and an obese, glucose-tolerant phenotype. ACE inhibition for 8 weeks produced weight loss. Furthermore, weight loss following ACE inhibitor treatment was specific to fat mass, while lean mass was unaffected.

The UKPDS study gave some insights regarding both the reduction in blood pressure and weight changes in the setting of type 2 diabetes. In total, 1148 participants with type 2 diabetes were treated with either captopril or atenolol. The average age was 56 years, and mean blood pressure at baseline was 160/94 mmHg. In the study, the two drugs were equally effective in lowering blood pressure to 144/83 mmHg in the captopril group and to 143/81 mmHg in the atenolol group. There was greater compliance in the captopril group compared to the atenolol group by 78% and 65% ($p = 0.0001$), respectively. Both groups were equally effective in reducing macrovascular end points as well as preventing deterioration in retinopathy or developing clinical grade albuminuria >300 mg/L. However, there was a difference in weight gain in the two groups. The participants in the atenolol group gained more weight than those participants in the captopril group, that is, 3.4 kg versus 1.6 kg over 9 years ($p = 0.020$).

14.5.2 Beta-Blockers

Beta-blockers have been used for blood pressure control as well as other setting such as heart rate control and migraine prophylaxis. There are various agents in this class that differ in their pharmacological properties. The first group comprises the nonvasodilating beta-1 selective blockers that preferentially inhibit cardiac beta-1 receptors as opposed to beta-2 receptors. Some examples are atenolol and metoprolol. Carvedilol is pharmacologically different and inhibits beta-1 and beta-2 receptors and alpha-1 receptors.

In the past, there have been reports of weight gain with beta-blocker therapy. This effect would be counterproductive in the overweight and obese population. There is now growing evidence that this effect is significant. Several mechanisms have been proposed, including reduction in resting energy expenditure, reduction in the thermic effect of food, reduction in exercise tolerance, increase in tiredness, reduction in nonexercise thermogenesis, inhibition of lipolysis, and exacerbation of insulin resistance. In addition to proposing mechanism for weight gain, Sharma et al. performed a systemic analysis of the literature. The median difference in weight between the beta-blocker groups and the control group was 1.2 kg and significant. There was no relationship between any demographic characteristic and beta-blocker-induced weight change; therefore, all patients appeared susceptible to weight gain when they received a beta-blocker.

Chronic beta-blocker therapy was also studied in two settings, a hypertension clinic and a diabetes clinic. Patients treated with beta-blockers had a higher weight gain compared with patients not treated with beta-blockers by 17.2 ± 3.2 kg ($p = 0.004$) and 9.2 ± 1.2 kg ($p = 0.0002$) in the hypertension clinic and diabetes clinic, respectively. There are some data to suggest propranolol may cause more weight gain than atenolol and metoprolol.

In addition to weight data, the resting energy expenditure (REE) has been studied in the setting of beta-blocker therapy to determine if there was a difference in selective and nonselective beta-blockers. Participants underwent a structured physical training program and a hypocaloric diet for a period of approximately 31 days. REE was measured by the indirect calorimetri method. Participants treated with selective beta-1 adrenoceptor blockers had a REE 1704 ± 283 versus nonselective beta-blockers 1974 ± 278; $p = 0.012$. There was also a difference in weight loss between selective versus nonselective beta-blockers −5.6 ± 2.4 vs −7.5 ± 2.7, respectively ($p = 0.048$).

14.5.3 Diuretics

Clinical trials have shown thiazide diuretics are effective tools for lowering blood pressure. Diuretics are an inexpensive option for blood pressure control. The Antihypertension and Lipid-Lowering Treatment to Prevent Heart Attack Trial (ALLHAT) was a randomized, double-blind, multicenter clinical trial sponsored by the National Heart, Lung, and Blood Institute. Participants were 33,357 people aged 55 years and older with hypertension and at least one other CHD risk factor were randomly assigned to receive chlorthalidone 12.5–25 mg a day, amlodipine 2.5–10 mg a day, or lisinopril 10–40 mg a day. The mean follow-up was 4.9 years, and there was no difference in the groups with regard to fatal or nonfatal myocardial infarctions. Five-year systolic blood pressures were significantly higher in the amlodipine (0.8 mmHg, $p = 0.03$) and lisinopril (2 mmHg, $p < 0.001$) groups compared with chlorthalidone, and 5-year diastolic blood pressure was significantly lower with amlodipine (0.8 mmHg, $p < 0.001$). For amlodipine versus chlorthalidone, secondary outcomes were similar except for a higher 6-year rate of HF with amlodipine (10.2% vs. 7.7%; RR, 1.38; 95% CI, 1.25–1.52). For lisinopril versus chlorthalidone, lisinopril had higher 6-year rates of combined CVD (33.3% vs. 30.9%; RR, 1.10; 95% CI, 1.05–1.16); stroke (6.3% vs. 5.6%; RR, 1.15; 95% CI, 1.02–1.30); and HF (8.7% vs. 7.7%; RR, 1.19; 95% CI, 1.07–1.31). The authors concluded that the chlorthalidone data supported first-line use of diuretics because of their efficacy compared to the other agents as well as lower cost.

In the Trial of Antihypertensive Interventions and Management, mildly hypertensive obese patients were noted to lose more weight when receiving chlorthalidone compared to atenolol or placebo. The mean weight reductions at 6 months in the three groups were 6.9, 3.0, and 4.4 kg, respectively. The weight loss was most pronounced at 6 months and persisted at month 24.

Despite its excellent blood pressure-lowering effect, thiazide diuretics have been shown to cause glucose dysregulation and may lead to overt diabetes in obese hypertensive patients. In the ALLHAT trial, chlorthalidone was associated with significantly higher incidence of diabetes compared to lisinopril in patients with metabolic syndrome (17.1% vs. 12.6%). In a prospective, randomized, open-label trial involving 240 obese, hypertensive patients with metabolic syndrome, the combination of low-dose hydrochlorothiazide plus losartan was found to significantly increase the risk of new-onset diabetes compared to verapamil plus trandolapril (27% vs. 11%).

14.5.4 Calcium Channel Blockers (CCBs)

Calcium channel blockers (CCBs) are effective drugs to control blood pressure in the setting of hypertension. They work by inhibiting intracellular migration of calcium into smooth muscle and myocardial cells, reducing arterial pressure through decrease in peripheral vascular pressure. In the setting of overweight and obesity, weight gain can be seen. However, this weight gain may be more due to fluid retention because CCB's blunt postural skin vasoconstriction, an autoregulatory mechanism that minimizes gravitational increases in capillary pressure and avoids fluid extravasation when standing, rather than a gain in fat mass. In a research project that measured leg weight in the setting of essential hypertension, subjects were treated with amlodipine 5 and 10 mg. Both doses showed an increase in leg weight. In the same study, when patients were treated with the ACEI enalapril, there was a reduction in the CCB-induced dose-dependent fluid accumulation.

Unlike the thiazide diuretics, calcium channel blockers do not have adverse metabolic effects and are not associated with increased risk of inducing diabetes. If a calcium channel blocker is needed in obese hypertensive patients, a nondihydropyridine calcium channel blocker may be more beneficial. This class can inhibit sympathetic activity, a known cause for hypertension in obese patients, and decrease hyperfiltration and microalbuminuria that are often seen in patients with metabolic syndrome.

14.5.5 Special Populations

The Eighth Joint National Committee (JNC8) set goals for people 18 years and older with diabetes. The initial pharmacological treatment goal in this group is to initiate pharmacological therapy at an SBP of 140 mmHg or greater or diastolic blood pressure of 90 mmHg or greater. The goal of treatment is SBP <140 and DBP < 90.0 mmHg. As discussed in the ACEI section above, both ACEI and beta-blockers were equally effective in reducing the emergence of macrovascular and microvascular complications; however, beta-blockers had undesirable weight gain. In the Appropriate Blood Pressure Control in Diabetes study, enalapril was compared to the CCB nisoldipine, and the ACE was found to have a highly significant reduction in the number of fatal MIs in a 5-year period compared to the CCB. Diuretics also have a role in treating hypertension in the setting of diabetes. In patient with diabetes, therapeutic regimens based primarily on thiazide diuretics were associated with a 33% decrease in CVD mortality in the hypertension detection and follow-up program.

14.6 Conclusions

Thirty percent to 75% of the cases of hypertension diagnosed in the western world can be directly attributed to obesity. As the prevalence of obesity increases, the prevalence of hypertension with its associated cardiovascular risk will increase as well. Obesity is an important cause of resistant hypertension, requiring a multipronged approach to effectively address the problem. The pathophysiology of obesity-related hypertension is not yet completely understood, but some proposed etiologies include blood volume overload, renin-angiotensin stimulation due to inappropriately high aldosterone levels, insulin resistance state, and overstimulation of the sympathetic nervous system.

Treating hypertension in the obese patients requires addressing obesity as part of the therapeutic plan. Lifestyle management focusing on decreasing sodium, alcohol, and caloric intake and increasing potassium and physical activities should be stressed. Weight loss medications may be necessary to achieve progressive or sustained weight loss. If weight loss is not possible, at least weight maintenance should be the goal.

ACE inhibitors or angiotensin receptor blockers are first-line antihypertensive agents for obese, hypertensive patients. These drugs lower blood pressure without worsening glucose or lipid metabolism. Nondihydropyridine calcium channel blockers are also drugs of first choice in this setting due to their favorable metabolic profiles. In clinical practice, antihypertensive monotherapy is seldom sufficient to control blood pressure. More than half of obese hypertensive patients are treated with two or more antihypertensive agents. Diuretics and beta-blockers are reasonable second- or third-line drugs if the defects warrant their use in a particular patient (hypervolemia, increased sympathetic activity, etc.)

Data on how to treat obese patients with resistant hypertension are scarce. These patients may require drugs that address multiple targets (RAAS, SNS, renal sodium excretion, and hypervolemia) as well as drugs that help with weight loss. Adding a mineralocorticoid antagonist may also be useful in these patients.

Reading List

Abernethy DR, Schwartz JB. Calcium-antagonist drugs. N Engl J Med. 1999;24(suppl A):S18–24.

ALLHAT Officers and Coordinators for the ALLHAT Collaborative Research Group. The Antihypertension and Lipid-Lowering Treatment to Prevent Heart Attack Trial. Major outcomes in high-risk hypertensive patients randomized to angiotensin-converting enzyme inhibitor or calcium channel blocker vs diuretic: The Antihypertensive and Lipid-Lowering Treatment to Prevent Heart Attack Trial (ALLHAT). JAMA. 2002;288(23):2981–97.

Bakris G, Molitch M, Hewkin A, et al. Differences in glucose tolerance between fixed-dose antihypertensive drug combinations in people with metabolic syndrome. Diabetes Care. 2006;29:2592.

Chan JM, Rimm EB, Colditz GA, et al. Obesity, fat distribution, and weight gain as risk factors for clinical diabetes in men. Diabetes Care. 1994;17(9):961–9.

Chobanian AV, Bakris GL, Black HR, et al. The seventh report of the Joint National Committee on prevention, detection, evaluation, and treatment of high blood pressure: the JNC 7 report. JAMA. 2003;289(19):2560–72.

Daskalopoulou SS, Rabi DM, Zarnke KB, et al. The 2015 Canadian Hypertension Education Program recommendations for blood pressure measurement, diagnosis, assessment of risk, prevention, and treatment of hypertension. Can J Cardiol. 2015;31(5):549–68.

Davis BR, Oberman A, Blaufox MD, et al. Effect of antihypertensive therapy on weight loss. The Trial of Antihypertensive Interventions and Management Research Group. Hypertension. 1992;19:393–9.

De Courten M, Ferrari P, Schneider M, et al. Lack of effect of long-term amlodipine on insulin sensitivity and plasma insulin in obese patients with essential hypertension. Eur J Clin Pharmacol. 1993;44:457–62.

DiNicolantonio JJ, Fares H, Asfandyar KN, et al. B-blockers in hypertension, diabetes, heart failure and acute myocardial infarction: a review of the literature. Open Heart. 2015;2:e000230:1–10.

Estacio RO, Jeffers BW, Hiatt WR, et al. The effect of nisoldipine as compared to enalapril on cardiovascular outcomes in patients with non-insulin-dependent diabetes and hypertension. N Engl J Med. 1998;338:645–52.

Franklin SS, Jacobs MJ, Wong ND, L'Italien GJ, Lapuerta P. Predominance of isolated systolic hypertension among middle-aged and elderly US hypertensives: analysis based on National Health and Nutrition Examination Survey (NHANES) III. Hypertension. 2001a;37(3):869–74.

Franklin SS, Larson MG, Khan SA, et al. Does the relation of blood pressure to coronary heart disease risk change with aging? The Framingham Heart Study. Circulation. 2001b;103(9):1245–9.

Go AS, Mozaffarian D, Roger VL, et al. American Heart Association Statistics Committee and Stroke Statistics Subcommittee. Heart disease and stroke statistics—2014 update: a report from the American Heart Association. Circulation. 2014;129(3):e28–e292.

Gondoni LA, Tagliaferri MA, Titon AM, et al. Effect of chronic treatment with beta-blockers on resting energy expenditure in obese hypertensive patients during a low-calorie and physical training program. Nutr Metab Cardiovasc Dis. 2003;13(4):232–7.

Goodfriend TL, Calhoun DA. Resistant hypertension, obesity, sleep apnea, and aldosterone: theory and therapy. Hypertension. 2004;43(3):518–24.

Hajjar I, Kotchen TA. Trends in prevalence, awareness, treatment, and control of hypertension in the United States, 1988–2000. JAMA. 2003;290:199–206.

Hall JE. Louis K. Dahl Memorial Lecture. Renal and cardiovascular mechanisms of hypertension in obesity. Hypertension. 1994;23(3):381–94.

Huang Z, Willett WC, Manson JE, et al. Body weight, weight change, and risk for hypertension in women. Ann Intern Med. 1998;128(2):81–8.

Hypertension Detection and Follow-up Program Cooperative Group. Five-year findings of the hypertension detection and follow-up program. JAMA. 1979;242:2562–71.

James PA, Oparil S, Carter BL, et al. 2014 evidence-based guideline for the management of high blood pressure in adults: report from the panel members appointed to the Eighth Joint National Committee (JNC 8). JAMA. 2014;311(5):507–20.

Kailasam MT, Parmer RJ, Cervenka JH, et al. Divergent effect of dihydropyridine and phenylalkylamine calcium channel antagonist classes on autonomic function in human hypertension. Hypertension. 1995;26:143–9.

Lee P, Kenge AP, Greenfield JR, et al. Metabolic sequelae of beta blocker therapy: weighing in on the obesity epidemic? Int J Obes. 2011;35(11):1395–403.

Leslie WS, Hankey CR, Lean MEJ. Weight gain as an adverse effect of some commonly prescribed drugs: a systemic review. Q J Med. 2007;100:395–404.

Messerli FH, Christie B, DeCarvalho JG, et al. Obesity and essential hypertension. Hemodynamics, intravascular volume, sodium excretion, and plasma renin activity. Arch Intern Med. 1981;141(1):81–5.

Morel Y, Gadient A, Keller U, et al. Insulin sensitivity in obese hypertensive dyslipidemic patients treated with enalapril or atenolol. J Cardiovasc Pharmacol. 1995;26:306–11.

Mozzafarian D, Benjamin EJ, Go AS, et al. Heart disease and stroke statistics-2015 update: a report from the American Heart Association. Circulation. 2015;131:e29–322.

Mul JD, Seeley RJ, Woods SC, et al. Angiotensin-converting enzyme inhibition reduces food intake and weight gain and improves glucose tolerance in melanocortin-4 receptor deficient female rats. Physiol Behav. 2013;121:43–8.

National Institutes of Health, National Heart, Lung and Blood Institute. Managing overweight and obesity in adults: systemic evidence review from the obesity expert panel, 2013. Bethesda: U.S. Department of Health and Human Services; 2013. p. 26–8.

Nguyen NT, Magno CP, Lane KT, et al. Association of hypertension, diabetes, dyslipidemia, and metabolic syndrome with obesity: findings from the National Health and Nutrition Examination Survey, 1999 to 2004. J Am Coll Surg. 2008;207(6):928–34.

Nwankwo T, Yoon SS, Burt V, Gu Q. Hypertension among adults in the US: National Health and Nutrition Examination Survey, 2011–2012, NCHS data brief, no. 133. Hyattsville: National Center for Health Statistics, Centers for Disease Control and Prevention, US Dept of Health and Human Services; 2013.

Palatini P, Parati G. Blood pressure measurement in very obese patients: a challenging problem. J Hypertens. 2011;29(3):425–9.

Pedrinelli R, Dell'Omo G, Melillo E, et al. Amlodipine, enalapril and dependant leg edema in essential hypertension. Hypertension. 2000;35:621–5.
Pickering T. Recommendations for the use of home (self) and ambulatory blood pressure monitoring. American Society of Hypertension Ad Hoc Panel. Am J Hypertens. 1996;9:1–11.
Pickering TG, Hall JE, Appel LJ, et al. Recommendations for blood pressure measurement in humans and experimental animals: part 1: blood pressure measurement in humans: a statement for professionals from the Subcommittee of Professional and Public Education of the American Heart Association Council on High Blood Pressure Research. Circulation. 2005;111(5):697–716.
Rahmouni K, Correia ML, Haynes WG, Mark AL. Obesity-associated hypertension: new insights into mechanisms. Hypertension. 2005;45(1):9–14.
Reaven GM, Lithell H, Landsberg L. Hypertension and associated metabolic abnormalities—the role of insulin resistance and the sympathoadrenal system. N Engl J Med. 1996;334(6):374.
Rocchini AP, Katch V, Kveselis D, et al. Insulin and renal sodium retention in obese adolescents. Hypertension. 1989;14(4):367–74.
Sacks FM, Svetkey LP, Vollmer WM, et al. Effects on blood pressure of reduced dietary sodium and the Dietary Approaches to Stop Hypertension (DASH) diet. N Engl J Med. 2001;344:3–10.
Sarzani R, Salvi F, Dessì-Fulgheri P, Rappelli A. Renin-angiotensin system, natriuretic peptides, obesity, metabolic syndrome, and hypertension: an integrated view in humans. J Hypertens. 2008;26(5):831–43.
Schmieder RE, Messerli FH. Does obesity influence early target organ damage in hypertensive patients? Circulation. 1993;87(5):1482–8.
Seventh Report of the Joint National Committee on Prevention. Detection, evaluation and treatment of high blood pressure (JNC 7) express. National Heart, Lung, and Blood Institute. Bethesda, Md. 2003. JAMA. 2003;289:2560–71.
Sharma AM, Pischon T, Hardt S, et al. B-adrenergic receptor blockers and weight gain. A systemic analysis. Hypertension. 2001;37(2):250–4.
Siu AL, U.S. Preventive Services Task Force. Screening for high blood pressure in adults: U.S. Preventive Services Task Force recommendation statement. Ann Intern Med. 2015;163(10):778–86.
Sjöström L, Lindroos AK, Peltonen M, et al. Lifestyle, diabetes, and cardiovascular risk factors 10 years after bariatric surgery. N Engl J Med. 2004;351:2683.
Spurgeon D. NIH promotes use of lower cost drugs for hypertension. BMJ. 2004;328:539.
Stamler R. Implications of the INTERSALT study. Hypertension. 1991;17(1 suppl):I16–20.
Steinberg HO, Chaker H, Leaming R, et al. Obesity/insulin resistance is associated with endothelial dysfunction. Implications for the syndrome of insulin resistance. J Clin Invest. 1996;97(11):2601–10.
Taylor BC, Wilt TJ, Welch HG. Impact of diastolic and systolic blood pressure on mortality: implications for the definition of "normal". J Gen Intern Med. 2011;26(7):685–90.
The fifth report of the Joint National Committee on detection, evaluation, and treatment of high blood pressure (JNC V). Arch Intern Med. 1993;153:154–83.
Torre JJ, Bloomgarden ZT, Dickey RA, et al. American Association of Clinical Endocrinologists Medical Guidelines for Clinical Practice for the diagnosis and treatment of hypertension. Endocr Pract. 2006;12(2):193–222.
Trovato GM, Pace P, Martines GF, et al. Stress, abdominal obesity and intrarenal resistive index in essential hypertension. Clin Ter. 2012;163(4):299–305.
Tu W, Eckert GJ, DiMeglio LA, et al. Intensified effect of adiposity on blood pressure in overweight and obese children. Hypertension. 2011;58:818.
UK Prospective Diabetes Study Group. Efficacy of atenolol and captopril in reducing risk of macrovascular and microvascular complications in type 2 diabetes: UKPDS 39. Br Med J. 1998;317:713–20.
Vasan RS, Beiser A, Seshadri S, et al. Residual lifetime risk for developing hypertension in middle-aged women and men: the Framingham Heart Study. JAMA. 2002;287:1003–10.

Weisinger RS, Begg DP, Chen N, et al. The problem of obesity: is there a role for antagonists of the renin-angiotensin system? Asia Pac J Clin Nutr. 2007;16(suppl 1):359–67.

Willett WC, Dietz WH, Colditz GA. Guidelines for healthy weight. N Engl J Med. 1999;341:427.

Wilson PW, D'Agostino RB, Sullivan L, et al. Overweight and obesity as determinants of cardiovascular risk: the Framingham experience. Arch Intern Med. 2002;162:1867.

Young JH, Klag MJ, Muntner P, et al. Blood pressure and decline in kidney function: findings from the Systolic Hypertension in the Elderly Program (SHEP). J Am Soc Nephrol. 2002;13:2776–82.

Zipes DP, Libby P, Bonow RO, Braunwald E, editors. Braunwald's heart disease: a textbook of cardiovascular medicine. 7th ed. Philadelphia: Saunders; 2005. p. 921–1012.

Chapter 15
Gonadal Dysfunction in Males with Overweight or Obesity, and Adiposopathy

J. Michael Gonzalez-Campoy

> **Pearls of Wisdom**
> - Very little high-level evidence is available about bariatric hypogonadism, or how isolated overweight or obesity cause hypogonadism in men.
> - Bariatric hypogonadism is a reversible process.
> - Successful management of overweight or obesity and their systemic complications will generally result in the resolution of bariatric hypogonadism, and sometimes in that of bariatric erectile dysfunction.
> - Treatment of hypogonadism in men with obesity is effective adjunct therapy to facilitate the initiation of lifestyle changes.
> - Use of pharmacological and surgical therapies to manage bariatric hypogonadism must be done in the context of each patient's overall health.

15.1 Introduction

This chapter discusses the relationship between overweight or obesity, adiposopathy, and hypogonadism in men, in the absence of comorbidities that are associated with one or both of these conditions. Therefore, the hypogonadism associated with either dysmetabolic syndrome or type 2 diabetes mellitus (T2DM) is not addressed in this chapter.

J. M. Gonzalez-Campoy
Minnesota Center for Obesity, Metabolism and Endocrinology, PA (MNCOME), Eagan, MN, USA
e-mail: drmike@mncome.com

J. M. Gonzalez-Campoy et al. (eds.), *Bariatric Endocrinology*,
https://doi.org/10.1007/978-3-319-95655-8_15

15.2 Definitions

15.2.1 Bariatric Hypogonadism Versus Hypogonadal Overweight or Obesity

True *bariatric hypogonadism* in men refers to hypogonadism resulting from the accumulation of excess fat mass. In this case, the development of overweight, obesity, and adiposopathy is etiological to the hypogonadism.

Although clinically similar to bariatric hypogonadism, *hypogonadal overweight or obesity* is the consequence of male hypogonadism and its systemic consequences. In this instance, gonadal dysfunction is etiological to overweight, obesity, and adiposopathy.

Hypogonadal overweight or obesity represents the other side of the pathological "coin" of bariatric hypogonadism. The importance of differentiating between these two conditions lies in how each will need to be managed. Therefore, the term bariatric hypogonadism facilitates the differentiation between these two etiopathogenic pathways that result in the simultaneous presence of overweight, obesity, adiposopathy, and hypogonadism in a male patient.

15.2.2 Bariatric Hypogonadism

Total testosterone [TT], free testosterone [fT], and nonsex hormone-binding globulin [SHBG]-bound testosterone [non-SHBG-bound T] are decreased in proportion to the degree of obesity in men. The decrease is similar for all three parameters. Overweight and obesity are associated with profound alterations in androgen secretion, transport, metabolism, and action. Androgen changes in overweight or obesity increase the susceptibility to develop comorbidities, especially T2DM and cardiovascular disease (CVD). In men with overweight or obesity, fertility can often be affected, in many cases very severely. This is the result of significant decreases in the sperm count. The infertility is correlated with increasing body mass index (BMI). Conversely, low T irrespective of symptoms is associated with obesity.

Overweight or obesity is frequently a cause of prediabetes. As is the case in patients with T2DM, hypogonadism in men with obesity is complex. Men with obesity actually can have primary, secondary, and tertiary hypogonadism at the same time, since obesity can produce endocrine alterations that impact, both directly and indirectly, the functions of the testis, the pituitary, and the hypothalamus. Furthermore, other obesity-related morbidities like obstructive sleep apnea (OSA) can also negatively impact male reproduction. This complexity has to be taken into consideration when evaluating the patient with overweight or obesity, as well as when selecting the appropriate management protocol.

In the management of bariatric hypogonadism, one must first determine if hypogonadism is indeed present. Then, one must determine if fertility is desired, and if so, determine if it is impaired. Finally, one must determine which interventions are safe and effective for a given patient, and in which order they must be instituted.

With the current pandemic of overweight and obesity, there are increasing numbers of children and adolescents affected. This can result in alterations in sexual development. Although some markers of puberty appear to indicate an early onset of puberty, others point in the opposite direction, to delayed puberty. However, more careful analyses show that testicular growth and pubertal progression through Tanner stages are normal in children with overweight or obesity. The endocrine story is not quite as reassuring. TT is normal during early pubertal development, but by Tanner stage 5, boys with overweight or obesity have reduced levels. SHBG levels in boys who are lean never change during pubertal development. On the other hand, boys who have overweight or obesity have a decline in SHBG levels during this period. By Tanner stage 5, boys with or without overweight or obesity have the same SHBG levels. Regarding fT, during early development [Tanner stages 1 and 2], fT is elevated in boys with overweight or obesity, but when they reach Tanner stage 5, their fT levels are low. Throughout pubertal development, estradiol (E_2) levels and E_2/T are elevated in boys with overweight or obesity. Finally, no measurable alterations in gonadotropin (Gn) levels are observed during the pubertal development of boys with overweight or obesity. In summary, by the end of their pubertal development, boys with overweight or obesity have an endocrine profile almost identical to that of men with overweight or obesity.

15.2.3 Hypogonadal Overweight or Obesity

Although less common, hypogonadal overweight or obesity is present as one of the consequences of pure male hypogonadism. When T deficiency is present, it induces expansion of fat mass and subsequent dysregulation of several functions controlled by adipose tissue. Among these endocrine consequences are a reduction in SHBG production, an increase in peripheral aromatase activity and, most importantly, an elevation of circulating leptin [Lep] levels. These alterations are important factors in initiating a vicious cycle that promotes increased adiposity, adiposopathy, overweight, or obesity, and ultimately leads to worsening of the hypogonadal state.

15.2.4 Bariatric ED

ED is common, and tends to be of greater severity, in men with overweight or obesity, whether ascertained by high BMI or high waist circumference. Lep is proinflammatory and increases directly and proportionally to the degree of adiposity. On the other hand, adiponectin is anti-inflammatory and its level is reduced in obesity. Therefore, it has been hypothesized that an adiposity-related chronic inflammatory status might be involved in the pathogenesis of ED in men with obesity.

15.3 Evaluation of Hypogonadism in Males with Overweight or Obesity

The diagnosis of male hypogonadism is one of exclusion. Many disorders share its main signs and symptoms, such as T2DM, CVD, vitamin D insufficiency, psychiatric disorders, and of course obesity. To complicate things, all of these conditions can result in the development of hypogonadism, and conversely, they can be the consequence of hypogonadism. Therefore, in order to make the diagnosis of hypogonadism in men with overweight or obesity, a comprehensive history and physical examination must be done. The goal is to determine the primary pathology which led to the development of the other.

Men with overweight or obesity have a progressive decrease in testosterone (T) levels with increasing body weight. Hypogonadotropic hypogonadism with reduced T levels, well into the hypogonadal range, is common in men with overweight or obesity. TT is low in 57.7% of these men, and fT is reduced in about a third. Men with hypogonadotropic hypogonadism have high HbA_{1c} levels and almost three-fold higher risk for CVD. ED and decreased libido are about seven times more common in these patients. TT should be measured, preferably in the morning, on two different days by liquid chromatography tandem mass spectrometry. SHBG can be decreased in men with overweight or obesity, so fT or bioavailable T [bT] should be calculated. Lutropin or luteinizing hormone (LH) and follitropin or follicle-stimulating hormone (FSH) should be measured to determine if pituitary and/or hypothalamic functions are affected.

Seventy-three percent of men with overweight or obesity reported at least one symptom of impaired sexual function. Compared to men without them, men with overweight or obesity reported at least one symptom of impaired sexual function more frequently [OR = 1.45; CI: 1.14–1.85].

Many men with OSA have overweight or obesity. The severity of biochemical androgen deficiency increases with greater hypoxemia in men with OSA and increasing adiposity in men with overweight or obesity. Therefore, men with overweight or obesity and OSA are likely to be at great risk for hypogonadism.

Table 15.1 summarizes the steps to determine if a man with overweight or obesity has hypogonadism. An assessment of the degree of adiposity (including biometric measurements) is paramount. The goal is to determine if the patient suffers from bariatric hypogonadism or, conversely, if the obesity is a consequence of hypogonadism. This distinction determines the course of management that should be followed.

15.4 Management

15.4.1 Efficacy and Safety of Testosterone Replacement Therapy (TRT) in Men with Overweight or Obesity

Several studies have demonstrated favorable effects of TRT in men with overweight or obesity. The current gold standard for TRT is the use of transdermal modalities

Table 15.1 Evaluation of the male with overweight or obesity and hypogonadism

H&P	Signs and symptoms
Family history	Positive paternal or maternal history of overweight or obesity
Patient history	High-caloric intake, meals rich in high-fructose syrup, sedentary lifestyle
Body habitus	Height, weight, waist circumference, fat pad with calipers, gynecomastia
Tegumentary	Loss of body hair, reduced shaving, hot flushes, sweats
Psychoneural	Depression, impaired cognition, poor concentration and memory, sleep disturbance, increased sleepiness
Musculoskeletal	Weakness, fatigue, reduced muscle bulk, osteopenia, or osteoporosis
Genitourinary	Testicular size with orchidometer, infertility, low sperm count, decreased libido, ED and/or LUTS, prostate cancer
Cardiorespiratory	CVD, OSA
Endocrine	TT levels below the normal range on at least two consecutive tests [<300 ng/dl, or according to some experts <270 ng/dl], LH levels, FSH levels, PRL levels. bT and fT levels can be calculated to confirm the presence of hypogonadism
Hematopoietic	Normochromic, normocytic anemia [due to a lack of erythropoietin stimulation by testosterone]

bT bioavailable testosterone, *CVD* cardiovascular disease, *ED* erectile dysfunction, *FSH* follitropin or follicle stimulating hormone, *fT* free testosterone, *H&P* History and Physical Examination, *LH* lutropin or luteinizing hormone, *LUTS* lower urinary tract symptoms, *ng/dl* nanograms per deciliter, *OSA* obstructive sleep apnea, *PRL* prolactin, *TT* total testosterone

such as gels, alcoholic solutions, or patches. Subdermal pellets, injectables, and oral formulations are also available. If the need to institute TRT is established, patients should be re-evaluated 3–6 months after onset or therapy. Because the T levels associated with the resolution of specific symptoms vary among symptoms and among individuals, the goal should be to attain a TT of 450–700 ng/dL. This range prevents reaching supraphysiological levels. However, in men with overweight or obesity and symptomatic bariatric hypogonadism, TRT is not to be automatically started. The reason for this is that sustained, significant weight loss can normalize gonadal function, obviating the need for TRT. TRT should not be considered as a weight loss therapy. The best indication for TRT in men with overweight or obesity is improvement in stamina, endurance, and muscular function in order to facilitate physical activity. TRT permits the patient to undertake physical activity regimens, which can result in weight loss. Improving lean muscle mass and muscle function leads to improved body composition and loss of fat mass.

The use of TRT in men with overweight or obesity and severe OSA initially worsens sleep-disordered breathing in a time-limited manner, irrespective of initial T concentrations. However, the negative effects of TRT on OSA are dose dependent. On the other hand, CPAP and weight loss increase blood T levels in men with OSA, or overweight or obesity, respectively. Therefore, one should initially use CPAP together with a weight loss program as the first line of management of the hypogonadism in men with overweight or obesity and OSA.

Multiple studies have demonstrated that TRT reduces fat mass and waist circumference in men with hypogonadism. These reductions are accompanied by body weight loss and a drop in the BMI. When used in men with overweight or obesity, and hypogonadism, TRT induces significant weight loss. The absolute decrease in weight is greater in men with a greater degree of adiposity. Based on this evidence and on the amelioration of multiple hypogonadism-related symptoms, it has been suggested that TRT should be an integral part of the management of overweight or obesity in men who also suffer from hypogonadism. The use of TRT is better justified as first line of management in men with hypogonadal overweight or obesity than in men with bariatric hypogonadism. In the former, the etiology lies in a deficiency in testicular steroidogenesis, and therefore, the replacement of T to normalize levels is more logical.

15.4.2 *Efficacy and Safety of Other Medications*

15.4.2.1 Aromatase Inhibitors

Since many men with overweight or obesity have elevated circulating estrogen levels, the use of aromatase inhibitors has been studied as a potential treatment of hypogonadotropic hypogonadism. Initially, testolactone was investigated and its use resulted in increases in serum LH and T levels, with concomitant reductions on serum E_2. Subsequently, letrazole was shown to produce similar results. However, in spite of its effects on endocrine parameters, letrazole had no impact on psychological function; body composition; capacity for physical activity; or glucose, lipid, and bone metabolism.

15.4.2.2 Clomiphene Citrate

A significant drawback of TRT in young men is that in elevating the circulating T levels, there may be suppression of the hypothalamus and pituitary. Thus, TRT leads to tertiary gonadal suppression and infertility. Therefore, other than for men with hypogonadal overweight or obesity where the cause is primary hypogonadism, treatment with clomiphene citrate should be considered. Although approved in the USA for the treatment of infertility in women, off-label use of clomiphene is appropriate for men. Clomiphene has been used in men since the 1960s. Clomiphene stimulates spermatogenesis by raising the endogenous serum FSH, LH, and T levels to initiate and maintain gametogenesis. There are improvements in the sperm count, sperm motility, and sperm morphology in response to clomiphene treatment.

15.4.3 *Bariatric Surgery in the Management of Hypogonadism in Men with Obesity*

In patients with stage 3 or higher obesity, bariatric surgery has a positive impact on their hypogonadotropic hypogonadism. Weight loss achieved 1 year after bariatric surgery leads to increases in TT, fT, SHBG, and FSH, as well as decreases in E_2 and PRL, but LH sometimes remains unchanged. The type of bariatric surgery does not appear to make a difference in the improvement of bariatric hypogonadism, with all types resulting in normalization or near normalization of testicular function.

15.4.4 Vitamin D in the Management of Hypogonadism in Men with Overweight or Obesity

Given that the relationship between overweight or obesity and reduced vitamin D levels is well established, and that vitamin D increases TT, bT, and fT levels, vitamin D supplementation should be considered as an inexpensive add on to the management of bariatric hypogonadism. Weight loss after bariatric surgery is associated with increases in vitamin D, but these increases do not normalize levels. Therefore, ingestion of at least 3000 IU vitamin D/day is needed to ensure sufficiency.

15.4.5 Lifestyle Modifications and Their Impact on Hypogonadism and Erectile Dysfunction in Men with Overweight or Obesity

Use of a meal-replacement regimen [Optifast®] results in improved plasma T levels. ED is also improved by nutritional intervention. A switch to the Mediterranean meal pattern improves erectile function as determined by the International Index of Erectile Function 5 [IIEF-5]. Physical activity improves circulating T levels, erectile function, and lower urinary tract symptoms (LUTS). Both TT and fT levels are increased by high-volume physical activity. Both high-volume and low-volume physical activities reverse ED and LUTS, as determined by the IIEF-5 and the International Prostate Symptom Scale, respectively.

15.4.6 Management of ED in Men with Overweight or Obesity

Use of a meal replacement regimen results in improved ED. Weight loss resulting from lifestyle changes tends to improve ED in many, but not all patients, and improvement in T levels does not predict resolution of ED. Bariatric surgery, on the other hand, improves ED in association with elevations in TT and fT levels. Phosphodiesterase inhibitors are appropriate therapy for ED in men with bariatric hypogonadism, if there are no contraindications.

15.4.7 *Management of Children and Adolescents with Overweight or Obesity*

Many of the alterations observed in men with overweight or obesity are not present in boys with overweight or obesity until the end of their pubertal development. One has time to undertake preventive measures to control excess adiposity in these patients. Hopefully, implemented in time, these measures should result in normal sexual function during adulthood.

15.5 Conclusion

15.5.1 *What We Want*

In bariatric endocrinology we want effective and safe management protocols that are appropriate for each individual patient, based on their medical status and lifetime goals.

15.5.2 *What We Know*

The degree of weight loss, either after bariatric surgery or due to a low-calorie meal plan, determines how well gonadal function is normalized. Similar data is not available yet for the long-term weight loss achieved through the implementation of a life-long chronic disease management program that includes pharmacotherapy.

15.5.3 *What We Need to Know*

To date, the data regarding the effects of overweight, obesity, and adiposopathy on male sexual function are at a suboptimal level of evidence. Larger, well-controlled studies are needed to both finish characterizing these alterations and to optimize their management. Just recently, the American Society for Reproductive Medicine issued an opinion on obesity and reproduction. However, even in this well-written document, there is scarce information on the reproductive disorders of men with overweight or obesity.

Table 15.2 Relationship between overweight or obesity and male hypogonadism

Tissue or cell type	Normal function	Overweight or obesity
Adipocytes	Produce Lep, produce low levels of E_2	Produce high levels of Lep, produce high levels of E_2
KISS neurons	Produce kisspeptin. Lep stimulates KISS neuron function	High E_2 levels, inflammation, and INS resistance inhibit KISS neuron function. Obesity inhibits Lep stimulation of KISS neuron function
GnRH neurons	Produce GnRH, kisspeptin stimulates GnRH neuron function	GnRH production is reduced. GnRH neuron response to kisspeptin may be impaired
Gonadotrophs	Produce LH and FSH, GnRH stimulates gonadotroph function	Gn production is reduced. Gonadotroph response to GnRH may be impaired
Leydig cells	Produce T and E_2, LH stimulates Leydig cell function	T and E_2 are reduced. Leydig cell response to LH is impaired. Obesity inhibits Lep stimulation of Leydig cell function
Sertoli cells	Regulates normal spermatogenesis, FSH and E_2 regulate Sertoli cell function	Spermatogenesis is impaired. Sertoli cell response to FSH may be impaired

E_2 estradiol, *FSH* follitropin or follicle-stimulating hormone, *Gn* gonadotropin, *GnRH* gonadorelin or gonadotropin-releasing hormone, *INS* insulin, *KISS* kisspeptin, *Lep* leptin, *LH* lutropin or luteinizing hormone, *T* testosterone

15.5.4 Summary

The management of the male patient with overweight or obesity, and adiposopathy, who presents with confirmed hypogonadism, starts with determining the root of the problem. If hypogonadism is a consequence of weight gain and adiposopathy, weight management should take precedence. On the other hand, if weight gain was caused by hypogonadism, then directly addressing the alteration[s] in the hypothalamic-pituitary-gonadal axis will resolve the hypogonadism and ameliorate the adipose tissue abnormalities.

Table 15.2 offers an oversimplified summary of the interrelationship between overweight or obesity and hypogonadism in men. Overweight or obesity, through direct effects, or as a result of the constituent adiposopathy, affects negatively, and in a variety of ways, every component of the hypothalamic-pituitary-testicular axis. Therefore, patients with overweight or obesity can simultaneously have primary, secondary, and tertiary hypogonadism. The clinical result is hypogonadism with impairment of both testicular steroidogenesis and spermatogenesis.

Reading List

Bendre SV, Murray PJ, Basaria S. Clomiphene citrate effectively increases testosterone in obese, young, hypogonadal men. Reprod Syst Sex Dis Curr Res. 2015;4(4):1–8.

Bhasin S, Cunningham GR, Hayes FJ, Matsumoto AM, Snyder PJ, Swerdloff RS, et al. Clinical practice guideline: testosterone therapy in men with androgen deficiency syndromes: an Endocrine Society clinical practice guideline. J Clin Endocrinol Metab. 2010;95:2536–59.

Botella-Carretero JI, Balsa JA, Gómez-Martin JM, Peromingo R, Huerta L, Carrasco M, et al. Circulating free testosterone in obese men after bariatric surgery increases in parallel with insulin sensitivity. J Endocrinol Investig. 2013;36:227–32.

Calderón B, Galdón A, Calañas A, Peromingo R, Galindo J, García-Moreno F, et al. Effects of bariatric surgery on male obesity-associated secondary hypogonadism: comparison of laparoscopic gastric bypass with restrictive procedures. Obes Surg. 2014;24(10):1686–92.

Corona G, Rastrelli G, Monami M, Saad F, Luconi M, Lucchese M, et al. Body weight loss reverts obesity-associated hypogonadotropic hypogonadism: a systematic review and meta-analysis. Eur J Endocrinol. 2013;168(6):829–43.

De Boer H, Verschoor L, Ruinemans-Koerts J, Jansen M. Letrozole normalizes serum testosterone in severely obese men with hypogonadotropic hypogonadism. Diabetes Obes Metab. 2005;7:211–5.

Dozio E, Barassi A, Dogliotti G, Malavazos AE, Colpi GM, D'Eril GVM, et al. Adipokines, hormonal parameters, and cardiovascular risk factors: similarities and differences between patients with erectile dysfunction of arteriogenic and nonarteriogenic origin. J Sex Med. 2012;9:2370–7.

Esposito K, Giugliano F, Di Palo C, Giugliano G, Marfella R, D'Andrea F, et al. Effect of lifestyle changes on erectile dysfunction in obese men: a randomized controlled trial. JAMA. 2004;291(24):2978–84.

George JT, Millar RP, Anderson RA. Hypothesis: kisspeptin mediates male hypogonadism in obesity and type 2 diabetes. Neuroendocrinology. 2010;91:302–7.

Grunstein RR, Handelsman DJ, Lawrenc SJ, Blackwell C, Caterson ID, Sullivan CE. Neuroendocrine dysfunction in sleep apnea: reversal by continuous positive airways pressure therapy. J Clin Endocrinol Metab. 1989;68:352–8.

Grunstein RR, Stenlof K, Hedner J, Sjöström L. Impact of obstructive sleep apnea and sleepiness on metabolic and cardiovascular risk factors in the Swedish Obese Subjects (SOS) Study. Int J Obes Relat Metab Disord. 1995;19:410–8.

Hammoud AO, Wilde N, Gibson M, Parks A, Carrell DT, Meikle AW. Male obesity and alteration in sperm parameters. Fertil Steril. 2008;90:2222–5.

Hammoud A, Gibson M, Hunt SC, Adams TD, Carrell DT, Kolotkin RL, et al. Effect of Roux-en-Y gastric bypass surgery on the sex steroids and quality of life in obese men. J Clin Endocrinol Metab. 2009;94:1329–32.

Han TS, Tajar A, O'Neill TW, Jiang M, Bartfai G, Boonen S, et al. Impaired quality of life and sexual function in overweight and obese men: the European Male Ageing Study. Eur J Endocrinol. 2011;164:1003–11.

Helo S, Ellen J, Mechlin C, Feustel P, Grossman M, Ditkoff E, et al. A randomized prospective double-blind comparison trial of clomiphene citrate and anastrozole in raising testosterone in hypogonadal infertile men. J Sex Med. 2015;12(8):1761–9. Epub 2015/07/16.

Hofstra J, Loves S, van Wageningen B, Ruinemans-Koerts J, Jansen I, de Boer H. High prevalence of hypogonadotropic hypogonadism in men referred for obesity treatment. Neth J Med. 2008;66(3):103–9.

Hoyos CM, Killick R, Yee BJ, Grunstein RR, Liu PY. Effects of testosterone therapy on sleep and breathing in obese men with severe obstructive sleep apnoea: a randomized placebo-controlled trial. Clin Endocrinol. 2012;77:599–607.

Isidori AM, Caprio M, Strollo F, Moretti C, Frajese G, Isidori A, et al. Leptin and androgens in male obesity: evidence for leptin contribution to reduced androgen levels. J Clin Endocrinol Metab. 1999;84:3673–80.

Khoo J, Tian H-H, Tan B, Chew K, Ng C-S, Leong D, et al. Comparing effects of low- and high-volume moderate intensity exercise on sexual function and testosterone in obese men. J Sex Med. 2013;10:1823–32.

Khoo J, Ling P-S, Tan J, Teo A, Ng H-L, Chen RY-T, et al. Comparing the effects of meal replacements with reduced-fat diet on weight, sexual and endothelial function, testosterone and quality of life in obese Asian men. Int J Impot Res. 2014;26:61–6.

Kolotkin RL, Zunker C, Østbye T. Sexual functioning and obesity: a review. Obesity. 2012;20:2325–33.

Liu PY, Yee B, Wishart SM, Jimenez M, Jung DG, Grunstein RR, et al. The short-term effects of high-dose testosterone on sleep, breathing, and function in older men. J Clin Endocrinol Metab. 2003;88:3605–13.

Loves S, Ruinemans-Koerts J, de Boer H. Letrozole once a week normalizes serum testosterone in obesity-related male hypogonadism. Eur J Endocrinol. 2008;158(5):741–7.

Loves S, de Jong J, van Sorge A, Telting D, Tack CJ, Hermus A, et al. Somatic and psychological effects of low-dose aromatase inhibition in men with obesity-related hypogonadotropic hypotestosteronemia. Eur J Endocrinol. 2013;169(5):705–14.

Mammi C, Calanchini M, Antelmi A, Cinti F, Rosano GMC, Lenzi A, et al. Androgens and adipose tissue in males: a complex and reciprocal interplay. Int J Endocrinol. 2012;2012:1–8.

Nguyen RHN, Wilcox AJ, Skjærven R, Baird DD. Men's body mass index and infertility. Hum Reprod. 2007;22(9):2488–93.

Pasquali R. Obesity and androgens: facts and perspectives. Fertil Steril. 2006;85(5):1319–40.

Patankar SS, Kaore SB, Sawane MV, Mishra NV, Deshkar AM. Effect of clomiphene citrate on sperm density in male partners of infertile couples. Indian J Physiol Pharmacol. 2007;51(2):195–8. Epub 2008/01/08.

Pellitero S, Olaizola I, Alastrue A, Martínez E, Granada ML, Balibrea JM, et al. Hypogonadotropic hypogonadism in morbidly obese males is reversed after bariatric surgery. Obes Surg. 2012;22:1835–42.

Pilz S, Frisch S, Koertke H, Kuhn J, Dreier J, Obermayer-Pietsch B, et al. Effect of vitamin D supplementation on testosterone levels in men. Horm Metab Res. 2011;43:223–5.

Practice Committee of the American Society for Reproductive Medicine. Obesity and reproduction: a committee opinion. Fertil Steril. 2015;104:1116–26.

Pramyothin P, Holick MF. Serum 25-hydroxyvitamin D levels after bariatric surgery. Clin Rev Bone Miner Metab. 2014;12:234–9.

Reis LO, Favaro WJ, Barreiro GC, de Oliveira LC, Chaim EA, Ferreira AU. Erectile dysfunction and hormonal imbalance in morbidly obese male is reversed after gastric bypass surgery: a prospective randomized controlled trial. Int J Androl. 2010;33:736–44.

Sallmén M, Sandler DP, Hoppin JA, Blair A, Baird DD. Reduced fertility among overweight and obese men. Epidemiology. 2006;17:520–3.

Soskić S, Stokić E, Isenović ER. The relationship between vitamin D and obesity. Curr Med Res Opin. 2014;30:1197–9.

Strain GW, Zumoff B, Kream J, Strain JJ, Deucher R, Rosenfeld RS, et al. Mild hypogonadotropic hypogonadism in obese men. Metabolism. 1982;31:871–5.

Strain GW, Zumoff B, Miller LK, Rosner W, Levit C, Kalin M, et al. Effect of massive weight loss on hypothalamic-pituitary-gonadal function in obese men. J Clin Endocrinol Metab. 1988;66:1019–23.

Traish AM. Testosterone and weight loss: the evidence. Curr Opin Endocrinol Diabetes Obes. 2014;21:313–22.

Vandewalle S, De Schepper J, Kaufman J-M. Androgens and obesity in male adolescents. Curr Opin Endocrinol Diabetes Obes. 2015;22:230–7.

Wu FCW, Tajar A, Beynon JM, Pye SR, Silman AJ, Finn JD, et al. Identification of late-onset hypogonadism in middle-aged and elderly men. N Engl J Med. 2010;363:123–35.

Young T, Peppard PE, Taheri S. Excess weight and sleep-disordered breathing. J Appl Physiol. 2005;99:1592–9.

Zumoff B. Hormonal abnormalities in obesity. Acta Med Scand. 1987;222(S723):153–60.

Zumoff B, Strain GW, Miller LK, Rosner W, Senie R, Seres DS, et al. Plasma free and non-sex-hormone-binding-globulin-bound testosterone are decreased in obese men in proportion to their degree of obesity. J Clin Endocrinol Metab. 1990;71:929–31.

Zumoff B, Miller LK, Strain GW. Reversal of the hypogonadotropic hypogonadism of obese men by administration of the aromatase inhibitor testolactone. Metabolism. 2003;52:1126–8.

Chapter 16
Gonadal Dysfunction and Infertility in Women with Obesity

J. Michael Gonzalez-Campoy

Pearls of Wisdom

- Overweight or obesity in women affect reproductive function, even in the absence of polycystic ovarian syndrome.
- Overweight or obesity affect the reproductive function of women at all levels, and in all facets of their lives, from ovarian function to the health of their progeny.
- Successful management of overweight or obesity and their systemic complications will generally result in the resolution of reproductive issues.
- Weight loss for the improvement of reproductive function should be multifaceted, ensuring that caloric intake is reduced but that the nutritional quality of the hypocaloric meal plan is improved, and supplementing it with increased physical activity.
- Bariatric surgery in women with obesity does not result in the resolution of all their reproductive problems.

16.1 Introduction

This chapter discusses gonadal dysfunction and infertility in women with overweight or obesity, and adiposopathy. Polycystic ovarian syndrome (PCOS) affects one in 20 women, and it is a leading cause of infertility. Yet, PCOS affects only a small number of women with overweight and obesity. In the absence of PCOS, there are changes associated with obesity that affect the gonadal axis in women. This chapter will address gonadal dysfunction in women with overweight or obesity who do not have PCOS.

J. M. Gonzalez-Campoy
Minnesota Center for Obesity, Metabolism and Endocrinology, PA (MNCOME), Eagan, MN, USA
e-mail: drmike@mncome.com

J. M. Gonzalez-Campoy et al. (eds.), *Bariatric Endocrinology*,
https://doi.org/10.1007/978-3-319-95655-8_16

16.2 Background

Overweight and obesity have been recognized as a cause of infertility since the time of Hippocrates. Overweight and obesity lead to a state of either relative or absolute insulin (INS) resistance. They also lead to the development of hypogonadotropic hypogonadism. The consequences of overweight or obesity on female reproduction are important, especially when increased abdominal adiposity is present. They include:

- Infertility
- Low assisted reproductive technologies (ART) efficacy
- Miscarriages
- Congenital abnormalities
- Obstetrical and neonatal complications
- Hormonal contraception inefficacy

Female overweight and obesity have been clearly related to poor reproductive outcomes in both natural and assisted conception. These effects are partially corrected by weight loss, which can be achieved by behavioral, medical, or surgical treatment.

16.3 Endocrine Alterations in Women with Overweight or Obesity

In women with overweight or obesity, endocrine alterations include the reduction of sex hormone-binding globulin (SHBG) (especially if increased abdominal adiposity is present), hyperleptinemia, decreased adiponectin secretion, INS resistance, hyperinsulinemia, increased gonadotropin and inhibin B levels, and elevated androgens levels (Table 16.1).

Table 16.1 Female reproductive endocrinology and changes in overweight or obesity

Tissue or cell type	Normal function	Obesity
β-cells	Produce INS	Through induction of INS resistance, INS production is increased
White adipocytes	Produce Lep	Obesity and elevated INS induce increased Lep production Adiponectin secretion is decreased
Liver	Produces SHBG	Increased INS decreases SHBG
GnRH neurons	Produce GnRH Lep regulates GnRH neuron function	Elevated Lep and T induce increased GnRH production
Gonadotrophs	Produce LH and FSH	LH production is increased, but FSH production is not
Ovary	Produces sex steroids Responsible for oogenesis	P_4 production is decreased and T production is increased Oogenesis is altered

Abbreviations: *FSH* follitropin or follicle-stimulating hormone, *GnRH* gonadotropin-releasing hormone, *INS* insulin, *Lep* leptin, *LH* lutropin or luteinizing hormone, *P4* progesterone, *SHBG* sex hormone-binding globulin, *T* testosterone

Premenopausal women with central obesity have higher testosterone (T) production and clearance than those with peripheral obesity. Women with overweight or obesity have reduced success rates per cycle, and this is associated with central adiposity. The risk of infertility in women with obesity is three times greater than in women who do not have obesity. Smoking increases the odds of infertility. ART success is compromised in women with obesity, and the efficacy of ART decreases with increasing fat mass.

16.4 Reproductive Issues in Women with Obesity

In women with overweight or obesity, an increase in the number of adipocytes results in a multitude of changes. There are increased levels of leptin (Lep), INS, and luteinizing hormone (LH) but not follicle-stimulating hormone (FSH). The net effect of these changes is to stimulate the partial development of follicles that secrete supraphysiological levels of T, but which rarely ovulate due to reduced progesterone (P_4) levels. These changes are enhanced by an INS-induced reduction in SHBG, which amplifies ovarian T production and action.

The negative effects of overweight or obesity on a woman's reproductive function are complex. Obesity in women who have a pregnancy negatively affects their progeny throughout their lives. An unhealthy maternal lifestyle leads to maternal obesity, which results in adiposopathy. Maternal adiposopathy causes an increase in maternal Lep levels. On the other hand, there is a reduction in placental and maternal leptin receptor (Lep-R) expression. The consequence of this is placental resistance to Lep, which in turn leads to increased fetal Lep levels. Impaired fetal growth can result in an increase in the number and size of adipocytes and an increase in INS resistance in adulthood. Adiposopathy leads to an altered hypothalamic-pituitary-ovarian axis in women with obesity. Obesity in turn is responsible for epigenetic changes that can lead to adiposopathy and other endocrine disorders in the progeny of these women. Treatment that results in the resolution of overweight or obesity and its accompanying adiposopathy leads to the normalization of these alterations. It is important to implement treatment for overweight or obesity, and adiposopathy, in advance of pregnancy. This improves the patient's overall health. It also improves the likelihood of a normal pregnancy and a healthy baby who will not suffer any maternal obesity-associated health issues in adulthood.

Reproductive alterations in women with overweight or obesity are not limited to the gynecological realm. In women with overweight or obesity, implantation, pregnancy, and live birth rates are reduced. Women with obesity who require ART have a lower ovarian response. There is a reduced number of mature oocytes, embryos, and ongoing day-3 embryos obtained from these patients. The lower ovarian response to ART in women with obesity may be due to alterations in the metabolism of amino acids, triglycerides, fatty acids, and carbohydrates in the embryos from these mothers.

Women with overweight or obesity who are pregnant have a threefold greater chance of suffering an early spontaneous abortion. The increased risk of early spontaneous abortion correlates with the degree of obesity. INS resistance is an important mechanism of action for the increased risk of spontaneous abortion in women with overweight or obesity.

The risk of congenital abnormalities is increased in pregnancies among women with obesity. In infertility medicine, the ultimate goal is a healthy 1-year-old baby. Therefore, anything that interferes with this goal should be considered when managing a woman and/or a couple.

16.5 Evaluation

As in any other clinical situation, a comprehensive history and physical examination are required to evaluate the gonadal axis in women with obesity. The major goal of the initial visit is to distinguish between pure obesity-related gonadal axis derangements and PCOS. A thorough reproductive history is necessary. Women with obesity have a 31% decrease in conception during the first years after stopping contraception. In these women, tobacco use increases the risk of delayed conception by over 11-fold. The proposed mechanism of action is the disturbance of the menstrual cycle. Factors involved are not restricted to adulthood, as obesity during childhood increases the risk of menstrual abnormalities in adulthood by 57%. Therefore, documenting a temporal profile of contraceptive use and tobacco use needs to be a part of the initial assessment.

Table 16.2 summarizes the steps to evaluate a woman with obesity in the context of reproductive function.

Table 16.2 Evaluation of a woman with obesity: emphasis on reproductive health

System	Signs and symptoms
History	Weight history History of tobacco use Dietary intake Family history of obesity Socioeconomic status
Body habitus	Height Weight Waist circumference Fat pad with calipers
Reproductive	Menstrual history Presence of infertility Contraceptive history History of failed ART Ovarian ultrasound
Endocrine	↑ LH levels Normal FSH levels ↑ INS levels ↑ Lep levels ↑ TT and other androgen levels ↓ E_2 and P_4 levels

Abbreviations: *ART* assisted reproductive technologies, E_2 estradiol, *FSH* follicle-stimulating hormone, *INS* insulin, *Lep* leptin, *LH* luteinizing hormone, *P4* progesterone, *TT* total testosterone

16.6 Management of Adiposopathy-Related Reproductive Problems

Management of adiposopathy-related reproductive problems in women includes four types of interventions:

1. Lifestyle modification
2. Psychological support measures
3. Medical therapy
4. Bariatric surgery

16.6.1 Lifestyle Modifications and Their Impact on Reproductive Function in Women with Overweight or Obesity

Chapters 19 and 20 in this textbook address nutritional interventions and physical activity for the management of overweight, obesity, and adiposopathy. The most cost-effective therapy for women with infertility and overweight or obesity is a hypocaloric meal plan. This increases SHBG. Nutritional management should have the dual goal of reducing caloric intake and improving the nutritional quality of meals. An example of this is that adequate intake of omega-3 fatty acids is associated with better embryo quality in patients with overweight or obesity. Additionally, patients should be made aware that although intensive physical activity yields faster results, it is the total periodic load of physical activity that will lead to improved metabolic health. They should be made aware that many less intensive activities, such as walking and gardening, can lead to improved overall and reproductive health. Furthermore, a combination of nutrition and physical activity can, in as little as 6 months, produce a weight loss that results in live births in 2/3 of women, compared to none in women without such a regimen. Another important lifestyle modification that will improve reproductive function is smoking cessation. Therefore, counseling of patients can be useful in addressing and improving multiple lifestyle factors.

16.6.2 Pharmacological Management of Reproductive Issues in Women with Overweight or Obesity

Chapter 21 in this textbook covers the pharmacological management of overweight, obesity, and adiposopathy. These therapies may be implemented in women who do not desire a pregnancy now. For women actively trying to achieve a pregnancy, metformin lowers insulin resistance in the liver and favorably impacts female reproduction. These benefits are amplified when metformin is used in combination with a hypocaloric meal plan. Resveratrol may be a useful compound to normalize SHBG levels in women with obesity.

16.6.3 Bariatric Surgery and Its Impact on the Reproductive Health of Women

Bariatric surgery, by significantly reducing weight and adiposity, and treating adiposopathy, improves the overall and endocrine health of women with obesity. There is also a beneficial effect on reproductive function, with decreased adverse maternal and neonatal outcomes in women who achieve a pregnancy after bariatric surgery, compared to women with obesity who did not have surgery.

16.7 Conclusions

16.7.1 What We Want

The goal of a reproductive endocrinologist treating a woman with infertility is to allow the patient to have a healthy 1-year-old child. Overweight and obesity interfere with this goal at multiple levels. The menstrual cycle is altered due to ovulatory dysfunction, and this leads to an increased risk for infertility and poor response to fertility drugs. Once there is a pregnancy, a woman with overweight or obesity faces an increased risk for miscarriage, both spontaneously and after infertility treatment. Labor is often complicated and can result in increased risk for neonatal morbidity and mortality. Therefore, maintaining normal endocrine ovarian function is important in ensuring the overall health of a woman. We want women with overweight or obesity to be able to achieve a pregnancy successfully. Weight management must be instituted as early as possible to help achieve this goal.

16.7.2 What We Know

Overweight, obesity, and adiposopathy in women have various deleterious consequences on the reproductive system. Women with overweight, obesity, and/or adiposopathy are affected in all facets of their lives. There are alterations in their reproductive capacity and the ability to safely carry a pregnancy. There is increased risk for obesity and other morbidities in their daughters. Treatment that results in a significant reduction of adiposity and reverts adiposopathy is associated with improvement and even normalization of female reproduction.

16.7.3 What We Need to Know

The immense majority of the information available on the reproductive function of women with overweight or obesity, and adiposopathy, is related to patients with

PCOS. Currently, there is very little high-quality information regarding the effects of adiposity or adiposopathy on the reproductive function of women. Large, well-designed studies are needed in order to provide conclusive guidance on the adequate management of women with obesity.

Reading List

Al-Safi ZA, Roth L, Chosich J, Bradford A, Polotsky A, Santoro N. Elevated insulin in obese women relates to low endogenous luteinizing hormone. Obstet Gynecol. 2014;123(Suppl 1):95S.

Bellver J, Busso C, Pellicer A, Remohi J, Simon C. Obesity and assisted reproductive technology outcomes. Reprod Biomed Online. 2006;12:562–8.

Bellver J, Melo MA, Bosch E, Serra V, Remohi J, Pellicer A, et al. Obesity and poor reproductive outcome: the potential role of the endometrium. Fertil Steril. 2007;88:446–51.

Bellver J, Ayllón Y, Ferrando M, Melo M, Goyri E, Pellicer A, et al. Female obesity impairs in vitro fertilization outcome without affecting embryo quality. Fertil Steril. 2010;93:447–54.

Bellver J, Pellicer A, García-Velasco JA, Ballesteros A, Remohí J, Meseguer M. Obesity reduces uterine receptivity: clinical experience from 9,587 first cycles of ovum donation with normal weight donors. Fertil Steril. 2013;100:1050–8.

Bellver J, De Los Santos MJ, Alamá P, Castelló D, Privitera L, Galliano D, et al. Day-3 embryo metabolomics in the spent culture media is altered in obese women undergoing in vitro fertilization. Fertil Steril. 2015;103:1407–15.e1.

Bolumar F, Olsen J, Rebagliato M, Saez-Lloret I, Bisanti L. Body mass index and delayed conception: a European Multicenter Study on Infertility and Subfecundity. Am J Epidemiol. 2000;151:1072–9.

Briffa JF, McAinch AJ, Romano T, Wlodek ME, Hryciw DH. Leptin in pregnancy and development: a contributor to adulthood disease? Am J Physiol Endocrinol Metab. 2015;308(5):E335–50.

Chadwick J, Mann WN. Medicine: airs, waters, places (an essay on the influence of climate, water supply and situation on health). In: Hippocratic writings. London: Penguin Classics; 1983.

Chow H-HS, Garland LL, Heckman-Stoddard BM, Hsu C-H, Butler VD, Cordova CA, et al. A pilot clinical study of resveratrol in postmenopausal women with high body mass index: effects on systemic sex steroid hormones. J Transl Med. 2014;12:223.

Christofolini J, Bianco B, Santos G, Adami F, Christofolini D, Barbosa CP. Bariatric surgery influences the number and quality of oocytes in patients submitted to assisted reproduction techniques. Obesity. 2014;22(3):939–42.

Clark AM, Thornley B, Tomlinson L, Galletley C, Norman RJ. Weight loss in obese infertile women results in improvement in reproductive outcome for all forms of fertility treatment. Hum Reprod. 1998;13:1502–5.

Crosignani PG, Ragni G, Parazzini F, Wyssling H, Lombroso G, Perotti L, et al. Anthropometric indicators and response to gonadotrophin for ovulation induction. Hum Reprod. 1994;9:420–3.

De Pergola G, Maldera S, Tartagni M, Pannacciulli N, Loverro G, Giorgino R. Inhibitory effect of obesity on gonadotropin, estradiol, and inhibin B levels in fertile women. Obesity (Silver Spring). 2006;14:1954–60.

Edison E, Whyte M, van Vlymen J, Jones S, Gatenby P, de Lusignan S, et al. Bariatric surgery in obese women of reproductive age improves conditions that underlie fertility and pregnancy outcomes: retrospective cohort study of UK National Bariatric Surgery Registry (NBSR). Obes Surg. 2016;26(12):2837–42. Epub 2016/06/19.

ESHRE Capri Workshop Group. Nutrition and reproduction in women. Hum Reprod Update. 2006;12:193–207.

Fedorcsak P, Dale PO, Storeng R, Ertzeid G, Bjercke S, Oldereid N, et al. Impact of overweight and underweight on assisted reproduction treatment. Hum Reprod. 2004;19:2523–8.

Kominiarek MA, Jungheim ES, Hoeger KM, Rogers AM, Kahan S, Kim JJ. American Society for Metabolic and Bariatric Surgery position statement on the impact of obesity and obesity treatment on fertility and fertility therapy endorsed by the American College of Obstetricians and Gynecologists and the Obesity Society. Surg Obes Relat Dis. 2017;13(5):750–7. Epub 2017/04/19.

Lake JK, Power C, Cole TJ. Women's reproductive health: the role of body mass index in early and adult life. Int J Obes Relat Metab Disord. 1997;21:432–8.

Lane M, Zander-Fox DL, Robker RL, McPherson NO. Peri-conception parental obesity, reproductive health, and transgenerational impacts. Trends Endocrinol Metab. 2015;26(2):84–90.

Le Goff S, Lédée N, Bader G. Obésité et reproduction: revue de la littérature. Gynecol Obstet Fertil. 2008;36:543–50.

Leary C, Leese HJ, Sturmey RG. Human embryos from overweight and obese women display phenotypic and metabolic abnormalities. Hum Reprod. 2015;30:122–32.

Linné Y. Effects of obesity on women's reproduction and complications during pregnancy. Obes Rev. 2004;5:137–43.

Lintsen AME, Pasker-de Jong PCM, de Boer EJ, Burger CW, Jansen CAM, Braat DDM, et al. Effects of subfertility cause, smoking and body weight on the success rate of IVF. Hum Reprod. 2005;20:1867–75.

Maggard MA, Yermilov I, Li Z, Maglione M, Newberry S, Suttorp M, et al. Pregnancy and fertility following bariatric surgery: a systematic review. JAMA. 2008;300(19):2286–96. Epub 2008/11/20.

Norman RJ, Noakes M, Wu R, Davies MJ, Moran L, Wang JX. Improving reproductive performance in overweight/obese women with effective weight management. Hum Reprod Update. 2004;10:267–80.

Nteeba J, Ganesan S, Keating AF. Progressive obesity alters ovarian folliculogenesis with impacts on pro-inflammatory and steroidogenic signaling in female mice. Biol Reprod. 2014;91(4):86, 1–11.

Ogbuji QC. Obesity and reproductive performance in women. Afr J Reprod Health. 2010;14:143–51.

Pasquali R. Obesity, fat distribution and infertility. Maturitas. 2006;54:363–71.

Pasquali R, Gambineri A, Biscotti D, et al. Effect of long-term treatment with metformin added to hypocaloric diet on body composition, fat distribution and androgen and insulin levels in abdominally obese women with and without the polycystic ovary syndrome. J Clin Endocrinol Metab. 2000;85:2767–74.

Pasquali R, Pelusi C, Genghini S, Cacciari M, Gambineri A. Obesity and reproductive disorders in women. Hum Reprod Update. 2003;9:359–72.

Ramsay JE, Greer I, Sattar N. ABC of obesity. Obesity and reproduction. BMJ. 2006;333:1159–62.

Roth LW, Allshouse AA, Bradshaw-Pierce EL, Lesh J, Chosich J, Kohrt W, et al. Luteal phase dynamics of follicle-stimulating and luteinizing hormones in obese and normal weight women. Clin Endocrinol. 2014;81(3):418–25.

Samojilik E, Kirschner MA, Silber D, Scneider G, Ertel NH. Elevated production and metabolic clearance rates of androgens in morbidly obese women. J Clin Endocrinol Metab. 1984;59:949–54.

Sharpe RM, Franks S. Environment, lifestyle and infertility – an inter-generational issue. Nature Cell Biol. 2002;4(Suppl):s33–40.

Tian L, Shen H, Lu Q, Norman RJ, Wang J. Insulin resistance increases the risk of spontaneous abortion following assisted reproduction technology treatment. J Clin Endocrinol Metab. 2007;92(4):1430–3.

Urano T, Inoue S. Recent genetic discoveries in osteoporosis, sarcopenia and obesity. Endocr J. 2015;62:475.

van der Steeg JW, Steures P, Eijkemans MJ, Habbema JD, Hompes PG, Burggraaff JM, et al. Obesity affects spontaneous pregnancy chances in subfertile, ovulatory women. Hum Reprod. 2008;23:324–8.

Wang JX, Davies M, Norman RJ. Body mass and probability of pregnancy during assisted reproduction treatment: retrospective study. BMJ. 2000;321:1320–1.

Wang JX, Davies MJ, Norman RJ. Obesity increases the risk of spontaneous abortion during infertility treatment. Obes Res. 2002;10:551–4.

Wass P, Waldenstrom U, Rossner S, Hellberg D. An android body fat distribution in females impairs the pregnancy rate of in vitro fertilization-embryo transfer. Hum Reprod. 1997;12:2057–60.

Wilkes S, Murdoch A. Obesity and female fertility: a primary care perspective. J Fam Plann Reprod Health Care. 2009;35:181–18531.

Zaadstra BM, Seidell JC, Van Noord PA, te Velde ER, Habbema JD, Vrieswijk B, et al. Fat and female fecundity: prospective study of effect of body fat distribution on conception rates. BMJ. 1993;3006:484–7.

Chapter 17
Neoplasia in Patients with Excess Fat Mass

Daniel L. Hurley

Pearls of Wisdom

- A healthy meal plan and regular physical activity have been associated with a lower incidence of obesity-related cancers.
- Increasing adiposity, defined by body mass index, is associated with increasing cancer incidence for many adult cancers, in both men and women who have overweight or obesity.
- Increased waist circumference is a better predictor of obesity-related cancers than body mass index.
- Adiposopathy, manifested by increased oxidative stress, tissue inflammation, insulin resistance, and an elevated waist circumference, leads to dysmetabolic syndrome, type 2 diabetes mellitus, and an increased risk of cancer.
- Avoiding adult weight gain and achieving weight loss may each confer protection against obesity-related cancers, particularly among women after the menopause who do not use hormone replacement therapy.

17.1 Introduction

The Centers for Disease Control and Prevention lists cancer as the second leading cause of death in the United States (US). An increase in fat mass (adiposity) in both men and women leading to overweight or obesity is associated with an increased risk of certain types of cancer. The number of cancers attributed to adiposity is

---

D. L. Hurley
Mayo Graduate School of Medicine, Mayo Clinic, Division of Endocrinology, Diabetes, Metabolism, and Nutrition, Rochester, MN, USA
e-mail: hurley.daniel@mayo.edu

J. M. Gonzalez-Campoy et al. (eds.), *Bariatric Endocrinology*,
https://doi.org/10.1007/978-3-319-95655-8_17

estimated at 20%, with increased risk of malignancy influenced by nutritional habits, weight gain, central body fat, and physical inactivity. Reports from the International Agency for Research into Cancer and the World Cancer Research Fund (WCRF) have shown strong evidence for an association between obesity and endometrial, esophageal, colorectal, postmenopausal breast, prostate, and renal malignancies. On the other hand, obesity is less commonly associated with leukemia, non-Hodgkin's lymphoma, multiple myeloma, malignant melanoma, and thyroid cancer. A prospective study in the United Kingdom identified 166,955 individuals with cancer during 7.5 years of observation from a cohort of 5.24 million adults without a previous diagnosis of cancer. In this study, an increased body mass index (BMI) was associated with a greater risk for cancers of the gallbladder, liver, colon, ovary, postmenopausal breast, cervix, endometrium, kidney, and thyroid, as well as leukemia. Adiposity in adult Canadians is reported to account for 7.7% of all adult cancers (9.7% in men and 5.9% in women). Obesity increased the risk of both overall cancer and specific cancers, to include cancers of the ovary, postmenopausal breast, pancreas, colon, rectum, kidney, and prostate as well as non-Hodgkin's lymphoma, leukemia, and multiple myeloma. A meta-analysis of 141 studies that included 282,137 cancer cases found that a BMI increase of 5 kilograms/meter^2 (kg/m^2) was associated with more frequent esophageal, colon, renal, and thyroid cancers in men and gallbladder, esophageal, endometrial, and renal cancers in women (Fig. 17.1). In an attempt to determine the degree of adiposity for obesity-related cancer risk, a cohort of 144,701 postmenopausal women in the Women's Health Initiative (WHI) trial were studied for the interaction between 17 cancer types, 6 anthropometric measures (weight, BMI, weight-to-height ratio, waist circumference [WC], waist-to-hip ratio [WHR], and waist-to-height ratio), and hormone replacement therapy (HRT) use. Colorectal, breast, endometrium, kidney, and all cancers combined were positively associated with all six anthropometric measures, whereas lung cancer among women who ever smoked tobacco was inversely associated with all measures except WHR. The ability to discriminate derived anthropometric cutoffs was generally poor, varied across cancer types (e.g., BMI cutoffs for breast and endometrium cancers were 30 kg/m^2 and 34 kg/m^2, respectively), and also depended on HRT use, with the indices cutoffs for predicting 5-year and 10-year cancer incidence higher among women who never used HRT.

In addition to excess adiposity, a sedentary lifestyle has been associated with increased cancer risk. Schmid and colleagues focused on a review of 43 observational studies on this topic, using random-effects meta-analysis and meta-regression for 68,936 cancer cases analyzed. The relative risk (RR) of colon cancer between the highest versus lowest levels of sedentary time, was 1.54 for television viewing time, 1.24 for occupational sitting time, and 1.24 for total sitting time. For endometrial cancer, the RR was 1.66 for television viewing time and 1.32 for total sitting time. A positive association with overall sedentary behavior was also noted for lung cancer (RR = 1.21), but sedentary behavior was unrelated to cancers of the breast, ovaries, prostate, esophagus, stomach, rectum, kidneys, and non-Hodgkin lymphoma.

	Cancer incidence (RR per 5 kg/m² increase)		Cancer mortality (RR for high BMI [>30, 35 or 40 kg/m²] vs. normal BMI)	
	♀	♂	♀	♂
Thyroid	1.14	1.33	–	–
Lung	0.80	0.76	0.81	0.67
Breast:				
Pre	0.92	–	2.12 (Pre and Post)	–
Post	1.12	–		
Esophagus:				
Adeno	1.51	1.52	2.64 (Adeno and Squamous)	1.94 (Adeno and Squamous)
Squamous	0.57	0.71		
Stomach	1.04	0.97	–	–
Liver	1.07	1.24	1.68	4.52
Gallbladder	1.59	1.09	2.13	1.76
Pancreas	1.12	–	2.76	2.61
Colon	1.09	1.24	1.46 (Colon and Rectum)	1.84 (Colon and Rectum)
Rectum	1.02	1.09		
Kidney	1.34	1.24	4.75	1.70
Endometrium	1.59	–	6.25	–
Ovary	1.03	–	1.51	–
Cervix	–	–	3.20	–
Prostate	–	1.03	–	1.34
Melanoma	0.95	1.17	–	–
Leukemia	1.17	1.08	–	–
Lymphoma	1.07	1.06	1.95	1.49
Multiple myeloma	1.11	1.11	1.44	1.71
All cancers			**1.88**	**1.52**

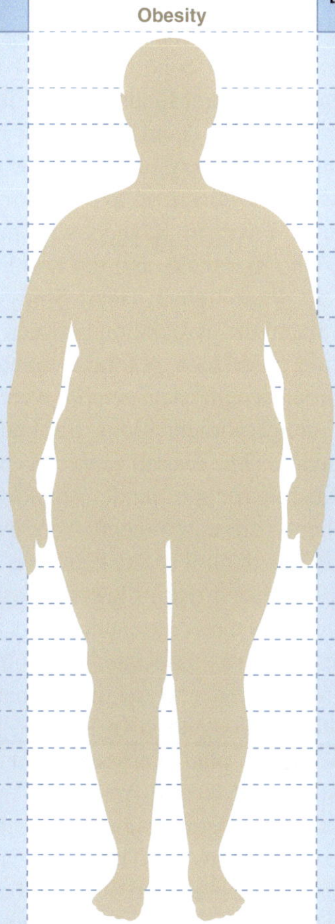

Fig. 17.1 The association between adiposity, adiposopathy, and cancer incidence and cancer-related mortality in the adult United States population. Left: the relative risk of cancer-specific incidence per 5-kg/m² increased weight increments. Right: the relative risk of cancer mortality in patients with a body mass index >30 kg/m² compared to individuals with a normal weight. Abbreviations: *RR* relative risk, *BMI* body mass index, kg/m² kilograms/meters². (From: Goodwin and Stambolic 2015; used with permission)

17.2 Observational and Epidemiological Data: Usefulness and Limitations

A plant-based meal plan with moderate alcohol consumption has been associated with a reduced risk of obesity-related cancer. The World Cancer Research Fund (WCRF) and American Institute for Cancer Research (AICR) released eight recommendations in 2007 related to healthy eating (to include increased plant foods, limited red and processed meats, and moderate alcohol consumption), adiposity, and physical activity targeted to prevent common cancers worldwide. These recommendations were operationalized during 7.7 years of follow-up in the Vitamins and Lifestyle Study cohort of 57,841 adults without prior diagnosis of cancer. Increased intake of plant foods and limiting foods that promote weight gain were strongly associated with decreased cancer mortality (hazard ratio [HR] 0.82, 95% confidence interval [CI] 0.67–1.00 and HR 0.82, CI 0.70–0.96, respectively). Cancer mortality was 10% lower on average for each additional recommendation met ($p < 0.001$), 61% lower in subjects who met at least five recommendations compared to those who met none, and did not differ by age or gender. A group of 2983 adults from the Framingham Heart Study Offspring Cohort were followed prospectively to evaluate the association between healthy behaviors consistent with the cancer prevention guidelines. A food frequency questionnaire, anthropometric measures, and self-reported physical activity were used to construct a seven-component score based on recommendations for body fatness, physical activity, and healthy eating behaviors. The overall score was not associated with obesity-related cancer risk after adjusting for age, gender, smoking, activity, and pre-existing conditions. However, when score components were evaluated separately, for every unit increment decline in the alcohol score, there was 29% lower risk of obesity-related cancers and 49–71% reduced risk of breast, prostate, and colorectal cancers. Each unit increment increase in the component scores for nonstarchy plant foods (fruits, vegetables, and legumes) was associated with 66% reduced risk of colorectal cancer. Consuming a Mediterranean-type dietary pattern has also been reported to be beneficial for health and longevity. In the US, high versus low conformity to a Mediterranean-type dietary plan was assessed in 214,284 men and 166,012 women in the National Institutes of Health-American Association of Retired Persons Diet and Health Study. Cancer-specific mortality declined by 17% in men and 12% in women during 5 years of follow-up. The beneficial effect of a Mediterranean dietary pattern on mortality may be mediated by a number of mechanisms, to include a low omega-6-to-omega-3 fatty acid ratio, dietary antioxidant intake reducing oxidative stress and chronic inflammation, and increased fiber consumption.

Of interest is the relationship between adiposity (excess fat mass), the dysmetabolic syndrome, and cancer. Overweight and obesity is commonly associated with the dysmetabolic syndrome, which is characterized by an increase in free fatty acids, triglycerides, glucose, and insulin resistance. Individual risk factors for the dysmetabolic syndrome have also been associated with increased cancer risk. Although the exact mechanism linking insulin resistance and cancer is unclear, hyperinsulinemia with increased insulin-like growth factor-1 (IGF-1) availability and oxidative stress appear to play a role in tumor initiation and progression. Oxidative stress occurs in the presence of hyperglycemia and increased free fatty acids and may disrupt mitosis of cells and result in deoxyribonucleic acid mutagenesis and carcinogenesis. There is an increasing body of evidence to support a connection between obesity, type 2 diabetes mellitus (T2DM), and cancer. An elevated risk of cancer was found in a cohort of 25,268 adults with obesity and

T2DM registered in the Swedish National Diabetes Register. In men with T2DM, both overweight and obesity were associated with increased risk of all cancer (HRs, 1.13 and 1.17), gastrointestinal cancer [HRs, 1.34 and 1.40), and colorectal cancer (HRs, 1.59 and 1.62). In women with T2DM, obesity was associated with increased risk of all cancers (HR, 1.30), gastrointestinal cancer (HR, 1.40), and postmenopausal breast cancer (HR, 1.39). The Framingham Heart Study Offspring Cohort has tracked impaired fasting glucose (IFG) and markers of insulin-glucose metabolism and cancer for over three decades with identification of 787 obesity-related cancers, including 136 colorectal, 217 breast, and 219 prostate cancers. The presence of IFG 10–20 years and 20 years before a cancer diagnosis was associated with 44% and 57% increased risk of obesity-related cancers, respectively. IFG was still associated with a 27% increased risk of cancer even with time-dependent variables and after adjusting for age, gender, smoking, alcohol, and BMI. A stronger association was present in subjects with the highest insulin (HR, 1.47) and hemoglobin A1C (HR, 1.54) levels. In the presence of IFG, a twofold increase in colorectal cancer risk was observed, but no increase in risk was seen for either breast or prostate cancer. Cancer risk may be lower among patients who have overweight or obesity and are metabolically healthy, compared to those with metabolic dysfunction, as seen in 3763 Framingham Heart Study adults. Subjects with increased adiposity (defined by BMI >25 kg/m^2 or a WHR >0.51 for men and >0.57 for women) with elevated fasting blood glucose (FBG) >125 mg/dL had a significant twofold increased risk of developing obesity-related cancer, whereas those with normal FBG had a 50% increased risk. Normal-weight adults with elevated FBG had no excess cancer risk. Of note, the effects of BMI and WHR were independent of one another. Women in this study with elevated FBG had a 2.6-fold increased risk of cervical, endometrial, and postmenopausal breast cancers, compared to women with normal FBG levels who had only a 70% increased cancer risk.

Adiposopathy is associated with a chronic inflammatory state and the development of malignancy. Visceral adipose tissue secretes a number of adipocytokines such as leptin, interleukin (IL)-6, IL-8, IL-1beta, and tumor necrosis factor (TNF)-alpha. These adipocytokines are linked to the Janus kinase (JAK)/STAT signal transduction in other tissues, which could result in an upregulation of a wide range of antiapoptotic, prometastatic, and proangiogenic genes. In addition, the gastrointestinal microbiome may be a potential risk factor for certain types of cancers. Altered microbial metabolism may contribute to the generation of procarcinogenic toxic metabolites, less nutrient availability resulting in metabolic dysregulation, and subclinical inflammation, all potentially contributing to tumor genesis. Finally, findings from a cohort of 368 adults who had historical exposure to a group of persistent organic pollutants and followed for 9 years suggested a potential relationship between pollutant residue in adipose tissue and the risk of cancer in men. However, in a 4-year National Health and Nutrition Examination Survey (NHANES), mortality associated with polychlorinated biphenyls and organochlorine pesticides was inversely related to high fat mass and positively related to low fat mass.

17.3 Prostate Cancer

The dysmetabolic syndrome has been associated with an increased risk of prostate cancer, although not in all studies. A biologic gradient seems to exist between the number of components of the dysmetabolic syndrome and both the risk of prostate cancer and a higher grade of cancer. Prostate-specific antigen (PSA) levels were followed at 2 and 4 years in a large study of 6426 men at risk for prostate cancer. Although only 3% of men had at least three components of the dysmetabolic syndrome, its presence was associated with an increased risk of high-grade prostate cancer ($p = 0.02$) and men with even two components of the dysmetabolic syndrome ($n = 724$, 11%) had a trend toward more aggressive prostate cancer. Of interest, men with more components of the dysmetabolic syndrome had significantly lower PSA levels ($p < 0.029$). The same gradient of risk with components of the dysmetabolic syndrome was seen in 2235 men undergoing prostate biopsy without prior cancer diagnosis, 22% of whom had the dysmetabolic syndrome. No individual dysmetabolic syndrome component was independently associated with cancer, but an increasing number of components was associated with a greater cancer risk and a higher grade of cancer, with the highest risk in those who had the dysmetabolic syndrome (odds ratio [OR], 1.54; $p = 0.002$ and 1.56; $p = 0.003$, respectively). Morote and colleagues found no difference in rates of biopsy-proven prostate cancer in 2408 men with and without the dysmetabolic syndrome (National Cholesterol Education Program, Adult Treatment Panel III [NCEP ATP III] definition) at 34.5% and 36.4%, respectively. However, the rate of high-grade prostate cancer (Gleason score 8–10) was significantly increased in those patients with the dysmetabolic syndrome compared to those without it (35.9% versus 23.9%, respectively; $p < 0.001$).

Meta-analyses have consistently demonstrated a small but statistically significant association between adiposity and prostate cancer. At the diagnosis of prostate cancer, low-grade prostate cancer has been reported to be less likely in men with obesity, whereas patients with obesity are more likely to have aggressive and advanced prostate cancer. A prospective cohort study analyzed data from 26,944 men aged 50–64 years and found that the incidence of prostate cancer was similar or slightly lower in men with obesity, compared to men without it, but more advanced disease was present in those with obesity. The proportion of Stage 3–4 cancer was 37% in the lowest BMI quartile and 48% in the highest BMI quartile ($p = 0.006$). Men with obesity and prostate cancer also had higher prostate cancer-specific mortality (HR, 1.48; $p = 0.002$) when comparing the highest and lowest quartiles of BMI. This association was attenuated, but not eliminated, by statistical adjustment for cancer stage. A study of 6729 men examined the association between adiposity and cancer grade in which prostate biopsies were largely independent of PSA levels between 2.5 and 10.0 ng/mL. Overall, 27% of men were of normal weight, 53% had overweight, and 20% had obesity. Multivariate analyses found obesity to be associated with a lower risk of low-grade prostate cancer (OR, 0.79; $p = 0.01$) and increased risk of high-grade prostate cancer (OR, 1.28; $p = 0.04$).

Two nested case-control studies assessed men undergoing radical prostatectomy for prostate cancer when matched to controls. After adjusting for age and PSA levels, men with obesity were more likely to present with higher grade Gleason grade 8–10 tumors (OR = 1.50; $p = 0.003$) and more aggressive cancer (OR = 1.30). A retrospective review analyzed 1213 men who underwent a transrectal ultrasound (TRUS)-guided prostate biopsy, 34% who had obesity and 28% positive for cancer. Men with obesity were less likely to have any abnormality on digital rectal examination (8.1% vs. 15.9%, $p < 0.001$), but had a larger prostate (49.2 vs. 42.9 mL, $p < 0.001$), a higher risk of biopsy-positive prostate cancer detection (OR, 1.45), and a higher rate of high-grade disease by Gleason score (OR, 1.50) compared to men without obesity. In a cross-sectional study of men receiving radiotherapy for prostate cancer, elevated BMI ($p = 0.054$) and WC ($p = 0.040$) were associated with an increased risk of high-grade cancer risk.

Adiposity has been associated with a decrease in serum PSA, and it has been postulated that hemodilution due to a greater body fat mass may lower PSA levels. Men with the dysmetabolic syndrome have reportedly lower serum PSA values relative to men of normal weight. Thus, there were concerns that PSA may be less accurate in detecting prostate cancer in men who have overweight or obesity. NHANES data showed that the dysmetabolic syndrome (defined by NCEP ATP III criteria) and higher FBG were the only factors independently associated with PSA levels in 3528 men, suggesting that the combined components comprising the dysmetabolic syndrome have a greater negative influence on PSA levels than do the individual components. Both non-Hispanic-whites and Mexican-American men with the dysmetabolic syndrome had significantly lower PSA values relative to those men without the dysmetabolic syndrome ($p = 0.01$). However, several recent papers report that PSA levels are not lower in men with obesity and would not reduce the accuracy for predicting prostate cancer risk. Results of TRUS-guided prostate biopsies of 854 Chinese men with PSA values <20 ng/mL were reviewed and showed no relationship between adiposity and PSA levels. In this study there was no difference in mean PSA values and adiposity, but the TRUS volumes were greater (63.2 mL and 51.6 mL, respectively; $p < 0.001$) and PSA density significantly lower in men with obesity ($p < 0.001$). A positive PSA density was associated with a fourfold increase (41.1% vs. 9.5%, $p < 0.001$) in prostate cancer risk, compared to only twice the risk in men of normal weight (18.8% vs. 9.7%; $p = 0.001$). In addition, recent studies of large numbers of Asian and Italian men suggest that PSA levels are not necessarily lower and do not impair the accuracy of assessing prostate cancer risk, regardless of the BMI category of adiposity. Whether or not PSA density by TRUS will be clinically useful in predicting the risk of prostate cancer in men with increased adiposity is unclear at the present time.

Obesity alters circulating levels of insulin and adiponectin, two hormones that have been implicated as possible mediators in carcinogenesis. A nested case-control study of 272 prostate cancer cases (Gleason score >7 or T3-T4 cancer) compared to age and race matched controls found no association between adiponectin or C-peptide and risk of aggressive prostate cancer, although the highest quartile of C-peptide, compared with the lowest quartile, was associated with increased cancer risk (OR, 1.41; CI, 0.72–2.78). Of interest, the role of body composition and oxidative stress was assessed by total thiol (glutathione) levels in multiple prostate biopsy specimens of patients with benign prostatic hyperplasia (BPH) or prostate cancer and compared to body composition as estimated by air plethysmography. A significant difference of thiol levels was observed between patients with BPH and cancer ($p < 0.05$), with a positive correlation observed between thiol levels, fat mass ($r = 0.76$; $p < 0.01$), and WC ($r = 0.49$; $p < 0.05$).

In a small retrospective study of patients who underwent radical prostatectomy for prostate cancer, no association was found between any measurements of adiposity (i.e., BMI, WC, and visceral fat) in men who developed cancer recurrence. The dysmetabolic syndrome was also not associated with prostate cancer recurrence in a slightly larger study, although there was an association between IFG and cancer recurrence (HR, 1.54; CI, 1.10–2.15). In a large retrospective cohort study of 11,152 men who underwent radical prostatectomy, obesity at the time of surgery was a significant predictor of biochemical recurrence-free survival (HRs, 1.30 and 1.45 for mild and moderate/severe obesity, respectively) and overall survival (HRs, 1.41 and 1.81, respectively), but did not predict prostate cancer-specific survival. Analysis of 522,736 men from 18 prospective cohort studies across six Asian countries found no significant association between prostate cancer mortality and overweight or obesity. Bonn reported a 47% increased rate of overall mortality in 4376 men who had localized prostate cancer and obesity (HR, 1.47; CI 1.03–2.10), but again, there was no significant association found for BMI and prostate cancer progression or prostate cancer-specific mortality. A weight gain >5% after diagnosis of cancer was associated with an almost twofold increased rate of prostate cancer-specific mortality, whereas a weight loss >5% was associated with significantly increased overall mortality, compared to maintaining a stable weight.

17.4 Breast Cancer

Adiposity is an established risk factor for postmenopausal breast cancer. Women who followed the WCRF/AICR cancer prevention recommendations were found to have a reduced incidence of postmenopausal breast cancer. In 30,797 women after the menopause, breast cancer risk was reduced by 60% in women who met at least five healthy WCRF/AICR recommendations compared with those who met none. Breast cancer risk reduction was due primarily to meeting recommendations related to body fatness and consumption of plant foods and alcohol. A systematic review and meta-analysis of 11 studies showed that women with obesity were at a greater risk of breast cancer than those without it. Menopause status may be a mitigating factor in breast cancer risk. Dual energy X-ray absorptiometry (DXA) was used in the WHI study to examine the association between body fat and breast cancer in 10,960 women past the menopause who did not have cancer at baseline evaluation. During a median follow-up of 12.9 years, body fat by DXA showed a strong positive association with breast cancer risk. Anthropometric indices for BMI (HR, 1.97; CI, 1.45–2.68), WC (HR, 1.97; CI,

1.46–2.65), and WHR (HR, 1.91; CI, 1.41–2.58) were all associated with the risk of breast cancer and did not differ from DXA-predicted cancer risk. A case-control study comparing Brazilian women with breast cancer to controls showed that sedentary women have a significantly higher risk of breast cancer (OR, 2.39; CI, 1.43–3.99), independent of percent body fat, and after adjusting for hormone-related risk factors and family history of breast cancer. The dysmetabolic syndrome has also been associated with breast cancer in women after the menopause.

Women with increased adiposity have been reported to have more aggressive breast cancer, shortened disease-free survival, and decreased longevity. Increased tumor size and lymph node metastasis are more common in patients with greater adiposity, and tumor subtypes appear to be more aggressive with a higher risk of distant metastasis. In contrast, a retrospective review of a prospectively maintained database was conducted on 523 patients with invasive breast cancer and found no differences in overall survival or in disease-free survival based on normal, overweight, and obesity BMI categories after a median duration of 49 months. Of interest, a study of 11,351 women from the California Cancer Registry suggested that the effect of adiposity on breast cancer mortality may vary across ethnic groups. In comparing non-Latina-whites, Latina's, Asian-Americans, and African-Americans, a BMI >40 kg/m^2 was associated with increased mortality in non-Latina-whites and Latina's, but not Asian-Americans or African-Americans. A high WHR was associated with increased mortality only in Asian-Americans. Pajares and colleagues performed a retrospective analysis of 5683 patients with breast cancer enrolled in four randomized clinical trials. Patients with class 2 obesity (BMI >35 kg/m^2) had a significantly increased risk of disease recurrence (HR, 1.26; CI, 1.00–1.59; $p < 0.05$), breast cancer mortality (HR, 1.32; CI, 1.00–1.74; $p = 0.05$), and overall mortality (HR, 1.35; CI, 1.06–1.71; $p < 0.02$). However, patients with class 1 obesity (BMI 30.0 to 34.6 kg/m^2) had similar prognoses for these parameters compared to individuals of normal weight (BMI <25 kg/m^2).

Elevated estrogen production by adipose tissue after menopause is one mechanism for cancer risk, due to a high level of aromatase activity and hormone-dependent tumors expressing both estrogen receptors (ER) and progesterone receptors (PR). In a study of 646 Iranian women, obesity was correlated with the tumor expression of both ER ($p = 0.004$) and PR ($p = 0.039$) and was also an independent predictor of a shorter disease-free survival after controlling for the ER/PR variables (HR, 3.33; CI, 1.26–9.02). Prospective cohort study outcomes in 2843 British women aged <40 years reported a significantly lower 8-year overall survival (HR, 1.65; $p < 0.001$) and distant disease-free interval (HR, 1.44; $p < 0.001$) in patients with obesity, independent of ER-positive status. Other authors have reported obesity and breast cancer recurrence and disease-specific or overall survival to be related or unrelated to ER-negative tumors, and related or unrelated to ER-positive tumors. Breast cancer stem cells make up only about 1–2% of the tumor mass and, yet, are the likely driver for much of breast cancer behavior. Adipocytes in the breast and other tissues produce estrogen as well as leptin, adiponectin, and adipokines with opposing endocrine and paracrine activities that may promote cancer growth. Inflammation in breast adipose tissue as indicated by macrophage accumulation may be an important pathologic factor responsible for both local aromatase activation and tumor genesis. Several studies have shown single-nucleotide polymorphism (SNP) in both the fat mass and obesity-associated gene (FTO) and the melanocortin-4 receptor gene (MC4R) to be linked to overweight and obesity. The association between obesity-related SNP and breast cancer risk was studied with SNP genotyping in patients with breast cancer compared to healthy women. When analyzed alone, FTO SNP did not show significant associations with breast cancer development, whereas MC4R SNP showed an increased risk ($p = 0.032$). The interaction of FTO and MC4R polymorphisms showed a strong association with breast cancer, having a 4.6-fold increased risk for women with these allele combinations, independent of both age and BMI.

Insulin resistance due to increased adiposity may also play a major role in cancer development due to insulin's mitogenic activity. In a case-cohort analysis of 22,494 women followed in the European Prospective Investigation into Cancer and Nutrition study for up to 15 years, of the dysmetabolic syndrome components, only high FBG was significantly associated with an increased risk of breast cancer in women after the menopause (HR 1.89; CI, 1.29–2.77), but not women before the menopause (HR, 0.80; CI, 0.52–1.22). Thus, insulin resistance has been shown to be the one component of the dysmetabolic syndrome consistently related to cancer risk. In 1607 Italian women followed for over 15 years with BMI and glucose data, the highest glucose tertile (tertiles defined as <84.0, 84.1–94.0, and >94.0 mg/dL) was related to greater breast cancer mortality compared to lower glucose values (HR, 2.6; CI 1.2–5.7). In a multivariate analysis of incident breast cancer cases from the WHI study, metabolically unhealthy women, defined by HOMA-IR or fasting insulin levels, were at a higher risk of breast cancer regardless of normal or overweight BMI status, whereas metabolically healthy and overweight women did not have an increased risk of breast cancer. An analysis of 621 women with local or regional breast cancer reported WC to be positively associated with all-cause mortality (HR, 2.99; CI, 1.14–7.86), but not breast cancer-specific mortality. In this study, WHR was positively associated with both all-cause mortality (HR, 2.10; CI, 1.08–4.05) and breast cancer-specific mortality (HR, 4.02; CI, 1.31–12.31). After adjustment for HOMA-IR score and C-reactive protein, risk estimates were attenuated and not statistically significant, suggesting that insulin resistance and inflammation may mediate the effects of central adiposity on breast cancer mortality.

17.5 Ovarian Cancer

Ovarian cancer is a fatal disease with a poor 5-year survival rate. Risk factors for ovarian cancer are not well established, but potential factors include age, infertility, positive family history, and adiposity. Wu and colleagues reported 30 incident ovarian cancers diagnosed from 11,258 women recruited into the Community-Based

Cancer Screening Program study and followed for a median 19.9 years. A BMI >27 kg/m^2 was associated with increased ovarian cancer risk (HR, 2.90; CI, 1.30–6.46), and a nested case-control study within the cohort identified an independent effect of adipokines on cancer risk. Several meta-analyses have shown a significant association between adiposity and ovarian cancer. In an updated meta-analysis of the Continuous Update Project, a nonlinear association (p-nonlinearity <0.0001) with ovarian cancer risk was present with increasing BMI ≥28 kg/m^2. The RR was 1.07 ($n = 28$ studies) for a five-unit increment in BMI and 1.06 ($n = 6$ studies) per 10-cm increase in WC. No association was found for weight gain, WHR, or hip circumference. Liu and colleagues conducted a meta-analysis of 26 observational studies on the association between adiposity and ovarian cancer, of which 13 were case-control studies (7782 cases and 21,854 controls) and 13 were cohort studies (5181 cases). These authors found that for all women, a greater BMI was associated with an increased risk of ovarian cancer, with a pooled RR of 1.07 and 1.28 for overweight and obesity BMI groups, respectively. However, in subgroup analysis, these associations were present only in women before, and not after, the menopause.

A pooled analysis of 15 case-control studies (13,548 cases and 17,913 controls) participating in the Ovarian Cancer Association Consortium evaluated the association between adiposity and ovarian cancer, histological subtype, menopausal status, and HRT use. An increased BMI at all ages was associated with increased cancer risk. Obesity appeared to increase the risk of the less common histological subtypes and did not increase the risk of high-grade invasive serous ovarian cancers. Among women after the menopause, the associations did not vary between women who did and did not use HRT. An international collaborative analysis of original data from 21 studies and 12,390 women with ovarian carcinoma explored associations between adiposity and histologic subtype. Overall, 54% of women ($n = 6715$) died during follow-up, and decreased overall survival was observed for women who had obesity (HR, 1.10 for BMI 30–34.9 kg/m^2; HR, 1.12 for BMI >35 kg/m^2). Results were similar for progression-free survival and ovarian cancer survival, and associations were the strongest for women with low-grade serous and endometrioid tumor subtypes. On multivariate analysis of 81 patients with low-grade ovarian cancer, obesity (HR, 2.8; CI, 1.05–7.3; $p = 0.04$) and primary tumor cytoreduction surgery (HR, 0.05; CI, 0.008–0.29; $p = 0.001$) were significant predictors of overall survival. However, obesity was not associated with worse disease-specific survival, suggesting other factors are also involved in cancer mortality. Two groups of women with increased adiposity (BMI 25.0–39.9 kg/m^2 and BMI >40 kg/m^2) showed no difference in overall survival after primary cytoreduction surgery, compared to normal-weight subjects, in a report of 620 women with advanced stage IIIC/IV epithelial ovarian cancer. This is in contrast to a retrospective review of 90 patients undergoing secondary cytoreduction surgery for recurrent ovarian cancer, where BMI in a multivariate analysis was an independent predictor of survival ($p = 0.02$).

17.6 Endometrial/Uterine Cancer

Epidemiological studies have related adiposity in childhood, adolescence/teens, and young adulthood with endometrial cancer risk. Weight gain after the teenage years was shown to be positively associated with endometrial cancer risk, and none of the younger weight associations persisted after adjustment for BMI in adulthood (HR 4.13, for adult BMI >35 versus BMI <25 kg/m^2). In women after the menopause, the association with BMI was significantly stronger among those not taking HRT. A review of anthropometrics in 51,948 women in the Nurses' Health Study found no independent association between WC or WHR and the risk of endometrial cancer after adjustment for BMI. A literature review and subsequent meta-analysis of 40 studies (20 prospective cohort studies and 20 case-control studies) involving 32,281,242 subjects were conducted to address the association between BMI and endometrial cancer. The estimated RR and OR of endometrial cancer was 1.34 and 1.43 for overweight and 2.54 and 3.33 for obesity groups, respectively. Wu and colleagues reported on 38 newly diagnosed uterine cancer cases from 11,258 women in the National Cancer Registry and Death Certification System. Multivariate analysis showed that alcohol intake, elevated triglycerides, years of endogenous estrogen exposure, and increased adiposity (HR 2.90 for BMI >27 kg/m^2; CI, 1.30–6.46) were associated with increased cancer risk. Subanalysis further showed an independent effect of adipokines on uterine cancer risk. Thus, adiposopathy, or adipose tissue dysfunction, is linked to the risk of cancer. A recent meta-analysis investigated the associations between circulating adiponectin, leptin, and the leptin/adiponectin ratio with endometrial cancer risk. Thirteen studies (five nested case-control and eight case-control studies) reported on a total of 1963 endometrial cancer cases and 3503 case controls. There was a decreased risk of cancer with elevated circulating adiponectin, decreased leptin/adiponectin ratio, and decreased leptin concentrations. An interesting study of genetic markers of the adiponectin gene reported on the genotype distribution of a single SNP [+276G > T (rs1501299)] marker, in an attempt to identify its impact on adiposity and endometrial cancer. Ninety women were treated surgically for endometrial cancer, and 90 women treated in parallel for uterine fibroids served as controls. SNP analysis was done in women who were lean, or had overweight or obesity, and who had endometrial cancer. The allele G was significantly more frequent and the allele T significantly less frequent in women with obesity, compared to lean controls. No correlations were present in either the lean or overweight groups.

Prolonged estrogen exposure is believed to be a major cause of endometrial cancer. Wang and colleagues assessed various menstrual and reproductive features (e.g., total number of menstrual cycles, age at menarche, and age at menopause) as markers of estrogen exposure on endometrial cancer risk in 482 cancer patients compared to 571 population controls. The total number of menstrual cycles was associated with endometrial cancer risk independent of adiposity, and the risk increased by 2.5% for every additional ten menstrual cycles. Age at menarche was also a significant risk factor, and this association remained statistically significant, although attenuated, after adjustment for obesity.

Trabert and colleagues examined whether metabolic factors, individually or combined, were associated with endometrial cancer in 16,323 cancer cases compared to 100,751 Medicare enrollees from the same registry. The dysmetabolic syndrome was identified using ICD-9-CM codes 1–3 years before the diagnosis of cancer. Endometrial cancer risk was associated with the dysmetabolic syndrome [OR, 1.39; CI, 1.32–1.47) and its component factors of overweight/obesity (HR, 1.95; CI, 1.80–2.11), IFG (HR, 1.36; CI, 1.30–1.43), high blood pressure (HR, 1.31; CI, 1.25–1.36), and high triglyceride levels (HR, 1.13; CI, 1.08–1.18). After adjusting for overweight/obesity, the increased risks associated with the other dysmetabolic syndrome factors remained. In patients with endometrial cancer, plasma levels of IL-8 were significantly elevated in patients with cancer compared to controls ($p < 0.001$). Visceral fat area as evaluated by ultrasound in this study was significantly larger compared to the control group ($p < 0.0001$), and a positive linear correlation was also found between plasma levels of IL-8 and visceral fat area.

IGF and IGF signaling proteins are associated with obesity, T2DM, hyperinsulinemia, and cell proliferation. Thus, the glycolytic pathway is a potential therapeutic target for the inhibition of tumor activity in cancer cells. Biological actions of IGF proteins are mediated by the IGF-1 receptor (IGF-1R), a transmembrane tyrosine kinase that is structurally associated with the insulin receptor. IGF-1R binds to the corresponding ligands, IGF-1, IGF-2, and insulin, inducing autophosphorylation which results in the activation of the phosphatidylinositol 3-kinase-AKT/mammalian target of rapamycin (mTOR) signaling pathway and promoting cell proliferation and suppressing apoptosis. Metformin use has been associated with significant reductions in cancer incidence, to include endometrial cancer. Metformin has been shown to inhibit cancer cell growth by activating adenosine monophosphate-activated protein kinase (AMPK), thereby inactivating mTOR and reducing mTOR effector activity. Metformin was also observed to downregulate IGF-1R and induce apoptosis in endometrial cancer cell lines. Chinese women with newly diagnosed T2DM were followed to assess endometrial cancer risk in patients who did ($n = 193,005$) and did not ($n = 285,916$) take metformin as T2DM therapy. A time-dependent approach was used to calculate endometrial cancer incidence, and during follow-up, 728 metformin ever-users and 2157 never-users developed endometrial cancer (HR, 0.675; CI, 0.614–0.742). Adjusted HRs for cancer in the low to high tertiles of cumulative duration of metformin therapy were 1.089, 0.707, and 0.313, respectively, with similar HR trends for cumulative dose of metformin (1.062, 0.620, and 0.376, respectively). The antiproliferative, molecular, and metabolic effects of metformin 850 mg daily was studied in 20 women with obesity and endometrial cancer. Metformin was administered for up to 4 weeks prior to surgical staging, and expression of the proliferation marker Ki-67, ER, PR, AMPK and downstream targets of mTOR pathway were measured. Based upon pre- and post-treatment comparison of endometrial tumors, metformin reduced cellular proliferation by 11.75% ($p = 0.008$), and 65% of patients responded positively to metformin as defined by decreased Ki-67 tumor staining. Metformin also decreased expression of phosphorylated-AMPK ($p = 0.00001$) and ER ($p = 0.0002$), but not PR expression. Metabolomic profiling indicated that metformin use induced a shift in lipid and glycogen metabolism that was more pronounced in the serum and tumors of responders versus nonresponders. Sivalingam and colleagues also studied presurgical administration of metformin (850 mg twice daily, median use 20 days) in patients with obesity and endometrial cancer either taking ($n = 28$) or not taking ($n = 12$) the drug. Sixty percent of patients had obesity, and 22 had either undiagnosed T2DM (FBG >7.0 mmol/L, $n = 4$) or insulin resistance (HOMA-IR >2.8, $n = 18$). In the metformin-treated group, Ki-67 was 12.9% lower at hysterectomy than at study recruitment.

Obesity is classically linked to type I or lower grade endometrial cancer. A retrospective review of the effect of adiposity on lymphovascular invasion was conducted in 1341 patients with endometrial cancer from a prospectively maintained uterine cancer database. A hysterectomy and salpingo-oophrectomy with or without lymph node dissection was performed in all patients. In multivariate analyses, higher BMI was independently associated with younger age at diagnosis and the presence of lower tumor grade and was not associated with lymphovascular invasion. Patients with endometrial cancer and adiposity are more likely to have stage I disease and <50% myometrial invasion than those at normal weight. The use of adjuvant therapy, disease recurrence, and cancer-specific survival have been reported not to vary by BMI status. However, BMI ($p = 0.016$), age ($p < 0.0001$), race ($p = 0.033$), and risk group ($p < 0.0001$) were predictive of all-cause mortality, suggesting a detrimental effect of adiposity independent of cancer-specific mortality. Others have also reported on increased all-cause mortality in patients with endometrial cancer and either increased adiposity or the dysmetabolic syndrome. A systematic review and random-effects meta-analysis of 18 studies reported significantly higher mortality with increasing BMI in patients with endometrial cancer. A single dose-response model in this review indicated a 9.2% increase in all-cause mortality correlated with a 10% increase in BMI ($p = 0.007$).

17.7 Esophageal and Gastric Cancer

Esophageal adenocarcinoma (EAC) is rapidly increasing in incidence in Western cultures, and Barrett's esophagus (BE) is the presumed precursor lesion. Risk factors for BE and EAC include adiposity, tobacco smoking, and gastroesophageal reflux disease (GERD). Despite these associations, most patients with EAC present with symptoms of dysphagia from late-stage tumors and only a small number of patients are identified by surveillance programs. Factors predicting progression from BE to EAC include dysplastic changes on esophageal histology and length of the involved BE segment. Locally advanced disease is generally managed with esophagectomy, often accompanied by neoadjuvant chemoradiation therapy or chemotherapy. Prognosis is based on tumor stage, and patients with early tumors have a good prognosis, while those with advanced disease have poor long-term survival.

Epidemiologic data have supported a strong association between excess adiposity and GERD. The prevalence of GERD in patients who have overweight or obesity is significantly higher than that in the general population. GERD is present in approximately one-third to one-half (range 15–65%) of patients with obesity who seek weight loss therapy. Central obesity, rather than elevated BMI, appears to be more closely associated, but the underlying mechanisms for GERD in patients with adiposity are not entirely clear and are likely multifactorial. Data from the Barrett's and Esophageal Adenocarcinoma Genetic Susceptibility Study used a genetic risk score as an instrument for lifetime adiposity to determine that BE risk increased by 12% and EAC risk increased by 16% for each kg/m^2 increase in BMI. To better evaluate the possible association between adiposity and EAC, a nationwide population-based Swedish study of patients with newly diagnosed esophageal ($n = 189$) and gastroesophageal junction adenocarcinoma ($n = 262$) were matched to controls ($n = 816$) and included data on BMI 20 years before study inclusion. BMI appeared to have the largest effect on gastroesophageal reflux (GER) frequency >3 times per week. However, there was no increased risk of cancer with BMI 20 years before inclusion, with or without adjustment for GER frequency, severity, or duration. Anthropometric data from 391,456 individuals from the European Prospective Investigation into Cancer and Nutrition Study was assessed over 11 years of follow-up by Steffen et al., who found that BMI was unrelated to EAC, while WC showed a strong positive correlation. Hardikar and colleagues also reported no relation between BMI and EAC risk, but noted a significant association with WHR. Thus, central adiposity, rather than total BMI, appears to be more important in the development of GER, BE, and EAC suggesting a possible metabolic etiology. Although 3-year follow-up in the Seattle Barrett's Esophagus Study did not find any correlation between the dysmetabolic syndrome and EAC risk, higher leptin levels had a positive association (HR, 2.51; CI, 1.09–5.81; $p = 0.03$) and adiponectin had a non-linear inverse association with EAC (HR, 0.34; CI, 0.14–0.82). To assess risk factors for the development of EAC in patients with T2DM, an EAC cancer cohort ($n = 1704$) was compared to a cohort group of patients with GERD and prior fundoplication ($n = 1132$). More subjects in the control cohort had obesity, and T2DM was more prevalent in the cancer cohort (31% vs. 15%; $p < 0.0001$). Logistic regression analysis adjusting for comorbidity and lifestyle factors found that T2DM was significantly associated with EAC as opposed to controls (OR, 2.2; CI, 1.7–2.8), and the association appeared to be independent of BMI. The dysmetabolic syndrome and Cancer Project pooled 578,700 prospective cohorts and used metabolic risk factors categorized into quintiles and transformed into Z-scores to create a composite dysmetabolic syndrome score. There were no significant associations between any metabolic factors and gastric cancer among men. Glucose (HR, 1.58), triglyceride levels, and the composite dysmetabolic syndrome score were associated with increased risk of gastric adenocarcinoma in women.

Excess adiposity is associated with an increased risk of gastric cancer. A large case-control study of Korean subjects (998 with gastric cancer, 313 with gastric dysplasia, and 1288 with normal endoscopic findings) analyzed the risk of gastric cancer and dysplasia with increasing adiposity in men and women. A BMI >25 kg/m^2

was associated with increased risk of early gastric cancer in men (OR, 1.66; $p < 0.02$) and gastric dysplasia in women (OR 2.089; $p < 0.05$), independent of *Helicobacter pylori* infection. A meta-analysis of 16 cohort and case-control studies identified that both overweight and obesity were associated with gastric cancer, especially for men (OR, 1.27; CI, 1.09–1.48). A summary of 41,791 subjects from 24 prospective studies found that increasing adiposity correlated with risk of cardia gastric cancer (RR, 1.21 and 1.82 for patients with overweight or obesity, respectively), but not with noncardia gastric cancer. A greater BMI does not appear to be associated with more advanced or invasive gastric cancer and does not seem to adversely impact disease-free survival or overall survival, with the possible exception of decreased survival in older (age >60 years) patients. There is a need to be aware of the possibility of other primary cancers in patients found to have gastric cancer. Takeuchi and colleagues followed 435 patients after surgical resection of gastric cancer and diagnosed other primary cancers in 25% ($n = 109$) of patients, 40 (9.2%) with synchronous and 76 (18.2%) with metachronous cancers. Colorectal cancer (22.8%) was the most common other primary cancer diagnosed. T2DM was found to be an independent risk factor for the occurrence of other primary cancers (OR, 2.22; $p = 0.011$) and was frequently observed with metachronous cancers ($p = 0.007$), whereas obesity was an independent risk factor for synchronous cancers (OR, 2.35; $p = 0.023$).

17.8 Pancreas Cancer

Gastric and hepatobiliary comorbidities, T2DM, and cancer share common risk factors to include increased adiposity and physical inactivity. Using genome-wide association studies, genotype and risk factor data from the Pancreatic Cancer Case Control Consortium were assessed in 2028 cases and 2109 controls to examine gene-obesity and gene-diabetes interactions in relation to pancreatic cancer risk. A significant interaction was observed with the chemokine signaling pathway and obesity, and near significant interaction between the calcium signaling pathway and T2DM. Thus, genetic variations in inflammatory response and insulin resistance may affect the risk of developing pancreatic cancer. The clinical relationship between adiposity and pancreatic cancer was assessed by a questionnaire in both an initial cohort ($n = 501{,}698$) and a subcohort who completed a second questionnaire ($n = 273{,}975$) over 10.5 years of follow-up. Compared to normal-weight individuals, persons overweight at any adult age had a greater risk of pancreatic cancer (HRs ranging from 1.15 to 1.53). Increased cancer risk was seen with weight gain after age 50 years and with a longer duration of excess adiposity (HR per 10-year increment of duration, 1.18; p-interaction = 0.01), especially in persons with T2DM. A retrospective, population-based, cohort study of 166,850 patients with T2DM were matched for age, gender, and locale to 166,850 controls without T2DM and followed for the risk of pancreatic cancer. Higher HRs for pancreatic cancer were seen in patients with T2DM, acute alcoholic hepatitis, acute pancreatitis, cholecystitis, and gastric ulcer compared to patients without T2DM or counterpart comorbidities.

17.9 Hepatobiliary Cancer

Hepatocellular carcinoma (HCC) is the most common histologic type of primary liver cancer, is the fifth most common cancer type, and the third highest cause of cancer death worldwide. Major risk factors for HCC include chronic hepatitis B (HBV) and C (HCV) virus infections, alcoholic liver disease, and nonalcoholic fatty liver disease (NAFLD). Most HCC occurs in the setting of liver cirrhosis from various causes, and approximately 20% of patients with NAFLD have nonalcoholic steatohepatitis (NASH) that may progress to cirrhosis. A 2012 meta-analysis (17 cohort, 18 case-control and cross-sectional, and 26 case series studies) reported an increased risk of HCC in the setting of NASH and cirrhosis (cumulative incidence between 2.4% and 12.8% over 3–7 years, respectively), although HCC risk was substantially lower in the cohorts with NASH versus HCV-related cirrhosis.

NAFLD is associated with the metabolic risk factors to include adiposity, T2DM, and dyslipidemia. Obesity in early adulthood (i.e., mid-20s to mid-40s) was a significant risk factor for HCC in a study comparing 622 newly diagnosed HCC cases with 660 age- and gender-matched healthy controls. Estimated ORs were significantly increased for the entire population (2.6; CI, 1.4–4.4), and for both men (2.3; CI, 1.2–4.4) and women (3.6; CI, 1.5–8.9) in this study. Each BMI unit increase at early adulthood corresponded to a 3.89-month decrease in age at diagnosis of HCC ($p < 0.001$), and there appeared to be a synergistic interaction between obesity and hepatitis virus infection. Data from an Italian HCC case-control study (185 cases and 404 controls) found that among subjects without HBV or HCV, the OR for those with more than two components of the dysmetabolic syndrome was increased over sixfold. However, a US NHANES study of 3846 subjects found that NAFLD was not a manifestation of the dysmetabolic syndrome, but rather a disease strongly associated with features of the dysmetabolic syndrome. Several studies have documented a significantly increased incidence of HCC in patients with obesity and T2DM. Demographics of patients with HCC referred to the Newcastle-upon-Tyne Hospitals found that NAFLD accounted for 35% of HCC cases in 2010, and metabolic factors to include obesity and T2DM were present in 66% of those patients. In 185 Italian subjects with HCC, T2DM and obesity were positively associated with cancer risk, with ORs of 4.33 (CI, 1.89–9.86) and 1.97 (CI, 1.03–3.79), respectively. A large US healthcare database study of patients with HCC identified NAFLD as the most common risk factor (59%), followed by T2DM (36%), and HCV infection (22%). Similar findings were reported in a German cohort, with NAFLD more common than alcoholic liver disease and chronic HBV and HCV infections. A meta-analysis of 26 studies (13 case-control and 13 cohort) found a 2.5-fold increased risk of HCC in patients with T2DM, independent of alcohol intake or viral hepatitis in studies that examined those factors. A more recent 2012 meta-analysis reported a twofold increased risk of HCC in patients with T2DM. Chen and colleagues identified older age (>65 years) and male gender as increased risk factors, but were unable to find any association between HCC and obesity or T2DM in 262 Taiwanese patients with HCC in a community endemic for HBV and HCV infections.

The potential mechanisms underlying the development of HCC in the presence of obesity and T2DM are not clearly delineated. It is possible that IGF-2 plays a role in hepatic carcinogenesis, as preneoplastic lesions express IGF-2 mRNA. IGF-1R is overexpressed in animal models of HCC, and IGF ligands exert their effects on HCC cells through IGF-1R. Levels of IGF-2R and TGF-beta, a growth inhibitor, are reduced in HCC tissue compared to adjacent normal liver. Another key mechanism involves peroxisome proliferator-activated receptor (PPAR) gamma. In vitro, PPAR gamma inhibits HCC, most probably by regulating pathways important in apoptosis. Metformin use has been associated with a reduced risk for certain cancers. In a Mayo Clinic case study of intrahepatic cholangiocarcinoma (612 cases and 594 matched controls) in patients with T2DM, the cancer risk in patients treated with metformin was significantly diminished by 60% (OR, 0.4; CI, 0.2–0.9; $p = 0.04$). Obesity and the dysmetabolic syndrome were not associated with increased cancer risk in this study. In addition, several studies have shown that obesity does not affect recurrence-free survival or overall survival in patients after surgical resection of HCC for up to 5 years of observation and either associated with HCV or without both HBV and HCV hepatitis.

17.10 Colorectal Cancer

Adiposity is associated with an increased risk of colon tumors, and the majority of sporadic colorectal cancers arise from adenomatous polyps. A 2012 meta-analysis showed that a BMI $\geq$25 kg/m^2 was associated with a 24% increased risk in colorectal adenomas. Among 1806 Caucasian and 378 African-American patients undergoing colonoscopy for average risk cancer screening, WC and WHR were associated with increased adenoma risk for both races. However, BMI was associated with adenoma risk only in Caucasians, and the authors speculated that these differences may be related to racial differences in body fat distribution. In a cross-sectional study of 19,361 Korean adults having colonoscopy, the dysmetabolic syndrome was associated with the prevalence of adenomatous polyps in both the proximal and distal colon. Increased prevalence ratios for any adenoma, comparing the 90th to 10th percentile, were also significant for FBG ($p = 0.04$), HOMA-IR, and hemoglobin A1C ($p = 0.02$). Interestingly, Trabulo and colleagues found no difference between adenomas and degree of adiposity in patients with the dysmetabolic syndrome. In contrast, a large cross-sectional study of 18,085 Korean adults found the prevalence of adenomas was increased in metabolically healthy individuals with obesity and in a dose-response manner with increasing categories of BMI ($p < 0.01$). In an analysis of 837 patients (467 men and 370 women) undergoing colonoscopy, 55% with colorectal adenoma or prior history thereof, significant differences were present for percent body fat, WC, and age among men with and without adenomas, but only age was significant among women. Kitahara and colleagues also found no impact of obesity on the incidence or follow-up recurrence of adenomas in women.

Colorectal cancer (CRC) is one of the leading causes of cancer death in men and women worldwide. Studies have shown a consistent association with adiposity and CRC in men, but the association has been weaker and inconsistent in women. In a large cohort of 239,658 young (ages 16–20 years) Swedish male military recruits followed for an average of 35 years, 885 cases of CRC occurred, to include 501 colon cancers and 384 rectal cancers. Compared with normal-weight controls, having overweight or obesity was associated with a 2.08-fold and 2.38-fold higher risk of CRC, respectively ($p < 0.001$). A large screening trial assessed the relationship between adiposity with colorectal adenomas and CRC among men and women, ages 55–74 years, randomly assigned to receive flexible sigmoidoscopy as part of the Prostate, Lung, Colorectal, and Ovarian Cancer Screening Trial. The authors prospectively evaluated the association between baseline BMI and the risk of incident distal adenoma ($n = 1213$), recurrent adenoma ($n = 752$), and incident CRC ($n = 966$). Men who had obesity had significantly higher risk of incident adenoma and CRC. No associations were observed for adenomas or CRC in women. Keskin and colleagues examined BMI, WC, WHR, and hip circumference in relation to CRC among 203,177 patients followed for 10 years. In men, CRC was associated with BMI, WC, and WHR, but all anthropometric measures were unrelated to CRC in women. However, in women using HRT, an inverse relation was suggested between CRC and WC and WHR, and a positive association with hip circumference, implying some modifying effect by HRT. Of note in this study, anthropometric variables were unrelated to rectal cancer for both genders. The inconsistency between CRC risk and obesity in women is likely related to the complex interactions between estrogen (i.e., pre- and postmenopausal status and HRT), body fat distribution, and the hormonal status of colorectal tumors. Emerging data suggest that the association between obesity and CRC is mediated by visceral fat rather than total body fat. For instance, WC and WHR have been reported to be more strongly associated with CRC than BMI in women. Visceral fat was also significantly higher in 191 women with CRC compared to 191 well-matched healthy controls studied by Lee and colleagues. Multivariate analysis revealed that the mean visceral fat area ≥67th percentile was associated with an increased CRC prevalence compared to subjects ≤33th percentile.

Adiposity does not seem to be associated with more advanced CRC stage or grade, as reported in 672 cancer patients from Winnipeg, Manitoba. However, obesity was an independent predictor of cancer recurrence after surgery in patients with stage 2 CRC, compared to subjects who did not have obesity ($p = 0.05$). In a study of 455 colon and 158 rectal cancer deaths, increasing age, higher BMI, and attained adult height were associated with increased risk of death from CRC. In addition, physical activity was associated with a 28% and 25% reduced risk of CRC and rectal cancer, respectively. Morality in a multiethnic cohort was captured over 6.0 ± 4.7 years observation among 4204 incident cases of invasive CRC. Study analysis detected little evidence for any adverse effect of excess adiposity on CRC-specific mortality, but all-cause survival was reduced in women. In contrast, the presence of the dysmetabolic syndrome was found to be an independent risk factor for disease-free survival (HR, 0.733; CI 0.545–0.987; $p = 0.041$), but not for overall survival. The dysmetabolic syndrome was present in 21% of 1069 CRC cases, and these patients were more likely to be older and with higher levels of FBG and triglycerides ($p < 0.05$ for all). Rickles and colleagues conducted a retrospective review of outcomes in patients with CRC following surgical resection. Visceral fat volume was measured by preoperative computerized tomography (CT) scans, and 111 patients had visceral obesity and 108 did not. BMI only weakly correlated with visceral fat volume, and patients had no difference in survival by BMI status. However, patients with CT identified visceral obesity had a 2.7-fold decrease in disease-free survival in stage 2 CRC.

Biochemical differences between visceral and subcutaneous adipose tissue metabolites were investigated by using mass spectrometry metabolomics and gene expression profiling in 59 subjects with CRC. Compared to subcutaneous fat, visceral fat displayed elevated markers of inflammation (i.e., inflammatory lipid metabolism, free arachidonic acid, phospholipases, and prostaglandin synthesis-related enzymes) as supporting evidence for the role of visceral fat in CRC. Expression levels of several genes related to the dysmetabolic syndrome were analyzed by real-time qPCR in two equivalent but independent sets of stage 2 CRC patients. The authors showed that a gene expression profile constituted by genes previously related to the dysmetabolic syndrome was significantly associated with clinical outcomes and able to identify both a low and high risk of relapse. Mendelian randomization was used to assess the association between BMI and cancer from 10,226 CRC cases and 10,286 controls of European ancestry. Mendelian randomization analysis using a weighted genetic risk score, derived from 77 genome-wide association studies, identified variants associated with high BMI. A greater number of BMI-increasing alleles were associated with a higher risk of CRC among women, but not in men. NDRG4, a novel candidate tumor suppressor, inhibits (PI3K/AKT) signaling, which is related to energy balance and carcinogenesis. NDRG4 mRNA levels from 226 patients with CRC were determined by real-time PCR, and decreased NDRG4 mRNA expression in tumors was significantly correlated with cancer differentiation, invasion, and metastasis. Obesity was adversely associated with disease-free and overall survival in tumors with reduced NDRG4 levels, but not in tumors with preserved NDRG4 levels. The authors postulated that host-tumor interactions might influence tumor aggressiveness and could stratify the prognostic value of obesity.

Current guidelines recommend that adults at average risk of CRC begin screening at age 50 years of age without consideration of other potential risk factors. Jung and colleagues recently addressed this issue in a cross-sectional study of 27,894 Koreans ≥30 years of age who underwent colonoscopy as part of a health screening program. Based upon the number needed to screen to identify one patient with advanced neoplasm, additional risk factors (i.e., male gender, smoking, the dysmetabolic syndrome, adiposity, and fatty liver) did not justify screening colonoscopies before 45 years of age. However, the number needed to screen for those 45–49 years old with additional risk factors was found to be lower than that for women after the menopause.

17.11 Other Obesity-Related Cancers

17.11.1 Renal Cell Cancer

Reasons for the recent global increase in the incidence of renal cancer are unclear, but have been speculated to be related to adiposity and hypertension. A recent review of the WHI clinical trials and the Multiple Risk Factor Intervention Trial (MRFIT) assessed these relationships. In the WHI trial ($n = 156{,}774$) using age-adjusted analyses, the risk for renal cancer increased across increasing systolic blood pressure and BMI categories ($p < 0.0001$ for both). In the MRFIT trial ($n = 353{,}340$), risk of death from renal cancer increased with increasing systolic blood pressure. Visceral fat area was determined by CT scanning prior to nephrectomy in 2187 Koreans with renal cell cancer. High visceral fat area (i.e., >50th percentile) was associated with longer cancer-specific ($p = 0.01$) and overall survival ($p = 0.03$), whereas the visceral fat-to-subcutaneous fat area ratio had no influence on survival. Different outcomes were seen in 577 renal cell cancer patients matched to 593 healthy controls at MD Anderson Cancer Center. Obesity at age 20 years ($p = 0.03$) and age 40 years ($p < 0.001$) and moderate ($p = 0.04$) and massive weight gain ($p = 0.01$) from age 20 to 40 years were all significantly associated with increased risk of renal cell cancer. Low physical activity was associated with a fourfold increased risk of cancer. The authors also found that among 190 SNP's in the mTOR pathway, six SNP's located in the AKT3 gene were significantly associated with increased risk for renal cell cancer.

17.11.2 Urothelial Cancer

In a retrospective analysis of 892 patients with primary invasive bladder cancer, greater adiposity and age were associated with an increased risk of disease recurrence, progression, cancer-specific mortality, and any-cause mortality ($p < 0.001$ for all). BMI remained an independent risk factor for all cancer outcomes after multivariate analyses for gender, carcinoma in situ, tumor size, number of tumors, and intravesical therapy. Another retrospective study of 972 patients with urothelial cancer and 1098 matched controls found a significant association with the dysmetabolic syndrome in women only ($p = 0.006$). T2DM ($p < 0.001$) and hypertriglyceridemia ($p = 0.032$) were also significantly associated with cancer risk. Cantiello and colleagues found that a worse pathological stage for urothelial bladder cancer was not associated with the dysmetabolic syndrome, but was associated with increased BMI and WC.

17.11.3 Thyroid Cancer

It appears that excess adiposity may be related to an increased risk of thyroid cancer, although the mechanism is unknown and there is inconsistency among clinical studies. Thyroid ultrasonography was performed as part of a routine health checkup in 15,068 subjects (8491 men and 6577 women), and fine-needle aspiration cytology was performed in 1427 patients based upon predefined criteria. The association between a high BMI and the prevalence of thyroid cancer was only seen in women ($p < 0.001$). There was no association with age or fasting serum insulin in either gender. From three independent case-control studies comparing 1917 pooled adults with papillary thyroid cancer and 2127 controls, an increased thyroid cancer risk was associated with greater BMI and percent body fat for both men and women. Patients who had overweight or obesity had ORs of 1.72 [CI, 1.48–2.00] and 4.17 [CI, 3.41–5.10], respectively. Compared with the lowest quartile of percent body fat, the ORs for the highest quartile were 3.83 [CI, 2.85–5.15] in women and 4.05 [CI, 2.67–6.15] in men. However, different outcomes were seen in 1216 patients with papillary thyroid cancer studied by Tresallet and colleagues, where patients who had overweight or obesity were not at a greater risk of cancer compared to those of normal weight. An association was seen between recurrent or residual loco-regional thyroid cancer and BMI (18.7% for obesity, 8.5% for overweight, and 9.8% for normal weight; $p = 0.03$). At the present time, neck palpation is the recommended initial screening for thyroid cancer in patients who have overweight or obesity.

17.12 Summary

Excess adiposity is implicated in carcinogenesis in many body tissues, and BMI is known to be associated with increased mortality for many cancers. However, little is known about the link between lifetime change in weight or BMI and cancer risk or mortality in adults. A recent meta-analysis of 50 prospective observational studies suggests that avoiding adult weight gain itself may confer protection against certain types of cancers, particularly among women not using HRT. For each 5-kg increase in adult weight gain, the summary relative risk was increased for CRC in men, renal cell cancer, postmenopausal endometrial cancer, and breast and ovarian cancer among postmenopausal women not using (or using low dose) HRT. Adult weight gain was unrelated to cancers of the prostate, pancreas, thyroid, CRC in women, and breast in premenopausal women and postmenopausal taking HRT.

The association between lifetime changes in BMI, calculated over different time periods, and cancer mortality was studied in a large cohort study of 8645 adults (baseline entry 1965–1990 with follow-up through 2008). Obesity at baseline was associated with a higher risk for any cancer mortality, for all subjects and women. Women with chronic obesity (i.e., obesity during the entire study period) had a higher risk of mortality from any cancer, to include breast, colorectal, and lung cancers. Although no significant association was seen between long-term annual change in BMI and cancer mortality, a decrease in BMI was associated with a lower mortality risk from any cancer.

Reading List

Agnoli C, Grioni S, Sieri S, et al. Metabolic syndrome and breast cancer risk: a case-cohort study nested in a multicentre Italian cohort. PLoS One. 2015;10(6):e128891.

Allott EH, Masko EM, Freedland SJ. Obesity and prostate cancer: weighing the evidence. Eur Urol. 2013;63:800.

Allott EH, Howard LE, Song HJ, et al. Racial differences in adipose tissue distribution and risk of aggressive prostate cancer among men undergoing radiotherapy. Cancer Epidemiol Biomark Prev. 2014;23(11):2404–12.

Arnold M, Colquhoun A, Cook MB, et al. Obesity and the incidence of upper gastrointestinal cancers: an ecological approach to examine differences across age and sex. Cancer Epidemiol Biomark Prev. 2015; pii:cebp.0753.2015. [Epub ahead of print].

Arrebola JP, Fernandez MF, Martin-Olmedo P, et al. Adipose tissue concentrations of persistent organic pollutants and total cancer risk in an adult cohort from Southern Spain: preliminary data from year 9 of the follow-up. Sci Total Environ. 2014;500–501:243–9.

Augustin LS, Dal Maso L, Franceschi S, et al. Association between components of the insulin-like growth factor system and endometrial cancer risk. Oncology. 2004;67:54–9.

Aune D, Navarro Rosenblatt DA, Chan DS, et al. Anthropometric factors and ovarian cancer risk: a systematic review and nonlinear dose-response meta-analysis of prospective studies. Int J Cancer. 2015;136(8):1888–98.

Bañez LL, Hamilton RJ, Partin AW, et al. Obesity-related plasma hemodilution and PSA concentration among men with prostate cancer. JAMA. 2007;298:2275.

Banez LL, Albisinni S, Freedland SJ, et al. The impact of obesity on the predictive accuracy of PSA in men undergoing prostate biopsy. World J Urol. 2014;32(2):323–8.

Bhaskaran K, Douglas I, Forbes H, et al. Body-mass index and risk of 22 specific cancers: a population-based cohort study of 5·24 million UK adults. Lancet. 2014;384:755.

Bhindi B, Locke J, Alibhai SM, et al. Dissecting the association between metabolic syndrome and prostate cancer risk: analysis of a large clinical cohort. Eur Urol. 2015;67(1):64–70.

Bieńkiewicz J, Smolarz B, Malinowski A. Association between single nucleotide polymorphism +276G > T (rs1501299) in ADIPOQ and endometrial cancer. Pathol Oncol Res. 2015;22:1–4. [Epub ahead of print].

Bonn SE, Wiklund F, Sjolander A, et al. Body mass index and weight change in men with prostate cancer: progression and mortality. Cancer Causes Control. 2014;25(8):933–43.

Calip GS, Malone KE, Gralow JR, et al. Metabolic syndrome and outcomes following early-stage breast cancer. Breast Cancer Res Treat. 2014;148(2):363–77.

Cantiello F, Cicione A, Autorino R, et al. Visceral obesity predicts adverse pathological features in urothelial bladder cancer patients undergoing radical cystectomy: a retrospective cohort study. World J Urol. 2014;32(2):559–64.

Capasso I, Esposito E, De Laurentiis M, et al. Metabolic syndrome-breast cancer link varies by intrinsic molecular subtype. Diabetol Metab Syndr. 2014;6(1):105.

Chaiteerakij R, Yang JD, Harmsen WS, et al. Risk factors for intrahepatic cholangiocarcinoma: association between metformin use and reduced cancer risk. Hepatology. 2013;57(2):648–55.

Chalasani N, Younossi Z, Lavine JE, et al. The diagnosis and management of non-alcoholic fatty liver disease: practice guideline by the American Association for the Study of Liver Diseases, American College of Gastroenterology, and the American Gastroenterological Association. Hepatology. 2012;55:2005–23.

Chalfin HJ, Lee SB, Jeong BC, et al. Obesity and long-term survival after radical prostatectomy. J Urol. 2014;192(4):1100–4.

Chang P, Friedenberg F. Obesity and GERD. Gastroenterol Clin N Am. 2014;43(1):161–73.

Chen CT, Chen JY, Wang JH, et al. Diabetes mellitus, metabolic syndrome and obesity are not significant risk factors for hepatocellular carcinoma in an HBV- and HCV-endemic area of Southern Taiwan. Kaohsiung J Med Sci. 2013a;29(8):451–9.

Chen Y, Liu L, Wang X, et al. Body mass index and risk of gastric cancer: a meta-analysis of a population with more than ten million from 24 prospective studies. Cancer Epidemiol Biomark Prev. 2013b;22(8):1395–408.

Chiu PKF, Teoh JYC, Chan SYS, et al. Role of PSA density in diagnosis of prostate cancer in obese men. Int Urol Nephrol. 2014;46(12):2251–4.

Cimino S, Favilla V, Russo GI, et al. Oxidative stress and body composition in prostate cancer and benign prostatic hyperplasia patients. Anticancer Res. 2014;34(9):5051–6.

Ciortea R, Mihu D, Mihu CM. Association between visceral fat, IL-8 and endometrial cancer. Anticancer Res. 2014;34(1):379–83.

Collaborative Group on Epidemiological Studies of Ovarian Cancer. Ovarian cancer and body size: individual participant meta-analysis including 25,157 women with ovarian cancer from 47 epidemiological studies. PLoS Med. 2012;9:e1001200.

Copson ER, Cutress RI, Maishman T, et al. Obesity and the outcome of young breast cancer patients in the UK: the POSH study. Ann Oncol. 2015;26(1):101–12.

Cramer DW, Vitonis AF, Bandera EV, et al. Obesity and risk of ovarian cancer subtypes: evidence from the Ovarian Cancer Association Consortium. Endocr Relat Cancer. 2013; 20(2):251–62.

Da Cunha PA, De Carlos Back LK, Sereia AFR, et al. Interaction between obesity-related genes, FTO and MC4R, associated to an increase of breast cancer risk. Mol Biol Rep. 2013;40(12):6657–64.

Dam-Larsen S, Franzmann M, Andersen IB, et al. Long term prognosis of fatty liver: risk of chronic liver disease and death. Gut. 2004;53:750–5.

De Pergola G, Silvestris F. Obesity as a major risk factor for cancer. J Obes. 2013;2013:291546.

Dixon JL, Copeland LA, Zeber JE, et al. Association between diabetes and esophageal cancer, independent of obesity, in the United States Veterans Affairs population. Dis Esophagus. 2015. https://doi.org/10.1111/dote.12402. [Epub ahead of print].

Dougan MM, Hankinson SE, Vivo ID, et al. Prospective study of body size throughout the life-course and the incidence of endometrial cancer among premenopausal and postmenopausal women. Int J Cancer. 2014;137(3):625–37.

Duggan C, Onstad L, Hardikar S, et al. Association between markers of obesity and progression from barrett's esophagus to esophageal adenocarcinoma. Clin Gastroenterol Hepatol. 2013;11(8):934–43.

Dyson J, Jaques B, Chattopadyhay D, et al. Hepatocellular cancer: the impact of obesity, type 2 diabetes and a multidisciplinary team. J Hepatol. 2014;60(1):110–7.

Eden JA. Menopausal status, adipose tissue, and breast cancer risk: impact of estrogen replacement therapy. Horm Mol Biol Clin Invest. 2013;14(2):57–63.

El-Serag HB. Hepatocellular carcinoma. N Engl J Med. 2011;365:1118–27.

El-Serag HB, Hampel H, Javadi F. The association between diabetes and hepatocellular carcinoma: a systematic review of epidemiologic evidence. Clin Gastroenterol Hepatol. 2006;4:369–80.

Ertle J, Dechêne A, Sowa JP, et al. Non-alcoholic fatty liver disease progresses to hepatocellular carcinoma in the absence of apparent cirrhosis. Int J Cancer. 2011;128:2436–43.

Fowke JH, McLerran DF, Gupta PC, et al. Associations of body mass index, smoking, and alcohol consumption with prostate cancer mortality in the Asia cohort consortium. Am J Epidemiol. 2015;182(5):381–9.

Gates MA, Rosner BA, Hecht JL, et al. Risk factors for epithelial ovarian cancer by histologic subtype. Am J Epidemiol. 2010;171:45–53.

George SM, Bernstein L, Smith AW, et al. Central adiposity after breast cancer diagnosis is related to mortality in the Health, Eating, Activity, and Lifestyle study. Breast Cancer Res Treat. 2014;146(3):647–55.

Gong TT, Wu QJ, Wang YL, et al. Circulating adiponectin, leptin and adiponectin-leptin ratio and endometrial cancer risk: evidence from a meta-analysis of epidemiologic studies. Int J Cancer. 2015;137(8):1967–78.

Goodwin PJ, Stambolic V. Impact of the obesity epidemic on cancer. Annu Rev Med. 2015;66:281–96.

Gunderson CC, Java J, Moore KN, et al. The impact of obesity on surgical staging, complications, and survival with uterine cancer: a Gynecologic Oncology Group LAP2 ancillary data study. Gynecol Oncol. 2014;133(1):23–7.
Gunter MJ, Xie X, Xue X, et al. Breast cancer risk in metabolically healthy but overweight postmenopausal women. Cancer Res. 2015;75(2):270–4.
Guo Z, Zhang J, Jiang JH, et al. Obesity does not influence outcomes in hepatocellular carcinoma patients following curative hepatectomy. PLoS One. 2015;10(5):e125649.
Han JM, Kim TY, Jeon MJ, et al. Obesity is a risk factor for thyroid cancer in a large, ultrasonographically screened population. Eur J Endocrinol. 2013;168(6):879–86.
Han J, Zhang L, Guo H, et al. Glucose promotes cell proliferation, glucose uptake and invasion in endometrial cancer cells via AMPK/mTOR/S6 and MAPK signaling. Gynecol Oncol. 2015;138(3):668–75.
Hardikar S, Onstad L, Blount PL, et al. The role of tobacco, alcohol, and obesity in neoplastic progression to esophageal adenocarcinoma: a prospective study of Barrett's esophagus. PLoS One. 2013;8(1):e52192.
Harima S, Hashimoto S, Shibata H, et al. Correlations between obesity/metabolic syndrome-related factors and risk of developing colorectal tumors. Hepato-Gastroenterology. 2013;60(124):733–7.
Hassan MM, Abdel-Wahab R, Kaseb A, et al. Obesity early in adulthood increases risk but does not affect outcomes of hepatocellular carcinoma. Gastroenterology. 2015;149(1):119–29.
Hastert TA, Beresford SAA, Patterson RE, et al. Adherence to WCRF/AICR cancer prevention recommendations and risk of postmenopausal breast cancer. Cancer Epidemiol Biomark Prev. 2013;22(9):1498–508.
Hastert TA, Beresford SAA, Sheppard L, et al. Adherence to the WCRF/AICR cancer prevention recommendations and cancer-specific mortality: results from the Vitamins and Lifestyle (VITAL) Study. Cancer Causes Control. 2014;25(5):541–52.
Haveman-Nies A, de Groot LP, Burema J, et al. Dietary quality and lifestyle factors in relation to 10-year mortality in older Europeans: the SENECA study. Am J Epidemiol. 2002;156(10):962–8.
Heo M, Kabat GC, Strickler HD, et al. Optimal cutoffs of obesity measures in relation to cancer risk in postmenopausal women in the Women's Health Initiative Study. J Women's Health. 2015;24(3):218–27.
Herlevic VC, Mowad R, Miller JK, et al. Breast cancer outcomes in a population with high prevalence of obesity. J Surg Res. 2015;198(2):371–6.
Jenabi E, Poorolajal J. The effect of body mass index on endometrial cancer: a meta-analysis. Public Health. 2015;129(7):872–80.
Jiralerspong S, Kim ES, Dong W, et al. Obesity, diabetes, and survival outcomes in a large cohort of early-stage breast cancer patients. Ann Oncol. 2013;24(10):2506–14.
Ju W, Kim HJ, Hankinson SE, et al. Prospective study of body fat distribution and the risk of endometrial cancer. Cancer Epidemiol. 2015;39(4):567–70.
Jung YS, Yun KE, Chang Y, et al. Risk factors such as male sex, smoking, metabolic syndrome, obesity, and fatty liver do not justify screening colonoscopies before age 45. Dig Dis Sci. 2015;61:1021. [Epub ahead of print].
Kamal M, Burmeister C, Zhang Z, et al. Obesity and lymphovascular! Invasion in women with uterine endometrioid carcinoma. Anticancer Res. 2015;35(7):4053–8.
Kantor ED, Udumyan R, Signorello LB, et al. Adolescent body mass index and erythrocyte sedimentation rate in relation to colorectal cancer risk. Gut. 2015:gutjnl-2014–309007. [Epub ahead of print].
Kaviani A, Neishaboury M, Mohammadzadeh N, et al. Effects of obesity on presentation of breast cancer, lymph node metastasis and patient survival: a retrospective review. Asian Pac J Cancer Prev APJCP. 2013;14(4):2225–9.
Keimling M, Renehan AG, Behrens G, et al. Comparison of associations of body mass index, abdominal adiposity, and risk of colorectal cancer in a large prospective cohort study. Cancer Epidemiol Biomark Prev. 2013;22:1383–94.

Kerimoglu OS, Pekin A, Yilmaz SA, et al. Effect of the percentage of body fat on surgical, clinical and pathological outcomes in women with endometrial cancer. J Obstet Gynaecol Res. 2015;41(3):449–55.

Keskin O, Aksoy S, Babacan T, et al. Impact of the obesity on lymph node status in operable breast cancer patients. J BUON. 2013;18(4):824–30.

Keum N, Greenwood DC, Lee DH, et al. Adult weight gain and adiposity-related cancers: a dose-response meta-analysis of prospective observational studies. J Natl Cancer Inst. 2015;107(2):djv088.

Kim JH, Chin HM, Hwang SS, et al. Impact of intra-abdominal fat on surgical outcome and overall survival of patients with gastric cancer. Int J Surg. 2014a;12(4):346–52.

Kim JH, Doo SW, Yang WJ, et al. Impact of obesity on the predictive accuracy of prostate-specific antigen density and prostate-specific antigen in native Korean men undergoing prostate biopsy. Int J Urol. 2014b;21(10):987–90.

Kim HJ, Kim N, Kim HY, et al. Relationship between body mass index and the risk of early gastric cancer and dysplasia regardless of Helicobacter pylori infection. Gastric Cancer. 2015a;18(4):762–73.

Kim SA, Kim KS, Lee YM, et al. Associations of organochlorine pesticides and polychlorinated biphenyls with total, cardiovascular, and cancer mortality in elders with differing fat mass. Environ Res. 2015b;138:1–7.

Kitahara CM, Berndt SI, de Gonzalez AB, et al. Prospective investigation of body mass index, colorectal adenoma, and colorectal cancer in the prostate, lung, colorectal, and ovarian cancer screening trial. J Clin Oncol. 2013;31:2450–9.

Klurfeld DM. Dietary fibre-mediated mechanisms in carcinogenesis. Cancer Res. 1992;52(7 suppl):2055s–9s.

Kluth LA, Xylinas E, Crivelli JJ, et al. Obesity is associated with worse outcomes in patients with T1 high grade urothelial carcinoma of the bladder. J Urol. 2013;190(2):480–6.

Knoops KT, de Groot LC, Kromhout D, et al. Mediterranean diet, lifestyle factors, and 10-year mortality in elderly European men and women: the HALE project. JAMA. 2004;292(12):1433–9.

Koh WP, Wang R, Jin A, et al. Diabetes mellitus and risk of hepatocellular carcinoma: findings from the Singapore Chinese Health Study. Br J Cancer. 2013;108:1182–8.

Kumar A, Bakkum-Gamez JN, Weaver AL, et al. Impact of obesity on surgical and oncologic outcomes in ovarian cancer. Gynecol Oncol. 2014;135(1):19–24.

Kwan ML, John EM, Caan BJ, et al. Obesity and mortality after breast cancer by race/ethnicity: the California breast cancer survivorship consortium. Am J Epidemiol. 2014;179(1):95–111.

Ladoire S, Dalban C, Roche H, et al. Effect of obesity on disease-free and overall survival in node-positive breast cancer patients in a large French population: a pooled analysis of two randomised trials. Eur J Cancer. 2014;50(3):506–16.

Lagergren J, Mattsson F, Nyren O. Gastroesophageal reflux does not alter effects of body mass index on risk of esophageal adenocarcinoma. Clin Gastroenterol Hepatol. 2014;12(1):45–51.

Lagiou P, Trichopoulos D, Sandin S, et al. Mediterranean dietary pattern and mortality among young women. Br J Nutr. 2006;96(2):384–92.

Larsson SC, Wolk A. Obesity and colon and rectal cancer risk: a meta-analysis of prospective studies. Am J Clin Nutr. 2007;86:556–65.

Lawrence YR, Morag O, Benderly M, et al. Association between metabolic syndrome, diabetes mellitus and prostate cancer risk. Prostate Cancer Prostatic Dis. 2013;16(2):181–6.

Lee SW, Kim JH, Yang HJ, et al. Association between obesity, prostate-specific antigen level and prostate-specific antigen density in men with a negative prostate biopsy. J Int Med Res. 2014a;42(3):821–7.

Lee JY, Lee HS, Lee DC, et al. Visceral fat accumulation is associated with colorectal cancer in postmenopausal women. PLoS One. 2014b;9(11):e110587.

Lee HW, Jeong BC, Seo SI, et al. Prognostic significance of visceral obesity in patients with advanced renal cell carcinoma undergoing nephrectomy. Int J Urol. 2015a;22(5):455–61.

Lee CH, Woo YC, Wang Y, et al. Obesity, adipokines and cancer: an update. Clin Endocrinol. 2015b;83:147–56.

Li C, Kong D. Cancer risks from diabetes therapies: evaluating the evidence. Pharmacol Ther. 2014;144(1):71–81.

Liesenfeld DB, Grapov D, Fahrmann JF, et al. Metabolomics and transcriptomics identify pathway differences between visceral and subcutaneous adipose tissue in colorectal cancer patients: the ColoCare study. Am J Clin Nutr. 2015;102(2):433–43.

Lin CC, Chiang JH, Li CI, et al. Independent and joint effect of type 2 diabetes and gastric and hepatobiliary diseases on risk of pancreatic cancer risk: 10-year follow-up of population-based cohort. Br J Cancer. 2014a;111(11):2180–6.

Lin XJ, Wang CP, Liu XD, et al. Body mass index and risk of gastric cancer: a meta-analysis. Jpn J Clin Oncol. 2014b;44(9):783–91.

Lindkvist B, Almquist M, Bjorge T, et al. Prospective cohort study of metabolic risk factors and gastric adenocarcinoma risk in the Metabolic Syndrome and Cancer Project (Me-Can). Cancer Causes Control. 2013;24(1):107–16.

Liu Z, Zhang TT, Zhao, JJ, et al. The association between overweight, obesity and ovarian cancer: a meta-analysis. Jpn J Clin Oncol. 2015;1–9. https://doi.org/10.1093/jjco/hyv150.

Lopez DS, Tsilidis KK, Hernandez M, et al. Racial and ethnic differences in the association of metabolic syndrome with prostate-specific antigen levels in U.S. Men: NHANES 2001–2006. J Men's Health. 2014;11(4):163–70.

MacInnis RJ, English DR, Hopper JL, et al. Body size and composition and colon cancer risk in women. Int J Cancer. 2006;118:1496–500.

MacLeod LC, Chery LJ, Hu EYC, et al. Metabolic syndrome, dyslipidemia and prostate cancer recurrence after primary surgery or radiation in a veterans cohort. Prostate Cancer Prostatic Dis. 2015;18(2):190–5.

Makarem N, Lin Y, Bandera EV, et al. Concordance with World Cancer Research Fund/American Institute for Cancer Research (WCRF/AICR) guidelines for cancer prevention and obesity-related cancer risk in the Framingham Offspring cohort (1991–2008). Cancer Causes Control. 2015;26(2):277–86.

Maskarinec G, Harmon BE, Little MA, et al. Excess body weight and colorectal cancer survival: the multiethnic cohort. Cancer Causes Control. 2015;26(12):1709–18.

Mazzarella L, Disalvatore D, Bagnardi V, et al. Obesity increases the incidence of distant metastases in oestrogen receptor-negative human epidermal growth factor receptor 2-positive breast cancer patients. Eur J Cancer. 2013;49(17):3588–97.

Miao Jonasson J, Cederholm J, Gudbjornsdottir S. Excess body weight and cancer risk in patients with type 2 diabetes who were registered in Swedish National Diabetes Register—Register-based cohort study in Sweden. PLoS One. 2014;9(9):e105868.

Michelotti GA, Machado MV, Diehl AM. NAFLD, NASH and liver cancer. Nat Rev Gastroenterol Hepatol. 2013;10(11):656–65.

Minami Y, Kawai M, Fujiya T, et al. Family history, body mass index and survival in Japanese patients with stomach cancer: a prospective study. Int J Cancer. 2015;136(2):411–24.

Minicozzi P, Berrino F, Sebastiani F, et al. High fasting blood glucose and obesity significantly and independently increase risk of breast cancer death in hormone receptor-positive disease. Eur J Cancer. 2013;49(18):3881–8.

Mitrou PN, Kipnis V, Thiébaut AC, et al. Mediterranean dietary pattern and prediction of all-cause mortality in a US population: results from the NIH-AARP Diet and Health Study. Arch Intern Med. 2007;167(22):2461–8.

Moller H, Roswall N, Van Hemelrijck M, et al. Prostate cancer incidence, clinical stage and survival in relation to obesity: a prospective cohort study in Denmark. Int J Cancer. 2015;136(8):1940–7.

Moore LL, Chadid S, Singer MR, et al. Metabolic health reduces risk of obesity-related cancer in Framingham study adults. Cancer Epidemiol Biomark Prev. 2014;23(10):2057–65.

Morote J, Ropero J, Planas J, et al. Metabolic syndrome increases the risk of aggressive prostate cancer detection. BJU Int. 2013;111(7):1031–6.

Morrison DS, Parr CL, Lam TH, et al. Behavioural and metabolic risk factors for mortality from colon and rectum cancer: analysis of data from the Asia-Pacific Cohort Studies Collaboration. Asian Pac J Cancer Prev APJCP. 2013;14(2):1083–7.

Murphy CC, Martin CF, Sandler RS. Racial differences in obesity measures and risk of colorectal adenomas in a large screening population. Nutr Cancer. 2015;67(1):98–104.

Nagle CM, Dixon SC, Jensen A, et al. Obesity and survival among women with ovarian cancer: results from the Ovarian Cancer Association Consortium. Br J Cancer. 2015;113(5):817–26.

Navarro M, Baserga R. Limited redundancy of survival signals from the type 1 insulin-like growth factor receptor. Endocrinology. 2001;142:1073–81.

Neumann K, Mahmud SM, McKay A, et al. Is obesity associated with advanced stage or grade of colon cancer? Can J Surg. 2015;58(2):140–2.

Neuzillet Y, Raynaud JP, Lebret T, et al. Obesity and hypogonadism are associated with an increased risk of predominant Gleason 4 pattern on radical prostatectomy specimen. Horm Mol Biol Clin Invest. 2015;22(3):101–9.

Ni J, Lou H, Zhu T, et al. Association between metabolic syndrome and prognosis of endometrioid carcinoma. Zhonghua Fu Chan Ke Za Zhi. 2014;49(10):768–71.

Nishikawa H, Arimoto A, Wakasa T, et al. The relation between obesity and survival after surgical resection of hepatitis C virus-related hepatocellular carcinoma. Gastroenterol Res Pract. 2013a;2013:430438.

Nishikawa H, Osaki Y, Takeda H, et al. Effect of body mass index on survival after curative therapy for non-B non-C hepatocellular carcinoma. J Gastrointestin Liver Dis. 2013b;22(2):173–81.

O'Neill S, O'Driscoll L. Metabolic syndrome: a closer look at the growing epidemic and its associated pathologies. Obes Rev. 2015;16(1):1–12.

O'Sullivan KE, Reynolds JV, O'Hanlon C, et al. Could signal transducer and activator of transcription 3 be a therapeutic target in obesity-related gastrointestinal malignancy? Journal Gastrointestinal Cancer. 2014;45(1):1–11.

Oh JJ, Jeong SJ, Lee BK, et al. Does obesity affect the accuracy of prostate-specific antigen (PSA) for predicting prostate cancer among men undergoing prostate biopsy. BJU Int. 2013;112(4):E265–71.

Ohwaki K, Endo F, Hattori K. Abdominal obesity, hypertension, antihypertensive medication use and biochemical recurrence of prostate cancer after radical prostatectomy. Eur J Cancer. 2015;51(5):604–9.

Okabayashi K, Ashrafian H, Hasegawa H, et al. Body mass index category as a risk factor for colorectal adenomas: a systematic review and meta-analysis. Am J Gastroenterol. 2012;107:1175–85.

Pajares B, Pollan M, Martin M, et al. Obesity and survival in operable breast cancer patients treated with adjuvant anthracyclines and taxanes according to pathological subtypes: a pooled analysis. Breast Cancer Res. 2013;15(6):R105.

Pan SY, Johnson KC, Ugnat AM, et al. Association of obesity and cancer risk in Canada. Am J Epidemiol. 2004;159:259.

Pappa T, Alevizaki M. Obesity and thyroid cancer: a clinical update. Thyroid. 2014;24(2):190–9.

Parekh N, Lin Y, Vadiveloo M, et al. Metabolic dysregulation of the insulin-glucose axis and risk of obesity-related cancers in the Framingham heart study-offspring cohort (1971–2008). Cancer Epidemiol Biomark Prev. 2013;22(10):1825–36.

Park J, Cho SY, Lee SB, et al. Obesity is associated with higher risk of prostate cancer detection in a biopsy population in Korea. BJU Int. 2013;114(6):891–5.

Parker AS, Thiel DD, Bergstralh E, et al. Obese men have more advanced and more aggressive prostate cancer at time of surgery than non-obese men after adjusting for screening PSA level and age: results from two independent nested case-control studies. Prostate Cancer Prostatic Dis. 2013;16(4):352–6.

Pena GG, Maia YC, Mendes MC, et al. Physical activity is associated with malignant and benign breast diseases in low-income Brazilian women. Nutr Cancer. 2014;66(4):707–15.

Pierobon M, Frankenfeld CL. Obesity as a risk factor for triple-negative breast cancers: a systematic review and meta-analysis. Breast Cancer Res Treat. 2013;137(1):307–14.

Pischon T, Lahmann PH, Boeing H, et al. Body size and risk of colon and rectal cancer in the european prospective investigation into cancer and nutrition (EPIC). J Natl Cancer Inst. 2006;98:920–31.

Pitsavos C, Panagiotakos D, Trichopoulou A, et al. Interaction between Mediterranean diet and methylenetetrahydrofolate reductase C677T mutation on oxidized low density lipoprotein concentrations: the ATTICA study. Nutr Metab Cardiovasc Dis. 2006;16(2):91–9.

Poorolajal J, Jenabi E, Masoumi SZ. Body mass index effects on risk of ovarian cancer: a meta-analysis. Asian Pac J Cancer Prev. 2014;15:7665–71.

Previs RA, Kilgore J, Craven R, et al. Obesity is associated with worse overall survival in women with low-grade papillary serous epithelial ovarian cancer. Int J Gynecol Cancer. 2014;24(4):670–5.

Rampal S, Yang MH, Sung J, et al. Association between markers of glucose metabolism and risk of colorectal adenoma. Gastroenterology. 2014;147(1):78–87.e3.

Renehan AG, Tyson M, Egger M, et al. Body-mass index and incidence of cancer: a systematic review and meta-analysis of prospective observational studies. Lancet. 2008;371:569–78.

Renne M, Conforti F, Camastra C, et al. Macrophage activation and patterns of inflammation in obese and non-obese women with breast carcinoma. Eur J Inflamm. 2014;12(1):197–200.

Rickles AS, Iannuzzi JC, Mironov O, et al. Visceral obesity and colorectal Cancer: are we missing the boat with BMI? J Gastrointest Surg. 2013;17(1):133–43.

Rocha GZ, Dias MM, Ropelle ER, et al. Metformin amplifies chemotherapy-induced AMPK activation and antitumoral growth. Clin Cancer Res. 2011;17:3993–4005.

Rogers CJ, Prabhu KS, Vijay-Kumar M. The microbiome and obesity-an established risk for certain types of cancer. Cancer J. 2014;20(3):176–80.

Rohan TE, Heo M, Choi L, et al. Body fat and breast cancer risk in postmenopausal women: a longitudinal study. J Cancer Epidemiol. 2013;2013:754815.

Rose DP, Vona-Davis L. Biochemical and molecular mechanisms for the association between obesity, chronic inflammation, and breast cancer. Biofactors. 2014;40(1):1–12.

Rubenstein JH, Shaheen NJ. Epidemiology, diagnosis, and Management of Esophageal Adenocarcinoma. Gastroenterology. 2015;149(2):302–17.e1.

Runge TM, Abrams JA, Shaheen NJ. Epidemiology of Barrett's esophagus and esophageal adenocarcinoma. Gastroenterol Clin N Am. 2015;44(2):203–31.

Sanfilippo KM, McTigue KM, Fidler CJ, et al. Hypertension and obesity and the risk of kidney cancer in 2 large cohorts of US men and women. Hypertension. 2014;63(5):934–41.

Sanyal A, Poklepovic A, Moyneur E, et al. Population-based risk factors and resource utilization for HCC: US perspective. Curr Med Res Opin. 2010;26:2183–91.

Scalera A, Tarantino G. Could metabolic syndrome lead to hepatocarcinoma via non-alcoholic fatty liver disease? World J Gastroenterol. 2014;20(28):9217–28.

Scarpa M, Ruffolo C, Erroi F, et al. Obesity is a risk factor for multifocal disease and recurrence after colorectal cancer surgery: a case-control study. Anticancer Res. 2014;34(10):5735–41.

Schmid D, Leitzmann MF. Television viewing and time spent sedentary in relation to cancer risk: a meta-analysis. J Natl Cancer Inst. 2014;106(7):dju098.

Schuler KM, Rambally BS, DiFurio MJ, et al. Antiproliferative and metabolic effects of metformin in a preoperative window clinical trial for endometrial cancer. Cancer Med. 2015;4(2):161–73.

Secord AA, Hasselblad V, Von Gruenigen VE, et al. Body mass index and mortality in endometrial cancer: a systematic review and meta-analysis. Gynecol Oncol. 2015. https://doi.org/10.1016/j.ygyno.2015.10.020. [Epub ahead of print].

Shiota M, Yokomizo A, Takeuchi A, et al. The feature of metabolic syndrome is a risk factor for biochemical recurrence after radical prostatectomy. J Surg Oncol. 2014;110(4):476–81.

Shu X, Lin J, Wood CG, et al. Energy balance, polymorphisms in the mTOR pathway, and renal cell carcinoma risk. J Natl Cancer Inst. 2013;105(6):424–32.

Simopoulos AP. Evolutionary aspects of diet, the omega-6/omega-3 ratio and genetic variation. Biomed Pharmacother. 2006;60(9):502–7.

Sivalingam V, McVey R, Gilmour K, et al. A presurgical window-of-opportunity study of metformin in obesity-driven endometrial cancer. Lancet. 2015;385(Suppl1):S90.

Smits MM, Ioannou GN, Boyko EJ, et al. Non-alcoholic fatty liver disease as an independent manifestation of the metabolic syndrome: results of a US national survey in three ethnic groups. J Gastroenterol Hepatol. 2013;28:664–70.

Sourbeer KN, Howard LE, Andriole GL, et al. Metabolic syndrome-like components and prostate cancer risk: results from the reduction by Dutasteride of prostate Cancer events (REDUCE) study. BJU Int. 2015;115(5):736–43.

Steffen A, Huerta JM, Weiderpass E, et al. General and abdominal obesity and risk of esophageal and gastric adenocarcinoma in the European prospective investigation into Cancer and nutrition. Int J Cancer. 2014;137(3):646–57.

Stevens VL, Jacobs EJ, Sun J, et al. No association of plasma levels of adiponectin and c-peptide with risk of aggressive prostate cancer in the Cancer prevention study II nutrition cohort. Cancer Epidemiol Biomark Prev. 2014;23(5):890–2.

Stine JE, Bae-Jump V. Metformin and gynecologic cancers. Obstet Gynecol Surv. 2014;69(8):477–89.

Stolzenberg-Solomon RZ, Schairer C, Moore S, et al. Lifetime adiposity and risk of pancreatic cancer in the NIH-AARP diet and health study cohort. Am J Clin Nutr. 2013;98(4):1057–65.

Taghizadeh N, Boezen HM, Schouten JP, et al. BMI and lifetime changes in BMI and cancer mortality risk. PLoS One. 2015;10(4):e0125261.

Takeuchi D, Koide N, Komatsu D, et al. Relationships of obesity and diabetes mellitus to other primary cancers in surgically treated gastric cancer patients. Int J Surg. 2014;12(6):587–93.

Tang H, Wei P, Duell EJ, et al. Genes-environment interactions in obesity- and diabetes-associated pancreatic cancer: a GWAS data analysis. Cancer Epidemiol Biomark Prev. 2014;23(1):98–106.

Thrift AP, Shaheen NJ, Gammon MD, et al. Obesity and risk of esophageal adenocarcinoma and Barrett's esophagus: a Mendelian randomization study. J Natl Cancer Inst. 2014;106(11).

Thrift AP, Gong J, Peters U, et al. Mendelian randomization study of body mass index and colorectal Cancer risk. Cancer Epidemiol Biomark Prev. 2015;24(7):1024–31.

Tilg H, Moschen AR. Mechanisms behind the link between obesity and gastrointestinal cancers. Best Pract Res Clin Gastroenterol. 2014;28(4):599–610.

Trabert B, Wentzensen N, Felix AS, et al. Metabolic syndrome and risk of endometrial cancer in the United States: a study in the SEER-Medicare linked database. Cancer Epidemiol Biomark Prev. 2015;24(1):261–7.

Trabulo D, Ribeiro S, Martins C, et al. Metabolic syndrome and colorectal neoplasms: an ominous association. World J Gastroenterol. 2015;21(17):5320–7.

Tran AQ, Cohen JG, Li AJ. Impact of obesity on secondary cytoreductive surgery and overall survival in women with recurrent ovarian cancer. Gynecol Oncol. 2015;138(2):263–6.

Tresallet C, Seman M, Tissier F, et al. The incidence of papillary thyroid carcinoma and outcomes in operative patients according to their body mass indices. Surgery. 2014;156(5):1145–52.

Trichopoulou A, Orfanos P, Norat T, et al. Modified Mediterranean diet and survival: EPIC-elderly prospective cohort study. BMJ. 2005;330(7498):991.

Tseng C-H. Metformin and endometrial cancer risk in Chinese women with type 2 diabetes mellitus in Taiwan. Gynecol Oncol. 2015;138:147–53.

Turati F, Talamini R, Pelucchi C, et al. Metabolic syndrome and hepatocellular carcinoma risk. Br J Cancer. 2013;108(1):222–8.

Vanni E, Bugianesi E. Obesity and liver cancer. Clin Liver Dis. 2014;18(1):191–203.

Vargas T, Moreno-Rubio J, Herranz J, et al. Genes associated with metabolic syndrome predict disease-free survival in stage II colorectal cancer patients. A novel link between metabolic dysregulation and colorectal cancer. Mol Oncol. 2014;8(8):1469–81.

Vidal AC, Howard LE, Moreira DM, et al. Obesity increases the risk for high-grade prostate cancer: results from the REDUCE study. Cancer Epidemiol Biomark Prev. 2014;23(12):2936–42.

Wang P, Kang D, Cao W, et al. Diabetes mellitus and risk of hepatocellular carcinoma: a systematic review and meta-analysis. Diabetes Metab Res Rev. 2012;28:109–22.

Wang Z, Risch H, Lu L, et al. Joint effect of genotypic and phenotypic features of reproductive factors on endometrial Cancer risk. Sci Rep. 2015;5:15582. https://doi.org/10.1038/srep15582.

White DL, Kanwal F, El-Serag HB. Association between nonalcoholic fatty liver disease and risk for hepatocellular cancer, based on systematic review. Clin Gastroenterol Hepatol. 2012;10:1342–1359.e2.

Wong J, Rahman S, Saeed N, et al. Effect of body mass index in patients undergoing resection for gastric cancer: a single center US experience. J Gastrointest Surg. 2014;18(3):505–11.
Wu MM, Chen HC, Chen CL, et al. A prospective study of gynecological cancer risk in relation to adiposity factors: cumulative incidence and association with plasma adipokine levels. PLoS One. 2014;9(8):e104630.
Xie Y, Wang YL, Yu L, et al. Metformin promotes progesterone receptor expression via inhibition of mammalian target of rapamycin (mTOR) in endometrial cancer cells. J Steroid Biochem Mol Biol. 2011;126:113–20.
Xie Y, Wang JL, Ji M, et al. Regulation of insulin-like growth factor signaling by metformin in endometrial cancer cells. Oncol Lett. 2014;8(5):1993–9.
Xu L, Port M, Landi S, et al. Obesity and the risk of papillary thyroid cancer: a pooled analysis of three case-control studies. Thyroid. 2014;24(6):966–74.
Xu S, Zhang GM, Guan FJ, et al. The association between metabolic syndrome and the risk of urothelial carcinoma of the bladder: a case-control study in China. World J Surg Oncol. 2015;13(1):5.
You J, Liu WY, Zhu GQ, et al. Metabolic syndrome contributes to an increased recurrence risk of non-metastatic colorectal cancer. Oncotarget. 2015;6(23):19880–90.
Yun KE, Chang Y, Jung HS, et al. Impact of body mass index on the risk of colorectal adenoma in a metabolically healthy population. Cancer Res. 2013;73(13):4020–7.
Zhang JQ, Geng H, Ma M, et al. Metabolic syndrome components are associated with increased prostate cancer risk. Med Sci Monit. 2015a;21:2387–96.
Zhang GM, Zhu Y, Dong DH, et al. The association between metabolic syndrome and advanced prostate cancer in Chinese patients receiving radical prostatectomy. Asian J Androl. 2015b;17(5):839–44.
Zheng J, Li Y, Zhu S, et al. NDRG4 stratifies the prognostic value of body mass index in colorectal cancer. Oncotarget. 2015. https://doi.org/10.18632/oncotarget.6182. [Epub ahead of print].

Chapter 18
Biopsychosocial Modifiers of Obesity

Domenica M. Rubino

Pearls of Wisdom

- From an adipocentric perspective, the physiological state of obesity induces paracrine and endocrine signals that contribute to a myriad of disease states. An individual's biopsychosocial state is a critical, albeit complex, modifier of and contributor to this signaling, although the mechanisms by which this occurs remain unknown.
- The "frame of blame" that emphasizes personal failure and responsibility for adiposity, neglecting scientific evidence, creates stigma and shame that is internalized by the individual and generates chronic psychological stress that can lead to altered mood and eating behavior in a vicious circle.
- The physiological interface between stress response, mood, behavior, chronic pain, and inflammation leads to altered neuroendocrine signaling of reward and appetite circuitry resulting in cravings and eating dysregulation affecting coping, mood, and activity in a vicious cycle.
- Negative early childhood experiences, impulsivity, untreated attention deficit disorder, food addiction, and night-eating syndrome increase the vulnerability for excess adiposity and mood disorders.
- A multidisciplinary approach for the treatment of obesity that recognizes the dynamic cyclical relationship between psychological, social, and physiological factors in the context of an individual's life is more likely to improve quality of life and behavioral change.

D. M. Rubino
Washington Center for Weight Management and Research, Arlington, VA, USA
e-mail: drubino@wtmgmt.com

J. M. Gonzalez-Campoy et al. (eds.), *Bariatric Endocrinology*,
https://doi.org/10.1007/978-3-319-95655-8_18

18.1 Introduction

A biopsychosocial approach to clinical care considers the biological, psychological, and social aspects of an individual's illness, accepts the circular nature of these influences, and recognizes the patient's subjective experiences as well as the relationship with the physician as critical elements of treatment. This chapter focuses on the confluence of physiology and psychology on the state and management of overweight, obesity, and adiposopathy. The recognition and understanding of the complexity, heterogeneity, and interdependence of factors impacting an individual's perception and struggle with weight is critical for the health care professional. The nature of research is to look for causality—a direct linear relationship of cause and effect. The applicability of this approach can be a challenge for a condition like obesity, upon which at any given time, there are a myriad of influences acting at once. Scientific evidence supports a bidirectional relationship between obesity and mood disorders and recognizes the influences of other psychological and social experiences as well. However, though the literature is extensive, it is heterogeneous. Limitations to establishing direction of causality include methodological heterogeneity in study design, criteria for diagnosis, and assessments. Despite the quest for causality, the author would suggest that an acceptance of a circular dynamic of influences (see below) is critical for the contextual clinical care of an individual with obesity (Fig. 18.1). This chapter focuses on some of the internal and external psychological experiences associated with obesity as embodied in the concepts of stigma, shame, body image, chronic pain, early childhood experiences, mood and physical illness, mood disorders, impulsivity, binge eating disorder (BED), and psychological changes after weight loss.

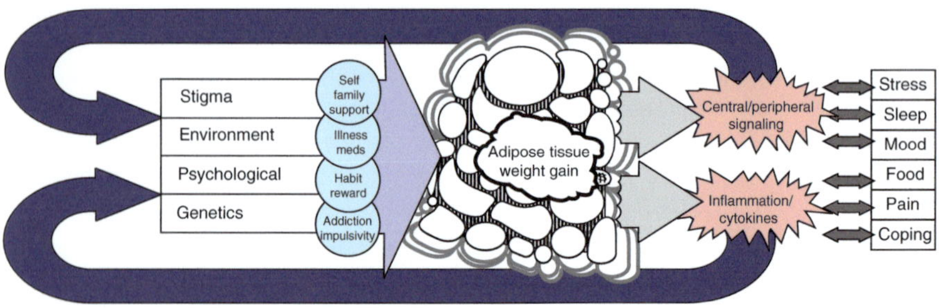

Fig. 18.1 Circular dynamic of influences affecting an individual's weight. Physiological response of weight gain (neuroendocrine signaling and inflammatory factors) interfaces with the context of an individual's experience reinforcing the drive to further weight gain. Stigma includes shame and social isolation. Psychological includes behavioral and emotional components. Genetics includes early childhood experiences

18.2 Stigma

I loathed my body and therefore functioned best when not thinking about it. My body was what was wrong with me. (patient quote from the Muse Project)

An awareness of the pervasive and insidious effect of fat stigmatization and its impact on an individual's health, psyche, and quality of life (QOL) is critical for the health professional. Fat stigma, defined as the negativity attached to having overweight or obesity, exists both externally to and within (internal) an individual. The individual with obesity lives within a "frame of blame" created by cultural and social norms that emphasize personal failure and responsibility for the excess weight. It is not unusual for a person with obesity to experience negative messaging in most aspects of his/her life, family, school, work, through the media, in health care, etc. In a society that focuses on the physical body as one's identity and an inability to hide the stigmatized part, the person with obesity may suffer tremendously.

The degree to which a person might experience fat discrimination varies among individuals. It ranges from outright teasing, bullying, directed criticism, decreased employment opportunities, and differential treatment by health care professionals, to indirect discrimination (such as public seating being too small, gowns that don't fit, "normal" size only, etc.). Additionally, the extent to which an individual is vulnerable to this discrimination varies. Feeling stigmatized can lead to altered behavior (direct effects) and/or increased psychosocial stress (indirect effects).

18.2.1 Altered Behavior

Experiencing stigma can impede weight loss directly or perpetuate weight gain. Studies have shown that people who feel judged about their size are less likely to participate in physical activity and more likely to avoid public settings like gyms, pools, or organized sports. Additionally, research has shown that individuals, who consider themselves overweight, will eat more following exposure to a video or magazine depicting stigmatization. Feeling stigmatized is associated with reports of comfort eating, binge eating, and severe calorie restriction in surveys, and can lead to habitual as well as biological cueing for emotional dysregulated eating patterns (see below). Weight-biased discrimination has been shown to affect binge eating behavior. Feeling stigmatized when visiting health care providers can also provide an impediment to obtaining health care potentially worsening comorbidities and quality of life as part of a vicious circle. Health care professionals should be aware of their own biases since individuals recognize physicians as the second most common source of stigma in their lives, and even those who work with obesity have been demonstrated to show high weight bias and a focus on personal responsibility.

18.2.2 Increased Psychosocial Stress

Research has shown that feeling stigmatized and being discriminated against creates a chronic stressed state for the individual. Chronic stress leads to weight gain, predominantly of visceral adipose tissue, and thought to be mediated by the hypothalamic-pituitary-adrenal axis (HPAA) and the sympathetic nervous system. Individuals who already have overweight or obesity may be more vulnerable to additional weight gain from stress. The weight gain mediated by stress-related chronic glucocorticoid elevation leads to alterations in food-seeking behavior, such as increased fat and sugar consumption. Studies have implied a role of cortisol exposure and metabolic impact. Middle-aged adults reporting stigmatization demonstrated increased A1C levels for a given waist circumference relative to those without stigmatization, and Asian Americans experiencing racial discrimination reported a higher body mass index (BMI) and rate of obesity. Additionally, stigma manifesting in socioeconomic stresses, bias affecting wage and career position, less access to health care, food insecurity, worse access to healthy food, or neighborhoods conducive to activity/exercise, and the built environment may aggravate stress in a given individual.

Unfortunately, these stigmas are believed, projected, and perpetuated by those with obesity. Internalized stigma or internalized weight bias (IWB) leads to doubt regarding the potential for success of a given intervention for weight loss (aggravated by physiological resistance to weight loss) and can lead to abandoning efforts or avoiding action altogether. These decreases in self-efficacy and self-esteem can impact every aspect of lifestyle intervention, including affecting the ability to see/feel success such as improvement in comorbid conditions compared to body weight measurements on the scale.

18.2.3 Eating Disorders

IWB is also associated with eating disorders. In a group seeking treatment for weight loss, an assessment for IWB found an increased prevalence in those with binge eating disorder (BED). This study found that the IWB correlated strongly with an increase in shape and weight concerns but not BMI per se. The authors proposed that the psychological context rather than the weight itself was important for IWB. These subjects were also found to have fat phobia, increased depression, and lower self-esteem, but that did not predict IWB. Others have proposed that IWB may be dynamic and show improvement with behavioral weight loss.

18.2.4 Depression, Social Isolation, and Suicide Risk

Stigma predicts a risk for depression, and females may be particularly vulnerable (see below, Depression). People may also cope with stigma by withdrawing and being more socially isolated. Social rejection and isolation impact psychosocial stress, and individuals with decreased social networks are more likely to be depressed. Markowitz et al. suggested that individuals with obesity may have less social support. Of note, perceived stress has been reported to be more damaging than objective isolation and is associated with neuroendocrine alterations in HPAA activation and inflammatory pathways, ultimately impacting health. Loneliness impacts many aspects of QOL, including physical and mental health. The combination of social isolation and stigma has been reported as an indicator of suicide risk, and obesity has also been reported as a risk factor for suicidal behavior, though this is debated. The potential coupling of these factors with depression may aggravate suicide risk.

18.3 Shame

Body-related shame, the painful emotion of perceiving one's self as flawed or bad, is complex and multifaceted. It integrates emotional, cognitive, behavioral, experiential, social, and physiological responses and is often experienced by individuals with obesity. Shame and stigma are interwoven, reinforcing experiences that embody the failure to get size and/or food "right" to fit into society, resulting in a loss of social status. This discrepancy (perceived or real) between "ideal" and one's actual weight status is associated with lower self-esteem and greater negative body-related emotions. Perceived weight discrepancy may be more important than actual weight discrepancy in creating a low self-esteem. It has been suggested that shame is more enduring than guilt, which may be more tied to behavior, and fleeting, i.e., "I am a bad person because I am overweight" versus "I am overweight because I don't exercise". Shame exists as a duality, with an individual experiencing shame internally (seeing the self as flawed and impacting affect regulation) and/or externally (belief that others see you as flawed and affecting social interaction). Both have been identified in a subgroup of individuals with obesity exhibiting levels of psychological distress. Shame has been reported to be associated with eating disorders including BED as well as depression, anxiety, and post-traumatic stress disorder (PTSD). In individuals with BED, shame is related to having shape and weight concerns, not BMI or number of episodes of binge eating.

Behavioral manifestations of shame include a tendency to hyper-focus on body-shape and/or weight concerns, including social comparison to body weights of others; avoidance (or withdrawal from) social interaction, size/shape information (scale, mirrors), body exposure (public pools/locker rooms), and/or intimacy. Compensation by overperformance (work, academics), self-destructive behaviors, concealment (needs, body, food), and difficulty seeking help have also been noted. Being "in control" by restricting food and desires is seen as the "ideal" and associated with an improved sense of self. Inability to maintain this control is then associated with shame and guilt. Fluctuations between pride and shame (in control vs. not) seen in individuals with eating disorders and obesity may create a vicious cycle by exacerbating shame, which then causes further disordered eating.

Though QOL improves after weight loss, many people remain *dissatisfied* with their body after weight loss, seeking plastic surgery in several areas. Explorations of individual variation in psychosocial outcomes after plastic surgery to remove excess skin using structured interviews revealed two themes: shame and lack of self-acceptance. Many subjects remained focused on the "future body," planning additional surgeries, more weight loss, and lacking acceptance of their current body. External shame (the sense that others do not accept you) persists in individuals with eating disorders in remission. Interventions directed toward treating shame, identification of the degree to which the lack of control is functioning as a major source of low self-esteem or distorted identity, and supporting social skills/interaction if an individual is socially isolated are useful in those who struggle with obesity, with or without an eating disorder. Group-based work may be helpful for those with shame, supporting self-acceptance and compassion through supporting and helping others.

18.4 Body-Weight/Shape Concerns and Perceptions

Psychosocial impairment can be found in subpopulations of individuals with obesity. It is mediated by variables such as presence of BED, poor physical health (see below), and negative body-weight/shape concerns. Identification and treatment of these variables are critical to improving QOL. Body-weight/shape concerns appear to have a greater impact on psychosocial impairment than BED. Negative-weight/shape concerns correlate more closely with psychosocial distress and body-related worrying correlates to negative affect with weight. An epidemiologic study of Australians examined the association between general psychological distress, life satisfaction, and social support, as assessed by questionnaires with body-weight/shape concerns, health status, and presence of BED. They documented that having body-weight/shape concerns was equally important as physical health status in mediating psychosocial functioning in both genders. They also documented that binge eating had no mediating effect. In men, binge eating was associated with a decrease in life satisfaction.

Many body-image studies do not include men because it was previously thought that men with obesity did not experience negative effects on their body image. Recent epidemiologic studies suggest that men with obesity do experience negative psychosocial effects and more research is needed.

"Chronic weight dissatisfaction" (a previously used term, now replaced by "body weight/shape concerns", reflecting a broader cognitive concept) has been reported to be associated with risk for type 2 diabetes mellitus (T2DM). A 5-year, longitudinal study of 9584 adults in the Aerobics Longitudinal study found that weight dissatisfaction was associated with increased risk for T2DM independent of BMI. Subjects who became more satisfied with their weight were more likely to become physically active with a trend toward improvement in T2DM risk. Physicians and health providers should take this into account and perhaps identify other motivators to promote health behavior change.

Fitness may play a role as a psycho-physiological modifier, improving self-esteem, body image, perceived weight satisfaction, and metabolic conditions. The degree to which a person is satisfied with their body weight seems to play a role in their choice of behaviors around motivation for change. Weight satisfaction has been reported to be associated with better lifestyle behaviors such as regular physical activity and consuming more fruits and vegetables. Weight satisfaction is also associated with *less* motivation to change in those who perceive their weight as positive, even if overweight. Weight dissatisfaction is associated with unhealthy behaviors such as snacking, binging, and smoking. Thus, weight dissatisfaction is not a motivator to achieve a healthier lifestyle. Focusing on body-weight/shape concerns in both males and females, and identifying potential modifiers of such concerns, may prove helpful to the individual with obesity.

18.5 Quality of Life

A patient's perception of their own well-being (physical and mental) and function as a consequence of a medical condition(s) is commonly measured in clinical research with the self-administered tool Health Related Quality of Life score. Most studies document that as BMI and comorbidities increase, quality of life (QOL) decreases. This association seems to be more prevalent in women and the elderly, where QOL scores typically show decreases in physical function and general health, but not mental scores. It has been shown that QOL is negatively impacted by mobility, pain, and lack of sleep. Chronic lack of sleep also leads to weight gain, metabolic syndrome, cardiovascular disease, alterations in immune function, inflammation, and mood disorders. QOL improves with weight loss.

18.6 The Physiological Interface of Stress, Mood, Behavior, Pain, and Food

18.6.1 Stress

The human adaptations to managing overwhelming environmental, physical, physiological, or emotional demands, in an effort to regain balance, are termed collectively as stress. The adaptive neuroendocrine mechanisms by which one maintains this allostasis, or new tentative physiological equilibrium, comes at a price. Allostatic load, or the cumulative excess of stress, weakens the human organism's ability to adapt and increases risk for illness and disease. The impact of stress on neurobiological pathways involved in reward circuitry, appetite, and addiction alters behavior and consequent physiology, leading to overeating and weight gain in vulnerable individuals.

There is an association between chronic stress and weight gain, predominantly from the accrual of visceral adipose tissue. Chronic stress leads to the subsequent risk for insulin resistance and abnormal regulation of glucose homeostasis induced by a dysregulated HPAA axis. The alterations in insulin regulation, together with the continued release of glucocorticoids, impact the hormonal circuitry regulating appetite (leptin, ghrelin, neuropeptide Y (NPY)) and change eating behavior (selection and intake of high calorie foods), promoting visceral adiposity, furthering this cycle. Ghrelin, a gastrointestinal hormone secreted before each meal, has been implicated in regulating mood and anxiety (see below). Additionally, persistent sympathetic activity may aggravate insulin resistance as well.

Increased feeding behavior leads to decreased anxiety and stress. The amygdala, prefrontal cortex (PFC), arcuate nucleus, and the hippocampus, under the regulation of corticotropin-releasing factor, NPY, and the noradrenergic system, all contribute to this effect of increased feeding. This highly integrated network impacts reward pathway activation. There is an increase in dopamine transmission and subsequent seeking of highly palatable (HP) food. This may be seen as a reward system, especially for food that is high in fat and sugar, potentially sensitizing this path for continued persistent activity. Given the involvement of this network in mediating limbic (emotions/memory) system function via the amygdala, hippocampus, and insula, as well as cognitive and executive functions via the PFC, it is clear how chronic stress might lead to alterations of eating behavior. It is also thought that exposure to, and consumption of, HP food, may not only act as a learned reward but also result in cue-triggered wanting (incentive salience) and increased sensitization to the *cue* itself, thereby augmenting potential induction of the response. Additionally, this heightened motivational response to the cue fluctuates with the physiological state.

18.6.2 Food and Behavior

The neurotransmitters serotonin, dopamine, opioids, and GABA play a role in the integration of mood, reward, pain modulation, eating behavior, and food consumption. Scientists have separated "wanting" (motivation to obtain) mediated by dopamine from "liking" or the hedonic/pleasurable part of the reward, mediated by opioids. Both of these systems work together to augment the seeking and experience of a given reward. Some scientists have suggested that this neurochemical circuitry, critical for drug and alcohol addiction, could easily play a role in overeating or "addictive" eating behaviors (coupling emotions and food/eating, habit, learning, and pleasure) in a vulnerable population in an obesogenic environment. People with drug and alcohol addiction in recovery have increased sugar cravings and weight gain. On a clinical level, some individuals who struggle with obesity do perceive this as an "addiction" or compulsion (see Food Addiction).

18.6.3 Mood and Food

An individual's physiological state is modified by mood (a temporary state of mind without obvious stimuli) and emotion (circumstantial feeling). Macht proposed five classes of emotion-induced changes of eating: (1) emotional control of food choice, (2) emotional suppression of food intake, (3) impairment of cognitive eating controls, (4) eating to regulate emotions, and (5) emotion-congruent modulation of eating. Emotional stress modifies intake depending on the type and intensity of stressor. This leads to an increase in palatable food consumption and weight gain, or the opposite, a decrease in intake and weight loss.

Depressed moods are associated with eating "comfort foods." In the short term, consumption of HP foods may lead to relief of the negative state. But, in the long term, consumption of HP foods leads to obesity, which can in turn lead to mood dysregulation. Mice chronically fed with a high-fat diet exhibit depressive-like and anxiety-like behavioral changes and heightened stress responses. When switched to normal meals, these mice demonstrate increased craving of HP foods and greater anxiety-like behavior. Meal plans high in saturated fat and low in polyunsaturated and monounsaturated fats have been associated with an increased incidence of depression. On the other hand, the Mediterranean meal pattern, which includes primarily unsaturated fats, is associated with a decrease in depression. Several studies have demonstrated a reduction in depression when omega-3 polyunsaturated fatty acids (PUFA) have been added to the meal plan.

Gastrointestinal hormones predominantly signal appetite, hunger, satiety, and energy homeostasis but are also involved in mood regulation. Ghrelin, produced in the stomach, signals hunger and energy homeostasis to the arcuate nucleus of the hypothalamus via vagal afferents that project to the nucleus solitarius tract. Additionally, ghrelin signals to mesolimbic dopaminergic pathways involved in reward/motivation pathways. Ghrelin receptors are capable of signaling to serotonin pathways, implicating a role for ghrelin to engage in crosstalk between mood and food. Several studies have suggested that ghrelin may modify stress and affect.

Leptin may play a role in mediating mood, given its main role in the neuroendocrine regulation of appetite and energy homeostasis in this circuitry. However, data regarding leptin and mood remain unclear, complicated by differential signaling within brain regions, and peripheral effects.

18.6.4 Inflammation, Food, and Mood

Obesity is associated with low-grade inflammation and an increase in inflammatory signals. Altered cytokines and interleukins, in turn, have been associated with mood disorders in animals and humans. Inflammatory pathways interface with, and modify, the regulation of the reward circuitry. This may manifest in altered food intake, craving, and overeating. Hypothalamic inflammation, as a consequence of an HP meal plan in animals, is associated with an increase in IL-6, TNFα, IKKb, and NFκB. Central inflammation at the level of the hypothalamus results in leptin and insulin resistance, altered behavior, weight gain, and glucose intolerance. Weight loss is associated with a decrease in inflammatory markers, such as C-reactive protein, TNFα, and IL-6. Cytokines vary in their effects on inducing or decreasing inflammation and may vary in the degree to which they contribute to obesity. Furthermore, insulin resistance has been proposed to affect insulin signaling at the level of the hypothalamus. Insulin resistance and its negative impact on mood are controversial, and research is currently underway to delineate its role.

18.6.5 Pain and Food

The individual factors that contribute to the management of pain and eating behavior changes are complex and likely involve alterations in reward circuitry. Food-induced analgesia involves the endogenous opioid system and can be modified by the opioid inhibitor naltrexone. Cyclooxygenase 2 selective inhibitors may have antidepressant effects and may cause nausea and/or decrease appetite. Mechanistically morphine works through two pathways in the brain—one for analgesia and one for the reward pathway—thought to be mediated by leptin, an adipose tissue hormone. Leptin seems to play a role in mediating the pain regulation network. Animals that are leptin deficient or inhibited experience the analgesic effect without the reward effect. Leptin may regulate pain and stress responses via its influence on dopamine neurotransmission. Allelic variation in the leptin gene showed differential responsiveness to dopamine (DA) release under a given pain stimulus. Thus, leptin is a hormonal signal linking pain modulation with DA circuitry affecting mood and eating.

18.7 Chronic Pain

The individual with obesity often suffers from chronic pain, with an increase in pain prevalence as BMI rises, especially at a BMI over 40 kg/m^2. Pain associated with obesity is multifactorial, involving genetic, metabolic, biomechanical, environmental, neuroendocrine, behavioral, social, and cultural contexts for a given individual. The combination of obesity and pain leads to a decrease in QOL and functional capacity and may make pain management more difficult. Pain is also a reciprocating condition. Pain aggravates, is aggravated by, and potentially interferes with the treatment of many of the comorbid conditions associated with obesity. These comorbid conditions include mood disorders, sleep disruption, low QOL, diabetes, and heart disease. The presence of pain may also interfere with weight loss, activity, and effecting lifestyle changes.

18.7.1 Mechanism(s) Linking Pain and Obesity

Several mechanisms link obesity and pain. Mechanical and structural factors affecting posture, vertical loading, joint misalignment, and altered ambulation result in muscular deconditioning and back and joint pain. Additionally, inflammatory effects of cytokines confer both local (e.g., degeneration in articular cartilage) and systemic (e.g., fibromyalgia) effects contributing to pain.

18.7.2 Specific Areas Affected by the Comorbid Conditions of Obesity and Pain

18.7.2.1 Osteoarthritis

Obesity is a significant risk factor (sevenfold) for osteoarthritis (OA) and is thought to be a consequence of both mechanical and inflammatory stresses. Biomechanical stress- and visceral fat-derived inflammatory factors both lead to joint degradation and pain. The pain is aggravated by inadequate muscle strength. Pain associated with OA affects mobility, self-efficacy, and function. Anatomically, abdominal obesity poses a greater risk for lower limb pain and doubles the risk for developing chronic pain, especially on the feet. Walking characteristics change as an individual alters his/her movement pattern to adapt to weight change, aggravating pain and limiting mobility. Obesity and overweight are associated with chronic low back pain and seeking care for low back, with risk proportional to increase in excess body weight.

18.7.2.2 Headache

There is a 5.3-fold increase in the relative risk of headaches in those with a BMI of ≥ 25 kg/m^2 compared to those with a BMI under 25 kg/m^2. However, an increased risk for migraine headaches in association with overweight or obesity remains controversial. Though the association with episodic migraine is not clear, there is increased risk of developing chronic migraine headaches in those with obesity, especially in younger adults. There is increased risk of weight gain attributed to the medications used for migraine headaches, such as gabapentin, beta-blockers, tricyclic antidepressants, and serotonin reuptake inhibitors (SSRI). Medication-related weight gain may aggravate comorbid conditions and lead to metabolic complications, thereby impacting QOL and self-esteem.

18.7.2.3 Fibromyalgia

Fibromyalgia (FM) is a constellation of symptoms including musculoskeletal pain, stiffness, point tenderness, fatigue, disordered sleep, cognitive impairment, and decreased QOL scores. FM strongly associates with depression. And there is a 40% increased prevalence of obesity in patients with FM. FM has a prevalence of 2–4% in the general population and rises to a prevalence of 5.1% in bariatric surgery candidates. FM is more prevalent in females. Patients with FM and higher BMI have lower QOL scores, corresponding to lower subscale scores in physical function.

Obesity aggravates the severity of the fibromyalgia symptoms and limits mobility. FM patients *without* obesity are twice as active as those with obesity. Both FM and obesity exhibit elevated cytokine levels implicating inflammation as playing a major role in the altered neurotransmitters and other neuroendocrine modulation of mood, symptoms, and behavior in these two diseases. There is improvement in baseline depression, pain, point tenderness, anxiety, sleep quality, body satisfaction, and QOL with medical or surgical weight loss in individuals with FM.

18.7.3 Behavioral Consequences of Pain

Chronic pain is associated with depression. The prevalence of physician-diagnosed major depressive disorder (MDD) in patients with back/neck pain is reported to be between 2.5% and 15.7%. In contrast, the rate of patient self-reported depression is in the range of 18–21%. Alterations in coping include changes in eating patterns combined with decreased movement, in a vicious cycle. Chronic pain is associated with hedonic hunger pathway stimulation (see Sect. 18.6). The Women's Health Initiative cohort showed that BMI and depression were independent predictors of pain and physical function over 3 years. Weight gain may be related to worsening depression.

18.7.3.1 Pain Experience and Behavioral Response

To gain better insight into the experience of pain in an individual with obesity, Janke and Kozak, utilizing small focus groups and structured interviews at a veterans' hospital, reported several central themes essential to understanding psychological barriers to weight loss interventions and pain management. Subjects described depression occurring with pain that made it difficult to cope, thwarted efforts to be active, prevented them from engaging socially, and affected eating behavior and food choices. Participants noted feelings of self-sabotage and shame related to using food to cope with pain. Food intake distracted them and helped manage the frustration of chronic pain. Some described eating as their only pleasurable activity. Many described the emotionally charged eating as a "binge" (even though clinical criteria were not assessed) with feelings of being out of control, eating large amounts of food, and finding temporary relief from pain. They then experienced a return of the pain with a depressed mood, in a vicious cycle. Subjects described "needing" foods high in sugar and fat to help the pain, even those who formerly (prior to pain onset) had healthy meal plans. Additionally, many experienced cravings for these foods and voiced a vulnerability and low self-efficacy to resist them. Being sedentary was the norm, and everyone described pain as making it difficult to move at all, even those who used to enjoy being regularly active. This limited movement, and awareness of it, aggravated their sense of shame, frustration with their body, negative self-image, social isolation, depressed mood, and low motivation to make changes. Furthermore, some participants noted that sometimes pain worsened with physical therapy and that this made it difficult to pursue other physical activity. Clearly, the interface between pain, low mood, limited activity, and coping with food needs to be better understood in an effort to help these individuals.

Chronic musculoskeletal pain, avoidance behaviors, decreased physical activity, and functional decline lead to weight gain in a vicious cycle for the individual with obesity (Fig. 18.2). Musculoskeletal pain (knee, hip, ankle, spine) associated with obesity directly impacts daily living and mobility (walking, standing, shopping, engaging in any activity that requires carrying one's body weight). Musculoskeletal pain becomes a barrier to engage in physical activity and even in perceptions about being physically active. Pain is associated with lower QOL and impaired psychosocial health. The frequent experience of musculoskeletal and joint pain, which may worsen after physical activity, and other discomforts such as dyspnea, cause many individuals with obesity to perceive physical activity as a negative. This makes it difficult to see the benefits of regular physical activity and leads to a more sedentary lifestyle. Given the necessity of increased energy expenditure for weight loss and weight-loss maintenance, it is critical to recognize the potential impediment of chronic pain.

Pain is uniquely subjective and has many facets, including physical, behavioral, psychological, and emotional, but several psychological responses to pain have been described to delineate quantifiable aspects. A "pain catastrophizing" scale (PCS) assesses the degree to which a person focuses on pain and feels helpless when experiencing pain. The *perceived ability to function, or not,* and the coping skills applied, are most pertinent to helping patients manage pain. Individuals who score high on this scale tend to engage in less physical activity. In those with a BMI between 38 and 61 kg/m^2, binge eating is reported more frequently, perhaps as a method of coping. *Self-efficacy* (the belief that one can perform a particular behavior) has been examined in patients with arthritis. Those who have high self-efficacy are less likely to score high on the PCS and more likely to participate in added physical activity. A randomized controlled trial examining the impact of pain-coping skills training and behavioral weight management demonstrated a reduction in negative psychological conditions, including a lower of PCS.

Kinesiophobia, or fear of movement, associated with chronic pain is seen in patients with increased BMI. In patients with musculoskeletal pain, muscle contraction results in an increase in generalized *pain,* whereas in normal volunteers, it results in generalized *analgesia.* In these patients with chronic pain, exercising the painful muscles did not result in analgesia. It is important to recognize the potential vicious cycle that may ensue for the patient with exercise-induced exacerbation of pain. Fear and avoidance of pain lead to decreased physical activity

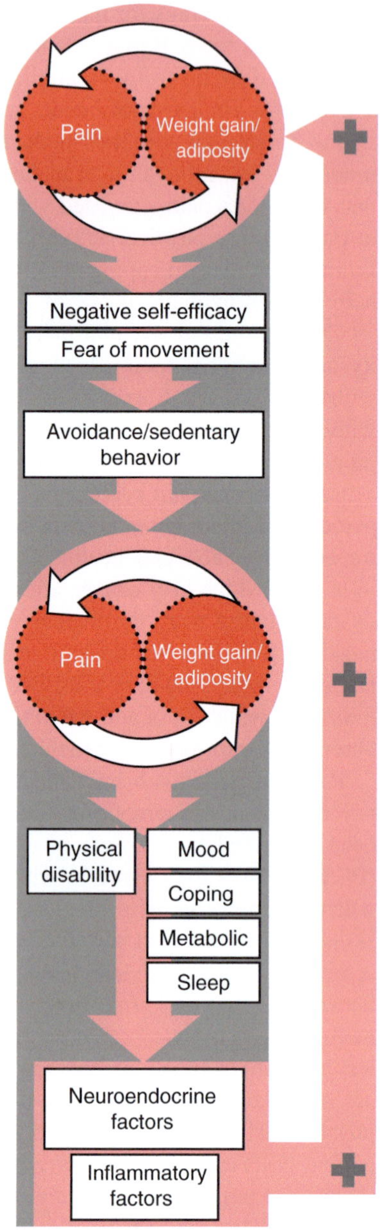

Fig. 18.2 The vicious cycle for the individual with obesity and chronic musculoskeletal pain includes negative self-efficacy and fear of movement, which leads to avoidance and sedentary behaviors, furthering weight gain. Weight gain leads to altered mood, sleep, coping, and metabolic abnormalities furthering physical disability. Neuroendocrine and inflammatory factors perpetuate this cycle

and in turn, decreased physical activity leads to more pain. Individuals with obesity and chronic low back pain have associated fear of movement that correlates with self-reported disability and physical performance. In older adults with obesity and lower back pain, decreased mobility is more related to fear around pain than actual decreased back strength.

18.7.4 Management

Physical therapy has a beneficial impact on weight loss and improvement in pain and performance in those with osteoarthritis in the extremities. Knee pain and mobility improve with weight training and nutritional intervention, independent of severity of joint damage on MRI. Supporting the development of pain-coping skills simultaneously with weight management can be beneficial long term. Assessing pain-related function and/or disability may be more helpful than a pain score per se. Encouraging movement and facilitating mobility is key to the management of chronic pain since many with pain remain inactive or have developed habits around being sedentary. Understanding the degree, to which an individual exhibits fear of movement, perceives helplessness due to pain, has altered coping, or has decreased self-efficacy, is critical to guiding management and facilitating outcome.

A program focused on strengthening and stabilizing the musculoskeletal system decreases depressive symptoms, joint pain, and the need for analgesic medication. It also improves mobility and is associated with increased self-efficacy for physical activity. Strengthening and stabilization of the musculoskeletal system also decrease inflammatory factors (IL-6, CRP), potentially protecting from further joint dysfunction. Modifying physical activity to small increments, including short sessions of weight bearing throughout the day, may help with pain management, improved endurance, and better attitudes regarding activity. Pain coping skills (distraction, relaxation, decreased sense of helplessness), when taught to individuals with knee OA in concert with a behavioral lifestyle intervention for weight, led to improved self-efficacy for physical activity, perceived function, and reduced pain. Use of mobile devices and accelerometers for weight management may help with promoting and supporting movement in those with obesity and chronic pain.

18.7.4.1 Pharmacotherapy

The use of pharmacotherapy for pain management is often essential to improve mobility and QOL and to achieve weight loss. However, potential weight gain from some of the commonly used pain medications is a concern. Analgesics such as gabapentin and pregabalin are associated with weight gain. One study showed 80% of patients taking gabapentin gained an average of 7% and no one lost weight. A weight gain of 7% can pose additional risk for furthering metabolic complications. Topiramate (approved for migraine) or zonisamide, if tolerated, can result in weight loss and may offer a possible alternative for pain management.

Opioids are effective for pain but are problematic and may be more so in an individual with obesity. Given the known risk for opioid dependence in the general population, there is concern that some individuals with obesity may have an increased genetic risk for addiction, making them more vulnerable. Also, opioid use can stimulate hunger and drive eating behavior in animals and humans, aggravating the potential for weight gain. Conversely, weight loss can occur with the use of naltrexone, an opioid antagonist, which is approved for use with bupropion as an obesity medication. Additionally, opioids may play a role in mediating insulin resistance. Normal-weight subjects who had first-degree relatives with obesity, when exposed to opioids, develop increased insulin resistance and fasting plasma glucose, compared to those without a first-degree relative. Furthermore, opioid hyperalgesia, increased sensitivity to pain occurring as a result of chronic use, may lead to greater opioid use as well as avoidance of physical activity. This perpetuates skeletal muscle weakness, inflammation, and pain in a vicious circle. Importantly, gastric bypass can affect absorption of pain medications, and increased use of opioids postoperatively is needed to control pain. Factors associated with this increased need are presurgery anxiety, smoking, and opioid use. Altered morphine absorption and increased morphine exposure during the postoperative period contribute to the risk for opioid dependency.

Antidepressants such as the serotonin-norepinephrine uptake inhibitors (SNRIs) duloxetine and venlafaxine have been used for relief from chronic pain; however, long-term use and higher doses are related to weight gain. Less than 30 weeks of use causes mild weight loss. Weight gain with prolonged use ranged from 2.5% to 9.9% in a review of 16 studies. There is a gender effect, with more women experiencing weight gain. SNRIs may be useful agents for an individual with obesity expressing several comorbid conditions such as coexisting depression, generalized anxiety, OA, FM, and/or diabetic neuropathy. A newer SNRI, milnacipran approved for fibromyalgia, is not associated with weight gain, and use greater than 3 months is associated with weight loss. Corticosteroids have been used acutely for pain flares either orally or via epidural injection. Intermittent acute use does not seem to be associated with weight gain; however, blood glucose increases in T2DM. Chronic corticosteroid use results in weight gain and worsens blood sugar control. Tricyclic medications such as amitriptyline and nortriptyline are known to result in weight gain for both acute and chronic use, though weight may stabilize with use of the latter after 4 months.

The effectiveness of pain medications is subject to an individual's sensitivity, response, and other potential side effects besides weight gain, such as alterations in mood, cognition, sleep, etc. Typically, we think of pain medication as chronic, but little is known about the potential advantage of using small doses of pain medications (such as opioids) to facilitate physical therapy or physical activity on an acute basis.

18.8 Early Childhood Experiences

Childhood experiences such as parental neglect/lack of support, abuse, trauma, depression, and school difficulties have been associated with an increased risk for obesity in adulthood, chronic illness, and depression. Several meta-analyses support the positive association of interpersonal violence in childhood from caregivers or peers and obesity in adulthood. All four types of childhood abuse—sexual, verbal, mental, and physical—have been associated with increased weight in adulthood. Any abuse increases the risk of obesity by 1.3 times, with a proportional increase in risk in those who experienced severe abuse. Adults reporting childhood abuse were 4 kg heavier than adults who reported no abuse during childhood. There is a proportional increase of abuse reports in those with BMI $\geq$40 kg/m^2, compared with those with a BMI $\geq$30 kg/m^2. There is a positive association between peer bullying and obesity. Gender, age, and baseline weight at time of bullying have been studied for possible increased susceptibility to weight gain, but no clear pattern has been identified. Evidence is inconsistent for an effect of community violence on the development of obesity. It has been proposed that community violence may be experienced differently than direct caregiver or peer violence and may be modified more directly by family.

Negative affect (emotional difficulties, anger, perceived stress), maladaptive coping, emotional/binge eating, stress, inflammation, and metabolic disturbance may be mediating factors in the relationship between childhood abuse and obesity. Experiencing violence in childhood is associated with stress eating and emotional coping in childhood. Waist circumference and central adiposity increase in those who experienced caregiver violence, implicating stress and inflammatory pathways, and potentiating future poor health. Depression, anxiety, personality disorders, and substance abuse in adulthood have been associated with a history of childhood abuse.

Weight gain has been proposed to serve an adaptive or self-protective function in women who have experienced childhood sexual abuse. Women may use their weight as a protection or barrier from sexual advances. Loss of this protection during weight loss may bring attention to one's body and trigger increased anxiety, impeding further loss or causing weight regain. Women who have a history of childhood sexual abuse have less weight loss and higher regain after being on a very low-calorie meal plan. These women report less body dissatisfaction.

Early childhood experiences shape psychological flexibility, sleep patterns, lifestyle choices, esteem, shame, self-blame, social relationships, trust, stress management, and ability for self-care and potentially impact future health as an adult.

18.9 Mood Disorders

18.9.1 Depression

Given the high prevalence of both depression and obesity and the known impact of each on metabolic disease, health, and well-being, understanding the relationship between the two offers opportunities for prevention and treatment. Most research has suggested a bidirectional relationship between obesity and depression, with more support for causality in the direction from obesity to depression. Depression, however, remains a risk factor for the development of obesity. Thus, baseline obesity is a risk for depression and depression is a risk for obesity. Causality *per se* may not be as important as the recognition that they can coexist, affect each other, and both should be treated. What is critical for the physician to understand is the complex, heterogeneous nature of both of the conditions and the biopsychosocial variables (see below) that modify a given clinical presentation, and therefore affect management.

Adolescence appears to be a vulnerable developmental period of increased risk for obesity (also see section on Early Childhood Experiences). Prospective and cross-sectional research examining this relationship from adolescence into early adulthood finds a bidirectional relationship between depression and obesity. However, there is also an inverse relationship, with less weight gain and obesity in those who were depressed. Baseline weight may make a difference—those with greater weight who developed depression were more likely to develop obesity, indicating a vulnerable subpopulation. Females may be more susceptible in childhood and adolescence to developing depression and obesity (bidirectional). The data for boys vary. Recent studies of adults found no difference for gender. There is a higher prevalence of depression in those seeking treatment for obesity, including bariatric surgery. Data are limited regarding the roles of race or education in affecting this relationship.

Biopsychosocial variables such as stigma, bias, poor physical function, pain, and low QOL moderate the expression of depression within an individual with obesity. Key modulators of the relationship between obesity and depression are the severity of obesity (BMI $\geq$ 30 kg/m^2), past history of childhood or physical abuse, family history of depression, poor physical health, perceived stigma, poor social support, and eating dysregulation. Additionally, younger persons between 25 and 64 years old may be at greater risk. Poor physical health, including general fatigue and pain that limits physical function, augments depressive symptoms, decreases QOL, and increases the risk for the development of depression in an individual with obesity. Physical activity may act as a bidirectional psycho-physiological modifier, improving self-efficacy, QOL, and commitment to further physical activity. Loneliness or perceived social isolation negatively impacts many aspects of QOL, including physical and mental health. Animal studies show a direct negative physiological response to social isolation, including a rise in sympathetic tone, HPAA activation, inflammatory and stress pathways, and altered activation of mesolimbic dopaminergic pathways. The quality and frequency of social relationships, and interpersonal effectiveness, mediate the relationship of depression to obesity and affect the response to a weight-loss intervention.

Given the heterogeneity of major depressive disorder (MDD), a group recently explored whether individuals with obesity might be more likely to show recurrent MDD as assessed by a structured clinical interview (defined as more than one episode in a 2-year period, with at least 2 months in between episodes), as opposed to a single episode. Individuals with a BMI $\geq$ 30 kg/m^2 were more likely to have recurrent MDD after adjusting for confounders. An altered structure of the hippocampus, which has been reported with recurrent MDD as well as increased visceral fat in middle-aged adults, may play a role.

Additional aspects are the use of antidepressants, quality of sleep, sleep disturbance (like apnea), level of physical activity, impediments to physical activity, eating disorders, family risks (for obesity, depression, or both), and severity of obesity (those with BMI ≥ 40 kg/m^2 may be at increased risk). Pharmacological treatment for mood disorders is associated with weight gain, but is out of the scope of this chapter. The use of antidepressant medications for chronic pain management and BED is discussed above.

The idea that there may be vulnerable subpopulations for obesity and/or depression is an important consideration. The identification of depression and its treatment is critical to the management of obesity. The awareness that depending on context depression may result in propensity for weight gain is equally important. We are just starting to assess the subphenotypes of obesity.

18.9.1.1 Illness

An additional important concern is the impact of co-occurring chronic diseases that can aggravate weight as well as potentiate cyclical effects on mood. Many chronic illnesses are worsened with the presence of depression and anxiety, often in a reciprocating way. Co-occurrence of a mood disorder (depression and anxiety) is thought to aggravate the chronic illness in both behavior and perception of intensity of illness. The co-occurrence may be more predictive of functional impairment than the severity of the chronic illness itself. Additionally, the more physical illnesses a person has, the less likely the mood disorder will be recognized.

In individuals with asthma, there is a higher prevalence of anxiety, panic disorder, psychological distress, and a sense of lack of control over their own health. The ability to choose appropriate self-management when given a clinical scenario was examined in a group of patients with chronic obstructive pulmonary disease. Those with anxiety and depression scored lower in choosing the appropriate action for a severe scenario despite having the knowledge. Subsyndromal depression and MDD are predictors of cardiovascular disease, myocardial infarction, morbidity, and mortality. Anxiety is also linked with increased morbidity and sudden death. A prospective study in a general medical clinic found that the degree of psychological distress was related to mortality from ischemic heart and pulmonary disease. Those having severe psychological distress had a mortality risk of 70%, compared to those with more moderate stress who had a mortality risk of 40%. Consistent with these findings, negative emotions such as social anxiousness were strongly related to increase the risk of heart disease. Additionally, a prospective study of patients after MI found that *perceived* "physical health" and depression were predictive of adherence to risk reduction behavior, but this was not so for "mental health."

A bidirectional relationship between depression and T2DM has been increasingly reported, although causality and risk have not been defined. The prevalence of depression has been reported to be twofold higher in individuals with T2DM compared to the general population, though risk assessment is methodologically limited. Depression and diabetes may be synergistic with reported higher functional disability, poor self-care, and earlier negative outcomes. Depression may precede the presentation of diabetes by years. Additionally, data from the Look AHEAD trial suggest that the combination of depressive symptoms and T2DM may confer a greater cardiovascular risk. The exact mechanisms are unknown, though a complex psychological and biological interface is likely. Given what appears to be a cyclical relationship between mood, illness, perceived impact of physical health, and psychological distress, an optimal approach would be to treat weight and the comorbidities simultaneously.

18.9.1.2 Suicide Risk After Bariatric Surgery

There is a fair amount of controversy regarding severe obesity as a risk factor for suicide. Importantly though, suicide post bariatric surgery is emerging as a concern, especially in view of the expected improvement of other serious comorbidities such as diabetes, cancer, and cardiovascular disease. In comparison to the general population (World Health Organization database) that estimates a suicide risk of 1.1 case per 10,000 individuals, post-bariatric surgery patients were found to have four times the risk. An even higher rate (6.6 times) of suicide after bariatric surgery has been documented. Men, between 45 and 54 years of age, have higher rates of suicide (13.7/10,000) compared to females (5.2/10,000). This compares to suicide rates in the general US population of 2.4 and 0.7 cases per 10,000 for men and women, respectively. The majority of suicides occurred 18 months to 5 years post surgery.

Depression is strongly associated with suicide. Also, previous suicide attempt and suicidal ideation are increased predictors for a completed suicide. Most studies report depressive symptoms as the most common potential factor for the suicide after gastric surgery. Additionally, impulsivity, history of child abuse, substance abuse, mood and borderline personality disorders, and loss of emotional coping through food ingestion are considered possible risk factors for depression and suicide. Lack of perceived success, such as weight regain or minimal weight loss, has also been suggested as a potential facilitator for depression and possibly suicide, as the same is true of re-emergence of medical illness such as diabetes or sleep apnea 3–7 years after surgery. Alcoholism appears to be an associated factor. There are concerns about the emergence of alcohol use disorder (AUD) during the second postoperative year after Roux-en-Y gastric bypass. Increased risk for AUD includes male gender, younger age, preoperative AUD, regular alcohol use, smoking, decreased interpersonal support, and recreational drug use. Additionally, altered alcohol metabolism postoperatively, resulting in higher and longer concentrations of blood alcohol than prior to bariatric surgery (gastric sleeve or Roux-en-Y gastric bypass) is a possible mechanism for AUD. Patients have self-reported greater sensitivity to alcohol, feeling more intoxicated with less alcohol consumed, as well as difficulty in limiting intake.

There is incomplete information regarding suicide post bariatric surgery. To understand suicide after bariatric surgery more information is needed, including method, time frame, amount of weight lost, attempts versus completed, and previous psychopathology. Furthermore, use of population comparators and controls differ among studies and have produced discrepant findings.

The lowering of ghrelin secretion by gastric bypass and sleeve gastrectomy contributes to depression and the potential for suicide. Partial gastrectomy for ulcer disease has been associated with increased suicide. Endocannabinoid 1 antagonists, removed from the market for depressive symptoms, lower ghrelin levels. Vagus nerve stimulation is used as a treatment for depression. Thus, possible mechanisms for increased depression include the interruption of the vagus nerve during surgery and alterations of other gastrointestinal hormones.

An increased risk (1.6×) of death—that may be emotionally or psychiatrically related, other than suicide, has been reported in post-bariatric surgery patients compared to a control group of individuals with severe obesity. Causes of death include accidents, poisonings, alcoholism (intoxication, cirrhosis, hepatitis), drug use, or lack of motivation in preventing nutritional deficiencies that result in death.

18.9.2 Anxiety

The link between obesity and anxiety remains unclear. Both conditions are common, with 25% of the population experiencing anxiety. Obesity can lead to the development of anxiety through weight-related stigma (public, private, internalized), discrimination, concerns about and dealing with comorbid health conditions, pressure regarding weight control, poor social networks, being isolated, lower socioeconomic stress, and sleep disturbance/apnea. Anxiety can lead to weight gain from altered coping styles (increased food and alcohol intake, decreased physical activity), cravings/appetite, chronic medical conditions, heritable traits, early childhood trauma, asthma, pain, worry about illness, insomnia, medications, and altered cortisol regulation. There is a positive risk of ~1.4 for anxiety in individuals, male and female, with obesity. In a study spanning 3 decades and using structured interviews, there was a 6.27-fold increased risk of generalized anxiety disorder (GAD) for an individual with a BMI $\geq$30 kg/m^2. There is an increased risk of lifetime diagnosis of anxiety disorder in women with a BMI $\geq$ 30 kg/m^2 and men with a BMI $\geq$ 40 kg/m^2 in a population-based study of 177,000 subjects. This risk was calculated after data were controlled for the diagnoses of diabetes, cardiovascular disease, and asthma but not other comorbid conditions of obesity, such as sleep apnea. The HUNT 11-year prospective cohort study examined anxiety and depression using the HADS (Hamilton Anxiety and Depression Scale) in ~25,000 adults. The HUNT study found that both males and females who developed anxiety and depression were heavier by a kilogram compared to those who did not develop them (controlling for smoking, alcohol, education level, economic difficulty). Excluding for comorbidities or use of antidepressants did not change the findings. PTSD was found to have the strongest association with obesity. Phobias also had a strong association with obesity, especially social phobia in women. Anxiety is contextual. Individuals altering their lifestyle to adapt to anxiety can develop obesity. And individuals with obesity who alter their lifestyle to lose weight can develop anxiety.

18.10 Impulsivity/Binge Eating Disorder

As a personality trait, impulsivity may put a person at risk for weight gain, especially food-related impulsivity. Two components of impulsivity have been suggested, which may apply to this risk: (1) being driven to obtain reward or having increased reward sensitivity with food which has neuroendocrinological basis or wiring and (2) tending to act rashly or spontaneously and disregarding consequences or exhibiting disinhibited behavior and loss of control. Either or both of these types of impulsivity can exist in an individual struggling with weight and can occur in other disorders such as binge eating disorder, attention deficit disorder, and addiction. Most studies do not distinguish between the two types of impulsivity when assessing food intake.

Binge eating disorder (BED) is the most common of the eating disorders, affecting 2–3.5% of adult men and women, respectively, of the general population. BED is defined as experiencing a loss of control over eating and consuming an abnormally large amount of food in a short period of time with three of the following features: consuming faster than normal; until uncomfortably full and when not hungry; alone due to embarrassment and feeling disgusted; and feeling depressed or guilty after eating the large amount of food at least once a week for more than 3 months. Within the subpopulation of individuals with obesity, BED is 2–10× more likely, with a greater prevalence in those with severe obesity and seeking medical and surgical treatment. BED co-occurs with associated metabolic conditions, mood disorders, chronic pain, and substance abuse.

Actual pathophysiology of binge eating disorder is unknown though a constellation of genetic/biological predispositions including reward sensitivity, impulsivity, mood regulation, sensitivity to external stimuli, and biopsychosocial factors seem involved in a complicated vicious cycle. Perception of loss of control has been associated with the most psychological distress.

BED is common in those seeking bariatric surgery with a reported prevalence of 5–25% of the population using structured interviews. Consensus varies regarding predicting outcomes of surgery based on preoperative BED. These studies are limited largely by variations in study methodology and diagnostic criteria (defining binge eating trait vs. disorder); the change in binge eating post-surgery (patients are unable to eat abnormally large amounts of food); assessment method (structured interviews or questionnaires); and other comorbid conditions such as mood, metabolic conditions, and eating style. Increased risk for poor outcome has been associated in individuals reporting loss of control and dysregulated eating patterns after surgery, who tend to demonstrate eating-disordered pathology with body-shape/weight concerns and psychological distress. Additionally, new forms of compulsive eating may emerge such as grazing and rumination with loss of control manifesting in weight regain.

People with obesity and BED may eat more under special conditions such as being in a fasted state, stressed or in a negative mood, or having been strongly exposed to food stimuli. Additionally, those with BED will eat more during the day regardless of instruction (whether told to binge or eat normally) independent of mood or level of hunger. Food exposure, especially to multi-item meals, led to more disinhibited eating perhaps because they are more stimulating and perceived as more rewarding.

Brain imaging, neurobehavioral paradigms, eye tracking, and/or EEG have been used to assess impulsivity with food in experimental approaches to delineate differences between individuals with obesity and BED. Due to the nature of the methodology, most of the studies are small (total n ~40), study conditions vary, and the results are inconsistent. In studies of individuals with obesity and no BED, functional MRI has suggested the activation of reward pathways in response to real food stimuli or food pictures in a fasted state compared to those of normal weight, especially with high-caloric food; however, some studies show only marginal differences between these groups, especially with a longer fasting period prior to exposure. The anatomical studies with positive results (increased reward pathways) differ in the representation of brain regions being activated, limiting conclusions. In individuals with obesity and BED, again results are highly variable, but overall, they suggest that reward sensitivity is dependent on homeostatic state. Increased attention to food and higher "wanting" scores were seen when satiated in obesity/BED subjects compared to normal controls.

In examining the second aspect of impulsivity, the question of do individuals with obesity show increases in rash-spontaneous behavior toward food, a recent review found no evidence for an increase in rash behavior in those with obesity alone—only in the sub group with BED. Researchers use EEG and eye-tracking methods to capture early subconscious processing to assess specific bias toward food versus nonfood stimuli. Individuals with obesity and BED showed increased beta activity on EEG and decreased inhibition to food cues compared to non-BED subjects. These results suggest that individuals with BED show an increased tendency to act impulsively toward food cues independent of internal state.

Negative affect; food cravings, particularly for sweets; and exposure to HP food are typical triggers for binge eating and are exacerbated under stress. Ghrelin may play a role in directing eating versus noneating responses to stress; stress exposure increases circulating ghrelin levels in human associated with acute response of cortisol to ACTH. Emotional eaters have lower baseline ghrelin levels compared to nonemotional eaters. Nonemotional eaters respond to food intake with a lowering of the ghrelin level but emotional eaters maintain ghrelin levels after food intake, suggesting that persistent ghrelin levels may contribute to continued food intake in response to stress.

18.10.1 Treatment

Cognitive behavioral treatment (CBT) for BED has been the treatment of choice for and has been associated with total remission in at least half of the persons treated. Additional improvements in QOL, psychosocial functioning, and depression have been seen. Interestingly, some work looking at the use of both behavioral weight management and CBT in those with BED indicates that the rapid responders (those who reduce the binge eating by >70% in the first 4 weeks) were more likely to achieve remission, decrease frequency of binge eating, and lose weight. A combined use of guided self-help via a workbook with a few CBT sessions (CBTgsh) has also shown to be effective for BED, with improvement in depression and functional impairment as well. A comparison of behavioral weight loss (BWL), CBTgsh, and individual psychotherapy (IPT) demonstrated that these psychological treatments were more effective as treatment for BED than behavioral weight loss alone, especially at 2-year follow-up. A low self-esteem at baseline seemed to minimize the response to BWL approach, whereas, the CBTgsh and IPT groups fared better, with IPT group faring the best, as expected. Overall, CBT, CBTgsh, and IPT are effective approaches for improving psychopathology and psychosocial functioning for 1–2 years in individuals with BED. These interventions do not result in weight loss but may prevent further weight gain.

Pharmacotherapy options for the treatment of BED are limited. Overall, some SSRIs (citalopram, escitalopram, and sertraline) have shown success compared to placebo in reducing binge eating severity and frequency with reduction in anxiety and obsession, and some modest weight loss ranging from 1 kg to 5.6 kg, respectively. Results examining the combination of fluoxetine and CBT have shown mixed results with improvement at 6 months but no effect at 2 years. The studies with SSRIs have been difficult to interpret due to high dropout rate, high placebo response rate, small sample sizes, short-term studies with minimal follow-up, and differential reporting outcomes. Rapid reduction of binge symptoms within the first 4 weeks also seems to predict overall response to fluoxetine. There remains a concern for long-term weight gain with the use of SSRIs. Topiramate, an anticonvulsant and migraine medication, has been shown to decrease binge frequency, severity of obsessions and compulsions, promote weight loss, and abstinence of binge eating compared to placebo. Use of topiramate has been limited by cognitive side effects. Atomoxitene, a selective norepinephrine uptake inhibitor, approved for attention deficit hyperactivity disorder (ADHD), has also been shown to reduce binge frequency, psychological symptoms, result in weight loss, and greater cessation of binge eating compared to placebo. Recently, lisdexamfetamine dimesylate, a dextroamphetamine prodrug, approved for the treatment of ADHD was approved for the treatment of moderate-to-severe BED with a reduction in impulsivity, binge-eating compulsions, and weight loss at 11 weeks compared to placebo, though limited to patients without cardiovascular or psychiatric conditions which were exclusionary for the trial. The side-effect profile is similar to that seen with use in patients with ADHD and effects of long-term use unknown. Effectiveness of the newer obesity medications, bupropion HCl/naltrexone, liraglutide, lorcaserin HCl, and phentermine/topiramate ER as treatment for the individual with BED remains unknown.

18.10.2 Attention Deficit Hyperactivity Disorder

ADHD is a comorbid condition occurring in adults with obesity with a risk factor of 1.8 or 1.6 with overweight, and several studies have suggested a prevalence ranging from 35% to 38% in those with a BMI ≥40 kg/m^2. ADHD typically co-exists with other mood disorders—depression, bipolar, anxiety as well as addictive disorders, alcoholism, and drug addiction. Family risk analyses link drug dependence and ADHD.

It is thought that the impulsivity, lack of organization, and novelty-seeking behaviors associated with ADHD can lead to poor dietary compliance and result in weight gain or inability to lose weight. Levy examined the effect of treating ADHD in adults diagnosed via semistructured clinical interviews on weight loss over 15 months. Diagnosis was supported by a childhood history of ADHD. Most subjects described a history of refractory attempts at weight loss. Comorbid conditions of sleep apnea, mood disorders, pain, gastroesophageal reflux disease, and BED were identified and treated *before* initiating ADHD treatment comprising primarily psychostimulants (dextroamphetamine/amphetamine, methylphenidate, and dexedrine) and atomoxetine if the psychostimulants were not effective or not tolerated. Subjects who refused or did not tolerate pharmacological therapy acted as the control group. Those who were treated for ADHD lost 12% of body weight compared to those not treated, who gained 3%. It was noted that as ADHD improved, weight loss occurred. Subjects in this study described more boredom with the dietary and exercise regimens, time management issues, restlessness, impulsiveness, and inconsistent focus in previous weight-loss attempts. Those treated described better assessment of when they were hungry—awareness of status of being hungry or full, less novelty seeking, better time management, persistence, overall less fatigue, more energy, and a decrease in binge eating. Whether the drugs act directly as appetite suppressants or support better regulation of behavior and application of healthier habits, or relieve the individual of the intensive cognitive efforts to comply is not clear. Bariatric surgery patients with untreated ADHD may be at risk for follow-up and compliance with necessary vitamin regimens. Overall, the research suggests that evaluating and treating ADHD in concert with weight-loss therapy may be valuable.

Impulsivity has been associated with obesity but it is difficult to clearly assess and separate roles of reward seeking from decreased inhibition or poor decision-making. Overeating takes many forms, and for some, it is a compulsive, "addictive" behaviorally driven activity. With the co-existence of binge eating disorder and ADHD, BED may mediate the link with overweight/obesity. Mechanistically, involvement of the dopaminergic pathways and altered regulation of arousal, attention, and reinforcement has been suggested. Does the "toxic environment" filled with sugar, fat, and salt act as a stimulant to a vulnerable population? Davis has suggested that for a person with ADHD, the impulsiveness and inattention coupled with a stimulatory environment may bring out addictive type of behaviors with food. She has also suggested that our overstimulated environment facilitates the expression of ADHD.

18.10.3 Food Addiction

Patients commonly self-describe the feeling of being "addicted" to food with a sense of loss of control, obsessive thoughts of food, cravings for sugar/fat, and persistence in the behavior despite negative consequences with psychological distress. Animal studies show that increased exposure to HP foods results in increased food seeking, consumption, and tolerance of electrical shock to attain HP food. The neuroendocrine overlap with reward, impulsivity, and addiction is thought to play a role.

The Yale Food Addiction Scale (YFAS) was developed as a diagnostic tool to assess addictive behaviors related to food. Use of this scale in clinical samples of individuals with obesity suggested that BED and a "food addicted" (FA) population may be distinct entities. Those who met both criteria (FA and BED, 40–60%) were found to have more depression, negative affect, emotional dysregulation, lower self-esteem, and greater binge eating frequency. Those with both criteria also had more disordered pathology with increased weight/body-shape concerns. fMRI studies in subjects with FA exposed to HP cues (without BED) show activation of neural networks associated with substance abuse. Individuals with obesity found to have FA presented with a greater severity of symptoms including impulsivity, emotional reactivity, and food cravings. Assessment of food addiction may help the clinician tailor the treatment to optimize outcomes.

18.10.4 Night-Eating Syndrome

An additional eating disorder that may be found in individuals with obesity and the constellation of stress and mood, eating, and sleep disturbances, is the night-eating syndrome (NES). NES was originally described as a triad of morning anorexia, eating ≥25% calories after 7 PM and insomnia in individuals who were unable to lose weight in a dietary and weight-loss intervention. NES was attributed to the stress of weight loss. Diagnostic criteria have been proposed, including evening hyperphagia (with awareness) with at least 25% of caloric intake after the evening meal and waking from sleep to eat ≥2 days a week; morning anorexia or skipping breakfast ≥4 days of the week; insomnia associated with the belief that eating is necessary to return to sleep; worsening evening mood; and impaired function or distress. Awareness of nocturnal ingestion is critical to differentiate this disorder from that of sleep-related eating disorder, a variant of parasomnia.

NES is associated with increased BMI. Furthermore, night eating, which leads to a weight gain of 4.3–4.5 kg over 3–6 years, precedes the development of obesity in 40% of night eaters with obesity. Obesity may occur earlier in life in those with NES. NES may be related to a change in circadian rhythm modulation, thought to be important in regulating weight (see below). Though there is a higher prevalence of NES among individuals with overweight or obesity, not everyone with NES is overweight. The reasons for these differences are not clear. Individuals with normal weight and NES may adapt behaviorally during the day with intensive physical activity, cognitive restraint, and more fear of weight gain. Furthermore, some individuals may be more vulnerable to night eating. Women with obesity and NES gained more weight (5.2 kg vs. 0.9 over 6 years) compared to those without NES.

Patients with NES lose less weight during intervention studies, but this may be due to the type of intervention. Comparing a 900-kcal liquid meal plan to a behavioral intervention with mild calorie restriction, physical activity, and psychoeducational sessions, the liquid meal plan intervention in those with NES resulted in 3 kg *less* weight loss than controls. There was no difference in the food-based behavioral group, i.e., those with NES did not fare worse than those without. Night eating may have impeded the overall calorie restriction in a liquid meal plan group. For those with NES, an approach with a multiple modality focus may be more useful, but more research is needed. The positive findings of the lifestyle approach suggest resetting of the circadian rhythm with redistribution of feeding, supported by dietary and behavioral strategies, as a benefit to those with NES.

Weight loss via both medical and surgical approaches results in improved NES behavior and symptomatology and lower night-eating questionnaire scores (NEQ) scores. The mechanism by which this occurs is unclear. Reduction in evening hyperphagia, ingestion, and frequency were seen in half of the subjects and persisted without concomitant improvement in binge-eating scores or depression. Pharmacological intervention with serotonin reuptake inhibitors (SSRIs) has shown improvement in NES symptoms and weight loss. Interestingly, subjects in an 8-week study reported improvement solely in night-eating behaviors without change in mood as assessed by Beck Depression Inventory II (BDI-II), implying an independent mechanism for NES. Further investigation using pharmacotherapy approaches with SSRIs, topiramate, and the new obesity medications is warranted.

Using cognitive behavioral techniques to rearrange timing of eating, work with the distress around night eating, and the concept of "I need to eat to sleep," there are improvements in QOL, decreased nocturnal ingestions and caloric intake, and improvements in BDI-II. CBT appears to be a viable option for treatment, though the studies are small and limited. Several case studies have utilized phototherapy as potential approaches for NES given the disturbed circadian and melatonin rhythms in this group.

Several possible mechanisms for impediment to weight loss in NES have been suggested. Conceptually, simply greater energy intake could be occurring in those with NES since several studies report caloric differences in the range of 300–600 kcal. Patients with NES report insomnia and increased nocturnal awakenings suggesting a possible contribution of a disturbed circadian rhythm. There is a decrease in sleep duration and efficiency and an increase in sleep latency in those with NES. Sleep disturbance may affect behavior, hunger/appetite, increased opportunity to eat, or daytime physical activity by a variety of mechanisms. The degree of sleep disruption is worsened by the co-existence of depression.

There is an association between moderate depression with an evening pattern of worsening, assessed utilizing the BDI. Major depression has been typically excluded from studies of NES, so a full picture of depression may not be known. Additional psychiatric disorders such as schizophrenia and bulimia have been reported to be associated with NES. NES has been associated with stress and anxiety. Progressive muscle relaxation has been used as a therapeutic approach and resulted in decreased night-eating episodes, better breakfast eating/morning hunger, and decrease in self-reported stress and anxiety.

Disturbances in cortisol, melatonin, and serotoninergic rhythms have been suggested to play a role in NES. Alteration in circadian rhythm resulting in late-night eating and a phase delay of 1.5 h has been reported in those with NES, but it is unclear if this is causally related. Chrono-disruption or the uncoupling of normal biological rhythms and its circadian-regulated behaviors, such as eating and sleeping, has been shown to negatively impact metabolic regulation and weight, perhaps through increase in inflammation at the level of the hypothalamus. Time of feeding synchronizes circadian rhythms, and whether resetting of these rhythms may be a potential treatment for NES is unknown.

Studies in both humans and mice that uncouple these rhythms, by altering caloric intake, timing and delaying sleep, result in weight gain, increased inflammation and metabolic abnormalities. The metabolic abnormalities include insulin resistance and alterations of lipid and glucose metabolism, cortisol rhythms, and leptin and melatonin secretion. Obesity itself may alter this rhythm as suggested by studies of mice fed a high-fat diet. Under this condition, there is altered circadian rhythm gene expression peripherally (liver, kidney) and centrally (nucleus tractus solitarius). There is also a potential functional effect where the mice are less able to readjust to light synchronization (simulated jet lag) after a high-fat diet. Better understanding of the cyclical relationships between obesity, altered rhythms, sleep, and mood may suggest new treatments.

18.11 Psychological Change with Weight Loss

Weight-loss intervention studies are not typically designed to examine psychological change as a primary outcome. In a recent meta-analysis exploring psychological impact of behavioral weight-loss interventions, there was improvement in psychological outcomes (vitality score on QOL, body image, self-esteem, and depressive symptoms), sometimes independently of weight loss. Of the four outcomes examined, improved QOL was the most strongly dependent on the amount of weight lost, with a loss of 5% or more being necessary to see this change. Greater improvements in QOL were seen with more than 10% weight loss. Interestingly, one study reported that postmenopausal women who noted a decline in social functioning after weight loss were more likely to regain weight later. This suggests the importance of understanding the impact of psychological outcomes on maintenance of weight loss. Improved body image scores were closely related to the amount of weight loss, though some studies did not find a direct relationship.

Weight-loss interventions, including surgical, pharmaceutical, and behavioral, lead to improvements in self-esteem and depression. Benefits to self-esteem are especially seen with behavioral intervention and are related to the degree of weight change, whereas, depression is significantly improved by surgical and pharmaceutical interventions and is *un*related to the degree of weight change. Another area of exploration is the concept of reciprocal actions, whereby a change in behavior begets change in another behavior. Weight loss leads to an improved body image, and in turn, the improved body image increases the chance of weight loss. Effects of self-acceptance, changing attitudes, improved self-esteem, and efficacy via a behavioral intervention focus may benefit an individual in addition to, or even without, weight loss and may be critical for long-term success. Increased social support and self-acceptance as an integral part of an intervention improve psychological well-being. The psychological support and the educational components including self-acceptance and promotion of health behaviors may lead to integration of these cognitive constructs and support persistence of these changes. Clearly, more research is needed to understand and improve psychological health and sustainability of healthy self-concepts.

In an effort to gain understanding of long-term psychological adaptation, structured interviews of individuals who had undergone bariatric surgery more than 5 years prior were performed. Many patients voiced the challenge of managing a totally transformed physical self while retaining the same relationships and environment. Perceiving this altered-self (often occurring rapidly) created psychological tension as individuals sought to redefine and reintegrate into the world. For many, the significant weight loss attracted attention to the body both externally and internally. Internally, many noted an increase in focus on the physical body, how one moves in space (still retaining habits of the larger body), awareness of the former body with the excess skin, and feelings of alienation. Additionally, for some as they became smaller, they felt more anxious and struggled with new feelings, realizing that the previous body had offered a sense of protection that they were now without.

The external awareness and response of others to their new body was often painful, with an increased sense of vulnerability, especially with the realization of differential treatment regarding appearance and body shape in relationships. Many individuals were able to increase physical function. They expressed feelings of emancipation and independence, finding a new ability to participate in activities in which they had not prior. Despite this joy, there was always the fear of regaining weight. Most experienced the initial restriction and structure around eating as positive to their sense of control. Later, there was a desire to have food be a more meaningful experience, being able to relax and enjoy it, and developing a sense of loss and emptiness around the food experience. Relapse and loss of control was typically associated with coping with emotional distress or lack of energy. Fear of weight regain was strong and related to shame and feelings of failure.

18.12 Treatment Approaches of Overweight or Obesity in the Context of the Psychological Need

The standard cognitive behavioral approach is to alter the context in which a behavior occurs with a goal to replace the maladaptive behavior with a healthier one. Typically, CBT is focused on using goal setting, self-monitoring to set calorie and weight targets, physical activity regimens, stimulus control, and skills-based therapy to develop well-trained daily habits. Variations of behavioral approaches have been emerging, including acceptance and commitment therapy (ACT) and mindfulness.

Individuals struggling with weight management are often caught between the chronic drive/desire to eat certain foods and the opposing desire of their own goals of a healthier lifestyle (being active, making healthy food choices, going to sleep, etc.). ACT is a therapeutic framework that focuses on developing psychological flexibility by promoting acceptance and tolerance of uncomfortable emotional feelings rather than avoiding them. The utilization of mindfulness techniques leads to an increased awareness of the self and one's thoughts without judgment. Additionally, this approach focuses on identifying one's values and committing to actions consistent with them. Often humans have several incompatible goals, clearly seen in behavior related to choices regarding being active and types of food. The struggle between short-term pleasure-seeking (hedonic) versus long-term health decisions is common. Much of human behavior is automatic or habitual and is often in conflict with long-term goals. This behavior can be easily triggered by environmental cues such as the sight or smell of certain foods and eating-associated activities such as watching TV or browsing the Internet. One is often not even aware of having made this choice, with immediate pleasure/comfort or habit being the determining factor. Increased awareness or "mindfulness" then becomes critical in governing behavioral choice. This in turn leads to behavior more consistent with our long-term goals/healthier choices. Mindfulness of being hungry or full can help with the decision-making around eating behavior. Perceptions of "hunger" can be complicated, with some persons experiencing this in response to cues/cravings for hedonic activities.

Individuals vary in their ability to tolerate negative internal experiences (sadness, anxiety, troubling thoughts, urges) and often try to extinguish them. This avoidance or repression can increase the distress level over time and lead to the development of maladaptive behaviors and potentially negative health outcomes. In the simplest example, a person participating in a weight-loss intervention who refrains from hedonically motivated eating may experience strong urges, feelings of deprivation, increased thoughts about food, and uncomfortable cravings. Women who are able to overcome urges to eat have greater weight loss at the end of 1 year than those who cannot overcome the urges. Similarly, those who experience negative feelings or sensations with physical activity (pain, sweating, boredom, anxiety, fatigue) are less likely to engage in physical activity goals than those who do not have the negative feelings. Limited tolerance for negative affect and the use of eating for emotional regulation is associated with regain and lapses in weight-control programs. It is early in the use of this methodology, and time is needed to prove long-term effectiveness but early work is promising.

An additional concept of behavioral change is the idea that taking action on one behavior increases the odds of changing another behavior. Implementation of one behavior increases the likelihood of a change in a second behavior, regardless of different populations or behaviors being implemented. The mechanisms for the change in a second behavior include: transfer effects of the learning process over to the new behavior(s); increased self-efficacy; habituation of one behavior, which allowed cognizance and change of other; a new found awareness of the other behaviors; and awareness and reduction of barriers to achieve the second behavior.

18.13 Conclusion

A comprehensive, biopsychosocial approach to treating the individual with obesity is warranted. The dynamic interface between physiological and psychological states may affect the response to the treatment of obesity. The clinician should understand that given the multifaceted, cyclical aspects of obesity, treating many components at the same time may be necessary to effect sustainable change. Recognition of contextual factors impacting a given individual, such as stigma, shame, pain, mood, coping, comorbid condition(s), and fear, increases trust in the physician-patient partnership and optimizes effectiveness.

Reading List

Allison KC, Grilo CM, Masheb RM, Stunkard AJ. Binge eating disorder and night eating syndrome: a comparative study of disordered eating. J Consult Clin Psychol. 2005;73:1107–15.

American Psychiatric Association. Diagnostic and statistical manual of mental disorders. 5th ed. Washington, DC: American Psychiatric Association; 2013.

Anderson SE, Cohen P, Naumova EN, Jacques PF, Must A. Adolescent obesity and risk for subsequent major depressive disorder and anxiety disorder: prospective evidence. Psychosom Med. 2007;69:740–7.

Arranz LI, Rafecas M, Alegre C. Effects of obesity on function and quality of life in chronic pain conditions. Curr Rheumatol Rep. 2014;16:390–8.

Ball K, Burton NW, Brown WJ. A prospective study of overweight, physical activity, and depressive symptoms in young women. Obesity. 2009;17:66–71.

Barefoot JC, Heitmann BL, Helms MJ, Williams RB, Surwit RS, Siegler IC. Symptoms of depression and changes in bodyweight from adolescence to mid-life. Int J Obes Relat Metab Disord. 1998;22(7):688–94.

Barlosius E, Philipps A. Felt stigma and obesity: introducing the generalized other. Soc Sci Med. 2015;130:9–15.

Biederman J. Attention-deficit/hyperactivity disorder: a selective overview. Biol Psychiatry. 2005;57(11):1215–20.

Blaine BE, Rodman J, Newman JM. Weight loss treatment and psychological well-being: a review and meta-analysis. J Health Psychol. 2007;12(1):66–82.
Borrell-Carrio F, Suchman AL, Epstein RM. The biopsychosocial model 25 years later: principles practice and scientific inquiry. Ann Fam Med. 2004;2:576–82.
Brewis AA. Stigma and the perpetuation of obesity. Soc Sci Med. 2014;118:152–8.
Brownley KA, Peat CM, La Via M, Bulik CM. Pharmacological approaches to the management of binge eating disorder. Drugs. 2015;75:9–32.
Brumpton B, Langhammer A, Romundstad P, Chen Y, Mai XM. The associations of anxiety and depression symptoms with weight change and incident obesity: The HUNT Study. Int J Obes. 2013;37:1268–74.
Burghardt PR, Love TM, Stohler CS, Hodgkinson C, Shen PH, Enoch MA, et al. Leptin regulates dopamine responses to sustained stress in humans. J Neurosci. 2012;32(44):15369–76.
Cacioppo JT, Hawkley LC, Norman GJ, Berntson GG. Social isolation. Ann N Y Acad Sci. 2011;1231(1):17–22.
Carels RA, Wott CB, Young A, Gumble A, Koball A, Oehlhof MW. Implicit, explicit and internalized weight bias and psychosocial maladjustment among treatment-seeking adults. Eat Behav. 2010;11:180–5.
Cleator J, Abbott J, Judd P, Sutton C, Wilding JPH. Night eating syndrome: implications for severe obesity. Nutr Diabetes. 2012;2:1–8.
Cortese S, Penalver CM. Comorbidity between ADHD and obesity: exploring shared mechanisms and clinical implications. Postgrad Med. 2010;122(5):88–96.
Cozzolino D, et al. The involvement of the opioid system in human obesity: a study in normal weight relatives of obesity people. J Clin Endocrinol Metab. 1996;81:713–8.
Dalle Grave R, Calugi S, Ruocco A, Marchesini G. Night eating syndrome and weight loss outcome in obese patients. Int J Eat Disord. 2011;44(2):150–6.
Davis C. Psychobiological traits in the risk profile for overeating and weight gain. Int J Obes. 2009;33:S49–53.
Davis C, Curtis C, Levitan RD, Carter JC, Kaplan AS, Kennedy JL. Evidence that 'food addiction' is a valid phenotype of obesity. Appetite. 2011;57(3):711–7.
de Zwaan M, Roerig DB, Crosby RD, Karaz S, Mitchell JE. Nighttime eating: a descriptive study. Int J Eat Disord. 2006;39(3):224–32.
Durso LE, et al. Internalized weight bias in obese patients with eating disorder: associations with eating disturbances and psychological functioning. Int J Eat Disord. 2012;45(3):423–7.
Faith MS, Butryn M, Wadden TA, Fabricatore A, Nguyen AM, Heymsfield SB. Evidence for prospective assocations among depression and obesity in population-based studies. Obes Rev. 2011;12:e438–53.
Forman EM, Butryn ML. A new look at the science of weight control: how acceptance and commitment strategies can address the challenge of self-regulation. Appetite. 2015;84:171–80.
Gallant AR, Lundgren J, Drapeau V. The night-eating syndrome and obesity. Obes Rev. 2012;13:528–36.
Gariepy G, Nitka D, Schmitz N. The association between obesity and anxiety disorders in the population: a systematic review and meta-analysis. Int J Obes. 2010;34:407–19.
Gearhardt AN, Phil M, White MA, Potenza MN. Binge eating disorder and food addiction. Curr Drug Abuse Rev. 2011;4(3):201–7.
Gearhardt AN, White MA, Masheb RM, Grilo CM. An examination of food addiction in a racially diverse sample of obese patients with binge eating disorder in primary care settings. Compr Psychiatry. 2013;54(5):500–5.
Gonzalez JS, Fisher L, Polonsky WH. Depression in diabetes: have we been missing something important? Diabetes Care. 2011;34(1):236–9.
Goss K, Allan S. Shame, pride and eating disorders. Clin Psychol Psychother. 2009;16:303–16.
Goss K, Allan S. The development and application of compassion-focused therapy for eating disorders (CTF-E). Br J Clin Psychol. 2014;53(1):62–77.
Gundersen C, Mahatmya D, Garasky S, Lohman B. Linking psychosocial stressors and childhood obesity. Obes Rev. 2011;12:e54–63.

Gustafson TB, Sarwer DB. Childhood sexual abuse and obesity. Obes Rev. 2004;5:129–35.
Hemmingsson E, Johansson K, Reynisdottir S. Effects of childhood abuse on adult obesity: a systematic review and meta-analysis. Obes Rev. 2014;15:882–93.
Henriksen CA, Mather AA, Mackenzie CS, Bienvenu OJ, Sareen J. Longitudinal associations of obesity with affective disorders and suicidality in the Baltimore epidemiologic catchment area follow-up study. J Nerv Ment Dis. 2014;202(5):379–85.
Herva A, et al. Obesity and depression: results from the longitudinal Northern Finland 1966 Birth Cohort Study. Int J Obes. 2006;30:520–7.
Hryhorczuk C, Sharma S, Fulton SE. Metabolic disturbances connecting obesity and depression. Front Neurosci. 2013;7:1–14.
Janke EA, Kozak AT. "The more pain I have, the more I want to eat": obesity in the context of chronic pain. Obesity. 2012;20(10):2027–34.
Jansen A, Havermans R, Nederkoorn C, Roefs A. Jolly fat or sad fat? Subtyping non-eating disordered overweight and obesity along an affect dimension. Appetite. 2008;51(3):635–40.
Johnson SS, Paiva AL, Mauriello L, Prochaska JO, Redding C, Velicer WF. Coaction in multiple behavior change interventions: consistency across multiple studies on weight management and obesity prevention. Health Psychol. 2014;33(5):475–80.
Kasen S, Cohen P, Chen H, Must A. Obesity and psychopathology in women: a three-decade prospective study. Int J Obes. 2008;32:558–66.
Katon WJ. Clinical and health services relationships between major depression, depressive symptoms, and general medical illness. Biol Psychiatry. 2003;54:216–26.
Kessler RC, Chiu WT, Demler O, Merikangas KR, Walters EE. Prevalence, severity, and comorbidity of 12-month DSM-IV disorders in the National Comorbidity Survey Replication. Arch Gen Psychiatry. 2005;62:617–27.
Kim MJ, Lim YR, Kwak HK. Dietary behaviors and body image recognition of college students according to the self-rated health condition. Nutr Res Pract. 2008;2:107–13.
King WC, et al. Prevalence of alcohol use disorders before and after bariatric surgery. JAMA. 2012;307(23):2516–25.
Kuk JL, Ardern CI, Church TS, Hebert JR, Sui X, Blair SN. Ideal weight and weight satisfaction: association with health practices. Am J Epidemiol. 2009;170:456–63.
Kushner RF. The burden of obesity: personal stories, professional insights. Narrat Inq Bioeth. 2014;4(2):129–33.
Lasikiewicz N, Myrissa K, Hoyland A, Lawton CL. Psychological benefits of weight loss following behavioural and/or dietary weight loss interventions. A systematic research review. Appetite. 2014;72(1):123–37.
Levy LD, Fleming JP, Klar D. Treatment of refractory obesity in severely obese adults following management of newly diagnosed attention deficit hyperactivity disorder. Int J Obes. 2009;33:326–34.
Lillis J, Kendra KE. Acceptance and commitment therapy for weight control: model, evidence, and future directions. J Contextual Behav Sci. 2014;3:1–7.
Luppino FS, de Wit LM, Bouvy PF, Stijnen T, Cuijpers P, Penninx BWJH, et al. Overweight, obesity, and depression. Arch Gen Psychiatry. 2010;67(3):220–9.
Macht M. How emotions affect eating: a five-way model. Appetite. 2008;50:1–11.
Markowitz S, Friedman MA, Arent SM. Understanding the realtion between obesity and depression: causal mechanisms and implications for treatment. Clin Psychol Sci Pract. 2008;15:1–20.
Marrero DG, et al. Depressive symptoms, antidepressant medication use, and new onset of diabetes in participants of the diabetes prevention program and the diabetes prevention program outcomes study. Psychosom Med. 2015;77(3):303–10.
McElroy SL, et al. Efficacy and safety of lisdexamfetamine for treatment of adults with moderate to severe binge-eating disorder, a randomized clinical trial. JAMA Psychiatry. 2015;72(3):235–46.
Meany G, Conceicao E, Mitchell JE. Binge eating, binge eating disorder and loss of control eating: effects on weight outcomes after bariatric surgery. Eur Eat Disord Rev. 2014;22:87–91.
Midei AJ, Matthews KA. Interpersonal violence in childhood as a risk factor for obesity: a systematic review of the literature and proposed pathways. Obes Rev. 2011;12:e159–72.

Mitchell JE, Crosby R, de Zwaan M, Engel S, Roerig J, Steffen K, et al. Possible risk factors for increased suicide following bariatric surgery. Obesity (Silver Spring). 2013;21(4):665–72.

Mond J, Mitchison D, Latner J, Hay P, Owen C, Rodgers B. Quality of life impairment associated with body dissatisfaction in a general population sample of women. BMC Public Health. 2013;13:920–31.

Mushtaq R, Shoib S, Shah T, Mushtaq S. Relationship between loneliness, psychiatric disorders and physical health? A review on the psychological aspects of loneliness. J Clin Diagn Res. 2014;8(9):WE01–4.

Narouze S, Souzdalnitski D. Obesity and chronic pain systematic review of prevalence and implications for pain practice. Reg Anesth Pain Med. 2015;40(2):91–111.

Natvik E, Gjengedal E, Raheim M. Totally changes, yet still the same: patients' lived experiences 5 years beyond bariatric surgery. Qual Health Res. 2013;23(9):1202–14.

Nigatu YT, Bultmann U, Reijneveld SA. The prospective association between obesity and major depression in the general population: does single or recurrent episode matter? BMC Public Health. 2015;15:350–6.

O'Reardon JP, Stunkard AJ, Allison KC. Clinical trial of sertraline in the treatment of night eating syndrome. Int J Eat Disord. 2004;35:16–26.

Palmeira AL, Markland DA, Silva MN, Branco TL, Martins SC, Minderico CS, et al. Reciprocal effects among changes in weight, body image, and other psychological factors during behavioral obesity treatment: a mediation analysis. Int J Behav Nutr Phys Act. 2009;9(6):1–12.

Pan A, et al. Bidirectional association between depression and obesity in middle-aged and older women. Int J Obes. 2012;36:595–602.

Parker K, Brennan L. Measurement of disordered eating in bariatric surgery candidates: a systematic review of the literature. Obes Res Clin Pract. 2015;9:12–25.

Pawlow LA, O'Neil PM, Malcolm RJ. Night eating syndrome: effects of brief relaxation training on stress, mood, hunger, and eating patterns. Int J Obes. 2003;27:970–8.

Perera S, Eisen R, Bawor M, Dennis B, de Souza R, Thabane L, et al. Association between body mass index and suicidal behaviors: a systematic review protocol. Syst Rev. 2015;4:52.

Peterhansel C, Petroff D, Klinitzke G, Kersting A, Wagner B. Risk of completed suicide after bariatric surgery: a systematic review. Obes Rev. 2013;14:369–82.

Pila E, Sabiston CM, Brunet J, Castonguay AL, O'Loughlin J. Do body-related shame and guilt mediate the association between weight status and self-esteem? J Health Psychol. 2015;20(5):659–69.

Preiss K, Brennan L, Clarke D. A systematic review of variables associated with the relationship between obesity and depression. Obes Rev. 2013;14:906–18.

Puhl R, Brownell KD. Ways of coping with obesity stigma: review and conceptual analysis. Eat Behav. 2003;4:53–78.

Puhl RM, Brownell KD. Confronting and coping with weight stigma: an investigation of overweight and obese adults. Obesity. 2006;14(10):1802–15.

Puhl RM, Heuer CA. The stigma of obesity: review and update. Obesity. 2009;17:941–64.

Rubin RR, et al. Four-year analysis of cardiovascular disease risk factors, depression symptoms, and antidepressant medicine use in the Look AHEAD (action for health in diabetes) clinical trial of weight loss in diabetes. Diabetes Care. 2013;36:1088–94.

Schag K, Schonleber J, Teufel M, Zipfel S, Giel KE. Food-related impulsivity in obesity and binge eating disorder—a systematic review. Obes Rev. 2013;14:477–95.

Schellekens H, Finger BC, Dinan TG, Cryan JF. Ghrelin signaling and obesity; at the interface of stress, mood and food reward. Pharmacol Ther. 2012;135:316–26.

Singh M. Mood, food, and obesity. Front Psychol. 2014;5:925

Sinha R, Jastreboof AM. Stress as a common risk factor for obesity and addiction. Biol Psychiatry. 2013;73(9):827–35.

Smith F, Farrants J. Shame and self-acceptance in continued flux: qualitative study of the embodied experience of significant weight loss and removal of resultant excess skin by plastic surgery. J Health Psychol. 2012;18(9):1129–40.

Sobel RM, Markov D. The impact of anxiety and mood disorders on physical disease: the worried not-so-well. Curr Psychiatry Rep. 2005;7:206–12.

Sominsky L, Spencer SJ. Eating behavior and stress: a pathway to obesity. Front Psychol. 2014;5:1–8.

Stunkard AJ, Grace WJ, Wolff HG. The night-eating syndrome: a pattern of food intake among certain obese paticnts. Am J Med. 1955;19:78–86.

Udo T, McKee SA, White MA, Masheb RM, Barnes RD, Grilo CM. Sex differences in biopsychosocial correlates of binge eating disorder: a study of treatment-seeking obese adults in primary care setting. Gen Hosp Psychiatry. 2013;35(6):1–13.

Ursini F, Naty S, Grembiale RD. Fibromyalgia and obesity: the hidden link. Rheumatol Int. 2011;31:1403–8.

Vamosi M, Heitmann BL, Kyvik KO. The relation between an adverse psychological and social environment in childhood and the development of adult obesity: a systematic literature review. International Association for the Study of Obesity. Obes Rev. 2010;11:177–84.

Van Zutven K, Mond J, Latner J, Rodgers B. Obesity and psychosocial impairment: mediating roles of health status, weight/shape concerns and binge eating in a community sample of women and men. Int J Obes. 2015;39:346–52.

Vincent HK, Adams MCB, Vincent KR, Hurley RW. Musculoskeletal pain, fear avoidance behaviors, and functional decline in obesity potential interventions to manage pain and maintain function. Reg Anesth Pain Med. 2013;38(6):481–91.

Webb C. Psychological distress in clinical obesity: the role of eating disorder beliefs and behaviors, social comparison and shame. Doctoral thesis, University of Leicester; 2000.

Williamson DF, Thompson TJ, Anda RF, Dietz WH, Felitti V. Body weight and obesity in adults and self-reported abuse in childhood. Int J Obes Relat Metab Disord. 2002;26(8):1075–82.

Wilson GT. Treatment of binge eating disorder. Psychiatr Clin N Am. 2011;34(4):773–83.

Wirth MD, Blake CE, Hebert JR, Sui X, Blair SN. Chronic weight dissatisfaction predicts type 2 diabetes risk: aerobic center longitudinal study. Health Psychol. 2014;33(8):912–9.

Wisse BE, Schwartz MW. Does hypothalamic inflammation cause obesity? Cell Metab. 2009;10:241–2.

Yankura DJ, Conroy MB, Hess R, Pettee KK, Kuller LH, Kriska AM. Weight regain and health-related quality of life in postmenopausal women. Obesity. 2008;16:2259–65.

Yen YC, Huang CK, Tai CM. Psychiatric aspects of bariatric surgery. Curr Opin. 2014; 27(5):374–9.

Young WB. Preventive treatment of migraine: effect on weight. Curr Pain Headache Rep. 2008;12:201–6.

Zhao G, Ford ES, Dhingra S, Li C, Strine TW, Mokdad AH. Depression and anxiety among US adults: associations with body mass index. Int J Obes. 2009;33:257–66.

Chapter 19
Medical Nutrition Therapy for Weight Management

Scott D. Isaacs

Pearls of Wisdom

- Nutrition and lifestyle changes are the backbone of weight management. The United States Preventive Services Task Force, in its 2014 recommendations, recommends referral for counseling by qualified healthcare professionals for all patients with overweight or obesity.
- A team approach to patient care should be used for the treatment of overweight, obesity, and adiposopathy. Qualified healthcare professionals must work closely with patients to implement and maintain a meal plan that fits their needs, capabilities, and motivation.
- Successful medical nutrition therapy must be individualized to meet specific patient energy-deficit requirements with consideration of medical, cultural, educational, religious, economic, and social needs.
- A healthy meal plan contains vegetables, fruits, low-glycemic carbohydrates, healthy proteins, and healthy fats.
- Medical nutrition therapy should be targeted to help each patient achieve realistic, achievable, sustainable, and incremental changes. Healthy eating and daily physical activity translate into weight loss, which in turn prevents weight gain or regain over the long term.

S. D. Isaacs
Atlanta Endocrine Associates, Atlanta, GA, USA

J. M. Gonzalez-Campoy et al. (eds.), *Bariatric Endocrinology*,
https://doi.org/10.1007/978-3-319-95655-8_19

19.1 Introduction

Overconsumption of calories from any macronutrient source, combined with aberrations in energy expenditure, is the primary contributing factor in the development and preservation of overweight and obesity. Multiple clinical practice guidelines emphasize medical nutrition therapy (MNT), physical activity, and behavior modification as necessary components of all obesity management approaches. From the most basic perspective, medical nutrition therapy is the avoidance of excessive calories from food and beverages that can have a negative impact on health. A healthy eating plan includes adequate quantities of macro- and micronutrients to provide an energy deficit and prevent nutritional deficiencies. Healthy eating must be sustained over a long period of time. The most effective and complete approach to MNT includes a healthy eating plan and lifestyle modification.

Few individuals meet national guidelines for healthy eating. The recommendation to consume a minimum of five fruits and/or vegetables daily is achieved by only 16–23% of people. Large portion sizes, restaurant meal consumption (especially fast foods), and drinking sugar-added beverages, all increase calorie intake and are associated with overweight, obesity, and adiposopathy. Many individuals choose popular fad diets with little or no scientific basis. Adherence to fad diets is often short lived, and these diets may be unhealthy. Sustained changes in eating patterns, meal plans, and choice of foods are more effective than a temporary restriction in calories. Instead of using the term "diet," instruct patients on meal planning and healthy eating patterns. The term "diet" implies restriction and deprivation whereas "healthy meal planning" is positive and empowering and emphasizes the significance of lifestyle change to produce improvements in health (See Table 19.1).

19.2 Fundamentals for Successful MNT

MNT should focus on decreasing fat mass and correcting adiposopathy. To be successful, MNT must be individualized for specific patient energy deficit requirements. Meal plans should be personalized to accommodate each patient's medical, cultural, educational, religious, economic, and social needs. Factors such as taste preference, attitudes, intentions, and knowledge should also be considered. Patients should be encouraged to maintain a healthy eating plan while adopting new behaviors to enforce a long-term lifestyle change. When possible, patients should involve their families in healthy eating behaviors, especially children.

There is no single type of medical nutrition therapy that will be an effective strategy for all patients. Therefore, in order to achieve success, macronutrient content and specific meal plan advice should be individualized to meet the specific needs of each patient. The literature has many articles comparing success rates of various meal plans and the importance of acquiring new skills and behaviors to implement

Table 19.1 Low-calorie meal plan

Calories:
1000–1500 kcal/day for women
1200–1600 kcal/day for men
500–1000 kcal/day energy deficit
Low energy-dense foods
Standard meal times with healthy low-calorie snacks
Behavior/lifestyle modification
Carbohydrates:
45–65% of calories
25–35 g of fiber daily
4.5–5 cups daily minimum vegetable and fruit intake
High-fiber whole grains
Limit simple carbohydrates (sugars and starches)
Carbohydrates in beverages (soda, juice, sweet tea, and sports drinks) should be replaced with water and low-calorie beverages
Reduced-fat dairy products such as yogurt and cottage cheese (carbohydrates and protein)
Proteins:
15–35% of calories
Plant proteins (beans, lentils, some nuts, broccoli, kale, and spinach)
Seafood, especially cold-water fatty fish
Reduced-fat dairy products
Reduced fat cheese (part-skim mozzarella, some goat cheeses, string cheese, and some soft cheeses)
Eggs
Lean or very lean cuts of animal protein, including skinless poultry
<6 ounces per day of animal protein
Fats:
25–35% of calories
Vegetable oils, seeds, avocados, olives, nuts, seeds, and seafood (MUFAs and PUFAs)
2 servings of cold-water fatty fish weekly (omega-3 fatty acids)
<7% of daily calories from saturated fats (butter and animal fats)
<1% of total calories from trans fats

Abbreviations: *kcal* kilocalories, *MUFAs* monounsaturated fatty acids, *PUFAs* polyunsaturated fatty acids

and maintain permanent lifestyle change. Several randomized trials have evaluated weight loss in subjects on meal plans with varying percentages of carbohydrates, proteins, and fat. Weight loss is similar for all meal plans, as well as ratings of satiety, hunger, and satisfaction with the meal plan.

Meal plans with the greatest likelihood of adherence have the greatest likelihood of success. For most patients, a meal plan that contains vegetables, fruits and low-glycemic carbohydrates, lean protein, and beneficial fats has the greatest likelihood of long-term adherence. In addition to a healthy eating meal plan, MNT should include strategies to reduce overeating, binge eating, and nonhunger eating (such as stress eating or eating due to boredom). MNT must be accompanied by adequate physical activity and adequate sleep. Patients should also be counseled to allow adequate time for recreation and relaxation for stress reduction and happiness.

A weight-maintenance program should be instituted immediately after successful weight loss to prevent weight regain. The program should consist of ongoing MNT, physical activity, lifestyle management, and pharmacotherapy when appropriate. Although losing weight is comparatively easy, the maintenance of weight loss is more difficult, especially if the patient is not adequately prepared to permanently adopt a new lifestyle. In a review of the literature, it was found that 80–95% of patients who lose weight with nutritional changes will regain it back within a few years. Multiple biological systems are activated when energy intake is reduced, increasing appetite and driving people to eat more caloric-dense foods. The challenge of MNT is to find ways to maintain energy balance despite these powerful biological mechanisms. At present time, interventions are limited and do not permanently correct the factors that prevent weight loss or lead to weight regain.

19.3 Setting Goals Based on Risk

Patients often have unrealistic weight loss goals. Counseling patients about attainable weight loss and food intake goals should focus on reducing excess fat mass and correcting adiposopathy more than actual body weight. Patients should be informed about the benefits of moderate initial weight loss in the range of 5–10% of body weight. Weight loss in this range can produce meaningful improvements in diabetes, dyslipidemia, obstructive sleep apnea, nonalcoholic fatty liver disease, and other comorbidities. Risks are further reduced with greater weight loss.

Healthy eating patterns and lifestyle change result in a 35% reduction in cardiovascular events and a 40% reduction in all-cause mortality over a 6-year period. Additionally, significant improvements in risk factors are achieved with 2–5% weight loss. A 5–10% weight loss leads to increased reductions in risk factors, and further reductions are achieved with 10–15% weight loss.

19.4 Low-Calorie Meal Plans

A low-calorie meal plan provides 1000–1500 kcal/day for women and 1200–1600 kcal/day for men, to allow for weight loss of 1–2 pounds per week and 5–10% weight loss within 6 months. Energy balance should be determined by measuring (using indirect calorimetry) or calculating energy requirements. A meal plan that contains a 500–1000 kcal/day energy deficit should be provided to the patient. A simple equation for estimating resting metabolic rate is 8 calories per pound for women and 10 calories per pound for men. A more precise method uses body weight, age, and height to estimate resting metabolic rate for patients with overweight and obesity:

- Men: 10 × weight (kg) + 6.25 × height (cm) – 5 × age (years) + 5
- Women: 10 × weight (kg) + 6.25 × height (cm) – 5 × age (years) – 161

The resting metabolic rate should be adjusted to total daily expenditure by using a multiplier of 1.2 for sedentary, 1.4 for low-to-moderate activity, and 1.6 for active individuals. Energy requirements decrease as an individual loses weight and should therefore be recalculated and the meal plan modified periodically to maintain a negative energy balance.

Low-calorie meal plans are relatively contraindicated in those with unstable psychiatric illness, eating disorders, substance abuse, pregnancy, or who are lactating. Patients with medical conditions that could be exacerbated with caloric restriction (unstable angina, recent cerebrovascular event, active malignancy) are not candidates for low-calorie meal plans. Potential side effects of low-calorie meal plans include hypotension, constipation, poor wound healing, hair shedding, cold intolerance, gallbladder disease, loss of muscle mass, depression, and irritability.

19.4.1 Beverages

Low-calorie meal plans can result in a mild diuresis. Patients may experience symptoms such as increased urination, lightheadedness, or dehydration. Patients should be encouraged to consume 2 L of water or low-calorie beverages daily, which replenishes fluids and maintains lipolysis. Artificial sweeteners should be limited or avoided. Caffeinated beverages should be limited to four cups daily. Consumption of water and low-calorie beverages was considered to be very important for weight loss by 40% of participants in the National Weight Control Registry. Warm beverages can stimulate the hypothalamus to decrease appetite more than cold beverages.

19.4.2 Alcohol

Small amounts of alcohol, especially red wine, have been shown to decrease the risk for a number of diseases. However, alcoholic beverages should be minimized or avoided within a low-calorie meal plan. Alcohol should be limited to two servings per day for men and one serving per day for women. Alcohol consumption results in the intake of extra calories. Drinking alcohol has been shown to increase hunger, decrease fullness, and increase total food intake primarily from energy-dense foods.

19.5 Very Low-Calorie Meal Plans

Very low-calorie (VLC) meal plans are indicated for patients with BMI >30 kg/m^2 who have significant comorbidities or who have not been successful achieving weight loss with other nutritional therapies. A VLC meal plan can be an effective short-term intervention (a few weeks to a few months) for motivated patients with severe obesity. VLC meal plans typically use meal replacement shakes and other foods and have a caloric intake of 500–800 kcal/day combined with medical monitoring along with intensive lifestyle coaching and education. In order to meet nutritional guidelines, it is essential to prescribe a VLC meal plan with careful food or meal replacement choices, adequate hydration, and vitamin and mineral supplements. Potassium supplementation may also be necessary in certain patients.

A VLC meal plan should begin with an informational session to select appropriate patients and to inform and educate about the expectations of the plan. Careful patient selection for VLC meal plans is important because weight regain and attrition rates have been found to be higher for patients on this meal plan.

VLC meal plans can produce rapid weight loss of 3–5 pounds per week and up to 45 pounds in 16 weeks. Patients treated with VLC meal plans achieve a mean weight loss of 21% at 24 weeks, or 52 pounds.

Side effects of VLC meal plans are generally minor and include lightheadedness, dizziness, headache, fatigue, cold intolerance, hair loss, nausea, muscle cramps, constipation, and diarrhea. More serious side effects include volume depletion, hypokalemia, and hyponatremia.

Gallstones, sometimes requiring surgery, occur in 10–25% of patients on VLC meal plans, although the risk for gallstones is already double to triple in persons 120% of their ideal body weight. Meal plans that are very low in fat and calories can result in the mobilization of cholesterol stores, slow down regulation of bile acid secretion, create bile that is supersaturated with cholesterol, and cause decreased gallbladder contraction. These conditions lead to biliary sludge and stone formation. Ursodeoxycholic acid 300 mg twice daily can be used for the prevention of gallstones during a low-calorie or VLC meal plan.

Serious ventricular arrhythmias have been described in patients on nutritionally inadequate liquid protein meals. However, there is no increase in the incidence of arrhythmias when high-quality meal replacements are used.

Contraindications to a VLC meal plan include pregnancy, active eating disorder, active substance abuse, or serious medical illness. Many medications including insulin, oral hypoglycemic agents, diuretics, warfarin, digoxin, antiseizure medications, and beta-blockers require dose adjustment during a VLC meal plan. VLC meal plans require medical monitoring for complications including volume depletion, hepatic transaminase elevation, electrolyte abnormalities, QT prolongation, and gallstone formation. Commercially available VLC meal plans include:

- Optifast
- Medifast
- Health Management Resources (HMR)

19.6 Meal Replacements

Meal replacements are portion-controlled servings of foods that are useful in the setting of a VLC meal plan and for people who have difficulty with self-selection or portion control. Commercially available meal replacements such as shakes, cereals, puddings, soups, bars, and entrees provide calorie- and portion-controlled replacements for higher calorie meals and snacks.

Meal replacements have a calming effect on appetite centers in the brain while lowering hunger and cravings, as assessed with functional magnetic resonance imaging (MRI). Meal replacements can produce initial greater weight loss, and greater total weight loss, compared to other meal plans. Meal replacements have also been found to enhance long-term maintenance of weight loss.

A study evaluating weight loss shakes compared nutritionally identical protein shakes that varied in viscosity. Subjects who drank thicker shakes reported decreased hunger and increased satiety compared to those who drank thinner shakes. The subjects who drank thicker shakes consumed fewer calories than those who drank the thinner shakes.

19.7 Micronutrient Supplementation During MNT

There is insufficient evidence to recommend supplemental vitamin intake above recommended dietary allowances in otherwise healthy patients. However, overt vitamin deficiencies may pre-exist in patients who consume meals poor in nutritional value. Meal plans should contain adequate nutrients from healthy foods so that vitamin and mineral supplementation is usually not necessary. Natural compounds in foods work individually or in combination to provide health benefits superior to dietary supplements or nutraceuticals. No supplement trial in healthy patients has been shown to reproduce the benefits of eating adequate amounts of healthy foods.

A large number of antioxidant and potentially anticarcinogenic phytochemicals are found in vegetables, fruits, whole grains, nuts, seeds, and fish including flavonoids, phenols, protease inhibitors, sterols, allium compounds, and limonene. These compounds are thought to play a role in the prevention of disease by detoxifying carcinogens in the blood, activating protective enzymes in the body and repairing and preventing cell damage that can lead to disease. Foods especially high in phytonutrients include whole grains, nuts, legumes, fruits (especially berries), and cruciferous vegetables.

Antioxidants are compounds that protect the body against cell damage from unstable molecules known as free radicals, which have been linked to both cancer and cardiovascular disease. Examples of antioxidants are lycopene; beta-carotene; carotenoids; and vitamins A, C, and E. Foods high in antioxidants include tomatoes (lycopene), berries (vitamin C, ellagic acid, anthocyanin), carrots (beta-carotene), spinach (carotenoids, lutein, and zeaxanthin) and other dark leafy vegetables, whole grains, flax, and sesame seeds (ligans, saponins).

Specific vitamin deficiencies should be screened for based on history and clinical findings. For example, elderly adults, patients who follow a vegetarian or vegan meal plan, and patients treated with metformin should be screened for vitamin B_{12} deficiency. Except in malabsorptive states, neurological symptoms, or pernicious anemia, vitamin B_{12} can be given as oral crystalline cobalamin 1000 mg per day. Patients at risk for vitamin D insufficiency include those with obesity, insufficient sunlight exposure, postmenopausal women, the elderly, and people with increased skin pigmentation. These patients should increase vitamin D intake from fortified foods and/or vitamin D supplements to at least 1000 IU per day. Vitamin D content in most foods is very low, with the exception of fatty fish and fortified foods.

Patients who consume meal replacements, or who have food restrictions, may require vitamin supplementation with a daily multivitamin. This is especially so if meal replacements are being used as exclusive nutrition in a VLC meal plan. Patients with malabsorption or who have undergone bariatric surgery (especially Roux-en-Y gastric bypass which is a malabsorptive procedure) are at especially high risk for vitamin deficiencies despite daily multivitamin supplementation.

19.8 Maintaining Energy Deficit

Regardless of the differences in macronutrient content of various meal plans, the overriding factor that leads to weight loss is a deficit in calories. Energy expenditure must exceed energy intake for weight loss to occur. Long-term adherence to the meal plan is vital. An effective healthy eating plan should be palatable, satiating, and sustainable.

Reduced-calorie meal plans should emphasize the satiation of appetite. Patients who follow overly restrictive meal plans may experience short-term weight loss but tend to have excessive hunger and feelings of deprivation, which can lead to deviations from the meal plan, or binge eating episodes. This leads to feelings of guilt and self-blame and can be viewed by both patient and physician as a "lack of willpower."

Patients should be instructed to consume three meals per day with healthy low-calorie snacks at variable times of the day if needed. It is recommended that total energy intake should be distributed evenly throughout the day, with greater caloric intake during the day, compared to overconsumption and grazing at night. Counseling patients to change eating patterns is a good way to get patients to start adopting healthy lifestyle behaviors. For example, if a patient usually does not eat breakfast, doing so can be an easy first step.

Appetite is affected by the taste, texture, volume, water content, and macronutrient composition of food as well as the palatability, texture, and whole food components. Consumption of foods with low energy density (vegetables, fruits, whole grains, reduced-fat dairy, low-fat proteins) decreases overall calorie intake and aids in losing and maintaining weight. Instruct patients to lower the energy density of meals by increasing the number of low-calorie high-volume foods and decreasing the number of high-calorie low-volume foods. This improves the ability to control hunger, which improves adherence to the meal plan. Lowering the energy density of meals compared to a prescribed low-fat meal plan results in more rapid weight loss at 6 months and greater weight loss at 12 months.

The texture of foods can have variable effects on appetite and satiety. Liquid (apple juice) has the weakest effect on appetite, while solid (apple) and semi-solid (applesauce) have the strongest effect. Both texture and taste affect energy consumption. People eat more food when it is both mashed and more savory.

19.9 Macronutrients

Macronutrients include carbohydrates, protein, and fat. When determining a meal plan, macronutrient quantity and quality should be considered. For example, emphasize starch or fiber over sugar, or unsaturated fats over saturated fats.

19.9.1 Carbohydrates

Carbohydrates should provide 45–65% of calories in a healthy eating meal plan. Healthy carbohydrates are high in both soluble and insoluble fibers, stanols, sterols, bioavailable micronutrients, and low in caloric density. Whole vegetables and fruits, whole grains, and low-fat dairy products are preferred over simple carbohydrates (sugars and starches) with a high glycemic effect. However, there is insufficient evidence to recommend a "low-glycemic" meal plan over other healthy meal plans. A typical patient should consume 6–8 servings of carbohydrates (90–120 g) per day with 3–4 servings coming from high-fiber foods such as vegetables, fruits, and whole grains.

Refined grains should be replaced with whole grains, which adds fiber and micronutrients. Added sugars should be limited to <100 kcal per day for women and <150 kcal per day for men. Carbohydrates in beverages such as soda, juice, sweet tea, and sports drinks should be replaced with water and low-calorie beverages.

Vegetable and fruit intake should be a minimum of 4.5–5 cups (2.5–3 cups of vegetables and 1.5–2 cups of fruit) daily for weight loss, prevention of chronic diseases, and health promotion. Fruits and vegetables can be frozen, canned (without added sugar), or fresh to allow flexibility.

Increased consumption of vegetables and fruits is recommended because these foods are low in calories, high in fiber and phytonutrients, and help with calorie control. There are a number of articles linking increased consumption of vegetables and fruits to a variety of health benefits. Vegetable and fruit consumption, especially cruciferous vegetables (cabbage, brussels sprouts, broccoli, cauliflower), green vegetables, citrus fruits, and other fruits and vegetables rich in vitamin C, has been associated with a decrease in the risk for coronary heart disease and stroke.

Grains that contain ≥1.1 g of fiber per 10-g serving of carbohydrates are considered high-fiber whole grains. The United States Department of Agriculture (USDA) recommends 5–8 ounces of grains daily, with at least half coming from whole grains.

Reduced-fat dairy products such as yogurt and cottage cheese are composed of both carbohydrates and high-quality protein. Patients should be counseled to replace high-fat dairy products with reduced-fat versions, although some reduced-fat yogurt products contain added sugar and may not be lower in calories than the full-fat variety.

19.9.2 Fiber

Fiber is a vital component of healthy nutrition and may play a role in disease prevention. Patients should consume 25–35 g of fiber per day coming from healthy foods rather than from supplements. Vegetables, fruits, legumes, and whole grains are superb sources of fiber but can vary in fiber composition (soluble vs. insoluble).

Soluble fiber, or viscous fiber including beta-glucan and pectin, lowers cholesterol levels by decreasing endogenous cholesterol production and increasing bile acid secretion. Sources of soluble fiber include beans, fruits, vegetables, and some grains (oats and barley). Insoluble fiber is contained in the roughage of vegetables or in the hull of grain and helps create a large well-formed easily passed stool. The more rapid transit is through the intestine, the lower the absorption of calories and nutrients. Fiber may also enhance satiety by delaying gastric emptying. Sources of insoluble fiber include whole grains (whole wheat bran) and some fruits and vegetables.

19.9.3 Proteins

Protein should comprise 15–35% of total calorie consumption as part of a healthy meal plan. Plant proteins such as those in beans, lentils, some nuts, broccoli, kale and spinach, and fish should be emphasized as important sources of protein because they are low in fat and contain soluble fiber and micronutrients. Animal protein, which contains saturated fat, should not exceed 6 ounces per day. Processed red meat should be limited to two servings per week. Lean or very lean cuts of animal protein should be chosen to help reduce saturated fat intake. Reduced-fat dairy products, eggs, fish, and skinless poultry are recommended as healthy sources of animal protein. Preferred types of cheeses include cottage cheese, part-skim mozzarella cheese, some goat cheeses, string cheese, and some soft cheeses.

19.9.4 Fats

Patients should consume 25–35% daily calories as healthy fats. The healthiest fats are mono- and polyunsaturated fats from liquid vegetable oils, seeds, nuts, and fish. Saturated fats such as butter and animal fats should be limited to <7% of daily calories. Trans fats should be avoided or reduced to <1% of total calories. Because fat is high in calories, reducing fat intake is associated with weight reduction. However, decreasing fat consumption can result in increased intake of carbohydrates and calories, often from added sugars or other refined sources. Patients should be counseled on ways to avoid this from happening.

Natural foods high in monounsaturated fats such as avocado, nuts (walnuts, macadamia nuts, and almonds), seeds, olives, and vegetable oils are recommended because they have been associated with improved health outcomes. These foods also contain phytonutrients such as polyphenols, which may confer added benefits. Liquid vegetable oils such as corn, soybean, sunflower, and safflower are high in linoleic acid, an essential omega-6 fatty acid. Canola and flaxseed oils contain the omega-3 fatty acid alpha-linoleic acid (ALA). Olive oil is high in monounsaturated fatty acids (MUFA).

Patients should consume a minimum of two servings of cold-water fatty fish (salmon or mackerel) weekly because they contain omega-three fatty acids. Omega-3 fatty acids are polyunsaturated fatty acids (PUFAs) derived from both animal and plant sources. Eicosapentaenoic acid (EPA) and docosahexaenoic acid (DHA) are omega-3 fatty acids that come from marine sources and have been shown to reduce the risk of cardiovascular disease.

19.10 Considerations for Patients with Comorbid Diseases

Optimal patient care in the management of chronic endocrine and metabolic diseases requires patient engagement and involvement of appropriate support mechanisms. Education is essential, and a team approach to patient care, directed by the clinical endocrinologist, is the optimal way to accomplish this goal. Registered nurses, registered dieticians, certified diabetes educators, physical activity coaches, and appropriate specialists each contribute to the care of these patients. Individual practices may vary on the personnel within the organization, but a referral network should be in place to assist in the care of these patients. Following are nutritional recommendations for selected endocrine and metabolic diseases.

19.10.1 Diabetes Mellitus

MNT should be prescribed to control blood glucose response to meals and normalize A1C levels. Forty-five percent to 65% of total calories should be carbohydrates including reduced-fat dairy products, vegetables, and fruits. Patients should consume 8–10 servings of vegetables and fruits daily and legumes appropriately. Patients with diabetes should avoid refined grains and limit simple sugars. Patients with diabetes may consume small amounts of artificial sweeteners. Patients with diabetes should consume 20–35 g of fiber daily, primarily from whole vegetables, fruits, and unprocessed grains. Patients with diabetes should consume protein at 0.8–1.0 g/kg/day.

Total fat intake should account for 30% of total daily calories with less than 7% of total daily calories from saturated fat. Polyunsaturated fatty acids such as vegetable oils high in omega-6 polyunsaturated fatty acids (PUFAs), soft margarine, salad dressings, mayonnaise, and some nuts and seeds are preferred sources of fat.

Patients on meal-time insulin or short-acting oral hypoglycemic agents (nateglinide, repaglinide) must synchronize medication administration and carbohydrate intake. Weight loss produces significant improvements in insulin sensitivity and blood glucose levels and may result in hypoglycemia if medications are not adjusted. Doses of sulfonylureas (glipizide, glyburide, glimepiride), short-acting oral hypoglycemic agents, and insulin may need to be reduced or discontinued as weight loss progresses.

19.10.2 Dyslipidemia

Adiposopathy results in elevated triglycerides and low high-density lipoprotein levels in the blood. The same nutritional interventions that help achieve weight loss also improve the lipid profile. A reduced-calorie meal plan consisting of fruits and vegetables (combined ≥5 servings/day), grains (primarily whole grains), fish, and lean meats is recommended. The intake of saturated fats, trans fats, and cholesterol should be limited. LDLC-lowering macronutrient intake should include plant stanols/sterols (~2 g/day) and soluble fiber (10–25 g/day).

The Mediterranean meal pattern incorporates most of these recommendations and is defined by seven elements:

- high consumption of legumes
- high consumption of grains and cereals
- high consumption of fruits and vegetables
- low consumption of meat and meat products and increased consumption of fish
- moderate consumption of milk and dairy products
- high-monounsaturated/saturated fat ratio
- low-to-moderate red wine consumption

The Mediterranean meal pattern leads to a drop in total cholesterol (−0.23 mmol/L) and LDL-C (−0.07 mmol/L), with variable impact on HDL-C and triglycerides. Compared to low-fat meal plans, the Mediterranean pattern produces improvements in total cholesterol, triglycerides, and overall cardiovascular risk after 2 years of use, with no significant differences in LDL-C or HDL-C.

19.10.3 Chronic Kidney Disease (CKD)

Patients with chronic kidney disease (CKD) should have a meal plan that is low in protein, potassium, sodium, and phosphorus. All patients with CKD should receive nutrition counseling from a qualified healthcare professional. Sodium intake should be limited to 2 g per day. Potassium intake should be limited to 2–3 g per day if hyperkalemia develops. Phosphate intake should be limited to 800 mg per day. In stage 1, 2, and 3 CKD, protein intake should be restricted to 12–15% of daily calorie intake or 0.8 g of protein per kilogram of body weight each day. In stage 4 CKD, protein intake should be further reduced to 10% of daily caloric intake or 0.6 g of protein per kilogram per day. For patients with stage 5 CKD or on renal replacement therapy, protein intake may be liberalized to 1.2–1.3 g per kilogram per day. Urinary protein losses in nephrotic syndrome should be replaced. At least 50% of protein intake should be from high biologic value sources to ensure adequate essential amino acids.

19.11 Behavioral and Psychological Aspects of MNT

Effective counseling during medical nutrition therapy is essential for patients to understand the importance of lifestyle change as an essential part of successful long-term weight loss. Motivational interviewing has become an important tool for enhancing patient self-management. Motivational interviewing promotes autonomy and creates motivation to change by setting self-defined goals. This approach guides rather than tells, and allows the patient to be in charge, focusing on strengths rather than weaknesses. Motivational interviewing is effective for weight loss by helping change underlying behaviors that influence health.

The three main aspects of motivational interviewing are ask, listen, and inform. Ask questions that are open-ended and invite the patient to consider how motivated they are to make a change. Patients should do the majority of the talking with practitioners listening reflectively and empathetically interjecting strategic and respectful reiterations of statements and feelings. This can provide positive feedback and instill confidence and optimism. Informing should always be done with permission in a collaborative manner. For example, one may ask a patient, "Would it be okay with you if we do this?" or "How do you feel about this?" Motivational interviewing should provide ongoing support and counsel, instead of being paternalistic and educational.

Behavior or lifestyle modification is a key aspect of MNT. Several observational and randomized controlled trials have shown that patients treated with behavior modification lose approximately 10% of initial weight. Patients must learn to implement new eating habits to supplant maladaptive behaviors that contributed to the development of excess body weight. Behavior modification should be used in conjunction with MNT and physical activity, as well as with pharmacotherapy or bariatric surgery. Behavioral modification strategies for MNT include self-monitoring, making specific nutrition goals (such as decreasing specific high-calorie foods), increasing physical activity, developing skills to cope, modification of the food environment, and enlisting social support.

Behavior modification treatments may be weekly group sessions led by registered dieticians, behavioral psychologists, or health educators. Most behavioral modification counseling should be delivered over the initial 16–26 weeks of MNT. Each session should include a structured curriculum beginning with a review of food and activity data. The health educator helps patients identify maladaptive eating behaviors, develop strategies to cope with identified problems, and adhere to a healthy meal plan. Maintaining food records as well as weekly homework assignments are important components of behavioral modification. Electronically delivered (telephone or Internet) behavior modification messages, which include personalized feedback, can be offered when face-to-face interventions are not possible.

Group behavioral modification treatment has been found to significantly result in weight loss, compared to individual treatment. Group treatment is cost-effective and allows for social support, comradery, healthy competition, and empathy. Selected individuals, especially those with mental or physical health concerns or those with a strong preference, are candidates for individualized therapy.

19.12 Self-monitoring and Using Technology

Food and activity logs, and other forms of self-monitoring, are effective tools to achieve weight loss. Self-monitoring requires recording all food and calories consumed in addition to related aspects of eating behavior, such as emotions, places, and times. Self-monitoring helps patients implement lifestyle modification as well as increasing accountability, self-awareness, and adherence. Self-monitoring helps patients identify and develop behavioral modification strategies to address maladaptive eating behaviors that may be induced by various environmental stimuli. Traditional food diaries have been largely replaced by electronic applications which can track calories consumed and energy expenditure and provide ongoing feedback.

Patients should be encouraged to weigh themselves at least three times per week. Frequent weighing improves weight loss, compared to subjects who weigh themselves infrequently.

19.13 Conclusion

MNT is the foundation for weight management. MNT is used in conjunction with physical activity, lifestyle improvements, and behavior modification. MNT should always be included when pharmacotherapy and/or bariatric surgery is used. A personalized low-calorie meal plan should provide appropriate quantities of macronutrients for an energy deficit of 500–1000 kcal daily, which will allow for weight loss of 1–2 pounds per week and 5–10% weight loss within 6 months. Essential micronutrients should be provided by nutritious foods that can be enjoyed within a healthy low-calorie meal plan. A VLC meal plan can be effective for highly motivated patients with severe obesity or for those who have not been successful with low-calorie meal plans. Meal replacements can be useful for VLC meal plans and for people who have difficulty with self-selection or portion control.

MNT must address a patient's food preferences, attitudes, intentions, and knowledge. MNT should also address medical, cultural, educational, religious, and social variables. Patients should be encouraged to adopt new behaviors to enforce long-term lifestyle change. Motivational interviewing is an important tool for patient self-management, by supporting autonomy and building motivation to change through self-defined goal-setting. Behavior modification should be used in conjunction with MNT. Group behavior modification treatment is more effective than individual treatment. Self-monitoring such as food and activity record keeping, and frequent weighing, should be employed to increase self-awareness and help motivate patients.

Reading List

Alhassan S, et al. Dietary adherence and weight loss success among overweight women: results from the A TO Z weight loss study. Int J Obes. 2008;32(6):985–91.

Allied Health Sciences Section Ad Hoc Nutrition Committee, Aills L, et al. ASMBS allied health nutritional guidelines for the surgical weight loss patient. Surg Obes Relat Dis. 2008;4:S73–108.

Alvarez-Leite JI. Nutrient deficiencies secondary to bariatric surgery. Curr Opin Clin Nutr Metab Care. 2004;7:569–75.

Anderson JW, et al. Structured weight-loss programs: a meta-analysis of weight loss at 24 weeks and assessment of effects of intensity of intervention. Adv Ther. 2004;21:61–75.

Apovian CM, et al. Endocrine society clinical practice guidelines on the pharmacological management of obesity. J Clin Endocrinol Metab. 2015;100(2):342–62.

Ashley JM, et al. Meal replacements in weight intervention. Obes Res. 2001;9(Suppl 4):312S–20S.

Asrih M, et al. Diets and nonalcoholic fatty liver disease: the good and the bad. Clin Nutr. 2014;33(2):186–90.

Bell EA, Rolls BJ. Energy density of foods affects energy intake across multiple levels of fat content in lean and obese women. Am J Clin Nutr. 2001;73:1010–8.

Berkey CS, et al. Sugar-added beverages and adolescent weight change. Obes Res. 2004;12:778–88.

Blackburn GL, et al. Ten-year self-management of weight using a meal replacement diet plan: comparisons with matched controls. Obes Res. 2003;11:A103.

Bloomberg RD, et al. Nutritional deficiencies following bariatric surgery: what have we learned? Obes Surg. 2005;15:145–54.

Brown T, et al. Systematic review of long-term lifestyle interventions to prevent weight gain and morbidity in adults. Obes Rev. 2009;10:627–38.

Brownell K. The LEARN program for weight management. Dallas: American Health Publishing; 2000.

Catenacci VA, et al. Low/no calorie sweetened beverage consumption in the National Weight Control Registry. Obesity (Silver Spring). 2014;22:2244–51.

DeBoer SW, et al. Dietary intake of fruits, vegetables, and fat in Olmsted County, Minnesota. Mayo Clin Proc. 2003;78:161–6.

Diabetes Prevention Program (DPP) Research Group. The Diabetes Prevention Program (DPP): description of lifestyle intervention. Diabetes Care. 2002;25:2165–71.

Dirks AJ, et al. Caloric restriction in humans: potential pitfalls and health concerns. Mech Ageing Dev. 2006;127:1–7.

Duffey KJ, et al. Differential associations of fast food and restaurant food consumption with 3-y change in body mass index: the Coronary Artery Risk Development in Young Adults Study. Am J Clin Nutr. 2007;85:201–8.

Ello-Martin JA, et al. Dietary energy density in the treatment of obesity: a year-long trial comparing 2 weight-loss diets. Am J Clin Nutr. 2007;85:1465–77.

Forde CG, et al. Texture and savoury taste influence on food intake in a realistic hot lunch time meal. Appetite. 2013;60:180–6.
Foster GD, et al. What is a reasonable weight loss? Patients' expectations and evaluations of obesity treatment outcomes. J Consult Clin Psychol. 1997;65(1):79–85.
Gonzalez-Campoy JM, et al. Clinical Practice Guidelines for Healthy Eating. Endocrine Practice. 2013;19(6):e1–e40.
Guthrie JF, et al. Role of food prepared away from home in the American diet, 1977–78 versus 1994–96: changes and consequences. J Nutr Educ Behav. 2002;34:140–50.
Hannum SM, et al. Use of portion-controlled entrees enhances weight loss in women. Obes Res. 2004;12:538–46.
Heymsfield SB, et al. Weight management using a meal replacement strategy: meta and pooling analysis from six studies. Int J Obes. 2003;27:537–49.
Hu T, et al. Effects of low-carbohydrate diets versus low-fat diets on metabolic risk factors: a meta-analysis of randomized controlled clinical trials. Am J Epidemiol. 2012;176(Suppl 7):S44–54.
Isner JM, et al. Sudden, unexpected death in avid dieters using the liquid-protein-modified-fast diet. Observations in 17 patients and the role of the prolonged QT interval. Circulation. 1979;60:1401–12.
Jensen MD, et al. 2013 AHA/ACC/TOS guideline for the management of overweight and obesity in adults: a report of the American College of Cardiology/American Heart Association Task Force on Practice Guidelines and the Obesity Society. Circulation. 2014;129(25 Suppl 2):S102–38.
Johnson BC, Kanters S, Bandayrel K, et al. Comparison of weight loss among named diet programs in overweight and obese adults: a meta-analysis. JAMA. 2014;312(9):923–33.
Joshipura KJ, et al. The effect of fruit and vegetable intake on risk for coronary heart disease. Ann Intern Med. 2001;134:1106–14.
King DE, et al. Turning back the clock: adopting a healthy lifestyle in middle age. Am J Med. 2007;120:598–603.
Kreitzman SN, et al. Safety and effectiveness of weight reduction using a very-low-calorie formulated food. Arch Intern Med. 1984;144:747–50.
Kris-Etherton PM, et al. Fish consumption, fish oil, omega-3 fatty acids, and cardiovascular disease. Circulation. 2002;106:2747–57.
Law MR, Morris JK. By how much does fruit and vegetable consumption reduce the risk of ischaemic heart disease? Eur J Clin Nutr. 1998;52:549–56.
LeCheminant JD, et al. A comparison of meal replacements and medication in weight maintenance after weight loss. J Am Coll Nutr. 2005;24:347–53.
Levitsky DA, et al. The more food young adults are served, the more they overeat. J Nutr. 2004;134:2546–9.
Liddle RA, et al. Gallstone formation during weight-reduction dieting. Arch Intern Med. 1989;149:1750–3.
Lloyd-Jones DM, et al. Consistently stable or decreased body mass index in young adulthood and longitudinal changes in metabolic syndrome components: the Coronary Artery Risk Development in Young Adults Study. Circulation. 2007;115:1004–11.
Lockwood DH, et al. Very low calorie diets in the management of obesity. Annu Rev Med. 1984;35:373–81.
Mattes RE, et al. Effects of food form and timing of ingestion on appetite and energy intake in lean young adults and in young adults with obesity. J Am Diet Assoc. 2009;109:430–7.
Mattes RD, et al. Beverage viscosity is inversely related to postprandial hunger in humans. Physiol Behav. 2001;74:551–7.
Mechanick JI, et al. American Association of Clinical Endocrinologists medical guidelines for the clinical use of dietary supplements and nutraceuticals. Endocr Pract. 2003;9:417–70.
Metzner CE, et al. Effect of a conventional energy-restricted modified diet with our without meal replacement on weight loss and cardiometabolic risk profile in overweight women. Nutr Metab. 2011;8:64.

Mifflin MD, et al. A new predictive equation for resting energy expenditure in healthy individuals. Am J Clin Nutr. 1990;51:241–7.
National Cholesterol Education Program; National Heart, Lung, and Blood Institute; National Institutes of Health. Third report of the National Cholesterol Education (NCEP) expert panel on detection, evaluation and treatment of high blood cholesterol in adults (adult treatment panel III) final report. Circulation. 2002;106:3143–421.
National Institutes of Health. Clinical guidelines on the identification, evaluation and treatment of overweight and obesity in adults. The evidence report. Obes Res. 1998;6(Suppl 2):51S–209S.
Ocher CN, et al. Treating obesity seriously: when recommendations for lifestyle change confront biological adaptations. Lancet Diabetes Endocrinol. 2015;3(4):232–4.
Paolini BM, et al. Meal replacement: calming the hot-state brain network of appetite. Front Psychol. 2012;5:249.
Reeves MJ, Rafferty AP. Healthy lifestyle characteristics among adults in the United States, 2000. Arch Intern Med. 2005;165:854–7.
Renjilian DA, et al. Individual versus group therapy for obesity: effects of matching participants to their treatment preferences. J Consult Clin Psychol. 2001;69:717–21.
Rollnick S. Motivational interviewing in health care. New York: Guilford Press; 2007.
Rolls BJ, et al. Effects of temperature and mode of presentation of juice on hunger, thirst and food intake in humans. Appetite. 1990;15(3):199–208.
Rolls BJ, et al. Changing the energy density of the diet as a strategy for weight management. J Am Diet Assoc. 2005;105:S98–103.
Rolls BJ, et al. Larger portion sizes lead to a sustained increase in energy intake over 2 days. J Am Diet Assoc. 2006;106:543–9.
Sacks FM, et al. Comparison of weight-loss diets with different compositions of fat, protein, and carbohydrates. N Engl J Med. 2009;360(9):859–73.
Schneeman BO. Gastrointestinal physiology and functions. Br J Nutr. 2002;88:S159–63.
Singh BN, et al. Liquid protein diets and torsade de pointes. JAMA. 1978;240:115–9.
Smith WM, Gallagher JJ. "Les torsades de pointes": an unusual ventricular arrhythmia. Ann Intern Med. 1980;93:578–84.
Steinberg DM, et al. Weighing every day matters: daily weighing improves weight loss and adoption of weight control behaviors. J Acad Nutr Diet. 2015;115(4):511–8.
Steinmetz KA, et al. Vegetables, fruit and cancer. II. Mechanisms. Cancer Causes Control. 1991;2:427–42.
Tuomilehto H, et al. Obesity and obstructive sleep apnea—clinical significance of weight loss. Sleep Med Rev. 2013;17(5):321–9.
U. S. Department of Agriculture. Dietary guidelines for Americans 2005. Available at: www.healtherus.gov/dietaryguidelines.
Very low-calorie diets. National Task Force on the Prevention and Treatment of Obesity, National Institutes of Health. JAMA. 1993;270: 967–74.
Wadden TA, et al. Very low calorie diets: their efficacy, safety, and future. Ann Intern Med. 1983;99:675–84.
Wadden TA, et al. One-year weight losses in the Look AHEAD study: factors associated with success. Obesity (Silver Spring). 2009;17:713–22.
Wooley SC, Garner DM. Dietary treatments of obesity are ineffective. Br Med J. 1994;309:655–6.
Yeomans MR, et al. Short term effects of alcohol on appetite in humans. Effects of context and restrained eating. Appetite. 2010;55:565–73.

Chapter 20
Physical Activity for Weight Management

Scott D. Isaacs

Pearls of Wisdom

- Habitual physical activity enhances the ability to achieve and maintain a lower body weight and has a demonstrated positive effect on promoting physical and mental health.
- Provide a physical activity prescription detailing the frequency, duration, intensity, and specific types of physical activity. The prescription should take into account the patient's mobility, cardiovascular conditioning, presence of diabetes, and/or other medical conditions.
- Adults should perform ≥150 min of moderate-intensity or ≥ 75 min of vigorous-intensity (or an equivalent combination) aerobic physical activity weekly. Include resistance activities ≥2 times per week.
- Initiate a physical activity with lower intensity and duration, with gradual progression to moderate- and higher-intensity physical activity as physical fitness improves.
- Use behavior modification strategies to accumulate increased nonexercise physical activity into daily activities in the home and workplace.

20.1 Introduction

Physical activity supports weight loss by enhancing the ability to achieve a negative energy balance through increased energy expenditure. There is an inverse correlation between physical activity and body weight. Although decreasing energy intake is more effective for weight loss, physical activity remains a significant element of

S. D. Isaacs
Atlanta Endocrine Associates, Atlanta, GA, USA

J. M. Gonzalez-Campoy et al. (eds.), *Bariatric Endocrinology*,
https://doi.org/10.1007/978-3-319-95655-8_20

energy expenditure and is fundamental to energy balance and weight management. There are several potential mechanisms for physical activity to facilitate weight loss and maintenance in addition to increased caloric expenditure including increased metabolic rate, increased lean body mass, and psychological factors.

Physical inactivity is the fourth leading risk factor for mortality worldwide and is responsible for 6% of deaths globally. Rates of physical inactivity are increasing in many countries. Sitting at work and too much screen time are major causes of inactivity. Physical inactivity is estimated to be responsible for 30% of ischemic heart disease, 27% of diabetes, and 21–25% of breast and colon cancers.

"Physical activity" and "exercise" are terms that define different concepts, although they are often used interchangeably. Physical activity is defined as any bodily movement produced by skeletal muscles that requires energy expenditure. Exercise is a subset of physical activity and is defined as "bodily exertion for the sake of developing and maintaining physical fitness." Exercise is typically structured, planned, and repetitive and has an objective of improving or maintaining physical fitness. Physical activity includes planned exercise as well as willful leisure time activities, compulsory occupational and household tasks in the context of everyday family, and community activities. Physical activity can be integrated into daily activities of living and through active travel such as walking or bicycling.

The term "physical activity" is preferred over the term "exercise" because physical activity encompasses a broader range of activities that can be performed for weight loss, physical fitness, and improved health. Although some people have an aversion to exercising, every person performs some level of physical activity as part of their daily life. Habitual increases of nonexercise physical activity accumulate to increase total energy expenditure.

20.2 Benefits of Physical Activity

There is a large body of conclusive scientific evidence demonstrating the health benefits of physical activity. There is a dose-response relationship with regard to the amount, duration, frequency, and intensity of physical activity. Some of the health benefits of physical activity include:

- Improved cardiorespiratory fitness
- Improved muscular strength
- Weight loss and maintenance
- Improved insulin sensitivity
- Improved glycemic control
- Lower blood pressure
- Decreased LDL-cholesterol
- Decreased triglycerides
- Increased HDL-cholesterol
- Reduced pain

- Improved bone density
- Decreased colon cancer
- Decreased breast cancer
- Decreased endometrial cancer
- Improved osteoarthritis
- Improved bone health
- Improved depression and anxiety
- Improved cognition
- Decreased cardiovascular disease
- Decreased stroke
- Decreased mortality

There is a consistent effect of physical activity (especially aerobic physical activity) as an adjunct to medical nutrition therapy for weight loss and maintenance. Physical activity has important metabolic effects that are independent of weight loss. There is a direct relationship between levels of physical activity and metabolic health including insulin resistance, diabetes, and metabolic syndrome. Progress has been made to elucidate the effects of physical activity as a method of reducing obesity and improving glucose tolerance; however, the specific exercise volume necessary to achieve optimal benefit is of considerable uncertainty and debate.

Physical activity can lessen age-related decline in bone mineral density. Weight-bearing and resistance activities (3–5 days per week, 30–60 min per session) help promote increased bone density. Studies have demonstrated that adults who are physically active are less likely to have a hip or vertebral fracture. Consistent physical activity (≥30–60 min daily) has been shown to lower risk for breast and colon cancers. Physical activity enhances skeletal muscle mass, strength, and power.

Physical inactivity is a risk factor for cardiovascular disease. There is a close relationship between the volume of physical activity and cardiovascular health. Physical activity improves cardiopulmonary fitness and improves favorable biomarkers for preventing cardiovascular disease. There is a graded inverse relationship between total physical activity and mortality. Even small amounts of physical activity show considerable reductions in mortality and improved health outcomes compared to sedentary control subjects.

Physical activity improves psychological functioning. Patients who perform regular physical activity perform better on tests of cognitive functioning and report improvements in anxiety and depression symptoms. Physical activity improves confidence and self-esteem and reduces response to stress. In a literature review of physical activity and improvement of depression, a dose-response relationship was established.

Prolonged sitting is associated with higher mortality and increased rates of cancer, cardiovascular disease, and type 2 diabetes, even among people who get regular physical activity. However, the deleterious effects associated with prolonged periods of inactivity are diminished in those who participate in higher levels of physical activity.

20.3 Skeletal Muscle as an Endocrine Organ

Along the same line as the functioning of adipose tissue as an endocrine organ, the skeletal muscle is also known to secrete a number of cytokines and other peptide hormones known as myokines. Myokines communicate locally within the myocyte in an autocrine or paracrine manner or in distant tissues in an endocrine manner. Myokines are important for communication between the muscle and adipose tissue, liver, and pancreatic cells. Myokines can have both beneficial and adverse effects functioning as mediators of inflammation or as mediators of exercise. Physical activity has a beneficial effect on the balance of myokines. Physical inactivity promotes an imbalance of myokines favoring a proinflammatory state leading to sarcopenia, accumulation of visceral fat, and development of many of the diseases associated with inactivity. It is thought that much of the protective effect of physical activity on chronic disease is attributed to the anti-inflammatory effect of myokines.

Myokines:

- Angiopoietin-like 4
- Brain-derived neurotrophic factor
- Fibroblast growth factor 21
- Follistatin-like 1
- Interleukin-6
- Interleukin-7
- Interleukin-15
- Irisin
- Leukemia inhibitory factor
- Myonectin
- Myostatin
- Vascular endothelial growth factor

20.4 General Guidelines for Physical Activity

Physical activity should be individualized to meet each patient's abilities, preferences, and progression. Physical activity includes planned exercise as well as transportation, occupational, household, sports, and recreational activities in the context of daily activities. Physical activity should include aerobic activities such as walking, walk-jog intervals, bicycle (routine or stationary), swimming, and other leisure sports or recreational activities. Aerobic activity can be individual endpoints for determining the intensity of physical activity such as fatigue, breathlessness, or heart rate.

Most government and academic organizations recommend that adults should accumulate a minimum of 150 min of moderate-intensity or preferably 75 min or more of vigorous-intensity (or an equivalent combination) aerobic physical activity weekly. As the intensity of a physical activity decreases, the duration should increase. Moderate-intensity physical activity of 300 min per week or 150 min of vigorous physical activity per week will provide additional health and weight loss benefits. Muscle strengthening activities with major muscle groups should be performed on 2 or more days per week.

The concept of accumulation refers to performing physical activity in multiple small bouts (≥10 min) throughout the day. A goal of 60 min of physical activity accumulated daily can be accomplished by adding together all the time during each bout (e.g., 3 bouts of 20 min or 2 bouts of 30 min). The benefits of physical activity are incremental; therefore, even if a patient is unable to achieve recommended levels of physical activity, there is still a benefit. Inactive adults will have a health benefit from any amount of physical activity. Plan to increase duration, frequency, and finally intensity as a goal for achieving the recommended levels.

The benefits of implementing a physical activity program outweigh the risks. At the recommended level of physical activity, musculoskeletal injury rates are low. To decrease the risk of musculoskeletal injuries, encourage a light start with gradual progression to more moderate and higher levels of physical activity. Pregnant or postpartum women should seek specific advice from their practitioner regarding specifics about physical activity; however, light- to moderate-intensity physical activity is generally recommended.

Physical activity is important irrespective of gender, race, ethnicity, or income level. Practitioners should use communication strategies and messaging tailored for various populations. Patients with disabilities should perform physical activity to the limits of their capacity adjusted for specific health risks or limitations. Physical activity should always be prescribed in conjunction with a reduced-calorie meal plan. Most individuals can easily consume quantities of food that are much greater than the increased energy expenditure from physical activity. Physical activity without a reduced-calorie meal plan is rarely effective for weight loss.

Physical activity recommendations for adults:

- Adults should do ≥150 min of moderate-intensity aerobic physical activity weekly or ≥ 150 min of vigorous physical activity weekly or an equivalent combination.
- Aerobic physical activity should be performed in bouts of ≥10 min.
- For additional health benefits, increase moderate-intensity to ≥300 min weekly or ≥ 150 min of vigorous-intensity physical activity weekly or an equivalent combination.
- Muscle-strengthening activities involving the major muscle groups should be done ≥2 days per week.

20.5 Physical Activity for Children and Youth

There is strong evidence that physical activity provides important health benefits in children and young people. Normal-weight children with high levels of physical activity have decreased adiposity compared to children with low levels of physical activity. In observational studies, higher levels of physical activity are associated with positive health indicators. Interventions to increase physical activity in overweight and obese children have been shown to have beneficial effects on weight and health. In experimental studies, physical activity improved cardiopulmonary fitness, muscle strength, bone health, and reduced symptoms of anxiety and depression.

Children and young people aged 5–17 years old should accumulate at least 60 min of moderate- to vigorous-intensity physical activity daily. Vigorous-intensity physical activity should be performed at least three times per week. Important health benefits have been documented in children and youth who perform at least 60 min of daily physical activity. Increasing physical activity beyond 60 min daily will provide additional health benefits. Doing less than the recommended amount of physical activity will still provide health benefits compared to doing nothing at all. The duration of physical activity should include all physical activity accumulated throughout the day, above and beyond normal daily activities. Children and young adults who are inactive should start slowly with a progressive increase in duration, intensity, and frequency until the recommended levels are achieved. Children and young adults should have ≤30 min of screen activities daily. Reduce nonactive time spent surfing the Internet, playing computer games, and watching television and videos to less than two hours per day and replace with more active behaviors.

Most physical activity for children and young people should be aerobic such as playing on playground equipment, running, jumping, playing games, and climbing trees. Pushing or pulling activities improve muscle strength and bone health in addition to aerobic benefits. Physical activity can also include sports, recreation, transportation, and physical education or planned physical activity in the context of school, community, and family activities. Youth should be encouraged to participate in a variety of activities to support healthy development and should be safe and enjoyable.

Physical activity recommendations for youth are universal; however, messaging and specific activities should be tailored to accommodate various population subgroups. Children younger than 5 years old benefit from increased physical activity; however, more research is needed to determine the amount of physical activity necessary for the greatest health benefits. Maintaining a high level of physical activity starting in childhood and continuing throughout adulthood improves long-term weight management as well as lower morbidity and mortality from cardiovascular disease and diabetes later in life.

Physical activity recommendations for children and young adults:

- Accumulate ≥60 min moderate- to vigorous-intensity physical activity daily.
- Physical activity >60 min daily provides additional health benefits.
- Vigorous physical activity ≥3 times per week.
- Most daily physical activities should be aerobic.
- Include activities to strengthen muscle and bone ≥3 times per week.

20.6 Physical Activity and Long-Term Weight Maintenance

Long-term weight maintenance is affected by compliance with a physical activity program. Randomized controlled trials demonstrate that ≥150 min of physical activity performed weekly is associated with 1–3% weight loss, which is considered to represent weight maintenance.

In a changing modern society, patients must learn to maintain physical activity in a variety of challenging situations such as inclement weather, shifting work schedules, and travel for work or pleasure. Suggest a travel plan for physical activity to include the use of hotel gyms, local walks, and active vacations (city walking tours, national parks, etc.). When standard facilities for physical activity are unavailable, patients may need to improvise. In inclement weather, walking at a shopping mall or in a gym can be suggested.

Patients with mild upper respiratory infections may continue light to moderate physical activity. Patients with influenza or influenza-like syndromes with fever should decrease or stop physical activity until they have recovered. An active lifestyle should be promoted from childhood throughout the adult years. For many people, walking is the best physical activity habit to adopt. A simple walking program for most individuals has clear weight maintenance and other health benefits. Vary the types of activities and pick ones that are enjoyable.

Use behavior modification strategies to encourage habitual physical activity. Patients must learn to implement new activity habits to replace sedentary behaviors. Behavior modification strategies for physical activity should be used in conjunction with medical nutrition therapy. Behavioral modification strategies for physical activity include self-monitoring, making specific physical activity goals such as brisk walking for 30 min 5 days a week, increasing physical activity in daily living such as taking the stairs or parking at the far end of the parking lot, developing skills to cope, and enlisting social support.

20.7 The Physical Activity Prescription

The physical activity prescription designates specific fitness-related activities for the purpose of weight loss and improved health. Each patient will have particular and unique needs for physical activity. The physical activity prescription should include behavioral modification to help motivate the patient and aid in long-term adherence. The dosage or volume of physical activity expressed in minutes or in kcal expenditure per week must be individualized for each physical activity prescription.

The physical activity prescription should include the following:

- Type of physical activity (running, walking, swimming, etc.)
- Frequency and duration of the physical activity (30–60 min, 5–6 times weekly)

- Intensity (light, moderate, vigorous)
- Special precautions regarding orthopedic, diabetes, cardiovascular, or other medical concerns

20.8 Types of Physical Activity

- Aerobic (brisk walking, bicycling, swimming, rowing, running, jumping rope)
- Anaerobic (lifting weights, sprinting, jumping)
- Strength/isotonic (lifting weights, bands, calisthenics)
- Flexibility (stretching)
- Balance (yoga)

The type of physical activity can be aerobic, anaerobic, strength, flexibility, and/or balance. The choice of physical activity can include traditional exercise activities as well as recreational, domestic, and occupational physical activity. Choosing the appropriate type of physical activity for patients is vital. Avoid high-impact physical activity that is difficult to maintain and has a higher risk for injuries. Patients should perform more than one type of physical activity and change up routines to keep it interesting.

Aerobic physical activity done for prolonged period of time is called endurance activity because it improves cardiopulmonary fitness. Even a single bout of endurance activity increases muscle insulin sensitivity; however, the effect is short-lived unless there are concomitant changes in body composition.

Anaerobic physical activity includes resistance activities with intense exertion such as lifting weights or bands, calisthenics, sprinting, or jumping. Anaerobic physical activity compliments aerobic physical activity and enhances fitness, lean body mass, strength, speed, and power. Resistance activities using free weights, equipment, or bands should be performed two to three times per week. Instruct patients to perform 8–10 sets consisting of 10–15 repetitions at moderate intensity to include legs, hips, back, trunk, chest, shoulders, and arms. The appropriate resistance can be provided with light hand weights, machines, elastic bands, or calisthenics. Perceived effort should be moderate to somewhat difficult. Lift and lower weights slowly to increase muscle strength and minimize injuries. As progress is made, instruct patients to slowly increase resistance (i.e., add 1–5 pounds) for continued improvements. Significant strength improvements generally take at least 6 weeks.

20.9 Duration

The duration of physical activity is generally prescribed in minutes. The duration of the physical activity should be 10–60 min per session. Physical activity may be accumulated with multiple small bouts performed at various times of the day or as one longer bout. The duration of physical activity should be above and beyond normal daily nonrecreational activities. Instruct patient to start with smaller amounts of physical activity and increase the duration as they improve fitness.

20.10 Frequency

The frequency is the number of times an activity is performed. Frequency is usually prescribed as episodes, sessions, or bouts each week. For best results, encourage habitual physical activity. Physical activity should be performed for at least 30–60 min on most days of the week (4–6 times each week).

20.11 Intensity

The intensity of physical activity represents how hard a person works to do the activity. Intensity may refer to a rate (i.e., walking or jogging speed) or magnitude of the effort necessary to perform physical activity. Moderate- to vigorous-intensity physical activity is recommended for weight management. Select activities that may be sustained for several minutes to an hour.

There is uncertainty as to whether the benefits of high-intensity physical activity are due to the greater amount of energy expenditure per unit of time or to other factors related to the actual intensity per se. In the Harvard Alumni Health Study, it was found that vigorous activities but not nonvigorous activities were associated with decreased all-cause mortality, although nonvigorous physical activity was shown to benefit other aspects of health. In a randomized controlled trial that evaluated the independent effects of exercise intensity on abdominal fat mass and insulin sensitivity, subjects in exercise groups achieved a 5–6% decrease in body weight and a 4- to 5-cm decrease in waist circumference in both low- and high-intensity exercise groups compared to control subjects. Equivalent amounts of exercise independent of intensity resulted in similar reductions in abdominal obesity. Improvement in 2-h glucose level was only seen in the high-intensity exercise group.

Physical activity is measured in metabolic equivalents (METs). One MET is the oxygen consumption at rest, which is assumed to be 3.5 ml of oxygen per kilogram per minute. Light-intensity physical activity is 0–3 METs, moderate-intensity physical activity is 3–6 METs, and vigorous-intensity physical activity is greater than 6 METs.

Light-intensity physical activity (0–3 METs):

- Walking less than 3 mph
- Water exercises
- Light gardening
- Cooking
- Light domestic or occupational activities

Moderate-intensity physical activity (3–6 METs):

- Walking 3–5 mph
- Hiking
- Skating (leisurely pace)
- Biking 5–9 mph level terrain
- Stationary bike, moderate effort
- Swimming, light-to-moderate effort
- Water aerobics
- Light calisthenics
- Yoga
- Gymnastics
- Stair climber machine
- Rowing machine
- Dancing (ballroom, ballet, line, etc.)
- Downhill skiing
- Playing on school playground equipment
- Gardening and yard work (raking, bagging leaves, digging, hoeing, light shoveling, or weeding)
- Moderate housework (scrubbing, hanging laundry, sweeping, washing windows, cleaning out the garage, moving light furniture, packing or unpacking boxes, walking and putting household items away, carrying out heavy bags of trash, or carrying water or firewood)
- Home repair
- Actively playing with children
- Moderate occupational activities

Vigorous-intensity physical activity (>6 METs):

- Speed walking
- Jogging or running
- Walking or hiking up a hill
- Bicycling more than 10 mph
- Roller skating at a brisk pace
- Skiing (active downhill, cross country)
- Jumping rope
- Martial arts (karate, judo, tae kwon do, jujitsu)
- Aerobic dancing
- Water jogging
- Swimming steady-paced laps
- Circuit weight training
- Vigorously playing with children
- Most competitive sports
- Home repair or construction with very hard physical labor
- Shoveling heavy snow
- Occupations that require extensive periods of running, rapid movement, lifting, and pushing or pulling objects

20.12 Volume

The volume of physical activity is characterized by the product of the duration, frequency, and intensity as well as the total longevity of the program. A dose-response relationship exists between the volume of physical activity and health indicators, with greater doses of physical activity associated with greater improvements. The volume of physical activity necessary for risk reduction varies with each condition. To reduce abdominal obesity, the lowest dose of physical activity is 150 min weekly with added reduction for >300 min weekly.

20.13 Pre-exercise Screening for Cardiovascular Disease

Patients who are at risk for cardiovascular disease (family history, obesity, diabetes, hypertension, and/or dyslipidemia) or those with known cardiovascular disease should have cardiovascular screening before initiating a physical activity program. Patients with undiagnosed or unstable disease could experience cardiac ischemia or arrhythmias due to the increased myocardial oxygen demands.

Initial screening for cardiovascular disease should start with a careful history and physical examination. Most organizations do not recommend that physicians routinely offer exercise stress testing to patients without symptoms or strong risk factors for cardiovascular disease. Patients at low-to-moderate risk may have an electrocardiogram as an initial screening modality.

The exercise stress test is a useful modality for coronary disease screening in asymptomatic but high-risk patients who want to initiate a physical activity program. Exercise testing is an established procedure that has been in widespread clinical use for several decades. Exercise testing is widely available and at relatively low cost. A cardiovascular stress test uses a treadmill or bicycle with electrographic and blood pressure monitoring. Pharmacological agents and the use of imaging modalities may also be used for disabled patients or other situations in which exercise testing is not possible.

20.14 Physical Activity for Special Populations

20.14.1 Severe Obesity

Low-impact physical activity is necessary to reduce orthopedic stress and injuries in patients with severe obesity. Non-weight-bearing physical activity can be recommended, such as water aerobics, swimming, and chair or floor exercises. High-impact physical activity should be avoided. Vigorous-intensity low-impact physical activity can be achieved with a stationary bike or elliptical machine. Emphasize the frequency and duration of physical activity over intensity. As patients with severe obesity lose weight and become more mobile, increase intensity as tolerated.

20.14.2 Poor Mobility

Physical activity should be encouraged for every person regardless of disability status. Patients with poor mobility due to neurologic, orthopedic, or other conditions should still perform physical activity to the best of their ability. Physical activity must be done in an environment that is safe and may need to have special equipment to meet specific needs. Adults with poor mobility should perform physical activity at least 3 days per week to improve balance and prevent falls.

20.14.3 Advanced Age

Maintaining physical activity throughout a lifetime promotes health and longevity. For adults with advanced age, physical activity includes transportation, occupational (if still working), household, sports, and recreational activities in the context of daily activities as well as planned exercise. The goal of physical activity is weight loss or maintenance, as well as improved functional health, cardiorespiratory and muscular fitness, and reduced depression and cognitive decline.

When possible, older adults should follow the same guidelines as adults of age 18–64 which include ≥150 min of moderate-intensity physical activity or ≥75 min of vigorous-intensity physical activity weekly. Muscle strengthening should be done on major muscle groups twice weekly. Physical activity also helps maintain muscle strength, endurance, bone mineral density, and joint mobility, all of which typically decline as people age. Considerations should be made for orthopedic and mobility issues. When recommended levels cannot be performed due to health conditions, individuals should be as physically active as their abilities and conditions allow. Chair exercises are an effective form of physical activity for patients in nursing homes or in wheelchairs.

20.14.4 Diabetes

Physical activity should be initiated as short sessions with careful glucose monitoring. Progress duration and intensity gradually, as tolerated. Although most patients have improved blood glucose readings, hypoglycemia or hyperglycemia can occur as a consequence of physical activity. Patients who take insulin secretagogues or insulin may require a reduction in dose. Patients should be instructed to consume a meal 1–3 h before physical activity and to take insulin >1 h before physical activity. Snacks and/or dose adjustments may be necessary for patients who take insulin or insulin secretagogues (glipizide, glyburide, glimepiride, nateglinide, or repaglinide) to accommodate for increased insulin sensitivity that occurs with physical activity. Some patients may need to consume small amounts of carbohydrates every 30 min during longer bouts of physical activity.

20.14.5 *Cardiovascular Disease*

Physical activity improves cardiovascular disease. Patients with occult or unstable coronary ischemia or arrhythmias may experience worsening of their condition with physical activity. Pre-exercise stress testing and medical supervision are necessary for patients with cardiovascular disease beginning a physical activity program. For patients post myocardial infarction, walking is the recommended initial type of physical activity. Patients with a history of a cardiac event need to take extra precautions and seek medical guidance before initiating a physical activity program and before striving to achieve increased levels of physical activity.

20.15 Conclusion

Physical inactivity is a leading risk factor for mortality worldwide. There are many scientific studies demonstrating the physical and mental health benefits of physical activity. Physical activity is beneficial for weight loss because it enhances the ability to achieve a negative energy balance by increasing energy expenditure. Physical activity also facilitates weight loss and maintenance through increased metabolic rate, increased lean body mass, and psychological factors. Habitual accumulated energy expenditure through physical activity allows long-term energy balance for achieving and maintaining weight loss. Even among people who participate in regular physical activity, prolonged sitting is associated with higher mortality and increased rates of cancer, cardiovascular disease, and type 2 diabetes. Physical activity promotes the production and favorable balance of anti-inflammatory myokines contributing to many of its metabolic benefits.

The physical activity prescription should be customized with consideration for any underlying health factors. The prescription should include details about the type, frequency, duration, and intensity of the physical activity. Adults should accumulate ≥150 min of moderate-intensity or preferably ≥75 min of vigorous-intensity (or an equivalent combination) aerobic physical activity weekly. Moderate-intensity physical activity of ≥300 min per week or >150 min of vigorous physical activity per week is preferred due to additional health benefits. Include resistance activities ≥2 times per week.

Children and young adults should have ≥60 min of physical activity daily. The majority of the physical activity for children and young people should be aerobic. Accumulate increased nonexercise physical activity into daily activities in the home and workplace.

Initiate a physical activity with lower intensity and duration with gradual progression to moderate- and higher-intensity physical activity as physical fitness improves. Patients with cardiovascular risk factors or those with known cardiovascular disease should have cardiovascular screening before initiating a physical activity program. For most patients with obesity, low-impact physical activity is preferred to reduce orthopedic stress and injuries. When physical activity is limited due to health conditions, adults should be as physically active as their condition and abilities allow. Patients must learn to implement new activity habits to replace sedentary behaviors. Use behavioral modification strategies such as self-monitoring, making specific goals, increasing physical activity in daily living, developing skills to cope, and enlisting social support.

Reading List

Adamson BC, et al. Effect of exercise on depressive symptoms in adults with neurologic disorders: a systematic review and meta-analysis. Arch Phys Med Rehabil. 2015;96:1329.

American College of Sports Medicine. ACSM's guidelines for exercise testing and prescription. 7th ed. Philadelphia, physical activity: Lippincott Williams & Wilkins; 2006.

Aviroop B, Oh PI, Faulkner GE, Bajaj RR, Silver MA, Mitchell MS, et al. Sedentary time and its association with risk for disease incidence, mortality, and hospitalization in adults: a systematic review and meta-analysis. Ann Intern Med. 2015;162:123–32, 146–147.

Balady GJ, Williams MA, Ades PA, et al. Core components of cardiac rehabilitation/secondary prevention programs: 2007 update: a scientific statement from the American Heart Association exercise, cardiac rehabilitation, and prevention committee, the council on clinical cardiology; the councils on cardiovascular nursing, epidemiology and prevention, and nutrition, physical activity, and metabolism; and the American Association of Cardiovascular and Pulmonary Rehabilitation. Circulation. 2007;115(20):2675–82.

Ballor DL, Keese RE. A meta-analysis of the factors affecting exercise-induced changes in body mass, fat mass and fat-free mass in males and females. Int J Obes. 1991;15(11):717–26.

Blair SN, et al. Changes in physical fitness and all-cause mortality. A prospective study of healthy and unhealthy men. JAMA. 1995;273(14):1093–8.

Brownell KD, Wadden TA. Etiology and treatment of obesity: understanding a serious, prevalent, and refractory disorder. J Consult Clin Psychol. 1992;60(4):505–17.

Caspersen CJ, et al. Physical activity, exercise, and physical fitness: definitions and distinctions for health-related research. Public Health Rep. 1985;100(2):126–31.

Clinical guidelines on the identification, evaluation, and treatment of overweight and obesity in adults—the evidence report. National Institutes of Health. Obes Res. 1998;6(Suppl 2):51S–209S.

Fletcher GF, Balady G, Blair SN, et al. Statement on exercise: benefits and recommendations for physical activity programs for all Americans. A statement for health professionals by the Committee on Exercise and Cardiac Rehabilitation of the Council on Clinical Cardiology, American Heart Association. Circulation. 1996;94(4):857–62.

Gibbons RJ, et al. ACC/AHA 2002 guideline update for exercise testing: summary article: a report of the American College of Cardiology/American Heart Association task force on practice guidelines (committee to update the 1997 exercise testing guidelines). Circulation. 2002;106(14):1883–92.

Haskell WL, et al. Physical activity and public health: updated recommendation for adults from the American College of Sports Medicine and the American Heart Association. Med Sci Sports Exerc. 2007;39(8):1423–34.

Hochberg MC, et al. American College of Rheumatology 2012 recommendations for the use of nonpharmacologic and pharmacologic therapies in osteoarthritis of the hand, hip, and knee. Arthritis Care Res (Hoboken). 2012;64(4):465–74.

Janssen I, Leblanc AG. Systematic review of the health benefits of physical activity and fitness in school-aged children and youth. Int J Behav Nutr Phys Act. 2010;7:40.

Janssen I. Physical activity guidelines for children and youth. Can J Public Health. 2007;98(Suppl 2):S109–21.

Jeon CY, et al. Physical activity of moderate intensity and risk of type 2 diabetes: a systematic review. Diabetes Care. 2007;30(3):744–52.
Laukkenen JA, et al. The predictive value of cardiorespiratory fitness combined with coronary risk evaluation and the risk of cardiovascular and all-cause death. J Intern Med. 2007;262(2): 263–72.
Lee IM, et al. Exercise intensity and longevity in men. The Harvard Alumni Health Study. JAMA. 1995;273(15):1179–84.
Lee IM, et al. Physical activity and all-cause mortality: what is the dose-response relation? Med Sci Sports Exerc. 2001;33(6 Suppl):S459–71. discussion S493–4.
Lee IM, et al. Physical activity and stroke incidence: the Harvard alumni health study. Stroke. 1998;29(10):2049–54.
Mayer J, et al. Relation between caloric intake, body weight, and physical work: studies in an industrial male population in West Bengal. Am J Clin Nutr. 1956;4(2):169–75.
Pate RR, et al. Physical activity and public health. A recommendation from the Centers for Disease Control and Prevention and the American College of Sports Medicine. JAMA. 1995;273(5):402–7.
Physical Activity Guidelines Advisory Committee (PAGAC). Physical Activity Guidelines Advisory Committee Report, 2008. Washington, DC, US department of Health and Human Services, 2008. Nutr Rev. 2009 Feb;67(2):114–20.
Poehlman ET, et al. Aerobic fitness and resting energy expenditure in young adult males. Metabolism. 1989;38(1):85–90.
Pratesi A, et al. Skeletal muscle: an endocrine organ. Clin Cases Mineral Bone Metabolism. 2013;10(1):11–4.
Raschke S, Eckel J. Adipo-Myokines: two sides of the same coin: mediators of inflammation and mediators of exercise. Mediat Inflamm. 2013;2013:1.
Ross R, et al. Effects of exercise amount and intensity on abdominal obesity and glucose tolerance in obese adults: a randomized trial. Ann Intern Med. 2015;162(5):325–34.
Schmid D, et al. A systematic review and meta-analysis of physical activity and endometrial cancer risk. Eur J Epidemiol. 2015;30:397.
Stevenson JD, Roach R. The benefits and barriers to physical activity and lifestyle interventions for osteoarthritis affecting the adult knee. J Orthop Surg Res. 2012;7:15.
Talbot LA, Morrell CH, Fleg JL, Metter EJ. Changes in leisure time physical activity and risk of all-cause mortality in men and women: the Baltimore longitudinal study of aging. Prev Med. 2007;45(2–3):169–76.
The President's Council on Physical Fitness and Sports. Physical activity and health. A report of the Surgeon General, US Department of Health and Human Services, Center for Disease Control and Prevention, National Center for Chronic Disease Prevention and Health Promotion. Ctr Dis Control Prev. Available at http://www.cdc.gov/nccdphp/sgr/sgr.htm.
Thune I, Furberg AS. Physical activity and cancer risk: dose-response and cancer, all sites and site-specific. Med Sci Sports Exerc. 2001;33(6 Suppl):S530–50; discussion S609–10.
Warburton D, et al. Evidence-informed physical activity guidelines for Canadian adults. Appl Physiol Nutr Metab. 2007;32:S16–68.
Wei M, et al. The association between cardiorespiratory fitness and impaired fasting glucose and type 2 diabetes mellitus in men. Ann Intern Med. 1999;130(2):89–96.
World Health Organization. Global recommendations on physical activity for health. 2010. ISBN: 9789241599979.
Zdziarski LA, et al. Chronic pain management in the obese patient: a focused review of key challenges and potential exercise solutions. J Pain Res. 2015;8:63–77.

Chapter 21
Pharmacotherapy for Weight Management

Elise M. Brett

Pearls of Wisdom

- Pharmacological management of patients with overweight, obesity, and adiposopathy starts with the avoidance of medications for comorbid conditions that promote weight gain or prevent effective weight loss.
- Offer patients pharmacotherapy as an adjunct in a weight loss program. Lifestyle changes are the key to long-term success.
- Reevaluate initial treatment strategies by 12 weeks. A lack of response by that time should prompt a search for barriers to weight loss and consideration of escalation in pharmacotherapy.
- Set realistic weight loss goals. Explain to patients the benefits of moderate weight loss. Tell the patients to expect a plateau, and the need for ongoing pharmacotherapy.
- Help patients understand that overweight and obesity are a continuum and together represent a chronic disease which needs long-term treatment. Explain that medications help achieve weight loss, and continued use helps prevent weight regain.

E. M. Brett
Icahn School of Medicine at Mount Sinai, Division of Endocrinology, Diabetes, and Bone Disease, New York, NY, USA
e-mail: elise.brett@mountsinai.org

J. M. Gonzalez-Campoy et al. (eds.), *Bariatric Endocrinology*,
https://doi.org/10.1007/978-3-319-95655-8_21

21.1 Introduction

Approaches and attitudes toward the patient with obesity have positively and considerably changed over the past 50 years, concomitant with the dramatic rise in obesity prevalence rates nationally and on a global scale. Not surprisingly, the early literature on obesity pharmacotherapy contains some disturbing statements. One paper from 1977 referred to patients with obesity as "miscreants" whose "overindulgence. .. makes it difficult to control their diabetes and obesity." Another described the high dropout rate in a clinical trial as being due to "the mental attitude of many who *allow* themselves to become overweight." In 1998, the National Institutes of Health defined obesity as a chronic disease, and since then, major medical societies including The Obesity Society in 2008, The American Association of Clinical Endocrinologists in 2012, and finally the American Medical Association in 2014 produced similar statements. In addition to recognizing that obesity is not simply a lifestyle choice, and thereby attempting to reduce the stigma and discrimination, a pragmatic dividend of elevating obesity to disease status is to facilitate prevention and treatment. Obesity is a risk factor for numerous other diseases, and the presence and degree of obesity negatively impact the treatment of obesity-related comorbidities. As a chronic disease, there should be greater coverage for prevention and treatment by government and private insurance companies, more physician engagement in treatment protocols, more funding for research, and the FDA may be more likely to approve drugs to manage it.

21.2 Rationale for Pharmacotherapy of Obesity

Pharmacotherapy can be an important adjunct to improved nutrition and lifestyle modification in inducing weight loss in select patients. There are certain factors that need to be recognized before considering the use of pharmacotherapy. One is the understanding that not only is obesity a disease but it is a *chronic* disease. It is rare that weight normalization occurs and rare to achieve "cure." In this way, its management can be thought of as analogous to the management of T2DM. It is therefore important to set some goals at the start of treatment. In research studies, successful outcomes have been defined in terms of absolute weight loss, percent loss of body weight, and improvement in associated conditions. The goal of treatment with medication is to reduce excess fat mass and restore normal adipocyte function. Adipose tissue is metabolically active. In many patients, adiposopathy develops as a complication of adiposity. Adiposopathy contributes to insulin resistance, increased free fatty acid release, other pathogenic endocrine and immune responses, and increased cardiovascular risk. A weight loss of ≥5% has been associated with improvements in glycemic control in patients with T2DM and reductions in the need for antidiabetic medications. In a large study involving subjects with prediabetes, weight loss of 5% decreased the risk of T2DM by 58%. Modest weight losses of 5–10% have also been shown to decrease triglycerides and increase HDL. In people with overweight/obesity and cardiovascular risk factors, even more moderate sustained weight losses of only 3–5% can produce clinically meaningful health benefits.

It is important to recognize that not all patients will respond to all antiobesity medications. Typically, if a response is going to be achieved, it will be detected in the first 3 months of therapy. According to product labels, all drug therapies should be initiated with a plan to discontinue the drug if a patient proves to be a nonresponder (i.e., typically if 5% of body weight is not lost in 3–6 months). It is not always clear why a patient does not respond to a particular agent, but if one agent is not effective, another with a different mechanism of action can be tried. At the present time, outside of fixed dose combination tablets, there is currently little published clinical data to support the use of combination therapies for weight loss, but this remains the standard of care in bariatric medicine practices and an exciting area for future investigation.

21.3 Historical Development of Pharmacotherapy for Obesity

The earliest widespread use of pharmacotherapy for weight loss involved the use of amphetamines in the late 1930s. While effective as weight loss agents, these drugs also caused euphoria and had serious addiction potential. Subsequently, amphetamine-like drugs were developed, which had similar weight loss effects without the potential for mood enhancing or abuse. These noradrenergic-releasing agents such as phentermine, benzphetamine, diethylpropion, and phendimetrazine were approved during 1959–1960 and are still available today. These drugs were not studied in long-term clinical trials, and are approved for short-term use, generally considered to be for up to 12 weeks. With the exception of phendimetrazine, these drugs have been studied in a limited number of trials of variable length and have demonstrated placebo-subtracted weight loss on the order of 3.0–3.6 kg. Similar to amphetamines, they can result in tachycardia, palpitations, agitation, dry mouth, difficulty sleeping, anxiety, and headache (Table 21.1).

Table 21.1 Weight loss agents approved for short-term use

Drug	Trade names	Schedule	Dose
Phentermine	Adipex-P® Ionamin®	IV	15 mg QD 30 mg QD 37.5 mg QD
Diethylpropion	Tenuate® Tepanil®	IV	25 mg TID 75 mg SR QD
Phendimetrazine	Bontril® Prelu-2® X-trozine® Plegine®	III	17.5–70 TID 105 SR QD
Benzphetamine	Didrex®	IV	25–50 mg TID

Abbreviations: *mg* **milligram,** *QD* **daily,** *TID* **three times a day,** *SR* **sustained release**

Unfortunately, the history of obesity pharmacotherapy is marked by safety concerns leading to several drug withdrawals over the past decade. This has led both physicians and the public to be wary about the use of currently available agents. In 1997, dexfenfluramine and fenfluramine, both serotonin-releasing agents and reuptake inhibitors, were withdrawn due to reports of valvular heart disease and pulmonary hypertension associated with their use. Dexfenfluramine was the first obesity agent to be studied and show efficacy in a long-term (1 year) clinical trial. Fenfluramine was often prescribed in combination with phentermine, which proved to be highly effective for many patients. The use of this combination therapy became popular and was commonly known as "Fen-Phen." Fen-Phen was also studied long term and was the first demonstration of the greater benefits of a combination therapy for obesity. The same year that these drugs were withdrawn, the FDA approved sibutramine, a tertiary amine whose metabolites are potent inhibitors of noradrenaline and serotonin reuptake, which reduces food intake and enhances satiety. Then, in 2010, sibutramine was withdrawn from the market. In The Sibutramine Cardiovascular Outcomes (SCOUT) trial, although the data set as a whole showed nonsignificant increases in nonfatal myocardial infarction and stroke in patients with known cardiovascular disease, there was a 16% increased risk of cardiovascular events, including nonfatal heart attack and nonfatal stroke comparing sibutramine to placebo. The next promising class of drugs to be suddenly discontinued after approval was the selective cannabinoid 1 receptor antagonists. Blockage of orexigenic endocannabinoids in the brain resulted in successful weight loss. Rimonabant was approved in Europe in 2008 and withdrawn later that year due to risk of depression and suicide. Subsequently, it was not approved in the USA, and the development of similar compounds was halted.

21.4 Challenges of Clinical Trials for Obesity Medications

The evaluation of obesity agents in clinical trials poses unique challenges. Dropout rates in obesity trials tend to be higher than in the evaluations of other drugs. This enhanced dropout rate may be due to difficulty with adhering to the lifestyle modification component of the trial or possibly patient perception of lack of essentiality of treatment. Dropout rates increase with longer duration of a study. High dropout rates lead to reduced statistical power and potential bias. To report the data despite high dropout rates, most studies use a modified intention-to-treat (mITT)-last observation carried forward (LOCF) analysis. mITT-LOCF analysis includes all randomized patients who received a least one dose of study drug or placebo and had at least one post-randomization weight measurement. If a subject's weight is not available at completion of the trial due to drop out, then the weight from the most proximal prior visit is used, and it is assumed that the outcome has not changed. LOCF is a single imputation method to address missing data points but can introduce bias in favor of treatment if there is an early treatment effect followed by early dropout due to an adverse effect of the drug or may underestimate the efficacy of a drug that is particularly effective in a subset of patients.

Besides the difficulty in interpreting the data, there are additional challenges to evaluating obesity drugs in clinical trials. Weight loss, even when pharmacologically assisted, typically plateaus at around 6–9 months. In all studies, increasing the duration of treatment does not necessarily lead to greater weight loss, but the effect of the drug changes from that of inducing weight loss to assisting in weight maintenance following weight loss. This is due to metabolic adaptations to weight loss which result from a decrease in spontaneous physical activity; reduced physical activity level in free-living individuals after weight loss; decreases in energy expenditure, which persist long after the period of dynamic weight loss; and changes in leptin and gut hormones such as ghrelin, peptide YY, gastric inhibitory polypeptide, pancreatic polypeptide, amylin, and cholecystokinin that persist long after weight loss and affect appetite and encourage weight regain.

All of the currently available weight loss agents have been studied in people with and without T2DM, and it is important to note that weight loss in patients with T2DM is typically less than with patients without T2DM. This may be due to several factors. First, if diabetes was previously uncontrolled and glycemic control improves with weight loss, glucosuria resolves and calories are no longer lost in the urine. It has also been shown that reductions in energy expenditure occur as glycemic control improves. Second, some medications such as sulfonylureas, meglitinides, and insulin put the individual at risk for hypoglycemia. It is necessary to eat on a regular basis, and it may be necessary to consume extra calories at times to avoid or treat a hypoglycemic event. In these patients, it is critical to frequently reevaluate the diabetes regimen during the weight loss period. Another class of diabetes medication, the thiazolidinediones, does not cause hypoglycemia but contributes to weight gain by causing fluid retention and increasing peripheral adipose. Psychological factors and reduced ability to exercise due to factors such as neuropathy or other comorbidities may also play a role in people with diabetes.

21.5 Available Medications for the Treatment of Obesity

Table 21.2 lists medications approved in the United States for long-term treatment of obesity.

21.5.1 Orlistat

The oldest drug studied and approved for long-term treatment of obesity including weight maintenance is orlistat. This medication was approved in 1999. It is a gastric and pancreatic lipase inhibitor that causes weight loss by inducing fat malabsorption. Approximately 30% of ingested fat is lost in the stool when orlistat is present. It is indicated for obesity management including weight loss and weight maintenance in patients with BMI ≥30 kg/m^2 or ≥27 kg/m^2 with other risk factors. Orlistat is available in a prescription formulation, which is dosed 120 mg TID, and it is also available over the counter in 60-mg capsule-dosed TID, which is sold under a

Table 21.2 Medications approved for long-term treatment of obesity (available data)

Drug	Orlistat	Phentermine-topiramate ER	Lorcaserin	Naltrexone-bupropion	Liraglutide
Trade name	Xenical® Alli®	Qsymia®	Belviq®	Contrave®	Saxenda®
Maximum age In studies (years)	75	70	65	70	78
Maximum study duration	4 years	108 weeks	52 weeks	56 weeks	3 years
Studied with antidepressants?	Yes	Yes	No	No	Yes
Effect on heart rate	No change or decrease 2–4 bpm	+1.2 bpm	−2.9 bpm	Initial increase +3.4 bpm first 20 weeks then decline <2.5 bpm	Increase +2–3 bpm
Mean effect on blood pressure	−5.3 SBP −2.6 DBP	−2.9 SBP −1.5 DBP	−1.4 SBP −1.2 DBP	−3.9 SBP −2.8 DBP	−6.9 SBP −2.9 DBP
Studied in type 2 diabetes	Yes	Yes	Yes	Yes	Yes
Range of reported placebo-subtracted weight loss in completers	1.9–3.19 kg	7.5–11.1 kg	3.6–3.8 kg	3.7–6.1 kg	5.8–6.0 kg
Range of reported percent weight loss in completers	7.6%	10.7–14.4%	5.5–8.2%	5.9–11.5%	6.7–9.2%
Controlled substance?	No	Schedule IV	Schedule IV	No	No
Possible drug interaction with alcohol	No	Yes	Yes	Yes	No

Abbreviations: *ER* extended release, *bpm* beats per minute, *SBP* systolic blood pressure, *DBP* diastolic blood pressure, *kg* kilogram

different brand name, Alli®. The drug is contraindicated in pregnancy and in patients with malabsorption, cholestasis, or known hypersensitivity. Despite its non-absorption, possible interactions with levothyroxine, warfarin, cyclosporine, and certain antiepileptics have been reported. Therefore, these drugs require dosing separation, and dose adjustments may be required. Due to the effects of orlistat on fat absorption, the risk for hyperoxaluria and oxalate nephrolithiasis is increased. Moreover, since fat-soluble vitamins may be malabsorbed, multivitamin supplementation, at least 2 h before or after the orlistat dose, is recommended.

In a pooled analysis of orlistat involving three trials of 1111 patients taking 120 mg TID vs. placebo, the mean change in body weight after 1 year ranged 7.9–9.4 kg. In 4 trials of subjects with T2DM, weight loss after 2 years ranged 3.89–6.19 kg, and more patients were able to avoid weight regain in the maintenance phase than those on placebo. Orlistat is associated with small reductions in blood pressure, total cholesterol, and blood glucose.

In the longest study of any weight loss agent, orlistat was studied in the Xenical in the Prevention of Diabetes in Obese Subjects (XENDOS) Study in which patients with normal glucose tolerance (79%) or impaired glucose tolerance (IGT) (21%) were randomized to orlistat 120 mg TID or placebo; 3305 subjects were randomized, and 52% of the treatment group vs. 34% of the placebo group completed the study. Subjects were prescribed an 800-kcal per day deficit diet containing 30% fat and were encouraged to walk an extra kilometer per day. Mean weight loss was 3.0 kg with placebo vs. 5.8 kg with the drug. After 4 years, the incidence rate of T2DM in the IGT group was 18.8% for the treatment group vs. 28.8% for placebo, corresponding to a 45% risk reduction.

Orlistat was also studied in a smaller trial of 254 patients with uncontrolled T2DM (A1C >8%) on oral agents, injectables, or insulin. Subjects were randomized to orlistat 120 mg TID vs. placebo and told to follow a 30% fat, 600-kcal per day deficit diet; 234 subjects completed the study. Weight decreased 9.5 kg in the treatment group vs. 2.7 kg in the placebo group after 1 year. A1C decreased 1.4% in the treatment group vs. 0.3% with placebo. Subjects in the treatment group also showed improvements in HOMA-IR, FPG, PPG, and CRP.

21.5.2 Phentermine-Extended Release Topiramate (PHEN/TPM)

In 2012, the FDA approved the combination drug PHEN/TPM. Topiramate is a carbonic anhydrase inhibitor. The drug was initially approved for the treatment of epilepsy in 1996 and subsequently migraine headaches in 2004 and was noted to cause weight loss in patients with obesity. The mechanism of action of topiramate in inducing weight loss is not known, but the carbonic anhydrase enzyme is present in mitochondria and involved in gluconeogenesis and lipogenesis. There is evidence in rats that topiramate increases metabolic rate by an unclear mechanism possibly involving uncoupling proteins. However, only one small study so far has looked at the effects of topiramate on metabolic rate in humans and it did not show any difference from placebo. As a combination capsule, phentermine is released in the morning and topiramate in the evening. The most common adverse effects are paresthesias, dry mouth, constipation, dysgeusia, and insomnia. Some patients also experience reversible memory loss or disturbance in attention due to the topiramate component or irritability, anxiety, or headache related to the phentermine. Topiramate can cause orofacial clefts in babies of mothers treated during pregnancy, and FDA required a risk evaluation and mitigation strategics (REMS) program for the drug; women of reproductive potential must be counseled to undergo pregnancy testing before starting treatment and monthly thereafter. The medication should be discontinued immediately if a woman becomes pregnant while taking it. It should not be used while breastfeeding. The drug is contraindicated during therapy with MAOI, history of glaucoma, and in untreated hyperthyroidism. The drug has been associated with risk for kidney stones.

PHEN/TPM is initiated at a dose of 3.75/23 mg for 14 days and then increased to 7.5/46 mg. It is recommended in the product label to reevaluate the patient after 12 weeks of treatment. If the patient has not lost at least 3% of body weight, then one should discontinue the drug or escalate the dose. One has the option to increase to 11.25/69 mg for 14 days followed by 15/92 mg and reevaluate after 12 weeks. If the patient has not lost 5% or more of initial body weight at that time, then treatment should be discontinued. According to the manufacturer, once at the top dose, the medication should be discontinued slowly by taking a dose every other day for 1 week prior to stopping altogether to avoid precipitating a seizure.

PHEN/TPM has been studied in three large clinical trials. It has been evaluated for up to 56 weeks and has been shown to be effective across all levels of BMI included in the trials. The mid-dose combination of both medications is more effective than the highest dose of either medication alone. In EQUATE, a 28-week randomized trial, the 7.5/46 mg and 15/92 mg doses of PHEN/TPM were compared to each of the individual components alone as well as placebo. The trial involved 34 centers and 756 subjects were randomized with 541 completing (71.6%) the trial. Subjects were counseled to reduce caloric intake by 500 kcal per day and to keep food diaries and increase physical activity as tolerated. Absolute weight losses were 8.3 kg in the 7.5/46 mg group and 9.0 kg in the15/92 mg group vs. 1.5 kg in the placebo group, 5.3 kg with phentermine alone, 4.7 kg with topiramate ER 46 mg, 6.0 kg with phentermine 15 mg, and 6.4 kg with topiramate ER 92 mg.

In EQUIP, a 56-week randomized controlled trial of subjects with BMI ≥35 kg/m^2 and without metabolic syndrome, subjects were randomized to placebo vs. PHEN/TPM 3.75/23 mg or PHEN/TPM 15/92 mg. Subjects were advised to follow a 500-kcal per-day deficit meal plan, were provided counseling based on the Lifestyle, Exercise, Attitudes, Relationships and Nutrition (LEARN) program, and advised to increase physical activity. The dropout rate was higher in the placebo arm at 47.1% than the study drug, which was 39% for 3.75/23 mg and 33.6% for 15/92 mg. Based on an ITT-LOCF analysis, patients receiving 15/92 mg, 3.75/23 mg, and placebo lost 10.9%, 5.1%, and 1.6% of body weight, respectively. Completers taking the highest dose lost 14.4% of body weight on 15/92. The percentages of patients losing ≥5%, ≥10%, and ≥15% were 66.7, 47.2, and 32.2 for the 15/92-mg dose, respectively.

In CONQUER, a randomized double-blinded placebo-controlled trial across 93 centers in the USA, subjects with a BMI 27–45 kg/m^2 and 2 or more comorbidities, elevated triglycerides, hyperlipidemia, elevated blood glucose including prediabetes, or large waist circumference were randomized to drug 15/92 mg vs. 7.5/46 mg vs. placebo. They were given a LEARN manual and instructed to reduce caloric intake by 500 kcal per day; Overall, 38% discontinued the study drugs, including 43% who discontinued placebo. Of the subjects who completed 1 year of treatment, they lost 12.9, 9.9, and 1.8 kg with the 15/92-mg dose, 7.5/46-mg dose, or placebo, respectively; 5% weight loss was experienced by 70%, 62%, and 21%; and 10% weight loss by 48%, 37%, and 7% with the 15/92-mg dose, 7.5/46-mg dose, or placebo, respectively. There were significant improvements in BP, waist circumference, lipids, glucose, CRP, and adiponectin in the treatment groups compared to placebo. The study included 388 patients with T2DM (baseline A1C 6.8%) treated with metformin or nutritional intervention alone.

A subgroup of subjects with prediabetes and/or metabolic syndrome were enrolled in SEQUEL, a 52-week extension of the CONQUER trial. After 108 weeks, the incidence rate of T2DM was 6.1, 1.8, and 1.3 for placebo, 7.5/46 mg, and 15/92 mg respectively. There were 70.5% and 78.7% risk reductions in progression to T2DM for the 7.5/46 mg and 15/92 mg doses, respectively. Greater weight loss was associated with a greater reduction in the incidence of T2DM. Dropout rates were low, with 84% of all subjects completing the trial. Weight loss in the treatment groups was maximal at 40 weeks and was largely maintained during the extension phase.

The drug has also been shown to be effective in patients with T2DM with suboptimal control. In a subsequent study, 210 patients with a baseline A1C of 8.7% and a mean duration of disease of 9 years were randomized to placebo vs. PHEN/TPM 15/92 mg dose. The majority of subjects were taking one or more oral agents for T2DM, and patients taking injectables were excluded; 79% of subjects enrolled completed the trial. Mean weight loss was 9.4% with drug vs. 2.7% with placebo by ITT-LOCF analysis. Mean A1C reductions were 1.2% for placebo vs. 1.6% for the study drug. There was a reduced need for antidiabetic medications in the treatment group.

21.5.3 Lorcaserin

Lorcaserin was approved by the FDA for weight loss in 2012. Its mechanism of action is selective serotonin 2C ($5\text{-}HT_{2C}$) receptor agonist. As a $5\text{-}HT_{2C}$ receptor agonist in the hypothalamus, it activates the pro-opiomelanocortin (POMC) system of neurons, which results in increased satiety and decreased hunger. Fenfluramine and dexfenfluramine targeted the 5-HT receptor but were not selective. It is thought that the valvular heart disease seen in association with their use was a result of $5\text{-}HT_{2B}$ receptor activation. Valvulopathy has not been seen with agents that activate $5\text{-}HT_{2A}$ or $5\text{-}HT_{2C}$ receptors.

The medication is dosed as 10 mg BID or in an extended-release preparation as 20 mg QD. Adverse effects of lorcaserin include headache, nausea, constipation, dizziness, fatigue, xerostomia, and dry eyes. Hyperprolactinemia and leukopenia have been reported. The pivotal clinical trials of lorcaserin excluded patients taking SSRI drugs due to the potential risk of serotonin syndrome when used in combination. The product label indicates that if 5% weight loss is not achieved by week 12, then the drug should be discontinued. The drug is contraindicated in pregnancy and should not be used during breastfeeding. Caution is advised in patients with depression and those with a prior history of valvular heart disease. The drug should be avoided in patients with severe liver injury or renal insufficiency.

Lorcaserin was studied in the Blossom trial, a 52-week randomized, double-blind, placebo-controlled multicenter trial in subjects with a BMI 30–45 kg/m^2 or 27–29.9 kg/m^2 with HTN, dyslipidemia, CVD, IGT, or sleep apnea. Subjects were randomized to lorcaserin 10 mg BID vs. 10 mg QD vs placebo. In this trial, the behavioral modification program was fairly intense with nutrition and physical activity counseling at weeks 1, 2, and 4 and monthly thereafter. Subjects were instructed to reduce caloric intake to 600 kcal below estimated requirements, to be physically active 30 min per day, and keep food diaries; 4008 patients were randomized, and 2224 (55.5%) completed the trial; 47.2% of subjects taking 10 mg BID vs. 40.2% taking 10 mg QD, lost 5% or more body weight, compared with 25% on placebo, based on mITT-LOCF analysis. Weight loss was 7.7 kg vs. 6.5 kg vs. 3.9 kg, and percent change in weight was −7.9% vs. −6.5% vs. −4.0%, for lorcaserin 10 mg BID, 10 mg QD, or placebo. There were small improvements in HDL and triglycerides in the treatment groups.

In BLOOM, another large multicenter trial, 3182 patients with a BMI ranging 30–45 or 27–45 kg/m^2 with at least one comorbidity were randomized to lorcaserin 10 mg BID vs. placebo. The behavior modification protocol was similar to BLOSSOM. Rates of completion were 55.4% in the lorcaserin group and 45.1% in the placebo group. At the end of 1 year, 47.5% of subjects in the lorcaserin treatment group lost 5% or more body weight compared with 20.3% in the placebo group, and 22.6% lost 10% or more compared to 7.7% with placebo. Average weight loss was 8.1 kg in the lorcaserin group vs. 3.3 kg in the placebo group. Patients in the lorcaserin group lost 8.2% of baseline weight. Glucose, insulin, cholesterol, CRP, and blood pressure improved with lorcaserin treatment, compared to placebo. This trial had an extended maintenance period. Patients who stayed on lorcaserin in year 2 experienced some regain but were better able to maintain their weight loss than patients switched to placebo who mostly regained.

Lorcaserin has also been studied in patients with T2DM in the BLOOM-DM trial. BLOOM-DM was a 1-year randomized trial that included 604 patients taking metformin, a sulfonylurea, or both (baseline A1C 7–10%) and BMI 27–45 kg/m^2 were randomized to lorcaserin 10 mg QD vs. 10 mg BID vs. placebo. Patients had to be able to participate in a moderate-intensity physical activity program. After 52 weeks, 37.5%, 44.7%, and 16.1% lost 5% or more body weight, while 16.3%, 18.1%, and 4.4% lost 10% or more by mITT-LOCF analysis, for lorcaserin 10 mg QD, lorcaserin 10 mg BID, or placebo. Weight change from baseline was −5% vs. −4.5% vs. −1.5% and − 5.0 vs. −4.7 vs. −1.6 kg for lorcaserin 10 mg QD, lorcaserin 10 mg BID, or placebo. A1C decreased by 0.9% with lorcaserin 10 mg BID vs. 1.0% with lorcaserin QD and 0.4% with placebo. Fasting glucose decreased 27 mg/dl, 28 mg/dl, and 11.9 mg/dl in the groups, respectively. The proportion of patients who achieved an A1C of <7% at 52 weeks was over 50% in both lorcaserin groups compared with 26.3% in the placebo group.

21.5.4 Naltrexone/Bupropion

Naltrexone HCL 8 mg/bupropion HCL 90 mg (NB) was approved by the FDA to treat obesity in 2014. Bupropion is a dopamine and norepinephrine reuptake inhibitor, which was originally approved as an antidepressant and then as a smoking cessation agent. Naltrexone is an opioid receptor antagonist used in the management of alcohol and opioid dependence. POMC-producing neurons in the arcuate nucleus of the hypothalamus release alpha-melanocyte-stimulating hormone and beta-endorphin. Alpha-MSH mediates the anorectic effect of POMC activation, whereas beta-endorphin causes autoinhibitory feedback by activating opioid receptors on POMC neurons. It is thought that the weight loss-inducing effects of bupropion may be attenuated by this beta-endorphin feedback loop. The addition of naltrexone may prevent the negative feedback on POMC neurons and thus potentiate the effects of the bupropion to increase alpha-MSH release and facilitate weight reduction. Adverse effects of NB may include nausea, constipation, headache, vomiting, dizziness, insomnia, dry mouth, and diarrhea. Bupropion can have mild pressor effects. NB is contraindicated in patients with uncontrolled HTN, seizure disorders, chronic opioid use, concomitant use of MAOI, and narrow-angle glaucoma. It should not be used during pregnancy or breastfeeding. Dosing of NB is as follows: the medication is titrated from 1 tablet daily for the first week adding one tablet per week up to 2 tablets BID starting on week 4. Dose reductions are recommended in patients with renal and hepatic impairment. The medication should not be taken with a high fat meal, as this may result in a significant increase in systemic exposure. Because bupropion is an antidepressant medication, there are warnings about increased risk of worsening depression and suicidal ideation and behavior. If the patient has not at least lost 5% of body weight by 12 weeks, the medication should be discontinued, as it is not likely to be effective.

In a 56-week multicenter study (CORI) , subjects with a BMI 30–45 or 27–45 kg/m^2 with controlled HTN or dyslipidemia or both were randomized to treatment with NB 32 mg, NB 16 mg, or placebo. The study excluded people with T2DM. Subjects were instructed to follow a meal plan with a 500 kcal per day deficit and advised to increase physical activity. Mean change in weight was 6.1%, 5.0%, and −1.3% with NB 32 mg, NB 16 mg, or placebo, respectively; 48%, 39%, and 16% of subjects lost >5% of their entry body weight with NB 32 mg, NB 16 mg, or placebo, respectively. There were improvements in waist circumference, insulin resistance, HDL, and triglycerides with the study drug, compared to placebo.

In another 56-week multicenter randomized placebo-controlled trial, (COR-BMOD), subjects with BMI 30–45 kg/m^2 or 27–45 kg/m^2 with HTN and/or dyslipidemia but not diabetes were randomized to NB or placebo. This studied involved an intensive behavior modification program with group meetings led by a dietitian, behavioral psychologist, or exercise specialist;202 subjects were randomized to placebo and 591 randomized to NB; 41.6% in the placebo and 42.1% in the treatment arm discontinued the study drug. At week 56, the placebo group lost 5.1% of body weight and the drug group lost 9.3% based on mITT-LOCF. Weight loss in completers was 7.3% with placebo + BMOD and 11.5% with NB32 + BMOD. The proportion of subjects losing ≥5% of weight based on mITT-LOCF was 42.5 vs. 66.4 and ≥10% was 20.2 vs. 41.5% for placebo vs. NB, respectively. With NB treatment, waist circumference, fasting plasma triglycerides, and insulin decreased, while HDL increased at week 56, compared to baseline measurements.

The medication has also been studied in patients with T2DM. In a 56-week, multicenter trial, subjects with T2DM and a BMI ranging 27–45 kg/m^2 and an A1c ranging 7–10% were randomized to NB 32 mg vs. placebo. The study excluded subjects taking insulin. They were instructed to follow a 500-kcal per day deficit diet and instructed to increase physical activity; 44.5% in the treatment group vs. 18.9% in the placebo achieved >5% weight loss. The rate of dropout was high: 47.8% in the NB group discontinued therapy compared with 41.2% in placebo group. Weight loss by mITT analysis was −5.0 kg vs. −1.8 kg in the placebo group and completers lost −5.9 kg vs. −2.2 kg. There was greater reduction in A1C in the treatment group −0.6% vs. −0.1% as well as modest improvements in HDL-c, triglycerides, and waist circumference. There was no difference in depressive symptoms.

21.5.5 Liraglutide

Liraglutide was approved for the treatment of chronic weight management in 2014 for people with a BMI of ≥30 or ≥27 kg/m^2 with HTN, T2DM, or dyslipidemia. The same drug has been used since 2010 for the management of T2DM at a lower dose. The medication is an analog of human GLP-1, an incretin hormone released from L-cells in the small intestine and colon in response to food intake, which is a physiological regulator of appetite. Liraglutide causes reduced appetite, increased satiety, and lower energy intake. The dose is given as a subcutaneous injection once daily and is titrated from 0.6 mg daily at weekly intervals to 3.0 mg daily. The package insert states that liraglutide should be discontinued if a patient has not lost 4% of body weight after 12 weeks of the 3.0 mg daily dose, or 16 weeks of therapy altogether. The most common adverse effects include nausea and vomiting, which are usually transient and occur mainly during the first 4 weeks of dose escalation. Liraglutide has a REMS for thyroid C-cell tumors because they developed in rats and mice exposed to the medication. The label states that the human relevance has not been determined. The drug is contraindicated in patients with a personal or family history of medullary thyroid cancer and in patients with multiple endocrine neoplasia type 2. Liraglutide has been associated with acute pancreatitis, including hemorrhagic and fatal. There is REMS in place for pancreatitis, and the drug was not studied in patients with a prior history of pancreatitis. Patients should be counseled about these potential risks. The drug is contraindicated in pregnancy and should not be used during breastfeeding. Caution is needed with a prior history of gastroparesis and cholelithiasis. Dehydration can occur. Injection site reactions can occur.

Liraglutide was shown to be effective for weight maintenance in the SCALE Maintenance Trial, a 56-week randomized double-blind placebo-controlled multicenter trial of liraglutide after a low-calorie meal plan. Trial participants without T2DM and with a BMI ≥30 or BMI ≥27 kg/m^2 with comorbidities of HTN or dyslipidemia, who had successfully lost ≥5% of body weight during a 4–12-week run-in of 1200–1400 kcal/day meal plan, were then randomized to liraglutide 3.0 mg (n = 212) vs. placebo (n = 210). Mean weight loss was 6.0% during the run-in period; 75% of subjects on liraglutide and 69.5% of the placebo group completed the trial. At week 56, the liraglutide group lost an additional mean of 6.2% of randomization weight compared with 0.2% for placebo; 81.4% of subjects on liraglutide vs. 48.9% on placebo maintained the weight loss induced by the low-calorie meal plan.

In SCALE Obesity and Prediabetes, a 56-week randomized placebo-controlled trial involving 3731 adult patients with BMI >30 or ≥27 kg/m^2 with dyslipidemia or HTN, patients were assigned to liraglutide or placebo and counseled regarding lifestyle modification. The trial excluded patients with T2DM but 61.2% had prediabetes; 71.9% of the liraglutide group vs. 64.4% of the placebo group completed 56 weeks. After 56 weeks, the liraglutide group lost 8.0 ± 6.7% (8.4 ± 7.3 kg) vs. 2.6 ± 5.7% (2.8 ± 6.5 kg) with placebo; 63.2% in the liraglutide group lost over 5% of body weight vs 27.1% in the placebo group; 33.1% in the liraglutide group lost 10% vs. 10.6% in the placebo group. A1C, FPG, and indices of insulin resistance were all better in the treatment group after 56 weeks. The incidence of prediabetes was lower in the treatment group. SBP and DBP decreased in the liraglutide group. Fasting lipids, CRP, PAI1, and adiponectin were also better in the treatment group.

A total of 1128 subjects from the trial above went on to complete 3 years of follow-up. At the end of the trial, mean weight loss was 6.1% in the liraglutide 3.0-mg group vs. 1.9% with placebo. By 160 weeks, 1.8% of the treatment group progressed to type 2 diabetes compared with 6.2% in the placebo group. By contrast, 36% in the placebo group regressed to normoglycemia vs. 66% in the treatment group.

In another 56-week multicenter trial, patients with overweight and obesity, with type 2 diabetes, were randomized to liraglutide 3.0 mg vs. liraglutide 1.8 mg vs. placebo and advised on a reduced-calorie diet and exercise program. Mean weight losses of 6.0% (6.4 kg), 4.7% (5.0 kg), and 2.0% (2.2 kg) were reported in the multiple imputation analysis in the 3.0-mg, 1.8-mg, and placebo groups, respectively. Reductions in HbA1C were the greatest in the liraglutide 3.0-mg group at −1.3, followed by −1.1 for the 1.8-mg group and −0.3% for the placebo group.

21.5.6 Lisdexamfetamine for Binge Eating Disorder

Five percent to 30% of patients with obesity may have binge eating disorder. Binge eating disorder is a type of eating disorder characterized by eating within a 2-h period an amount of food that is definitely larger than most people would eat under similar circumstances associated with a sense of a lack of control over eating during the episode. The diagnosis is made in people who have at least one episode per week for at least 3 months. Recently, lisdexamfetamine, a CNS stimulant, was the first drug approved for the treatment of moderate-to-severe binge eating disorder. It has been shown in a meta-analysis to show tolerability and efficacy in reduction in binge eating frequency and obsessive thought and compulsions regarding binge eating. It is not approved for weight reduction, but weight reduction compared to placebo is typically in the range of 5–6%. Adverse effects include headaches, sleep disturbance, gastrointestinal upset, and decreased appetite. The recommended starting dose is 30 mg/day to be titrated in increments of 20 mg at approximately weekly intervals to achieve the recommended target dose of 50–70 mg/day. The drug is absolutely contraindicated in pregnancy.

21.5.7 Supplements Marketed for Weight Loss

There are numerous dietary supplements marketed for weight loss. Stimulants such as caffeine (found in herbal supplements cola nut, guarana, and mate), especially when combined with ephedra (ma huang), result in mild weight loss. However, the sale of ephedra was banned in 2004 due to reports of tachycardia, stroke, and sudden cardiac death. Most herbal supplements with purported efficacy on metabolic rate, appetite suppression, carbohydrate absorption, fat absorption, and laxative or diuretic effect have not been shown to have any benefit and may be associated with risk. One in particular that deserves mention is HCG, which is typically prescribed as an injection along with a 500-kcal per day meal plan. There is no proven efficacy for a direct effect of HCG itself, and the FDA has issued safety alerts on its use. The only supplement that may have mild benefit for safe weight loss is fiber, which may help increase satiety and slow digestion.

21.6 Adjustment of Pharmacotherapy for Other Associated Diseases

Before starting pharmacotherapy for overweight or obesity, the physician must consider whether the patient's current medical regimen first would benefit from adjustment. For example, beta-blockers may inhibit energy expenditure and weight loss by multiple mechanisms including a negative chronotropic cardiac effect, antagonism of epinephrine, the development of respiratory insufficiency, and triggering depression. If a beta-blocker is being used to treat HTN, it may be beneficial to switch to an alternative weight-neutral agent. If the use is for migraine prevention, then switching to a carbonic anhydrase inhibitor would likely facilitate weight loss. Carbonic anhydrase inhibitors are also used for the treatment of epilepsy and, if adequate, would be preferred to valproate and carbamazepine for seizure prevention, which typically cause weight gain.

Diabetes medications have quite varied effects on body weight. Thiazolidinediones and sulfonylureas are associated with weight gain up to 2.8 kg. However, the weight gain with TZD may be less concerning than with SU since it may be partly just due to fluid retention and the medication is associated with a shift from visceral to subcutaneous adipose along with an improvement in insulin sensitivity. Insulin typically causes weight gain. Pramlintide when added to insulin can help reduce appetite and insulin doses and limit this weight gain. GLP-1 receptor agonists as a class-effect reduce appetite by mechanisms discussed above and are associated with weight loss. SGLT-2 inhibitors result in glucosuria and therefore calorie loss via the kidneys and typically cause some weight loss. Metformin increases plasma GLP-1, stimulates fatty acid oxidation and may increase PYY, and has been associated with weight losses up to 2.5 kg. Alpha-glucosidase inhibitors slow carbohydrate absorption and especially with a high-carbohydrate "eastern" diet have been associated with weight loss. When reasonable, for glycemic control, in the absence of other contraindications, medications that are associated with weight loss should be used first.

Atypical antipsychotics are the other class of medications that are associated with increased adiposity and adiposopathy. The mechanism is not known. Clozapine and olanzapine are the highest risk (average weight gain is around 4 kg) followed by quetiapine. The lowest risk is seen with aripiprazole, lurasidone, and ziprasidone.

Antidepressant therapy may also need to be reconsidered. Amitriptyline, mirtazapine, and paroxetine are associated with weight gain, whereas fluoxetine and bupropion are associated with weight loss.

It is important to assess the patient's motivation for weight loss. The drug will only help facilitate weight loss in a motivated patient. All of the drugs have the potential to have adverse effects. The physician needs to discuss potential side effects with the patient and together decide which the patient may be willing to tolerate.

Meal planning may also play a role in the effectiveness of pharmacotherapy. For example, the patient who follows a very low fat meal plan will not likely benefit from orlistat. On the other hand, the patient who follows a very high fat meal plan will not likely tolerate the drug.

It is critical to consider the other drugs that the patient is already taking. Those requiring narcotics must avoid NB. A patient taking a GLP-1 receptor agonist or DPP-4 inhibitor for T2DM will need to discontinue these agents when liraglutide 3.0 mg is added. One must also consider cardiovascular risk and potential effects on heart rate and blood pressure with the different agents. A patient with or at high risk for cardiovascular disease may best avoid phentermine or other amphetamine-like drugs.

One can also consider potential additional benefits of the components of the agents, as many have other indications, although in their form as a weight loss agent they lack specific study and approval as such. For example, the patient who currently smokes may benefit from NB. A patient who suffers from depressed mood already treated with bupropion might make an easy transition to NB. Patients with migraines may obtain benefit from PHEN/TPM. In the patient with T2DM not currently taking a similar agent, liraglutide may be considered a preferred choice.

21.7 Conclusion

While obesity and its comorbidities plague our society, pharmacotherapy for weight loss is underutilized. The underutilization of pharmacotherapy for weight management is due to past safety concerns, low patient acceptance, payer issues, and lack of physician training in nutrition, behavioral modification therapy, and obesity management.

Endocrinologists are well positioned to take the lead in improving weight management in this country. Patients present to us for weight-related complications all the time. We are already managing the comorbidities and we can take advantage of this opportunity to focus specifically on the weight issues as well. This is an exciting time as we now have a variety of safe and effective treatment options to offer.

Reading List

Allison DB, Gadde KM, Garvey WT, Peterson CA, Schwiers ML, Najarian T, et al. Controlled-release phentermine/topiramate in severely obese adults: a randomized controlled trial (EQUIP). Obesity. 2011;20:330–42.

Aronne LJ, Wadden TA, Peterson C, Winslow D, Odeh S, Gadde KM. Evaluation of phentermine and topiramate versus phentermine/topiramate extended-release in obese adults. Obesity. 2013;21:2163–71.

Astrup A, Carraro R, Finer N, Harper A, Kunesova M, Lean MEJ, et al. Safety, tolerability and sustained weight loss over 2 years with the once-daily human GLP-1 analog, liraglutide. Int J Obes. 2012;36:843–54.

Bartels CL, Miller SJ. Dietary supplements marketed for weight loss. Nutr Clin Pract. 2003;18(2):156–69.

Davies MJ, Bergenstal R, Bode B, Kushner R, Lewin A, Skjoth TV, et al. Efficacy of liraglutide for weight loss among patients with type 2 diabetes. JAMA. 2015;314:687–99.

Derosa G, Cicero AF, D'Angelo A, Fogari E, Maffioli P. Effects of 1-year orlistat treatment compared to placebo on insulin resistance parameters in patients with type 2 diabetes. J Clin Pharm Ther. 2012;37(2):187–95.

Domecq JP, Prutsky G, Leppin A, Sonbol MB, Altayar O, Undavalli C, et al. Drugs commonly associated with weight change: a systematic review and meta-analysis. J Clin Endocrinol Metab. 2015;100(2):363–70.

Expert Panel on the Identification, Evaluation, and Treatment of Overweight and Obesity in Adults (US). Clinical guidelines on the identification, evaluation, and treatment of overweight and Obesity in adults. Bethesda: National Institutes of Health, National Heart, Lung, and Blood Institute; 1998.

Fidler MC, Sanchez M, Raether B, Weissman NJ, Smith SR, Shanahan WR. Anderson CM for the BLOSSOM clinical trial group: a one-year randomized trial of lorcaserin for weight loss in obese and overweight adults: the BLOSSOM trial. J Clin Endocrinol Metab. 2011;96:3067–77.

Gadde KM, Allison DB, Ryan DH, Peterson CA, Troupin B, Schwiers ML, et al. Effects of low-dose, controlled-release, phentermine plus topiramate combination on weight and associated comorbidities in overweight and obese adults (CONQUER): a randomized, placebo-controlled, phase 3 trial. Lancet. 2011;377:1341–52.

Garvey WT, Ryan DH, Bohannon NJ, Kushner RF, Rueger M, Dvorak RV, et al. Weight-loss therapy in type 2 diabetes: effects of phentermine and topiramate extended release. Diabetes Care. 2014a;37(12):3309–16.

Garvey WT, Ryan DH, Henry R, Bohannon NJV, Toplak H, Schwiers M, et al. Prevention of type 2 diabetes in subjects with prediabetes and metabolic syndrome treated with phentermine and topiramate extended release. Diabetes Care. 2014b;37:912–21.

Gonzalez-Campoy JM, Richardson B, Richardson C, Gonzalez-Cameron D, Ebrahim A, Strobel P, et al. Bariatric endocrinology: principles of medical practice. Int J Endocrinol. 2014;2014:917813.

Greenway FL, Fujoka K, Plodkowski RA, Mudaliar S, Guttadauria M, Erickson J, et al. Effect of naltrexone plus bupropion on weight loss in overweight an dobese adults (COR-I): a multicenter, arandomised, double-blind, placebo-controlled, phase 3 trial. Lancet. 2010;376:595–605.

Haddock CK, Poston WS, Dill PL, Foreyt JP, Ericsson M. Pharmacotherapy for obesity: a quantitative analysis of four decades of published randomized clinical trials. Int J Obes Relat Metab Disord. 2002;26(2):262–73.

Hollander P, Gupta AK, Plodkowski R, Greenway F, Bays H, Burns C, et al. Effects of naltrexone sustained-release/bupriopion sustained-release combination therapy on body weight and glyccmic parameters in overweight and obese patients with type 2 diabetes. Diabetes Care. 2013;36:4022–9.

Jensen MD, Ryan DH, Apovian CM, Ard JD, Comuzzie AG, Donato KA, et al. 2013 AHA/ACC/TOS guideline for the management of overweight and obesity in adults: a report of the American College of Cardiology/American Heart Association Task Force on Practice Guidelines and The Obesity Society. J Am Coll Cardiol. 2014;63(25 Pt B):2985–3023.

Mechanick JI, Garber AJ, Handelsman Y, Garvey WT. Association of Clinical Endocrinologists' position statement on obesity and obesity medicine. Endocr Pract. 2012;18(5):643.

O'Meara S, Riemsma R, Shirran L, Mather L, TerRiet G. A systemic review of the clinical effectiveness of orlistat used for the management of obesity. Obes Rev. 2004;5:51–68.

O'Neil PM, Smith SR, Weissman NK, Fidler MC, Sanchez M, Zhang J, et al. Randomized placebo-controlled clinical trial of loracserin for weight loss in type 2 diabetes mellitus: the Bloom-DM study. Obesity. 2012;20:1426–36.

Pi-Sunyer X, Astrup A, Fujioka K, et al., for the SCALE Obesity and Prediabetes NN8022–1839 Study Group. A randomized, controlled trial of 3.0 mg of liraglutide in weight management. N Engl J Med. 2015;373:11–22.

Smith SR, Weissman NJ, Anderson CM, Sanchez M, Chuang M, Stubb S, et al. Multicenter, placebo-controlled trial of lorcaserin for weight management. NEJM. 2010;363:245–56.

Sumithran P, Prendergast LA, Delbridge E, Purcell K, Shulkes A, Kriketos A, et al. Long-term persistence of hormonal adaptations to weight loss. N Engl J Med. 2011;365(17):1597–604.

Torgerson JS, Hauptman J, Boldrin MN, Sjöström L. XENical in the prevention of diabetes in obese subjects (XENDOS) study: a randomized study of orlistat as an adjunct to lifestyle changes for the prevention of type 2 diabetes in obese patients. Diabetes Care. 2004;27(1):155–61.

TOS Obesity as a Disease Writing Group, Allison DB, Downey M, Atkinson RL, Billington CJ, Bray GA, et al. Obesity as a disease: a white paper on evidence and arguments commissioned by the Council of the Obesity Society. Obesity. 2008;16:1161–77.

van Can J, Sloth B, Jensen CB, Flint A, Blaak EE, Saris WHM. Effect of the once-daily GLP-1 analog liraglutide on gastric emptying, glycemic parameters, appetite and energy metabolism in obese, non-diabetic adults. Int J Obes. 2013;162:1–10.

Wadden TA, Foreyt JP, Foster GD, Hill JO, Klein S, O'Neil PM, et al. Weight loss with naltrexone SR/bupropion SR combination therapy as an adjunct to behavior modification: the COR-BMOD trial. Obesity. 2011;19:110–20.

Wadden TA, Hollander P, Klein S, Niswender K, Woo V, Hale PM, et al. Weight maintenance and additional weight loss with liraglutide after low-calorie-diet-induced weight loss: the SCALE maintenance randomized study. Int J Obes. 2013;37:1443–52.

Chapter 22
Bariatric Procedures

J. Michael Gonzalez-Campoy

Pearls of Wisdom

- There are nonpharmacological treatments to achieve weight loss in patients with overweight, obesity, and adiposopathy. These treatments include bariatric surgical procedures, other invasive procedures, and noninvasive interventions.
- Bariatric surgical restrictive and malabsorptive procedures have evolved to provide effective weight loss in patients with significant burden of disease, while minimizing the risk of complications. They treat adiposity and adiposopathy, revert their complications, and improve mortality.
- The bariatric endocrinologist needs to have awareness of a patient's previous surgical procedures and provide life-long monitoring for complications, ongoing treatment for weight management, and continued surveillance for the re-development of adiposopathy.
- There are emerging procedures for weight loss, which do not involve intestinal interventions and which offer alternatives to the traditional bariatric surgery procedures.
- All patients who undergo nonpharmacological interventions for weight loss should be carefully selected and reminded that overweight and obesity still need to be managed indefinitely. Procedures have a finite effect, and the duration of the benefit is variable.

J. M. Gonzalez-Campoy
Minnesota Center for Obesity, Metabolism and Endocrinology, PA (MNCOME), Eagan, MN, USA
e-mail: drmike@mncome.com

J. M. Gonzalez-Campoy et al. (eds.), *Bariatric Endocrinology*,
https://doi.org/10.1007/978-3-319-95655-8_22

22.1 Introduction

In 1901, Dr. Peters published "*Resection of the pendulous, fat abdominal wall in cases of extreme obesity,*" which was his account of one patient who had excision of a large volume of fat from the abdomen in May 1899, by Dr. Kelly at Johns Hopkins. This may be the first published "bariatric surgery" procedure.

Weight loss surgery began in the 1950s with the introduction of various intestinal bypass procedures, each designed to shorten the digestive tract. Intestinal bypass procedures involved creating an anastomosis of the proximal to the most distal intestine, which bypassed a large amount of the absorptive capacity of the small intestine. Weight loss from intestinal bypass was caused purely by the malabsorption of food, and many patients did poorly because of this, developing diarrhea, dehydration, and severe electrolyte imbalances. Table 22.1 provides the major developments in bariatric surgery of the twentieth century.

Table 22.1 Historical development of bariatric and metabolic surgical procedures in the twentieth century

Year	Procedure	Author
1952	105-cm small bowel resection	Henrikson
1953	End-to-end jejuno-ileostomy with ileo-cecostomy	Varco
1963	End-to-side jejuno-transverse colostomy (jejuno-colic shunt)	Payne and DeWind
1963	Partial ileal bypass	Buchwald
1965	End-to-side jejuno-ileostomy	Sherman
1966	End-to-side jejuno-cecostomy	Lewis, Turnbull, and page
1967	Gastric transection with loop gastro-jejunostomy	Mason and Ito
1969	Classic "14 + 4" end-to-side jejuno-ileostomy	Payne and DeWind
1971	End-to-end jejuno-ileostomy with ileo-sigmoidostomy	Scott
1971	Partial gastric transection, greater curve conduit	Mason and Printen
1977	End-to-side jejuno-ileostomy with anti-reflux valve (plication)	Forestieri
1977	Horizontal gastric stapling with loop gastro-jejunostomy	Alden
1977	Horizontal gastric stapling with Roux-en-Y gastro-jejunostomy	Griffen
1978	Bilio-intestinal bypass	Lavorato
1978	Gastric band	Wilkinson
1979	Biliopancreatic diversion	Scopinaro
1979	Horizontal gastric stapling, greater curve conduit	Gomez
1979	Gastric partitioning	Pace and Carey
1979	Total horizontal gastric stapling with gastro-gastrostomy	LaFave and Alden
1981	Gastroplasty with vertical stapling	Fabito
1981	Silastic ring vertical gastroplasty	Laws
1981	Vertical banded gastroplasty	Mason
1983	Vertical gastric stapling with Roux-en-Y gastro-jejunostomy	Torres, Oca, and Garrison

Table 22.1 (continued)

Year	Procedure	Author
1986	Adjustable silastic gastric band	Kuzmak
1986	Biliopancreatic diversion with duodenal switch	Hess
1987	Vertical gastric stapling with Roux-en-Y gastro-jejunostomy with long biliopancreatic limb	Torres and Oca
1988	Sleeve gastrectomy	Hess
1988	End-to-end jejuno-ileostomy with ileo-gastrostomy	Cleator and Courlay
1991	Vertical gastric division with interposed Roux-en-Y gastro-jejunostomy and proximal silastic ring	Fobi
1993	Duodenal switch with cross-stapling of the duodenum	Marceau
1993	Laparoscopic vertical banded gastroplasty	Hess and Hess
1993	Laparoscopic nonadjustable gastric band	Broadbent
1993	Laparoscopic adjustable gastric band	Belachew//Forsell
1993	Laparoscopic Roux-en-Y gastric bypass	Wittgrove and Clark
1997	One anastomosis gastric bypass/mini gastric bypass	Rutledge
1998	Duodenal switch with division of the duodenum	Hess and Hess
1999	Laparoscopic biliopancreatic diversion with duodenal switch	Gagner
1999	Laparoscopic vertical sleeve gastrectomy (as the first stage to subsequent Roux-en-Y gastric bypass for extreme body mass index)	Gagner

One of these early procedures, the partial ileal bypass developed by Henry Buchwald in the 1960s ameliorates the development of severe malnutrition and remains a treatment choice for patients with severe hypercholesterolemia.

In 1965, Dr. Edward E. Mason and Dr. Chikashi Ito at the University of Iowa developed the original gastric bypass for weight reduction which led to fewer complications than the intestinal bypass. This ushered a new era in weight loss surgery.

In 1983, Dr. Mason became the founding president of the American Society for Bariatric Surgery (ASBS). Over the years, bariatric surgery has been documented to be effective for the treatment of metabolic diseases, especially type 2 diabetes mellitus, in addition to its effectiveness in reducing fat mass. A meta-analysis published in 2004 by Buchwald and colleagues documented that most patients who undergo bariatric surgery have sustained improvements not only in glycemia but also dyslipidemia, blood pressure, and sleep apnea. There is now documentation of a significant reduction in the burden of each of the complications of obesity with bariatric surgery procedures (Table 22.2). Accordingly, the name of the organization was changed on August 15, 2007, from ASBS to the American Society for Metabolic and Bariatric Surgery (ASMBS). In Europe, the International Federation for the Surgery of Obesity and Metabolic Disorders (IFSO) made a similar decision in choosing its name.

This chapter will review bariatric operations for the management of obesity, and other nonpharmacological interventions which are currently available or in development to treat patients with overweight, obesity, and adiposopathy.

Table 22.2 Outcomes of bariatric surgery on some obesity comorbidities

Obesity-related condition	Outcome after bariatric surgery
Asthma	69–82% improved
Cardiovascular disease	82% risk reduction
Depression	47–55% reduced
Diabetes mellitus, type 2	82–98% resolved
Dyslipidemia	63% resolved
Dysmetabolic syndrome	80% resolved
Gastroesophageal reflux disease	72–98% resolved
Gout	72–77% resolved
Hirsutism in women	75–79% resolution
Hypertension	52–92% resolved
Migraine headaches	57% resolved
Mortality from obesity-related cancers	60% reduction
Mortality from diabetes mellitus, type 2	92% reduction
Mortality from heart disease	56% reduction
Mortality, overall, 5–7 years	40–89% reduction
Nonalcoholic fatty liver disease	37% resolution
Obstructive sleep apnea	74–98% resolved
Osteoarthritis	41–76% resolved
Polycystic ovarian syndrome	100% resolution of menstrual irregularity
Pseudotumor cerebri	84–96% resolved
Quality of life	95% of patients improved
Urinary stress incontinence	44–88% resolved
Venous stasis dermatitis	95% resolution of stasis ulcerations

22.2 Bariatric Operations for Management of Obesity

Bariatric procedures achieve weight loss by causing intestinal malabsorption, restricting gastric capacity to produce fullness, or a combination of both. In addition to changing nutrient volumes and absorption, each procedure brings about changes in the signaling system that regulates energy balance, favoring weight loss. In the sections that follow, some of the bariatric procedures will be discussed. With the advent of laparoscopy and flexible endoscopy, and refinements in surgery derived from them, there are additional procedures available to manage obesity with significantly decreased morbidity. The bariatric and metabolic surgery procedures available, recently in disfavor, or in development, as of 2016 include:

- Adjustable gastric band (AGB)
- Biliopancreatic diversion (BPD)
- Biliopancreatic diversion with duodenal switch (BPD-DS)
- Duodenojejunal bypass (DJB)
- Loop Duodeno-jejunal bypass with sleeve gastrectomy (LDJB-SG)
- Endoluminal sleeves (ES; duodeno-jejunal bypass sleeve and gastro-duodeno-jejunal bypass sleeve)

- Intragastric balloons (IGB)
- Jejunoileal bypass (JIB)
- Mini gastric bypass (MGB)
- One anastomosis gastric bypass (OAGB)
- Percutaneous gastrostomy (PG)
- Roux-en-Y gastric bypass (RYGB)
- Single anastomosis duodeno-ileostomy (SADI)
- Single anastomosis gastro-ileostomy (SAGI)
- Single anastomosis sleeve ileostomy (SASI)
- Stomach intestinal pylorus sparing surgery (SIPS)
- Transoral gastroplasty (TOGA)
- Vertical banded gastroplasty (VBG)
- Vertical sleeve gastrectomy (VSG)

Most bariatric surgery is now done with laparoscopy, and procedures that once were designed for open laparotomy are now done with minimal trauma and shortened hospital stays.

The American Association of Clinical Endocrinologists and the ASMBS have produced clinical practice guidelines for the evaluation and management of patients who undergo bariatric surgery. The guidelines are updated periodically. The criteria for referral to bariatric surgery have changed over time and will likely continue to change in the future. Any patient with a body mass index (BMI) of 40 kilograms/meter^2 (kg/m^2) should be referred for weight loss surgery if refractory to medical nutrition therapy, lifestyle changes to increase physical activity, and pharmacotherapy. Patients with a BMI of 35 kg/m^2 and two or more metabolic complications of obesity may be considered for a weight loss procedure.

22.2.1 Malabsorptive Procedures

22.2.1.1 JIB

JIB involved dividing the proximal jejunum at a length of 30–45 cm. The proximal end of the jejunum was anastomosed, end-to-side or end-to-end, to the terminal 10 cm of the ileum. The distal end of the jejunum became a blind loop. Severe malabsorption caused rapid weight loss (Fig. 22.1). Patients who weighed over 345 pounds at the time of surgery lost a mean of 127 pounds at the end of 1 year of surgery.

The severe malnutrition caused by JIB required reversal of the procedure or conversion to a different bariatric procedure frequently. Additionally, bacterial overgrowth in the excluded blind loop caused the arthritis-dermatitis syndrome, thought to be an immune complex-mediated process related to bypass enteritis. After more than 10 years, 19% of patients had severe irreversible complications that outweighed the benefit of the procedure, including hepatic fibrosis.

JIB was abandoned, and most patients who had this procedure have died or had the procedure reversed. However, there are still patients who may present with

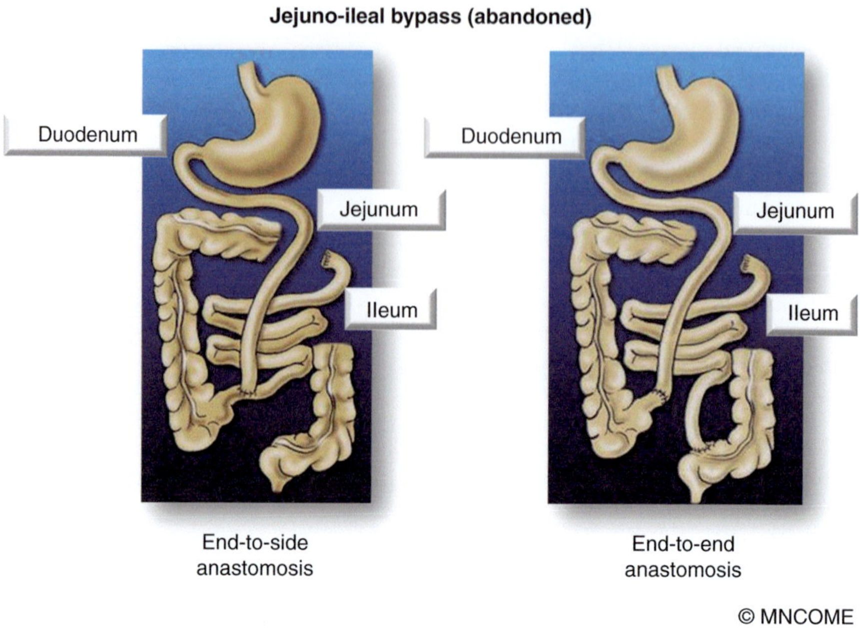

Fig. 22.1 Jejunoileal bypass. Jejunoileal bypass was abandoned because complications outweighed benefits. Twenty-five percent of patients developed mild hepatic dysfunction, 5% of patients developed full-blown cirrhosis, and 1–2% of patients ended with liver failure. Most patients developed chronic diarrhea with anal burning, electrolyte abnormalities, dehydration, and a low quality of life. Protein depletion, calcium malabsorption, renal lithiasis, cholelithiasis, and vitamin B12 deficiency developed frequently. Only one-third of patients had a benign course. (Copyright Minnesota Center for Obesity, Metabolism and Endocrinology, PA (MNCOME))

advanced liver disease, a history or renal lithiasis, progressive kidney failure, arthritis, chronic diarrhea, fatigue, and joint pain. A history of weight loss surgery in the 1960s or 1970s should prompt consideration of having had JIB.

22.2.1.2 PG Device

A percutaneous gastrostomy device to treat obesity is marketed with the name of Aspire Assist® (Fig. 22.2). In the phase 1 trial with this device, there was 18.6% weight loss in 1 year. There were no adverse effects on eating behavior. There was no compensation for aspirated calories. Patients did not experience binge eating.

In the registration trial for Aspire Assist®, 207 patients with class 2 or higher obesity were randomized to lifestyle counseling alone or lifestyle counseling and treatment with the device. At 52 weeks, the average weight loss was 12.1% of entry total body weight, or 31.5% of excess body weight. At the end of the study, 58.6% of patients using the device had lost at least 25% of their excess body weight. This compares to 15.3% of patients who did not use the device. In the registration trial,

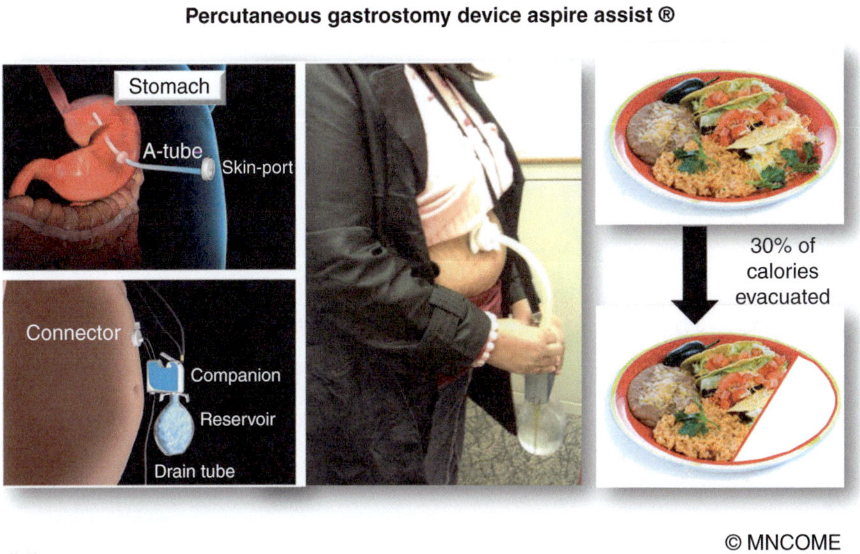

Fig. 22.2 Percutaneous gastrostomy device. The Aspire Assist System® is a weight loss device that comprises an endoscopically placed percutaneous gastrostomy tube and an external device to facilitate drainage of about 30% of the calories consumed in a meal. (Copyright Minnesota Center for Obesity, Metabolism and Endocrinology, PA (MNCOME))

abdominal pain in the perioperative period and periostomal granulation in the postoperative period were the most common side effects, each affecting over 40% of patients. Serious adverse events occurred in 3.6% of patients, including peritonitis, severe abdominal pain after the tube placement, and abdominal pain from a prepyloric ulcer 53 weeks after tube placement from friction with the intragastric portion of the tube.

22.2.1.3 ES

The Valentx ES and EndoBarrier® by GI Dynamics are under development for the treatment of obesity. As of 2017, neither is available in the US market.

The ES are made of polymer material that is impervious to moisture or acidity. They are delivered into the stomach with endoscopy. They each have unique ways of getting anchored to the mucosa in a circumferential attachment. The Valentx ES is designed to be anchored at the esophago-gastric junction. EndoBarrier® is designed to be anchored in the duodenal bulb. The sleeves create an inner passage within the stomach or intestine—a lumen within a lumen.

When food enters the stomach, it is exposed to the normal gastric digestive processes with EndoBarrier®. With the Valentx ES, food enters the inner channel before exposure to the gastric digestive processes. Upon entering the duodenum, food enters the inner lumen of the EndoBarrier®, and it continues within the lumen

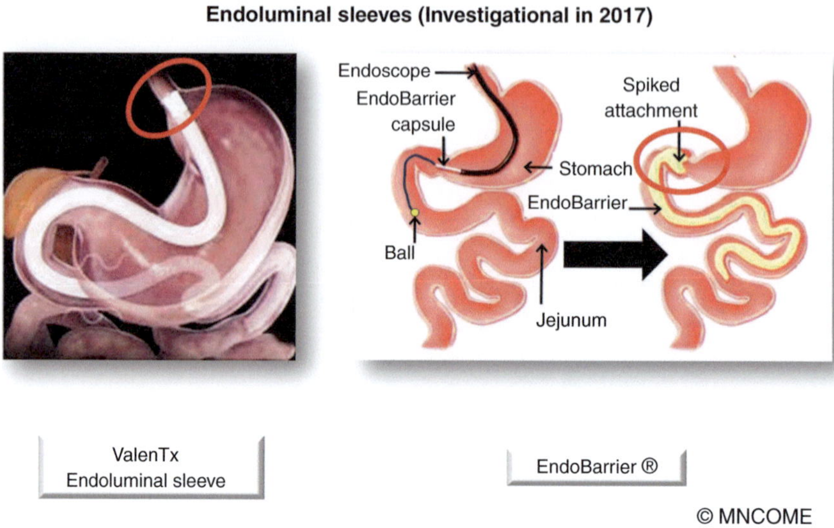

Fig. 22.3 Endoluminal sleeves. There are two endoluminal sleeves under investigation for the treatment of obesity. EndoBarrier® by GI Dynamics and the Valentx sleeve. Both are inserted with upper endoscopy and are anchored to the mucosa creating a false lumen. The ValenTx endoluminal sleeve anchors at the esophago-gastric junction. The EndoBarrier® anchors at the pyloric junction. The red circles highlight the attachment sites. Food is delivered in the ileum where it finally comes into contact with the digestive juices. This results in malabsorption of nutrients with weight loss. (Copyright Minnesota Center for Obesity, Metabolism and Endocrinology, PA (MNCOME))

of the ValenTx ES. Food does not come into contact with bile or pancreatic digestive enzymes. The length of the inner sleeves may be varied, but the design is to bypass the duodenum and jejunum. The common channel begins at the end of the sleeve and may be changed depending on individual need (Fig. 22.3).

Both companies have generated preliminary results documenting effective weight loss, with improvements in metabolism. The benefits of this approach are that it does not alter normal gastrointestinal anatomy, that malabsorption is reversible by removing the sleeve, and that it may be safely redeployed. The technical challenge is to anchor the sleeves without incurring damage to the structures they become attached to.

22.2.2 Restrictive Procedures

22.2.2.1 VBG (Stomach Stapling)

Mason developed VBG in 1980. A small vertical pouch is created by stapling the stomach. The pouch is separated from the fundus of the stomach by the staple line. The pouch size is less than 50 ml. The pouch outlet is reinforced by a narrow band of polypropylene mesh passed through a circular window, also created by stapling.

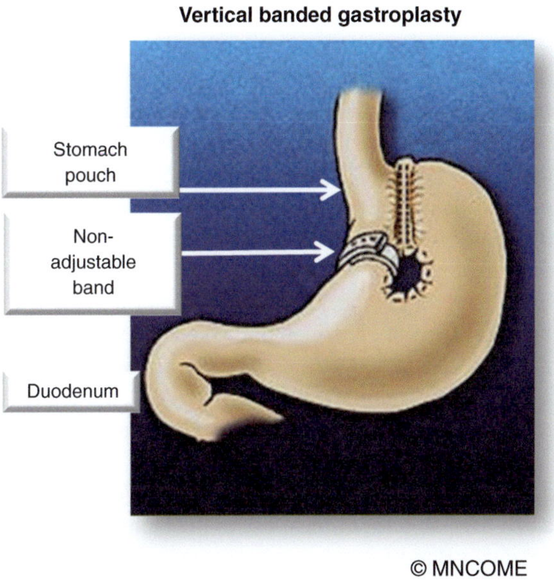

Fig. 22.4 Vertical banded gastroplasty. The stomach is partially divided by stapling. A nonadjustable band is placed around the stomach inlet. The resulting stomach pouch restricts intake. The pouch outlet is 1 cm in diameter, further restricting the passage of food into the rest of the stomach and the intestines. (Copyright Minnesota Center for Obesity, Metabolism and Endocrinology, PA (MNCOME))

The stomach pouch has a 1-cm diameter exit. The pouch limits the amount of food that may be ingested. The narrow exit slows passage of food onto the remainder of the stomach (Fig. 22.4).

VBG preserves the pyloric sphincter, and there is no dumping syndrome (rapid gastric emptying). VBG does not have a risk of ulcers, anemia, or malnutrition. Weight loss with VBG is less sustained than with malabsorptive procedures. Eighty percent of VBG patients achieve some degree of weight loss and 30% of VBG patients achieve normal weight. Ten years after surgery, only 10% of patients maintain weight loss of at least 50% of their total excess weight at the time of their initial surgery. Most patients regain weight.

The disadvantages of this procedure are that patients must adhere to their meal plan, which, for most, is impossible to continue over time. The band creates a fixed diameter exit and cannot be adjusted. Foods high in fiber or with a denser consistency are difficult to eat, and patients may experience emesis and severe epigastric pain if the food bolus was not properly chewed. Rapid ingestion of food also results in these symptoms. Highly refined foods, on the other hand are easy to eat. Weight regain comes from a shift to foods easier to eat. When needed, reversal of a VBG is complex. The polyurethane bands used in the 1980s and 1990s created scarring, which makes the takedown procedure more difficult. And removal of the staple lines makes it impossible to return the stomach to its native anatomy. High revision rates and conversions of VBG to RYGB made ongoing use of VBG less desirable.

Other complications of VBG include disruption of the staple line, stomal fibrosis, gastroesophageal reflux, and incisional ventral hernia.

22.2.2.2 AGB

The application of an external band around the stomach (gastric banding) was first done in 1978 by Wilkinson. This was a nonadjustable 2-cm wide strip of Marlex mesh placed around the upper third of the stomach. Various versions of gastric banding are reported in the literature. Slippage of the stomach was common, and band erosions and strictures led to intractable vomiting, severe food intolerances, and dilatation of the esophagus. The proximal pouch would gradually dilate, and weight regain frequently happened.

In 1985, Hallberg and Forsell first described the use of an inflatable gastric band in humans. In 1986, Kuzmak published his early experience with an inflatable band, which allowed for adjustments of the diameter of the stomach outlet. Weight loss was better, and complications were reduced, using the adjustable gastric band, compared to the nonadjustable bands used earlier.

Kuzmak's band was commercialized as the LAP-BAND® system and became available in the United States in 2001. The Forsell Swedish Adjustable Gastric Band became available for clinical use in the United States in 2007 and came to market as the Realize Band®.

AGB reduces the stomach inlet and achieves an average 50% excess weight loss (EWL). It takes 2–3 years to achieve this weight loss, compared to 12–18 months with other bariatric procedures. Patients require close follow-up and adjustments of the band's inner diameter based on patient's weights and symptoms (Fig. 22.5).

AGB have a reoperation rate of 5% per year. The main complication of AGB is band slippage and cephalad gastric prolapse through the band. This prolapse leads to gastric obstruction or proximal gastric pouch dilatation. Refinement of surgical techniques has made this problem less prevalent. Band erosion, esophageal dilatation, and malfunction of the reservoir or tubing are other complications of AGB.

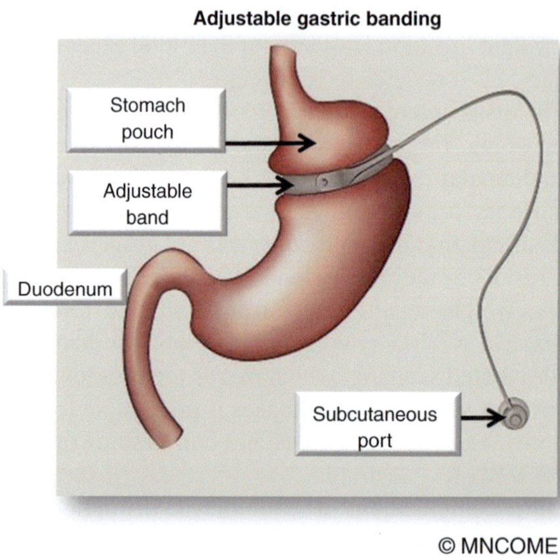

Fig. 22.5 Adjustable gastric banding. The adjustable band placed around the upper stomach allows for its inner diameter to be adjusted by adding or subtracting volume through the subcutaneous port. (Copyright Minnesota Center for Obesity, Metabolism and Endocrinology, PA (MNCOME))

22.2.2.3 VSG and LVSG

VSG evolved from prior procedures. In 1976, Tretbar described an extension of the fundoplication (for the treatment of acid reflux) that created a tubular structure in the stomach. Weight loss was observed after this procedure (Fig. 22.6).

Hess used this concept of a tubular stomach and modified it from an extended plication to an actual longitudinal or vertical gastrectomy. He performed the first open sleeve gastrectomy in March 1988, as a part of BPD-DS.

In 1999, the first laparoscopic approach to the BPD-DS was developed. Gagner implemented the laparoscopic BPD-DS in humans but noted a high complication rate in patients with a higher BMI. He subsequently developed the technique of staging the intestinal bypass procedure by performing the laparoscopic vertical sleeve gastrectomy (LVSG) first, as an initial stage. From 2001 to 2003, seven patients with a BMI of 58–71 kg/m^2 underwent a first-stage LVSG. The average EWL was 37 kg (33% EWL), and this allowed for a safer second stage. These preliminary results quickly popularized LVSG as a safer laparoscopic option for the higher BMI group.

Many of the patients who had lost enough weight with the LVSG did not require a secondary procedure. LVSG as a standalone procedure gained popularity over the past decade. LVSG is technically less demanding than RYGB or BPD-DS, is associated with minimal morbidity, avoids the use of foreign material like the VBG or gastric band, and has fewer long-term problems. At 5 years, the EWL is between 33% and 85%. Weight regain or insufficient weight loss is the cause for conversion from LVSG to RYGB or BPD-DS.

LVSG can cause staple line leaks and strictures. Leaks may not heal spontaneously since the remaining gastric tube operates at high pressure.

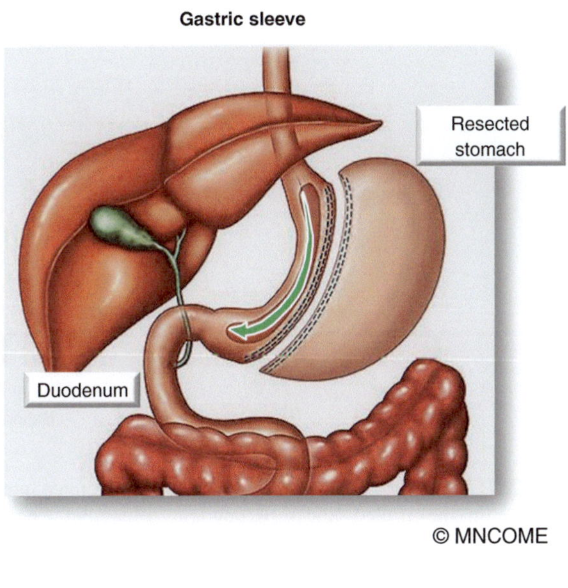

Fig. 22.6 Gastric sleeve. Excision of the stomach vertically results in a narrow gastric passage (green arrow) with preservation of the lower esophageal and pyloric sphincters. (Copyright Minnesota Center for Obesity, Metabolism and Endocrinology, PA (MNCOME))

22.2.2.4 IGB

In 1985, the Garren-Edwards Gastric Bubble was approved by the US Food and Drug Administration (FDA) for temporary use as a weight loss device. Significant complications and limited weight loss, especially when compared to bariatric surgery procedures, led to discontinuation of the bubble in 1988 and FDA withdrawal of approval in 1992.

The concept that occupying volume within the stomach restricts food intake was not abandoned, and there are now three IGB for commercial use in the United States (Fig. 22.7). In 2015, the Food and Drug Administration approved the ReShape® Duo Integrated Dual Balloon System and the ORBERA® gastric balloon for clinical use. These balloons are placed endoscopically, inflated with saline, and left in place in the stomach for up to 6 months.

With the ReShape® Balloon, there was a 14.3-pound weight loss (6.8% of total body weight) at 6 months. At 12 months, the patients kept off 9.9 pounds. With the Orbera® IGB, the US pivotal study demonstrated an average EWL of 38.4% at 6 months. Worldwide, there are over 277,000 placements.

The Obalon Balloon System® is a swallowed (does not require endoscopy) intragastric balloon system approved for up to 6 months of use for weight loss. It is for adults with BMI of 30–40 kg/m² who have failed to lose weight through nutritional and physical activity interventions. In the US registration trial, done at 15 sites, two-thirds of patients had meaningful weight loss and 89% of weight loss was

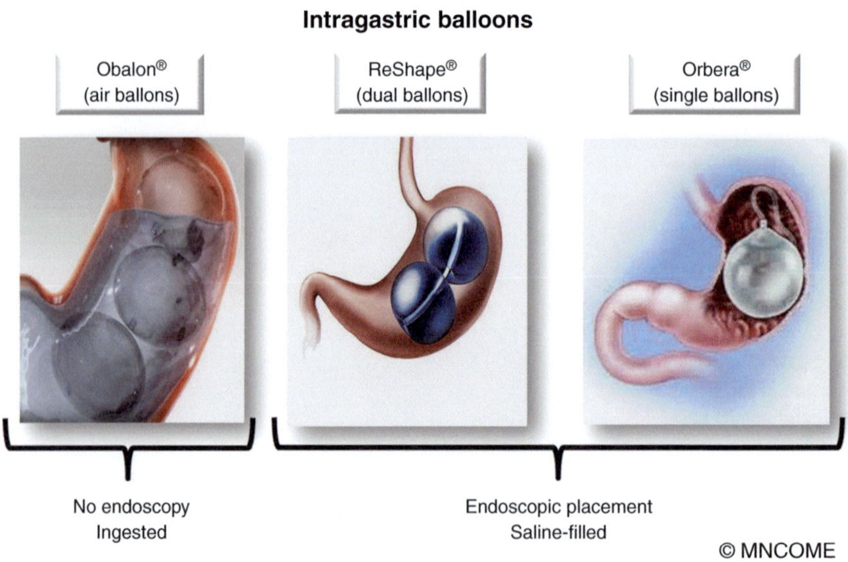

Fig. 22.7 Intragastric balloons. As of 2017, there are three intragastric balloon systems available for use in the United States. (Copyright Minnesota Center for Obesity, Metabolism and Endocrinology, PA (MNCOME))

kept off for 6 months after the removal of the balloons. There was a serious adverse device event rate of 0.3% (n = 1/336). One, two, or three balloons may be in the stomach at a time. Figure 22.7 summarizes the three IGB options.

For all IGBs, the common adverse events are abdominal pain and nausea. Gastritis, ulceration, early retrieval, gastroesophageal reflux, vomiting, bowel obstruction, severe dehydration, renal insufficiency, and cardiac arrhythmia have all been documented at a level below 1% in association with IGB use.

The FDA has issued two warnings regarding IGB. There are reports of pancreatitis and hyperinflation. The rate of pancreatitis was reported as 0.07–0.1%. Hyperinflation, the spontaneous increases in the size of IGB, occurred at a rate of 0.02% and 0.04%.

There have been four deaths of patients with IGB in the United States since 2015. This rate of four in an estimated 10,651 implants gives a mortality rate of 0.037%. They were associated with esophageal or gastric perforation.

22.2.2.5 Gastric Plication and TOGA

Gastric plication surgery is also called laparoscopic greater curvature plication, gastric imbrication, and pseudo sleeve surgery. The result is similar to that of a VSG, with significant restriction of the stomach volume. In gastric plication, the stomach is sown on itself rather than being resected. Gastric plication has the benefit of meaningful weight loss without removing part of the stomach or rearranging the small intestine. It results in less weight loss and health benefits than the more established VSG, RYGB, BPD-DS, and AGB procedures.

TOGA research and development was halted indefinitely because in clinical trials the procedure did not reach set targets. Further, the company that makes the TOGA system, Satiety, Inc., faced a lawsuit from a patient who suffered an esophageal rupture during the procedure, which dampened enthusiasm for the concept. The transoral approach to gastric surgery remains a focus of clinical interest.

22.2.3 Mixed Procedures

22.2.3.1 BPD

In a BPD procedure, the distal two-thirds of the stomach are excised, and the proximal one third remains as a stomach pouch. There is restriction of stomach volume, but the pouch still allows for food to enter the stomach unrestricted. The stomach pouch is anastomosed side to end directly to the final segment of the ileum, completely bypassing the duodenum, jejunum, and proximal ileum. A common channel remains, in which bile and pancreatic digestive juices mix prior to entering the colon. Weight loss occurs since most of the calories and nutrients are routed into the colon where they are not absorbed (Fig. 22.8).

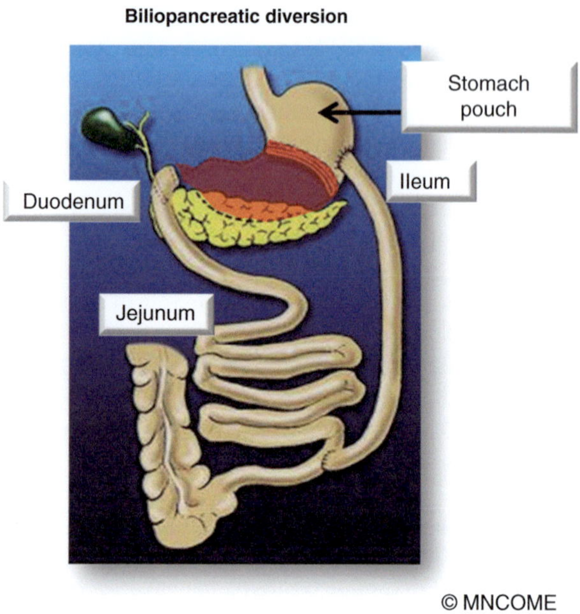

Fig. 22.8 Biliopancreatic diversion. A partial distal gastrectomy is performed including the pyloric sphincter. The area in red represents the part of the stomach that is excised in this procedure. Biliopancreatic drainage is preserved. The alimentary channel is restricted to the terminal ileum. (Copyright Minnesota Center for Obesity, Metabolism and Endocrinology, PA (MNCOME))

In a historical review of 2241 patients, EWL after 1 year averages 75%, most patients maintain the lost weight off over 21 years, there is 98% remission of diabetes 10 years after surgery, and both hypertension and dyslipidemia improve.

BPD causes long-term diarrhea, anemia, protein malnutrition (in 30% of patients), dumping syndrome, peripheral neuropathy, Wernicke's encephalopathy, and osteoporosis (calcium malabsorption). This procedure is not done any more because of the need for long-term nutritional follow-up.

22.2.3.2 BPD-DS, SADI, and SIPS

BPD-DS is a modification of the BPD procedure. In BPD-DS, the greater curvature of the stomach is excised with a longitudinal cut. The entire lesser curvature remains, and the pylorus is preserved. The duodenum is transected distal to the pylorus but proximal to the sphincter of Odi. The distal portion of the duodenum is turned into a blind loop, which takes the secretions of the biliary tree and pancreas and carries them distally. The proximal portion of the duodenum is anastomosed end-to-end to the distal ileum. The pancreas and biliary tree still drain normally into the duodenum. Digestive juices do join meals in a common channel at the distal ileum. In BPD-DS, preservation of the pylorus and the first portion of the duodenum helped solve the problem of dumping symptoms and marginal ulcers seen with the BPD (Fig. 22.9).

All patients who undergo a BPD-DS are required to take supplemental vitamins and minerals to compensate for the malabsorption. Anemia and osteoporosis commonly develop over time. Despite supplementation, in around 2% of patients, severe

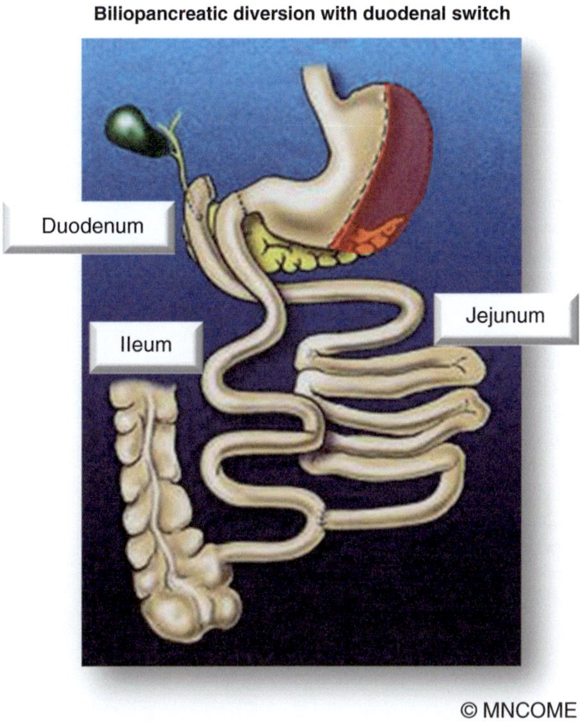

Fig. 22.9 Biliopancreatic diversion with duodenal switch. A vertical gastrectomy is performed by preserving the lower esophageal and pyloric sphincters. The area in red represents the part of the stomach that is excised in this procedure. Biliopancreatic drainage is preserved. The alimentary channel is restricted to the terminal ileum. (Copyright Minnesota Center for Obesity, Metabolism and Endocrinology, PA (MNCOME))

malabsorption develops. This causes nutritional deficiencies which require reversal of the procedure. Gallstone formation is common with rapid weight loss. If a prophylactic cholecystectomy is not done, ursodeoxycholic acid should be prescribed to decrease the risk of gallstones.

In 2007, Torres developed the loop technique, which reduced two anastomoses down to one and bypassed less of the intestine. This became known as the SADI procedure. The SADI procedure is safer than the BPD-DS, with less risk of malnutrition, diarrhea, and vitamin deficiencies.

Roslin Cottam refined the technique further, creating the SIPS procedure. The SIPS procedure bypasses the intestine even less, decreasing the potential for long-term problems even more.

SADI and SIPS are useful for patients who have had a prior VSG with inadequate weight loss, or weight regain. In the past, these patients had a conversion to a standard RYGB. The SADI and SIPS procedures allow for further weight loss without undue risk of nutritional deficiencies.

22.2.3.3 RYGB, MGB, OAGB, SAGI, and SASI

The first gastric bypass surgery was performed by Ito and Mason at the University of Iowa in 1967. The current RYGB represents an evolution over time (Fig. 22.10). RYGB completely bypasses the stomach and duodenum. The stomach is divided

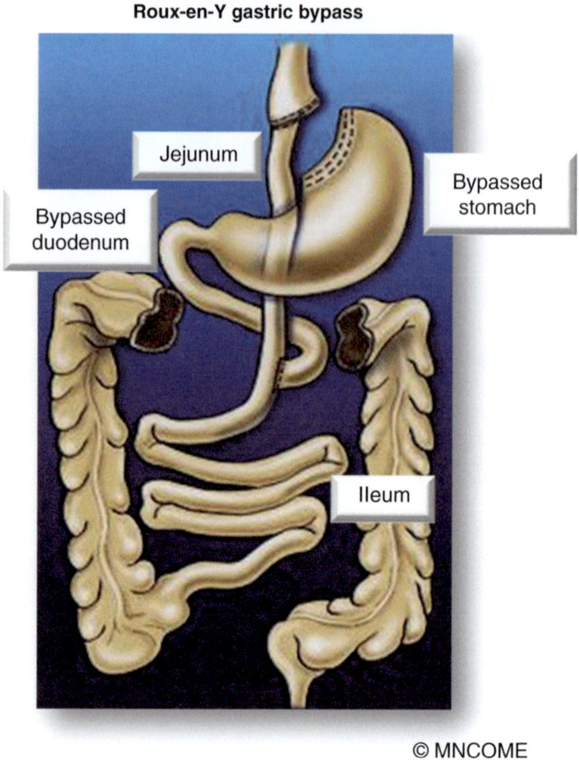

Fig. 22.10 Roux-en-Y gastric bypass. The stomach is transected as proximally as possible at the cardia. The proximal jejunum is transected, and the distal end is anastomosed to the stomach peduncle. The body of the stomach, pancreas, and biliary tree drain normally. The proximal end of the jejunum is anastomosed back to the small intestine, and the lengths of the biliopancreatic limb and the common channel may be varied. (Copyright Minnesota Center for Obesity, Metabolism and Endocrinology, PA (MNCOME))

close to the lower esophageal sphincter, isolating the cardia and leaving enough tissue to create an anastomosis. A very small upper pouch is created, and a much larger lower "remnant" remains. The small intestine is divided and the distal end is advanced upward to connect to the upper gastric pouch, creating an alimentary channel. The stomach, pancreas, and biliary tree drain normally into the duodenum and the jejunum, proximal to the transection. This biliopancreatic channel is then anastomosed end to side to the small intestine. From this anastomosis site, where the biliopancreatic and alimentary channels join, there is a common or digestive channel.

There are several versions of the RYGB procedure. The most common, the proximal RYGB is done by dividing the jejunum 45 cm below the stomach outlet. The Roux (distal) limb of the intestine is advanced upward to make an anastomosis with the small upper gastric pouch. The Y-intersection is formed at the upper end of the small intestine by an anastomosis to the proximal end of the jejunum to the distal jejunum or ileum. The procedure accomplishes:

- Isolation of the gastric cardia
- Exclusion of the distal stomach
- Exclusion of the duodenum and proximal jejunum
- Exposure of the distal jejunum to undigested food
- Partial vagotomy (performed during the transection of the stomach)

The Y-intersection can be placed anywhere along the length of the small intestine, distal to the division of the duodenum. The more distal along the small intestine that the Y-intersecion is placed, the lower the surface area to absorb nutrients. More distal Y-intersection placement produces greater degrees of weight loss but higher risks of malabsorption. In the distal RYGB, the Y-connection is formed much closer to the distal end of the small intestine, usually 100–150 cm from the ilio-colic valve. Fat and carbohydrate malabsorption reduces caloric intake. Various minerals and the fat-soluble vitamins are not adequately absorbed either. The unabsorbed food passes into the large intestine where it is exposed to the bacterial flora of the colon. Irritants and malodorous gases are frequently a consequence of this. These larger effects on nutrition are traded for a relatively modest increase in total weight loss.

The first laparoscopic RYGB (LRYGB) was done in 1994 by Wittgrove. Most RYGB is now done with laparoscopy. Laparoscopy also brought the opportunity to modify the original RYGB.

MGB was developed by Rutledge as a modification of the Billroth II procedure and introduced in 1997. The stomach is divided longitudinally along the lesser curvature to create a vertical gastric passage. As opposed to a VSG, the vertical gastric passage is disconnected from the pylorus. The bypassed stomach is what remains attached to the pylorus instead. A 3-cm wide antecolic end-to-side gastro-jejunostomy is performed 200-cm distal to the ligament of Treitz. The anastomosis may be placed further distal, at 250 cm, for patients with an extreme BMI (Fig. 22.11).

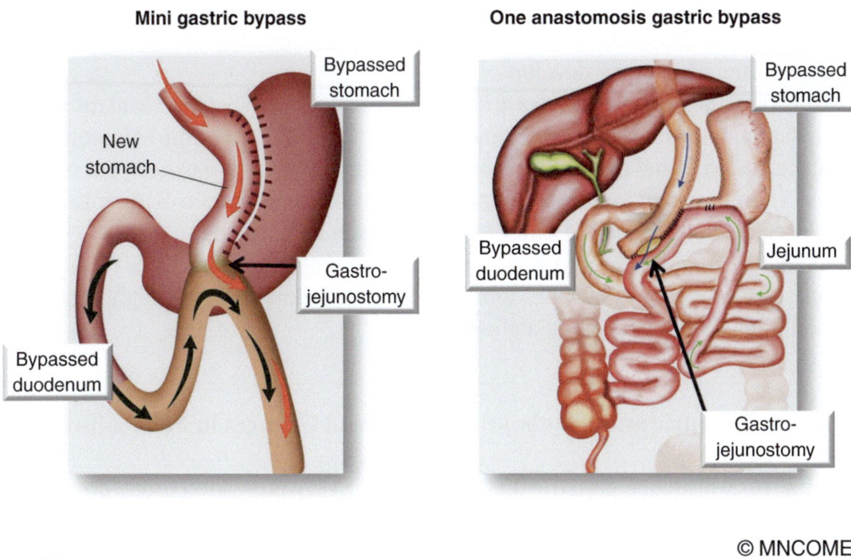

Fig. 22.11 Mini gastric bypass and one anastomosis gastric bypass. In both of these procedures, a gastric passage is created. The bypassed stomach remains in continuity with the pylorus. A gastro-jejunostomy is done. In mini gastric bypass, the anastomosis is done end to side. In one anastomosis gastric bypass, the anastomosis is done side to side. (Copyright Minnesota Center for Obesity, Metabolism and Endocrinology, PA (MNCOME))

In 2002, Carbajo introduced OAGB. In this procedure, there is an antecolic side-to-side anastomosis of the jejunum in the biliopancreatic limb to the gastric pouch. This facilitates emptying of the biliopancreatic juice toward the efferent limb and prevents reflux. The common limb must always be 300 cm to prevent any malabsorption (Fig. 22.11).

SAGI and SASI are laparoscopic procedures, which also modify the RYGB. SAGI was introduced in 2016 by De Luca. In OAGB, the measurement of the afferent limb starting at the ligament of Treitz may result in insufficient absorptive surface of the intestine of the remaining efferent limb. SAGI addresses this concern by constructing the gastrointestinal anastomosis at a fixed distance from the ileocecal valve (i.e., 300 cm).

SASI was introduced by Santoro in 2006. In the initial publication, the term "digestive adaptation with intestinal reserve" was used. In a second publication, the procedure was referred to as "sleeve gastrectomy with transit bipartition." SASI involves a sleeve gastrectomy followed by a side-to-side gastro-ileal anastomosis. In SASI, there is dual gastric emptying, both through the normal pyloric channel and through the gastro-ileal anastomosis (bipartition). In SASI, nutrient transit is maintained in the duodenum, avoiding blind loops and minimizing malabsorption. A lateral enteroanastomosis connects both segments at 80 cm proximal to the cecum.

Data from 33,117 RYGB operations done in 106 US Centers of Excellence documents a 0.11% mortality rate within 30 days of the procedure (364 deaths). The 90-day mortality rate is 0.3%. Short-term complications of surgery include infection, venous thromboembolic disease, hemorrhage, development of ventral or intra-abdominal hernias, and bowel obstruction. Additionally, anastomotic leaks, strictures, and ulcers may develop.

Nutritional deficiencies after gastric bypass occur in 30% of patients. Malabsorption of the fat-soluble vitamins A, D, E, and K, and vitamin B12, are quite common. Iron-deficiency anemia and calcium malabsorption often occur after gastric bypass procedures. Therefore, life-long oral supplementation of iron, vitamin B12, folate, and calcium are recommended to avoid specific nutrient deficiencies.

Other late complications of RYGB include dumping syndrome, since food passes directly into the small intestine, food intolerance, failure to lose weight, need for reoperation, and esophageal dilatation.

22.2.3.4 Bariatric and Metabolic Surgeries and Changes in Metabolism

As of 2016, worldwide bariatric and metabolic surgery utilization broke down as:

- 48% for VSG
- 42% for RYGB
- 8% for AGB
- 2% for BPD-DS

The effects of these procedures are summarized in Tables 22.3 and 22.4.

Bariatric surgical procedures are superior to intensive medical management in achieving long-term glycemic control and in meeting lipid and blood pressure goals.

Table 22.3 Characteristics of surgical procedures for the treatment of obesity

	Malabsorptive Procedures	Restrictive Procedures		Mixed Procedures
	Biliopancreatic diversion	Adjustable gastric banding	Vertical sleeve gastrectomy	Roux en-Y gastric bypass
Benefit	Rapid improvement in glucose regulation Weight-independent effects on glucose regulation are the greatest	No anastomosis No nutritional deficiencies Potentially reversible	Weight-independent effect on glucose Endoscopic surveillance is possible Nutritional deficiencies uncommon	Rapid improvement in glucose regulation Weight-independent effects on glucose regulation are the greatest
Immediate complications	Anastomotic leak Anastomotic ulcer Gastro-gastrointestinal stenosis Gastro-jejunal stenosis Internal hernia	Band erosion Band infection Band slippage Esophageal dilatation Esophagitis GERD Port infections Stomal obstruction	Gastric leaks GERD (severe, recurrent) Intraoperative bleeding	Anastomotic leak Anastomotic ulcer Gastric remnant distention Gastro-gastrointestinal stenosis Gastro-jejunal stenosis Internal hernia
Long-term complications	Fat malabsorption Hypoglycemia Kidney stones Nutrient deficiencies Osteoporosis Renal failure	Dysmotility Ineffective for weight loss Reoperation rate is high	Vitamin B12 deficiency Weight regain	Gallstones Hypoglycemia Micronutrient deficiency Ventral hernia Weight regain
Contraindications	Cirrhosis, class C Need for surveillance endoscopy Portal hypertension with varices	Previous weight loss surgery Portal hypertension with varices Chronic steroid use	Portal hypertension with varices Severe GERD	Cirrhosis, class C Portal hypertension with varices
Reversal or Revision for failure (highest percent)	5.7%	24%	1.5%	35%
Excess weight loss	76%	44%	66%	50%
BMI change	−18	−7.1	−10.9	−16.7

BMI body mass index, *GERD* gastroesophageal reflux disease

Table 22.4 Changes in metabolic parameters with the bariatric procedures most commonly done

	Malabsorptive Procedures	Restrictive Procedures		Mixed Procedures
	Biliopancreatic diversion duodenal switch	Adjustable gastric banding	Vertical sleeve gastrectomy	Roux en-Y gastric bypass
Excess weight loss	82%	44%	66%	50%
Mean weight loss	30–40%	15–30%	20–30%	25–35%
BMI change	−18	−7.1	−10.9	−16.7
Sleep apnea remission	98%	45%	80%	76%
Diabetes remission	98%	59%	81%	78%
Dyslipidemia remission	99%	36%	67%	61%
Hypertension remission	83%	56%	78%	66%
Hunger	n/a	n/a	n/a	↓
Satiety	n/a	n/a	n/a	↑
Food intake	n/a	↓	↓	↓
Sweet preference	n/a	n/a	↓	↓
Fat preference	n/a	n/a	↓	↓
Energy expenditure	n/a	↓	↓	↑
Gastric emptying	→	→	↑	↑
Bile acids	↑	→↑	→↑	↑
Gut microbiome	Altered	Altered	Altered	Altered
Ghrelin	↓↓	↓→↑	↓↓	↓→↑
Glucagon-like peptide-1	↑	→↓	↑	↑
Peptide YY	↑	↑	↑	↑
Oxyntomodulin	↑	→	↑	↑
GIP	↓	→	→↑	↓→↑
Cholecystokinin	n/a	n/a	→	→
Pancreatic polypeptide	↓	→	→	→
Amylin	n/a	→	→	↓
Glucagon secretion	↑	n/a	n/a	↓→↑
Postprandial insulin secretion	↑	→↓	↑	→↓
Hepatic insulin sensitivity	↑	↑	↑	↑
Muscle insulin sensitivity	↑	↑	↑	↑
Plasma glucose	↓	↓	↓	↓
Hemoglobin A1C	↓3.8%	↓1.8%	↓2.9	↓2.9%
Glucose effect	Weight-independent	Weight-dependent	Weight-independent	Weight-independent
Triglycerides	↓	↓	↓	↓

Table 22.4 (continued)

	Malabsorptive Procedures	Restrictive Procedures		Mixed Procedures
	Biliopancreatic diversion duodenal switch	Adjustable gastric banding	Vertical sleeve gastrectomy	Roux en-Y gastric bypass
LDL-C	↓	↓↑	↓	↓
HDL-C	→	→	↑	↑
Resistin	n/a	↑	↓	→
Leptin	↓	↓	↓	↓
Adiponectin	↑	↑	→	↑
Leptin-to-adiponectin ratio	↓	↓	↓	↓

Multiple arrows denote equivocal data
BMI body mass index, *GIP* glucose-dependent insulinotropic polypeptide, *HDL-C* high-density lipoprotein–cholesterol, *LDL-C* low-density lipoprotein–cholelsterol, *n/a* no data available

Bariatric surgery is also effective in preventing type 2 diabetes mellitus, as demonstrated in the Swedish Obesity Subjects Study.

In addition to this, the risk of death is decreased by bariatric surgery. In the Veteran's Affairs system, retrospectively analyzed data documented that at the end of the 14-year study period, there were a total of 263 deaths in the surgical group (mean follow-up, 6.9 years) and 1277 deaths in the matched control group (mean follow-up, 6.6 years). This corroborates previous observations of decreased mortality with bariatric surgery.

Adiposity is the accumulation of fat mass (poundage). Adiposopathy is the derangement of adipose tissue function and structure that develops with the accrual of excess fat mass. Bariatric surgery is an effective treatment of both adiposity and adiposopathy.

Leptin levels are directly proportional to fat mass. Adiponectin levels are inversely proportional to fat mass. The leptin-to-adiponectin ratio (see Chap. 3 in this textbook) is a reflection of adipose tissue health. A low leptin-to-adiponectin ratio implies good adipose tissue health and function. A high leptin-to-adiponectin ratio implies adiposopathy has developed. Trending the leptin-to-adiponectin ratio of an individual patient over time allows for an assessment of adipose tissue health longitudinally. All bariatric procedures lower leptin and raise adiponectin levels over time—they lower the leptin-to-adiponectin ratio. Thus, all bariatric procedures treat adiposopathy.

22.3 Other Interventions for Management of Obesity

In addition to gastrointestinal procedures to achieve weight loss, the traditional bariatric surgical procedures, there are now several alternatives. As a group, these interventions are new to the market, and the volume of data on each of them is modest.

22.3.1 *Gastric Electrical Stimulation (GES)*

The idea that GES may help weight loss has not translated into a useful clinical application. GES for the treatment of obesity should induce satiety by modulation of the gut-brain neural axis. With GES, behavior modification could be facilitated to overcome problems with nonadherence. GES has a low surgical risk and has the advantage of allowing for adjustments to the pacer device on demand.

Transneuronix, Inc., a Mount Arlington, New Jersey company, was founded in 1995. Transneuronix developed the TRANScend® implantable gastric stimulator (IGS). The first study of GES for the treatment of obesity in humans occurred in 2002 and used the TRANScend IGS. By 2006, there were open-label studies of over 300 patients treated with GES. At >12 months, on average, there was a loss of 20% of EWL in these patients.

The Screened Health Assessment and Pacer Evaluation (SHAPE) trial was started by Transneuronix in May 2004. It was a US multicenter, double-blind randomized controlled trial of GES, designed to detect the difference in excess weight loss between patients who received GES and a placebo group who did not (sham treatment). With SHAPE under way, Medtronic acquired Transneuronix in 2005 and assumed a leadership role in the field. However, in December 2005, Medtronic announced that the preliminary results of the SHAPE trial did not meet the efficacy endpoint of a difference in mean EWL at 1 year (%EWL: 11.8 ± 17.6 vs. 11.7 ± 16.9, respectively). This led to withdrawal of the device.

22.3.1.1 Appetite Suppression Induced by Stimulation Trial (ASSIST)

Early in 2005, Medtronic launched ASSIST, a feasibility trial to determine the safety and efficacy of the Medtronic Enterra® IGS for weight loss (Fig. 22.12). The study was done in subjects diagnosed with type 2 diabetes with a body mass index between 32 and 45 kg/m^2 (ClinicalTrials.gov Identifier: NCT00200018). The primary objectives of ASSIST were to assess and report the incidence of device-, procedure-, and therapy-related adverse events associated with GES for the treatment of obesity in subjects with type 2 diabetes and to demonstrate that subjects who receive GES have a minimum mean EWL of 10% and EWL is at least 5% more than the mean loss in the control group at 12 months post implant. Secondary diabetes control objectives were included in the study. The first subject was implanted on June 7, 2005. A total of 25 subjects were implanted during the course of the study. The longest duration of follow-up was 22 months. The ASSIST data were locked on December 12, 2007. The last subject follow-up visit was conducted on April 18, 2007.

The ASSIST study was not powered for hypothesis testing. Neither the control (GES current OFF) nor the treatment group (GES current ON) had statistically significant percent EWL between baseline and 12 months. The between-group difference in percent EWL between baseline and 12 months ($p = 0.061$) was not

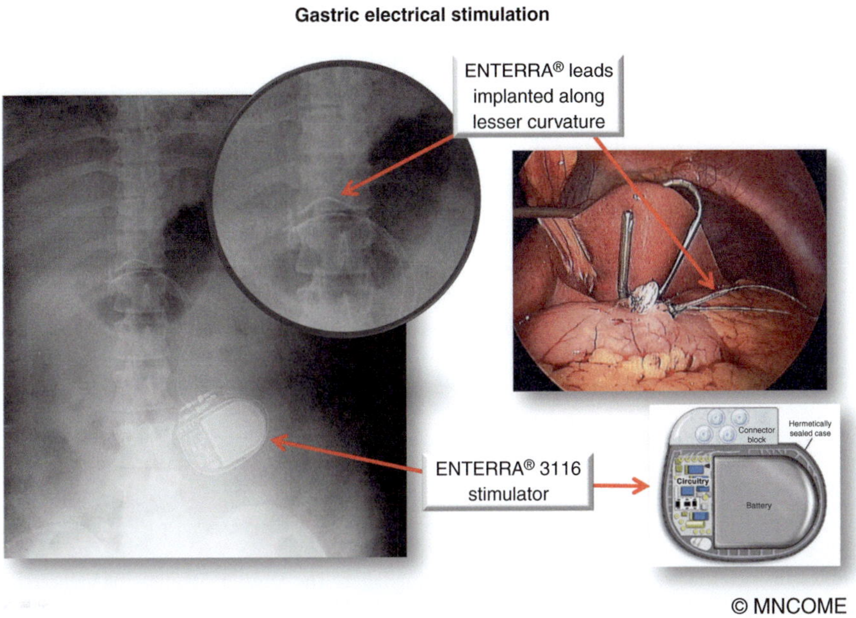

Fig. 22.12 GES. The Enterra® implantable gastric stimulator is an example of the stimulators that have been used for gastric electrical stimulation. Enterra was originally developed for the treatment of gastroparesis and was used in ASSIST. The leads are implanted into the lesser curvature of the stomach. The stimulator pack is placed in the upper abdomen. (Copyright Minnesota Center for Obesity, Metabolism and Endocrinology, PA (MNCOME))

statistically significant (Fig. 22.13). The results of this trial were not published in the peer-reviewed literature. The device remains in the market and has evolved, but it is not used for weight management. The only use for it now is the treatment of gastroparesis.

22.3.1.2 GES Devices under Development

Tantalus®, recently renamed Diamond®, and Exilis® are other implantable gastric stimulators under development.

The surgical procedure for implantation of Diamond® is more complex than Transcend and involves the placement of several electrodes on the stomach. The first study with Diamond® was reported in 2006 along with four subsequent studies. Data are reported on a total of about 100 patients. Outcome measures are variable. There is 20% EWL, or actual weight loss of about 4.5 kg, at 12 months. With GES, there is improvement in glycemic control in patients with diabetes. The improvements in glycemia are not explained by weight loss, since they begin before any significant weight loss may be achieved. Electrical stimulation with Diamond® exerts metabolic control, but the mechanism for this is not defined.

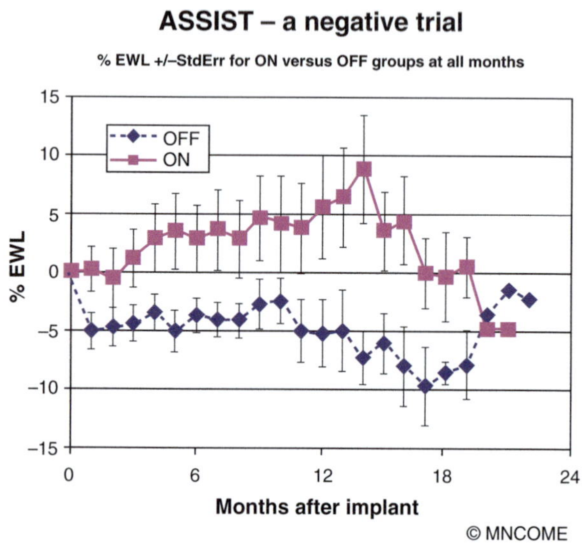

Fig. 22.13 ASSIST – a trial of gastric electrical stimulation. The Appetite Suppression Induced by Stimulation Trial (ASSIST) was conducted from June 7, 2005, through April 18, 2007. It used the Enterra® implantable gastric stimulator. In this study, gastric stimulation led to weight gain, not weight loss. The control group had better glycemic control than the group with gastric electrical stimulation. EWL Excess weight loss, StdErr Standard error. (Copyright Minnesota Center for Obesity, Metabolism and Endocrinology, PA (MNCOME))

A trial with Exilis® started in March 2013. The trial data have not been reported. Altogether, GES for weight loss remains experimental in the United States, but commercialization has begun in Europe.

22.3.2 *Vagal Blockade*

The Maestro® system, from EnteroMedics of St. Paul, Minnesota, consists of a rechargeable neuroregulator device implanted into the lateral chest wall. Flexible leads from the neuroregulator device are placed laparoscopically around the vagus nerve. Electrical pulses act to suppress neural signals, leading to fullness and decreasing the drive to feed. The system also includes a mobile charger, a transmit coil, and an AC recharger, as well as a laptop computer loaded with clinician programmer software and a programmer cable. Clinicians can modify therapy parameters and schedules and can obtain diagnostic information through the programmer.

The system is indicated for adults with a BMI of 40 kg/m^2, or more. Adults with a BMI of 35 kg/m^2 and at least one obesity-related comorbidity are also eligible.

In the registration trial, called ReCharge, average excess weight loss in patients randomly assigned to VBLOC came to 24.4% at 12 months, compared with 15.9% for patients randomly assigned to sham implants, for a difference of 8.5%; 52.5% of VBLOC patients had excess weight loss of at least 20%; 38.4% had excess weight loss of at least 25%.

22.3.3 *Gastric Artery Embolization*

Gastric anatomy lends itself not only to surgical procedures but also to percutaneous radiological interventions for weight loss. The gastric fundus is the major source of ghrelin. The arterial supply of the fundus comes mostly from the left gastric artery (LGA).

In March 2013, Kipshidze presented data on LGA embolization (LGAE), which was performed on five patients in Tbilisi, Georgia. LGAE was done with 300–500 u particles. Three of the patients had abdominal pain for a few hours after the embolization, but two did not. Six months post-embolization, the BMI decreased from 43 kg/m^2 at baseline to 35 kg/m^2. The average weight loss at 6 months was 45 pounds. Ghrelin levels dropped up to 29% from the baseline. These findings have been replicated in a phase 1 US trial on five patients.

22.3.4 *Oral Volume Restricting Device*

Scientific Intake was founded in 2003. It offers SmartByte®, a noninvasive, clinically validated, medical device to treat overweight and class I (mild) obesity (BMI 27–35 kg/m^2) (Fig. 22.14). The principle behind the device is that restriction of oral volume during feeding results in smaller bites, which slows intake, resulting in satiety with less food. Using the device ends gulping and wolfing of food. It allows for more appreciation of the taste (savoring), smell, and texture of meals. The device gained FDA approval for weight management in the spring of 2017.

Screenings of the upper and lower dentures are made in the office and shipped to the company. The company creates an oral device unique to each patient. Each SmartByte® device is designed to fit perfectly into the roof of mouth, anchored on the back maxillary molars. The device is to be inserted at the beginning of a meal and withdrawn at the end of the meal.

Each SmartByte® contains a smart chip within it. The chip senses temperature changes and therefore registers usage. Each device comes with a reader which is synchronized to the device using bluetooth technology. The reader downloads usage data and transfers it to the SmartByte® app which may be downloaded into any hand-held device. The app in turn transmits usage data, and weight data entered by

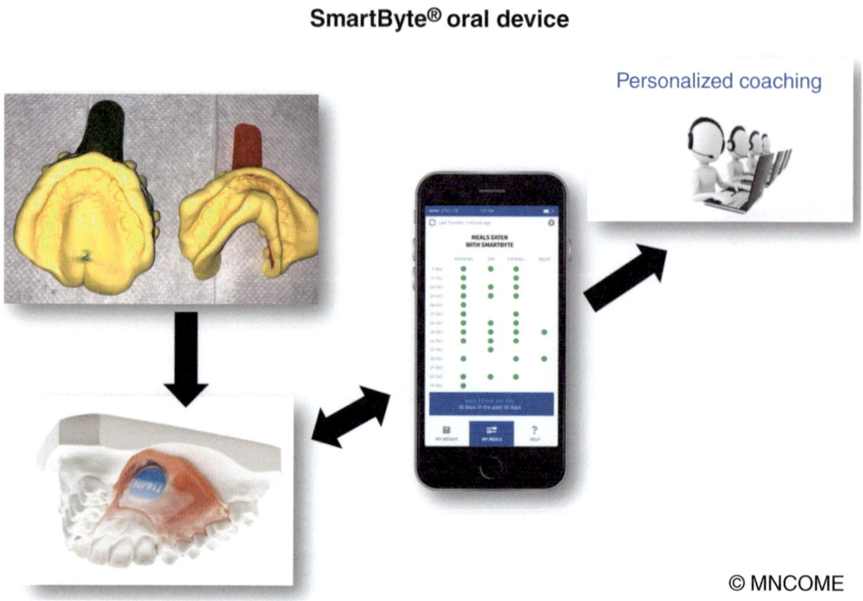

Fig. 22.14 SmartByte® Oral Device. The SmartByte® Oral Device is made by Scientific Intake. Using the device during meals restricts oral volume, forces smaller bites, prolongs mastication, and brings about fullness with less quantities of food. It is the only device approved by the Food and Drug Administration in the United States for weight management that does not require an actual invasive procedure for deployment. The device is simply inserted into the roof of the mouth at the beginning of each meal and removed once the meal is ingested. (Copyright Minnesota Center for Obesity, Metabolism and Endocrinology, PA (MNCOME))

the patient, to the company's cloud. The data are then made available to a personal coach hired by the company to support effective behavior modification for each patient.

In the registration trial, 76 patients were fitted with their own SmartByte® device. They each received individualized video lifestyle instruction. The prespecified per protocol (PP) population ($N = 40$) required sensor-verified use of the device ≥7 times per week for 14 of 16 weeks. The overall device usage rate required from each patient was ≥33%. At week 16:

- 12 (30%) achieved ≥5% weight loss
- 16 (40%) achieved ≥4%
- 21 (52.5%) achieved ≥3%.

Week 16 mean loss for the PP population was 2.93%, and among 36 participants who did not meet PP criteria, it was 1.45%. Among 76 intent-to-treat subjects, two subjects reported three mild-to-moderate device-related adverse events, resolving spontaneously (one hard palate abrasion and two tongue lacerations).

The SmartByte® device is the only device for weight loss that does not require an invasive procedure.

22.4 Cosmetic Plastic Surgery and Body Contouring Procedures

Overweight and obesity lead to physical, metabolic, and psychological complications. When patients successfully lose weight, there almost invariably continues to be self-consciousness of the redundant skin. The following procedures are available to recontour after weight loss:

- Arm lift (Brachioplasty): Surgery to remove excess hanging skin from the upper arm between the elbow and shoulder. The incision is along the posterior aspect of the arm.
- Body lift (Torsoplasty): Surgery to remove and lift sagging skin around the buttocks, thighs, hips, and abdomen. It combines a lower body lift (buttocks, thighs, and hips) and abdominoplasty into a single procedure. The incision extends around the entire body. A total body lift includes the arms, back, and breasts as well.
- Breast lift (Mastopexy) and breast augmentation (augmentation mammoplasty): Surgery and body contouring procedure to lift a sagging breast and enhance natural breast volume. Breast size is often reduced with weight loss since breasts are mainly composed of adipose tissue.
- Breast reduction in men (for gynecomastia and lipomastia): Surgery to remove loose chest skin and female-like breast contours in men. Incision lines can be an issue.
- Face lift (Rhytidectomy) or neck lift (Platysmaplasty): A face lift is a surgery to remove extra skin and tighten muscles of the neck and face. If surgery is performed under the jaw line and in the neck area only, it is known as a neck lift.
- Liposuction (Lipoplasty): Cosmetic procedure used to remove small amounts of fatty tissue from the hips, thighs, buttocks, and abdomen to sculpt a more desirable body shape. It is often combined with body lift surgery. Liposuction is not for weight loss but for sculpting the body's shape and contour.
- Panniculectomy: Surgery to remove the excess skin and fat that hangs from the stomach after weight loss. Panniculectomy involves tightening the abdominal muscles. It may be covered by health insurance.
- Tummy-Tuck (abdominoplasty): Surgery to remove excess skin and fat from the middle and lower abdomen and tighten muscles in the abdominal wall. The effect is to create a more slender waistline and flatter stomach. The incisions go from hip to hip and around the umbilicus.

22.5 Conclusion

Bariatric procedures which were originally developed for weight loss are now also universally regarded as an effective treatment for the physical and metabolic derangements that come with overweight and obesity. The bariatric endocrinologist should have familiarity with all of the procedures that are available for weight loss. Bariatric procedures are effective and have become increasingly safe. Taken together, they provide effective treatment for adiposity and also for adiposopathy.

Weight loss procedures must be recommended for selected patients who are truly refractory to medical management of overweight or obesity and who have significant burden of disease, including adiposopathy. It must be emphasized that having a procedure, or using a device, does not cure the disease. Rather, overweight and obesity are life-long diseases that will require ongoing care well beyond the perisurgical window. These bariatric procedures, like pharmacotherapy, are tools to achieve a better state of health. And having a bariatric procedure does not preclude ongoing use of pharmacotherapy, as appropriate.

Reading List

Abdelbaki TN, Huang CK, Ramos A, Neto MG, Talebpour M, Saber AA. Gastric plication for morbid obesity: a systematic review. Obes Surg. 2012;22(10):1633–9. Epub 2012/09/11.

Anton K, Rahman T, Bhanushali A, Patel AA. Bariatric left gastric artery embolization for the treatment of obesity: a review of gut hormone involvement in energy homeostasis. AJR Am J Roentgenol. 2016;206(1):202–10. Epub 2015/12/25.

Apovian CM, Shah SN, Wolfe BM, Ikramuddin S, Miller CJ, Tweden KS, et al. Two-year outcomes of vagal nerve blocking (vBloc) for the treatment of obesity in the ReCharge trial. Obes Surg. 2016;27:169. Epub 2016/08/11.

Arterburn DE, Olsen MK, Smith VA, Livingston EH, Van Scoyoc L, Yancy WS Jr, et al. Association between bariatric surgery and long-term survival. JAMA. 2015;313(1):62–70. Epub 2015/01/07.

Baker MT. The history and evolution of bariatric surgical procedures. Surg Clin North Am. 2011;91(6):1181–201, viii. Epub 2011/11/08.

Bays HE, Gonzalez-Campoy JM, Bray GA, Kitabchi AE, Bergman DA, Schorr AB, et al. Pathogenic potential of adipose tissue and metabolic consequences of adipocyte hypertrophy and increased visceral adiposity. Expert Rev Cardiovasc Ther. 2008a;6(3):343–68. Epub 2008/03/11.

Bays HE, Gonzalez-Campoy JM, Henry RR, Bergman DA, Kitabchi AE, Schorr AB, et al. Is adiposopathy (sick fat) an endocrine disease? Int J Clin Pract. 2008b;62(10):1474–83. Epub 2008/08/07.

Bays HE, Laferrere B, Dixon J, Aronne L, Gonzalez-Campoy JM, Apovian C, et al. Adiposopathy and bariatric surgery: is 'sick fat' a surgical disease. Int J Clin Pract. 2009;63(9):1285–300. Epub 2009/08/21.

Beckman LM, Beckman TR, Sibley SD, Thomas W, Ikramuddin S, Kellogg TA, et al. Changes in gastrointestinal hormones and leptin after roux-en-Y gastric bypass surgery. JPEN J Parenter Enteral Nutr. 2011;35(2):169–80. Epub 2011/03/08.

Benjamin SB, Maher KA, Cattau EL Jr, Collen MJ, Fleischer DE, Lewis JH, et al. Double-blind controlled trial of the Garren-Edwards gastric bubble: an adjunctive treatment for exogenous obesity. Gastroenterology. 1988;95(3):581–8. Epub 1988/09/01.

Buchwald H, Rucker RD. The history of metabolic surgery for morbid obesity and a commentary. World J Surg. 1981;5(6):781–7. Epub 1981/11/01.

Buchwald H, Moore RB, Lee GB, Baltaxe H, Amplatz K, Frantz ID, et al. Five years experience with the use of partial ileal bypass in the treatment of hypercholesterolemia and atherosclerosis. Isr J Med Sci. 1969;5(4):760–5. Epub 1969/07/01.

Buchwald H, Avidor Y, Braunwald E, Jensen MD, Pories W, Fahrbach K, et al. Bariatric surgery: a systematic review and meta-analysis. JAMA. 2004;292(14):1724–37. Epub 2004/10/14.

Carbajo MA, Luque-de-Leon E, Jimenez JM, Ortiz-de-Solorzano J, Perez-Miranda M, Castro-Alija MJ. Laparoscopic one-anastomosis gastric bypass: technique, results, and long-term follow-up in 1200 patients. Obes Surg. 2017;27(5):1153–67. Epub 2016/10/27.

Carlsson LM, Peltonen M, Ahlin S, Anveden A, Bouchard C, Carlsson B, et al. Bariatric surgery and prevention of type 2 diabetes in Swedish obese subjects. N Engl J Med. 2012;367(8):695–704. Epub 2012/08/24.

Cha R, Marescaux J, Diana M. Updates on gastric electrical stimulation to treat obesity: systematic review and future perspectives. World J Gastrointest Endosc. 2014;6(9):419–31. Epub 2014/09/18.

Chouillard E, Schoucair N, Alsabah S, Alkandari B, Montana L, Dejonghe B, et al. Laparoscopic gastric plication (LGP) as an alternative to laparoscopic sleeve gastrectomy (LSG) in patients with morbid obesity: a preliminary, short-term, case-control study. Obes Surg. 2015;26:1167. Epub 2015/10/21.

Coffin B, Maunoury V, Pattou F, Hebuterne X, Schneider S, Coupaye M, et al. Impact of intragastric balloon before laparoscopic gastric bypass on patients with super obesity: a randomized multicenter study. Obes Surg. 2017;27(4):902–9. Epub 2016/09/25.

De Luca M, Himpens J, Angrisani L, Di Lorenzo N, Mahawar K, Lunardi C, et al. A new concept in bariatric surgery. Single anastomosis gastro-Ileal (SAGI): technical details and preliminary results. Obes Surg. 2017;27(1):143–7. Epub 2016/07/20.

Edmundowicz SA, Shelby S. A new gastric balloon for weight loss that eliminates the need for endoscopy—good news for the bariatrician. Endoscopy. 2017;49(2):108–9. Epub 2017/02/02.

Gonzalez-Campoy JM, Richardson B, Richardson C, Gonzalez-Cameron D, Ebrahim A, Strobel P, et al. Bariatric endocrinology: principles of medical practice. Int J Endocrinol. 2014;2014:917813. Epub 2014/06/06.

Gunn AJ, Oklu R. A preliminary observation of weight loss following left gastric artery embolization in humans. J Obes. 2014;2014:185349. Epub 2014/10/29.

Henrikson V. Kan tunnfarmsresektion forsvaras som terapi mot fettsot? Can small bowel resection be defended for therapy for obesity? Nord Med. 1952;47:744.

Hogan RB, Johnston JH, Long BW, Sones JQ, Hinton LA, Bunge J, et al. A double-blind, randomized, sham-controlled trial of the gastric bubble for obesity. Gastrointest Endosc. 1989;35(5):381–5. Epub 1989/09/01.

Ikramuddin S, Korner J, Lee WJ, Connett JE, Inabnet WB, Billington CJ, et al. Roux-en-Y gastric bypass vs intensive medical management for the control of type 2 diabetes, hypertension, and hyperlipidemia: the diabetes surgery study randomized clinical trial. JAMA. 2013;309(21):2240–9. Epub 2013/06/06.

Ikramuddin S, Blackstone RP, Brancatisano A, Toouli J, Shah SN, Wolfe BM, et al. Effect of reversible intermittent intra-abdominal vagal nerve blockade on morbid obesity: the ReCharge randomized clinical trial. JAMA. 2014;312(9):915–22. Epub 2014/09/04.

Kirby DF, Wade JB, Mills PR, Sugerman HJ, Kellum JM, Zfass AM, et al. A prospective assessment of the Garren-Edwards Gastric Bubble and bariatric surgery in the treatment of morbid obesity. Am Surg. 1990;56(10):575–80. Epub 1990/10/01.

Kourkoulos M, Giorgakis E, Kokkinos C, Mavromatis T, Griniatsos J, Nikiteas N, et al. Laparoscopic gastric plication for the treatment of morbid obesity: a review. Minim Invasive Surg. 2012;2012:696348. Epub 2012/07/20.

Kramer FM, Stunkard AJ, Spiegel TA, Deren JJ, Velchik MG, Wadden TA, et al. Limited weight losses with a gastric balloon. Arch Intern Med. 1989;149(2):411–3. Epub 1989/02/01.

Kumar N, Sullivan S, Thompson CC. The role of endoscopic therapy in obesity management: intragastric balloons and aspiration therapy. Diabetes Metab Syndr Obes Targets Ther. 2017;10:311–6. Epub 2017/07/26.

Mahdy T, Al Wahedi A, Schou C. Efficacy of single anastomosis sleeve ileal (SASI) bypass for type-2 diabetic morbid obese patients: gastric bipartition, a novel metabolic surgery procedure: a retrospective cohort study. Int J Surg. 2016;34:28–34. Epub 2016/10/21.

Mason EE. Vertical banded gastroplasty for obesity. Arch Surg. 1982;117(5):701–6. Epub 1982/05/01.

Mason EE. Development and future of gastroplasties for morbid obesity. Arch Surg. 2003;138(4):361–6. Epub 2003/04/11.

Mason EE. History of obesity surgery. Surg Obes Relat Dis. 2005;1(2):123–5. Epub 2006/08/24.

Mason EE, Ito C. Gastric bypass in obesity. Surg Clin North Am. 1967;47(6):1345–51. Epub 1967/12/01.
Mechanick JI, Kushner RF, Sugerman HJ, Gonzalez-Campoy JM, Collazo-Clavell ML, Guven S, et al. American Association of Clinical Endocrinologists, the Obesity Society, and American Society for Metabolic & Bariatric Surgery Medical guidelines for clinical practice for the perioperative nutritional, metabolic, and nonsurgical support of the bariatric surgery patient. Endocr Pract. 2008;14(Suppl 1):1–83. Epub 2008/09/06.
Mechanick JI, Youdim A, Jones DB, Garvey WT, Hurley DL, McMahon MM, et al. Clinical practice guidelines for the perioperative nutritional, metabolic, and nonsurgical support of the bariatric surgery patient—2013 update: cosponsored by American Association of Clinical Endocrinologists, the Obesity Society, and American Society for Metabolic & Bariatric Surgery. Endocr Pract. 2013;19(2):337–72. Epub 2013/03/27.
Musella M, Milone M, Deitel M, Kular KS, Rutledge R. What a mini/one anastomosis gastric bypass (MGB/OAGB) is. Obes Surg. 2016;26(6):1322–3. Epub 2016/04/20.
Ochner CN, Gibson C, Shanik M, Goel V, Geliebter A. Changes in neurohormonal gut peptides following bariatric surgery. Int J Obes. 2011;35(2):153–66. Epub 2010/07/14.
Rutledge R. Naming the mini-gastric bypass. Obes Surg. 2014;24(12):2173. Epub 2014/09/24.
Ryan DH, Parkin CG, Longley W, Dixon J, Apovian C, Bode B. Efficacy and safety of an oral device to reduce food intake and promote weight loss. Obes Sci Pract. 2018;4(1):52–61. Epub 2018/02/27.
Sandler BJ, Rumbaut R, Swain CP, Torres G, Morales L, Gonzales L, et al. Human experience with an endoluminal, endoscopic, gastrojejunal bypass sleeve. Surg Endosc. 2011;25(9):3028–33. Epub 2011/04/14.
Sandler BJ, Rumbaut R, Swain CP, Torres G, Morales L, Gonzales L, et al. One-year human experience with a novel endoluminal, endoscopic gastric bypass sleeve for morbid obesity. Surg Endosc. 2015;29(11):3298–303. Epub 2015/01/30.
Santoro S, Malzoni CE, Velhote MC, Milleo FQ, Santo MA, Klajner S, et al. Digestive adaptation with intestinal reserve: a neuroendocrine-based operation for morbid obesity. Obes Surg. 2006;16(10):1371–9. Epub 2006/10/25.
Santoro S, Castro LC, Velhote MC, Malzoni CE, Klajner S, Castro LP, et al. Sleeve gastrectomy with transit bipartition: a potent intervention for metabolic syndrome and obesity. Ann Surg. 2012;256(1):104–10. Epub 2012/05/23.
Schauer PR, Bhatt DL, Kirwan JP, Wolski K, Aminian A, Brethauer SA, et al. Bariatric surgery versus intensive medical therapy for diabetes—5-year outcomes. N Engl J Med. 2017;376(7):641–51. Epub 2017/02/16.
Sjostrom L, Peltonen M, Jacobson P, Sjostrom CD, Karason K, Wedel H, et al. Bariatric surgery and long-term cardiovascular events. JAMA. 2012;307(1):56–65. Epub 2012/01/05.
Sullivan S. Aspiration therapy for obesity. Gastrointest Endosc Clin N Am. 2017;27(2):277–88. Epub 2017/03/16.
Therapeutics MLoDa. ReShape and Orbera—two gastric balloon devices for weight loss. Med Lett Drugs Ther. 2015;57(1476):122–3. Epub 2015/08/26.
Thompson CC, Abu Dayyeh BK, Kushner R, Sullivan S, Schorr AB, Amaro A, et al. Percutaneous gastrostomy device for the treatment of class II and class III obesity: results of a randomized controlled trial. Am J Gastroenterol. 2017;112(3):447–57. Epub 2016/12/07.
Tretbar LL, Taylor TL, Sifers EC. Weight reduction. Gastric plication for morbid obesity. J Kans Med Soc. 1976;77(11):488–90. Epub 1976/11/01.
Vyas D, Deshpande K, Pandya Y. Advances in endoscopic balloon therapy for weight loss and its limitations. World J Gastroenterol. 2017;23(44):7813–7. Epub 2017/12/07.
Weiss CR, Kathait AS. Bariatric embolization: a new and effective option for the obese patient? Expert Rev Gastroenterol Hepatol. 2017;11(4):293–302. Epub 2017/03/10.
Weiss CR, Akinwande O, Paudel K, Cheskin LJ, Holly B, Hong K, et al. Clinical safety of bariatric arterial embolization: preliminary results of the BEAT obesity trial. Radiology. 2017;283(2):598–608. Epub 2017/02/15.

Index

J. M. Gonzalez-Campoy et al. (eds.), *Bariatric Endocrinology*,
https://doi.org/10.1007/978-3-319-95655-8

X

Y

MIX
Papier aus verantwortungsvollen Quellen
Paper from responsible sources
FSC® C105338

If you have any concerns about our products,
you can contact us on
ProductSafety@springernature.com

In case Publisher is established outside the EU,
the EU authorized representative is:
Springer Nature Customer Service Center GmbH
Europaplatz 3, 69115 Heidelberg, Germany

Printed by Libri Plureos GmbH
in Hamburg, Germany